Contents

version 9 – last updated for print 9/11/2024

Note: If you have trouble with the abbreviations used in this book, please go to **quackquackmed.com/abbr**.

This book is dedicated to my mother, Mrs Jo Loo – thank God for you :)

Acute coronary syndrome

D: spectrum of acute myocardial ischaemia or infarction

STEMI: ECG+ve [*ST-elevation*], trops+ve	**NSTEMI:** ECG inconclusive [normal or other Δ], trops+ve	**Unstable angina:** normal ECG, *normal trops*

STEMI criteria – ≥20 min s/smx, ECG features in ≥2 contiguous leads
- 2.5 mm ST elevation in V2-3 in men ≤40yo, or ≥ 2.0 mm in men >40yo
- 1.5 mm ST elevation in V2-3 in women
- 1 mm ST elevation in other leads   • new LBBB (always pathological)

S/Smx: angina at rest (>20 min) not relieved by GTN. Gripping/heavy pain, a/w nausea, sweating, dyspnea, palpitations, etc

Ix: ECG, ABG, bloods (**trops**, FBC, lipids, HbA1c, U&E, LFT, TFT), CXR, echo, blood glucose

Mx

All: Aspirin 300 mg, O2 if sats <94%, **paracetamol** 1g PO/IV [morphine if severe pain only], **GTN** 1 spray (caution hypotension), ± ondansetron 4 mg IV

STEMI: (1) <12h of smx AND (2) is PCI possible within 2h?	**PCI possible within 2h** — no — **Fibrinolysis**
	- Prasugrel
	  - clopidogrel if pt is on PO anticoag
	  - ticagrelor if pt is high risk bleeding
	- Obtain radial access (preferred to femoral)
	- UFH + bailout GPIIb/IIIa inhibitor
	- PCI: Drug eluting stent
		Fibrinolysis
		- Alteplase etc
		  + antithrombin
		- Thereafter, ticagrelor
		- If no ECG resolution after 60-90 min, PCI

If pt presents >12h but has ongoing smx of STEMI or has cardiogenic shock, consider sending for PCI anyway

NSTEMI (1) GRACE ≤3% or >3%?	**Low risk (≤3% 6mo mortality):** fondaparinux & ticagrelor **Int/high risk (>3%):** - If unstable: PCI immediately (see STEMI PCI) - If stable, PCI within 72h + give fondaparinux, prasugrel or ticagrelor, and UFH

GRACE score predicts all-cause mortality 6mo after discharge for ACS

Unstable angina & 2' prevention (lifelong): (6As) aspirin 75 mg od, another antiplatelet *for 12mo* (eg clopidogrel), atorvastatin 80 mg od, ACEI (eg ramipril), atenolol (or bisoprolol), aldosterone antagonist for HF (eg eplenerone)

Other notes
- MI a/w cocaine use: add IV benzodiazepine, ?avoid βB
- Diet: Mediterranean style diet. No rec for omega-3 or fish
- Exercise: 20-30 min daily
- Sex: ok to resume in 4w.
- PDE-5 inhibs (sildenafil) can be used 6mo after MI. Avoid in pts prescribed nitrates and nicorandil

Complications "DREAD": death, rupture of myocardium, edema, arrhythmia and aneurysms, Dressler's syndrome

Post-MI ACS risk stratification using Killip classes

I: no clinical signs of HF	6%
II: lung crackles + S3	17%
III: frank pulmonary edema	38%
IV: cardiogenic shock	**81% 30d mortality**

P: ~10% morbidity. ↑ risk for future events

R: • Unmodifiable: ↑age, males, FHx
• Modifiable: smoking, DM, HTN, hypercholesterolaemia, obesity

P: • Atherosclerosis in coronary vessels 2/2 endothelial dysfunction (smoking, HTN, hyperglycaemia)
• Plaque formation causes physical blockage → ↓blood flow to myocardium → ischaemia & angina
• Plaque rupture may cause complete occlusion → myocardial infarction

ECG cardiac territories

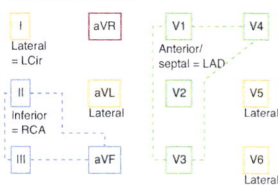

I Lateral = LCir	aVR	V1 Anterior/ septal = LAD	V4
II Inferior = RCA	aVL Lateral	V2	V5 Lateral
III	aVF	V3	V6 Lateral

V1-6, aVL = Proximal LAD

Posterior STEMI:
• Reciprocal V1-3 changes
  - ST depression
  - tall, broad R waves
  - upright T waves
• Confirmed by ST elevation and Q waves in posterior leads (V7-9)

Inferior MIs are a/w AV block

DDx:
• Global T wave inversion: think non-cardiac cause
• Pericarditis: global ST elevation
• PE: sinus tachy (most common), S1Q3T3

Mean arterial pressure = average arterial pressure throughout systole & diastole
MAP = DBP + 1/3(SBP - DBP)

Hypertension

Stage 1 HTN Clinic BP ≥140/90 **ABPM ≥135/85**	Stage 2 HTN Clinic BP ≥160/100 ABPM ≥150/95	Stage 3 HTN Clinic BP ≥180/120 = HTN crisis

Treat if ———————— Treat ————————
<80yo AND • target organ damage
• established CVD, AKI/CKD, T2DM
• 10y cardiovascular risk ≥10%

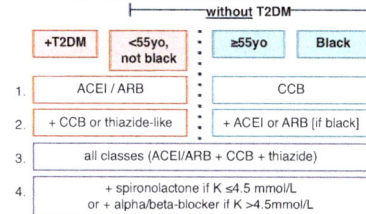

—————————— without T2DM ——————————

	+T2DM	<55yo, not black	≥55yo	Black
1.	ACEI / ARB		CCB	
2.	+ CCB or thiazide-like		+ ACEI or ARB [if black]	
3.	all classes (ACEI/ARB + CCB + thiazide)			
4.	+ spironolactone if K ≤4.5 mmol/L or + alpha/beta-blocker if K >4.5mmol/L			

D: persistently raised BP

R: obesity, metabolic syndrome, ↓exercise, ↑alcohol, DM, black ancestry, >60yo, FHx (HTN, CKD), sleep apnoea

Aetiology:
• Essential HTN - no specific cause
• Secondary HTN
  - **Primary hyperaldosteronism**
  - Renal disease, eg glomerulonephritis, renal artery stenosis
  - Endocrine disorders, eg Cushing's, phaeochromocytoma, acromegaly
  - Drugs, eg steroids, COCP
  - *Others:* pregnancy, coarctation of the aorta

Other notes on Mx:
• DM: ACEI/ARB best
• CKD: ACEI/ARB first line. Furosemide useful in GFR<45 - monitor for dehydration
• Isolated systolic hypertension - treat same way as normal HTN

Diagnosing hypertension
• If clinic BP ≥140/90, measure again after 5 min, measure on both arms, and check cuff placement
• Use ambulatory BP monitoring (ABPM) to Dx (clinic BP - white coat syndrome)
• Alternatively, home BP monitoring – 2 readings in the morning, 2 at night, for 4-7d

Ix: Fundoscopy, urine dipstick, ECG, bloods (FBC, U&Es, HbA1c, lipids, etc)

Hypertensive retinopathy
• Grade I: barely detectable arterial narrowing
• II: obvious narrowing + focal irregularties
• III: flame haemorrhages, dot and blot haemorrhages, hard and soft exudates, cotton wool spots
• IV: papilloedema

Antihypertensives: side effects

ACE-inhibitors: dry cough (15%; usually in 1st year of starting), angioedema, hyperkalaemia, first dose hypotension
• If dry cough develops, switch to **ARB**
• Avoid in pregnancy & breastfeeding
• CI/caution in renovascular disease (eg bilateral renal artery stenosis) and aortic stenosis, hereditary idiopathic angioedema
• May cause ↑creatinine (up to 30% acceptable)

CCBs: Verapamil - constipation, hypotension, bradycardia, flushing; caution in HF
• Diltiazem - hypotension, ↓HR, ankle swelling, caution in HF
! DO NOT give verapamil & diltiazem with βB - may result in heart block
• Amlodipine, nifedipine, etc - flushing, HA, ankle swelling, reflex tachycardia. No issues with HF.

Thiazide-like diuretics: hypoK, hypoNa, *hyper*Ca, gout, impaired glucose tolerance, impotence
• Rarely, pancreatitis, ↓platelets, agranulocytosis, photosensitivity rash

Continued on 01.09

Ischaemic heart disease

D: inadequate blood supply to the myocardium. **Angina** = chest pain due to reduced blood flow to the myocardium

R: age, smoking, CAD, HTN, ↑chol, DM, IVDU, male, sedentary lifestyle.

P: • Atherosclerosis in coronary vessels 2/2 endothelial dysfunction (smoking, HTN, hyperglycaemia)
• Plaque formation causes physical blockage → ↓blood flow to myocardium → ischaemia & angina

S/smx:
• Stable angina (all 3 features)
   - chest pressure / constriction <20min
   - provoked by exertion
   - relieved by rest or GTN
• Atypical angina in women, DM, older people - 2 of 3 + GI discomfort, dyspnea, nausea

Ix: ECG, bloods (Hb, lipids, HbA1c)
• If stable angina cannot be excluded by clinical Ax alone, consider
   - CT coronary angiography
   - non-invasive functional imaging
   - 3rd invasive coronary angiography

Mx: • Sublingual **GTN** for relief of smx (or before activities known to cause angina)
   - 1 dose + rest → if no relief, take 2nd dose → if no relief, call 999
• **Aspirin** 75 mg OD, unless pt is already on antiplatelet (eg clopidogrel)
• **Statin**, eg atorvastatin
• **β-blocker and/or CCB**
   - don't give βB to asthmatics
   - if CCB used as monotherapy, give verapamil or diltiazem
   - if CCB combined with βB, use amlodipine, nifedipine, etc
• Long-acting nitrate (eg isosorbide mononitrate), nicorandil, ivabradine or ranolazine
• In pts with DM, consider ACE inhibitor
• Lifestyle changes
   - Smoking cessation, limit alcohol
   - Cardioprotective diet
   - Wt loss & exercise
• DVLA: if angina occurs at rest, do not drive (no need to notify DVLA)

Atrial fibrillation

D: supraventricular tachyarrhythmia causing uncoordinated and ineffective contractions of the atria
÷ new onset, paroxysmal, persistent AF

R: age, ↑↑alcohol, smoking, HTN, ↑chol, HF, T2DM, obesity, other heart disease, hyperthyroidism, etc

A: [SMITH] sepsis, mitral valve pathology, IHD, thyrotoxicosis, HTN / P: anatomical, histological Δ in atria due to underlying heart disease, resulting in conductive Δ.

S/Smx: **palpitations, irregularly irregular pulse**, SOB, CP, fatigue, dizziness, syncope

Ix: ECG, bloods (FBC, clotting profile, U&E, TFT, U&Es - including Mg)

Mx:
Haemodynamically **unstable**
(SBP<90, HR>150, syncope, CP etc)
→ electrical cardioversion (cv)

Stable + onset <48h
• Rate control: βB or CCB digoxin
• Heparinise, and early rhythm control with electrical cv or pharmacological cv

Onset >48 / uncertain onset
• Rate control: βB or CCB digoxin
• If rhythm control considered, must anticoag for ≥3w before cv, then elective electrical cv
• OR, transoesophageal echo (TOE) to r/o left atrial appendage thrombus – can heparinise and cardiovert asap
• Catheter ablation if wishes to avoid antiarrhythmics
   - Femoral access → radiofrequency to burn off cardiac origin of aberrant electrical activity
   - Requires anticoagulation 4w before and during procedure
   - Even after catheter ablation, risk of stroke remains – consider anticoag
   - Risk of cardiac tamponade, stroke, pulmonary vein stenosis; 50% recur within 3mo and may need multiple procedures

Mx (continued)
• Consider rhythm control if reversible cause, HF 2/2 AF, new-onset (<48h), atrial flutter manageable with ablation
• Electrical cv synchronised to **R wave** to prevent inducing VFib
• Pharmacological cv: flecanide or amiodarone (latter if structural heart disease present)

• Anticoagulation for all pts: use CHADSVASc score to calculate risk of stroke & ORBIT score for risk of bleeding
   - if ≥1 (M) or ≥2 (F): DOAC indefinitely
   - warfarin only if mechanical heart valves or severe mitral stenosis
   - DOAC/warfarin for stroke/TIA + AF

CHA2DS2VASc score
• Age   65-74yo =1   ≥75yo =2
• Sex   Male =0   Female =1
• Heart failure =1
• Hypertension =1
• Stroke/TIA/VTE =2
• Vascular disease (prior MI, PAD) =1
• Diabetes =1

ORBIT score
• Age   ≥75yo   =1
• Bleeding Hx (GI bleed, ICH,
  haemorrhagic stroke)   =2
• GFR <60 mL/min   =1
• Tx with antiplatelets   =1

Complications: stroke/TIA (5x ↑risk compared to non-AF pts), bradycardia, hypotension, heart failure, death, etc
• Amiodarone - risk of thyroid issues

Advanced life support

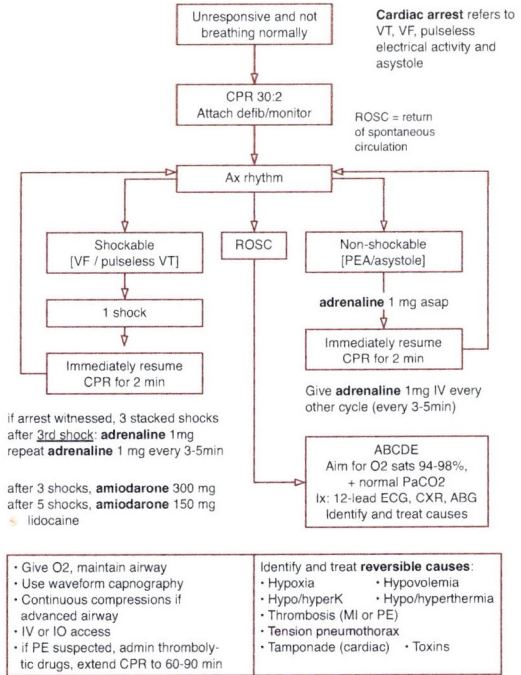

Unresponsive and not breathing normally

CPR 30:2
Attach defib/monitor

Ax rhythm

Shockable [VF / pulseless VT]
1 shock
Immediately resume CPR for 2 min

ROSC

Non-shockable [PEA/asystole]
adrenaline 1 mg asap
Immediately resume CPR for 2 min

Give **adrenaline** 1mg IV every other cycle (every 3-5min)

if arrest witnessed, 3 stacked shocks
after 3rd shock: **adrenaline** 1mg
repeat **adrenaline** 1 mg every 3-5min

after 3 shocks, **amiodarone** 300 mg
after 5 shocks, **amiodarone** 150 mg
lidocaine

Cardiac arrest refers to VT, VF, pulseless electrical activity and asystole

ROSC = return of spontaneous circulation

ABCDE
Aim for O2 sats 94-98%, + normal PaCO2
Ix: 12-lead ECG, CXR, ABG
Identify and treat causes

• Give O2, maintain airway
• Use waveform capnography
• Continuous compressions if advanced airway
• IV or IO access
• if PE suspected, admin thrombolytic drugs, extend CPR to 60-90 min

Identify and treat **reversible causes**:
• Hypoxia   • Hypovolemia
• Hypo/hyperK   • Hypo/hyperthermia
• Thrombosis (MI or PE)
• Tension pneumothorax
• Tamponade (cardiac)   • Toxins

Ax of rhythm via defib or ECG monitor
• **VF and VT**: ventricular tachyarrhythmia causing unsynchronised and ineffective contractions of the ventricles
• **Pulseless electrical activity** (PEA): ECG detects some rhythm (eg sinus tachy), but no there is no detectable pulse (eg on the carotids)
   ↳ electrical activity of heart present, but no mechanical activity
• **Asystole**: cessation of electrical and mechanical activity of the heart
   - Usually occurs as decompensation of VT, VF or PEA - terminal rhythm
   - Poor prognosis unless 2/2 choking or pacemaker failure
   - Neurological deficits even if pts survive

Ventricular fibrillation

D: ventricular tachyarrhythmia causing unsynchronised and ineffective contractions of the ventricles ("quiver")

R: CAD, acute MI, HOCM, long/short QT, Brugada, ventricular pre-excitation (e.g. WPW), e- imbalance, drugs, infxn

A: (see risk factors) / P: anatomical, histological Δ in cardiac tissue (esp scarring) due to underlying heart disease, resulting in conductive Δ.

S/Smx: **tachycardia**, **hypotension**, (pre)syncope, airway compromise, impaired consciousness, chest discomfort, dyspnea, etc

Ix: **ECG**, FBC, clotting profile, U&E, **TFT**, CXR, TTE, etc
→ ECG: wide QRS complex, differentiated from other VTachs by irregularly irregular pattern

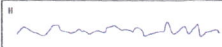

Mx: **DC cardioversion stat** ± amiodarone or lidocaine.
· Long-term: ICD, anti-arrhythmic meds

P: ICD results in better outcomes

Ventricular pre-excitation: Slurring of R wave due to abnormal AV conduction pathway, which activates the ventricles before the normal electrical impulse conducts down the AV node or Bundle or His. Accessory pathway, e.g. WPW.

Ventricular tachycardia

D: broad-complex tachycardia originating from ventricular ectopic focus
· QRS >120ms, rate >100 bpm
· Monomorphic VT (most commonly caused by MI)
· Polymorphic VT: one subtype is torsade de pointes (2/2 prolongation of QT interval)

Causes of prolonged QT interval:
· Congenital
· Drugs - amiodarone, TCAs, fluoxetine, chloroquine, terfenadine, erythromycin
· Electrolyte abn: hypoCa, hypoK, hypoMg
· Acute MI   · Myocarditis
· Hypothermia   · SAH

Ix: ECG, echo, bloods (trops, U&Es)

Mx if unstable
· S/smx: SBP <90, HF, chest pain, syncope, etc
· Immediately cardiovert (DC) - treat under ALS algorithm

Mx if stable
↳ Amiodarone - loading dose then 24h infusion
↳ Lidocaine, procainamide
+ ICD if drug therapy fails or if impaired LV function

Mx of TdP: Mg sulphate

! DO NOT use verapamil

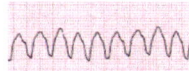

Bradycardia: peri-arrest

D: abnormally slow HR causing haemodynamic compromise; defined <50 bpm

R: medications, >70yo, recent MI, surgery

A: sinus node dysfunction, conduction system disease (including AV block), escape rhythms, AV dissociation, etc

S/smx: dizziness, syncope, fatigue, exercise intolerance, dyspnea, jugular venous distention (+ a-waves)

Ix: ABG, bloods (TFTs, U&Es, trops), 12-lead ECG, Holter monitoring, exercise testing or event monitor, echo

Mx of peri-arrest bradycardia
· O2 - aim for 94-98%
· ↳ **Atropine** boluses to total 3 mg
  - 500 mcg boluses
  - CI in pts with heart transplant
  - If bradycardia 2/2 to βB or CCB, give glucagon
  - If 2/2 to digoxin, call expert help
· Transcutaneous pacing
· ↳ Isoprenaline / adrenaline / dopamine
- Consider if risk of asystole or no response to atropine
- Drug options if pacing unavailable
- Risk factors for asystole: recent asystole, Mobitz II AV block, complete heart block, ventricular pauses >3s

Valsava manoeuvre
· Forced expiration against a closed glottis
· Can be used to terminate episode of supraventricular tachycardia or normalise middle-ear pressures

Tachycardia: peri-arrest

D: ↑HR, generally >100 bpm
· Broad complex
  - Regular: assume VT
  - Irregular: AF + bundle branch block, AF with ventricular pre-excitation, TdP
· Narrow complex
  - Regular: SVT
  - Irregular: probably AF (see 01.02)

Regular narrow complex tachycardia
= **supraventricular tachycardia**
· = tachycardia not ventricular in origin
· QRS <80ms, usually HR 150-220
· Causes: AV nodal re-entry tachy (AVNRT) or AV re-entry tachy, junctional tachycardia, etc

Ix: ECG, bloods (U&Es, trops, etc)

Mx:
Stable SVT
· Valsava manoeuvre (eg blowing into empty plastic syringe)
· Carotid sinus massage
Unstable SVT
· Adenosine IV
  - Rapid IV bolus of 6mg
  - No effect, give 12 mg
  - No effect, give further 18 mg
  ! CI in asthmatics - give verapamil
· Electrical cardioversion
Long term Mx
· β-blockers   · Radio-frequency ablation

Pacemakers

Temporary pacemakers
- used in haemodynamically unstable bradycardia not responding to atropine
- acute anterior MI
- trifascicular block prior to surgery

Implanted cardioverter defibrillator (ICD)
· Indicated for
  - complete AV block
  - Mobitz type II AV block
  - persistent AV block after anterior MI
  - symptomatic bradycardias (eg sick sinus syndrome)
  - heart failure
  - drug-resistant tachyarrythmias
· Ventricular pacing and sensing ICDs are most commonly used
· Show up in ECG with pacing spike

Cardiac enzymes

· Most commonly used: **troponin**
  - rises 4-6h after start of cardiac damage
  - peaks at 12-24h
  - returns to normal after 7-10d
· Most useful for reinfarction: **CKMB**
  - begins to rise 2-6h
  - peaks at 16-20h
  - returns to normal after 2-3d

Others (less specific)
· Myoglobin
  - begins to rise 1-2h (rises first)
  - peaks at 6-8h
  - returns to normal after 1-2d
· CK   - begins to rise 4-8h
        - peaks at 16-24h
  - returns to normal after 3-4d
· AST - begins to rise 12-24h
        - peaks at 36-48h
  - returns to normal after 3-4d
· LDH - begins to rise 24-48h
        - peaks at 72h
  - returns to normal after 8-10d

diagrams from Wikipedia

Usual settings for ECG:
voltage: 10 mV
speed: 25 mm/s

Normal range
- PR: 120-200 ms
- QRS: 80-100 ms
- QTc:
  360-440 ms in M
  360-460 ms in F

P

↑P wave amplitude
- Cor pulmonale

Broad, notched (bifid) p waves
- Often most pronounced in lead II
- ≈ Left atrial enlargement
- Mitral stenosis

No P wave – atrial fibrillation

PR

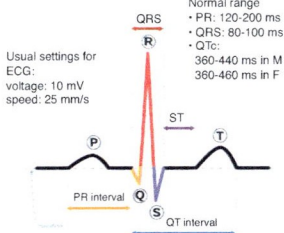

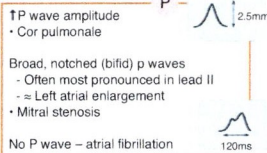

Prolonged PR interval
↳ >200 ms (5 small squares)
- Ischaemic heart disease
- Digoxin toxicity
- Hypokalaemia
- Rheumatic fever
- Aortic root pathology
- Lyme disease
- Sarcoidosis
- Myotonic dystrophy
- Idiopathic   · Athletes

Short PR interval
- Wolff-Parkinson-White (δ wave)

Atrioventricular blocks
- 1st degree heart block
  - PR >200 ms
- 2nd degree heart block
  - Type 1 (Mobitz I, Wenckebach): progressively prolonging PR until dropped beat occurs
  - Type 2 (Mobitz II): constant PR interval between dropped beats
- 3rd degree heart block = complete
  - dissociation between P waves and QRS complexes
  - if arising post MI, think RCA lesion

QRS

QRS complex
↳ normal: 80-100 ms
- Broad complex tachycardia (>100-120 ms) – assume to be ventricular tachycardia until otherwise proven
- Narrow complex tachycardia – likely supraventricular in origin
  - atrioventricular nodal re-entry tachycardia (AVNRT)
  - atrioventricular re-entry tachycardia (AVRT)
  - junctional tachycardia

ST

ST elevation
- MI (ie STEMI)
- Pericarditis / myocarditis
  ↳ diffuse ST elevation + PR depression
- Normal variant ("high take off")
- Left ventricular aneurysm
- Prinzmetal angina (coronary artery spasm)
- Takotsubo cardiomyopathy
  ↳ difficult to differentiate from MI
- Subarachnoid haemorrhage (rare)

ST depression
- MI (ie NSTEMI)
- 2/2 abnormal QRS (LVH, LBBB, RBBB)
- Digoxin
- Hypokalaemia
- Cardiac syndrome X

T

T wave changes
↳ represents ventricular repolarisation
- T wave "inversion" is normal in aVR and V1
- Peaked T waves
  - Hyperkalaemia
  - MI
- Inverted T waves
  - MI
  - Digoxin toxicity
  - Subarachnoid haemorrhage
  - Arrhythmogenic right ventricular cardiomyopathy
  - Pulmonary embolism (S1Q3T3)
    ↳ most commonly presents with sinus tachycardia
  - Brugada syndrome

Note: QTc = correct QT interval; estimates the QT interval at a standard HR of 60 bpm

Left bundle branch block (LBBB)
- Slow or absent conduction through LBB → longer time for LV to fully depolarise
- Causes: acute MI, aortic stenosis, hypertension, etc
  ↳ a new LBBB is always assumed to be an MI until otherwise proven
- "WiLLiaM"
  - W in V1 and
  - M in V6

Right bundle branch block (RBBB)
- Slow or absent conduction through RBB → longer time for RV to fully depolarise
- Causes: normal variant (esp with ↑age), RV hypertrophy, pulmonary embolism, MI, etc
- "MaRRoW"
  - M in V1 and
  - W in V6

Left axis deviation (LAD)
≈ QRS +ve in lead I
  QRS -ve in leads II, III, aVF
- Causes
  - left anterior hemiblock
  - LBBB   - inferior MI
  - Wolf-Parkinson-White, where there is a right-sided accessory pathway
  - Hyperkalaemia
  - Congenital: ASD

Right axis deviation (RAD)
≈ QRS -ve in lead I
  QRS +ve in leads II, III, aVF
- Causes
  - RV hypertrophy
  - left posterior hemiblock
  - lateral MI
  - cor pulmonale
  - pulmonary embolism
  - WPW, where there is a left-sided accessory pathway
  - normal in infants <1yo

Bi-fascicular block
- RBBB + left anterior or posterior hemiblock
  ↳ RBBB + left axis deviation
  ↳ RBBB + right axis deviation

Tri-fascicular block
- RBBB + left hemiblock + 3rd degree heart block
  ↳ PassMed says 1st degree heart block but LITFL says true trifascicular block is with 3rd degree heart block

Left ventricular hypertrophy
- sum of S wave in V1 + R wave in V5 or V6 >40 mm

Right ventricular hypertrophy
- Left atrial enlargement
  - bifid P wave in lead II with duration >120 ms
- Right atrial enlargement
  - tall P waves in leads II and V1 which exceed 25 ms

Hypothermia
- Bradycardia
- J wave (Osborne wave) – small hump at the end of QRS complex
- 1st degree heart block
- Long QT interval
- Atrial and ventricular arrhythmias

Digoxin
- Down-sloping ST depression
- Flattened / inverted T waves
- Short QT interval
- Arrhythmias, eg AV block, bradycardia

Normal variants in athletes
- Sinus bradycardia
- Junctional escape rhythm
- First degree heart block
- Second degree, Mobitz I

Wolff-Parkinson-White syndrome
- D: Congenital cardiac condition arising from an accessory pathway between the atrium and ventricle
  - type A (left-sided pathway)
  - type B (right-sided)
- R: Ebstein anomaly, other cardiac defects, HOCM, ?FHx
- A/P: Accessory pathway can lead to atrioventricular re-entry tachycardia (AVRT) → can degenerate to AF/VF
- S/smx: pt may be asymptomatic, or present with palpitations, dizziness, dyspnea, chest pain, etc
- Ix: ECG (short PR interval, δ wave = wide QRS with slurred upstroke, LAD/RAD) ± echo, electrophysiology
  - type A: dominant R wave in V1
  - type B: nope
- Mx:
  - radiofrequency ablation of accessory pathway - safe and effective
  - medical: sotalol, amiodarone, flecainide
    ↳ avoid sotalol in coexistent AF

Wellen's syndrome
- = pattern that arises due to high-grade stenosis in the left anterior descending coronary artery
- Needs to be referred for PCI asap as very high risk of progression to ACS
- ECG
  - biphasic or deep T wave inversion in V2-3
  - minimal ST elevation
  - no Q waves

Junctional escape rhythm
= isolated QRS complexes
  - usually with rate 40-60 bpm
  - usually narrow (<120 ms)
  - no relationship between QRS complexes and preceding atrial activity
- aka junctional rhythm
- Arise when rate of supraventricular impulses is less than impulses arising from the AV node

Long QT syndrome

D: congenital or acquired condition that is characterised by a prolonged QT interval

QTc is prolonged if
> 440ms in men (>2.2 big sq)
> 460ms in women (>2.6 big sq)

Causes of long QT
- Congenital - Jervell-Lange-Neilsen, Romano-Ward
- Anti-arrythmics: amiodarone, sotalol, class 1a antiarrhythmics
- TCAs, SSRIs (esp citalopram)
- Antipsychotics, eg haloperidol
- Chloroquines   · Terfenadine
- Erythromycin   · Ondansetron
- E- disturbances, eg ↓Ca, ↓K, ↓Mg
- Myocarditis   · Hypothermia
- SAH / big brain bleeds

S/Smx: commonly presents in **young** people with **cardiac arrest** or **unexplained syncope**
- Freq misDx as epilepsy.
- **Cardiac syncope**: premonitory smx such as palpitations, CP, dyspnea → syncope (+ pallor, cyanosis) → recovery (flushing)
- ❗ Identify **trigger** (in LQTS1 & 2, excitement, ↑adrenergic tone; in LQTS3, rest, bradycardia; in acquired, drugs, electrolyte imbalance, etc)

Ix: ECG, bloods (K, Mg, Ca). Consider Holter monitor, exercise tolerance test, ECG, genetic testing

Mx: ❋ lifestyle mod, βB (propranolol or metaprolol)
- avoid extreme exertion; expert evaluation, avoid QT-prolonging drugs, avoid electrolyte imbalance
- ❋ ICD in pts who have had prev cardiac arrest + smx despite βB
Mx of TdP: IV Mg sulphate

P: asmx pts may have normal life expectancy.
- Smx + ≥1 syncopal episodes – risk of recurrent syncopal episodes.
- Smx + cardiac arrest – ↑↑ risk; survival enhanced by βB and ICD

Short QT syndrome

D: inheritable condition that is characterised by a shortened QT interval
- defined as QTc ≤330ms or
- <360ms and one of the following
  · Hx of cardiac arrest or syncope
  · FHx of sudden cardiac death ≤40yo
  · FHx of SQTS

A: e- imbalances (↑K, ↑Ca), hyper-thermia, acidosis, endocrine disorders

S/Smx: · lone AF in the absence of structural heart disease
- ventricular arrhythmias and sudden cardiac arrest
- ± palpitation, syncope, AF.
- May be asmx, picked up on screening
Mean age at Dx is 23yo, more in males

Ix: ECG, bloods (K, Mg, Ca). Consider Holter monitor, exercise tolerance test, ECG, genetic testing

Mx: mainstay is ICD (although pts may get inappropriately shocked due to difficulties in interpreting ECG) ± hydroquinidine (↑QT)

Brugada syndrome

D: inherited cardiac disease with a typical ECG pattern

Epidemiology: ↑prevalence (≥0.2%; ≥1 in 500) in Iran and Thailand

A: disorder of myocardial Na channels, causing variable repolarisation
- characteristic J-point elevation, downward ST in V1-2, "saddle-back"

Dx/Ix – ECG
- Most pts are asmx, identified coincidentally or based on Fhx
- Na-channel blockers can be used to provoke and confirm Dx
- Smx: cardiac arrest, VTach, VF

Mx: in smx pts, ICD + quinidine or ablation

Atrial flutter

D: a supraventricular tachy-arrhythmia characterised by a succession of rapid atrial depolarisation waves

R: ↑age, valvular dysfunction, atrial septal defect, atrial dilation

S/smx: · Palpitations
- Fatigue or lightheadedness
- JVP pulsation with rapid flutter or cannon waves

Ix: ECG – "saw-tooth" appearance best seen in leads II, III, aVF, V1
- 2:1 atrioventricular block is common, where ventricular rate is characteris-tically at 150 bpm

Mx: · similar to that of AF
- More sensitive to cardioversion – lower energy levels may be used
- Definitive Mx: radiofrequency ablation of the tricuspid valve isthmus

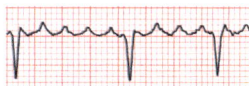

V1
V2
V3

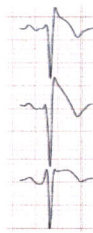

diagrams from Wikipedia

Shock

In general,
- D: life-threatening acute circulatory failure causing cellular and tissue hypoxia
- Mx: ❗ ABCDE ❗
- 2x wide-bore cannulas asap
- Take bloods:
  ◊ ABG/VBG
  ◊ G&S & X-match if need to give blood
  ◊ trops – cardiogenic shock
  ◊ blood cultures – septic shock
- IV fluids – 500 mL fluid bolus + other fluids according to response
- Other Mx according to type of shock

Cardiogenic shock
- Shock 2/2 pump failure (ie heart cannot pump blood around the body)
- A: MI, arrhythmias, toxic substances (eg alcohol, other drugs), heart trauma, chest trauma, etc
- S/smx: ↓BP, ↑HR, ↑RR
- Ix: trops, ECG, echo
- Mx: as above, and
- Consider loop diuretic if heart failure
- Consider vasopressors / ionotropes – specialist Mx
- P: very high mortality if occurring 2/2 MI

Hypovolaemic shock
- Shock 2/2 decreased intravascular volume
- Haemorrhagic shock classified by volume of blood loss
  ◊ Class I: <750 mL   ◊ II: 750-1500 mL
  ◊ III: 1500-2000 mL   ◊ IV: >2000 mL
- A: haemorrhage, dehydration, GI loss, third-spacing (eg hypoalbuminaemia)
- S/smx: ↓BP, ↑HR, ↑RR
- May have obvious wound or bleeding, but internal bleeding may not be obvious
- Ix: bloods (esp group & save + X-match), may need exploratory surgery or scopes to identify source of bleeding if not apparent
- Note that Hb may not be an accurate reflection of acute blood loss – treat clinically
- Mx: as above ± major haemorrhage protocol if necessary

Obstructive shock
- Shock 2/2 obstruction of blood flow → hypoperfusion of tissues distal to obstruction
- A: tension pneumothorax, cardiac tamponade
- Mx: remove obstruction

Distributive shock
- Shock 2/2 failure of vasoregulation
- Further ÷ septic shock, anaphylactic shock, and neurogenic shock

Septic shock
- Systemic immune response to infection (including cytokine storm) results in ↑ peripheral vasodilation
- S/smx: as per sepsis – ↑temp, warm peripheries, ↑RR, ↑HR, WBC <4 or >12
- Ix: blood cultures, ABG/VBG (for lactate), measure UO; other bloods as necessary, look for source of infxn if unknown (eg CXR, urine MC&S)
- Mx: as above + IV abx

Anaphylactic shock [see more 15.01]
- Systemic IgE-mediated hypersensitivity reaction – massive degranulation of mast cells → ↑↑inflammation and vasodilation
- S/smx: ↓BP, ↑HR, ↑RR
  - Systemic smx: facial & throat swelling, hives, difficulty breathing
- Ix: clinical Dx, treat asap
- Mx: **adrenaline 1:1000 IM injection**
  ◊ Adults and >12yo: 0.5 mL (500 mcg)
  ◊ 6-12yo: 0.3 mL (300 mcg)
  ◊ 6mo-6yo: 0.15 mL (150 mcg)
  ◊ <6mo: 0.1-0.15 mL (100-150 mcg)
  - Repeat every 5min if necessary
  - IM injection into anterolateral aspect of thigh (if using Epipen – "orange to the thigh, blue to the sky", count "3 elephants")
  - If refractory (non-responsive after 2 doses of IM adrenaline), consider use of IV adrenaline infusion (expert only)

Neurogenic shock
- Shock 2/2 interruption of autonomic nervous system
- A: spinal cord transection
- S/smx: ↓BP, ↓HR, ↑RR, **warm flushed skin**; other smx depend on level of transection
  - ↓HR due to ↑vagal response with no opposing sympathetic system
  - if above C3, pt may go into respi arrest
- Ix: MRI whole spine
- Mx: vasopressors, atropine, refer to neurosurgeons

"Nacho+": Neurogenic, anaphylactic, cardiogenic, hypovolaemic, obstructive, other misc causes (eg mitochondrial failure)
[mnemonic from *Deranged Physiology*]

	Mitral stenosis	Mitral regurgitation	Aortic stenosis	Aortic regurgitation
Aetiology	· Rheumatic heart disease (99%)	· Rheumatic heart disease · Infective endocarditis · Valve prolapse · Papillary muscle rupture · Marfan syndrome · SLE · LV dilatation (functional MR)	· Rheumatic heart disease · Calcified bicuspid valve (50-60yo) · Calcified tricuspid valve (≥70yo)	· Rheumatic heart disease · Infective endocarditis · Syphilitic cardiomyopathy · Bicuspid valve · Rheumatic · Hypertension arthritis · Aortic dissection · Ankylosing · Marfan syndrome sypondylosis
S/smx	· SOB, fatigue · Pulmonary oedema, haemoptysis · Right heart failure	· SOB and fatigue · LV failure – orthopnea, paroxysmal nocturnal dyspnoea	· SOB · Syncope / pre-syncope · Angina	· SOB, fatigue · Palpitations
Timing Position Manoeuvre Quality Radiation	· Mid-diastolic · Apex · On LHS, on expiration · Rumbling (low-pitched) · None	· Pansystolic · Apex · (none) · Blowing quality · Axilla	· Ejection systolic · Aortic area · (none) · Crescendo-decrescendo · Carotid area	· Early diastolic · Left lower sternal edge · Sitting up, on expiration · Breath-like (high-pitched) · None
Associated features	Opening snap (indicates mitral valve leaflets are still mobile), tapping apex, AF, loud 1st HS (∵ closure of mitral valve), mitral facies, low volume pulse	3rd HS (∵ rapid ventricular filling), thrusting/displaced apex, quiet 1st HS (∵ ↓closure of mitral valve), AF, audible 'click' in valve prolapse	4th HS (∵ poorly compliant ventricle), heaving apex, **slow-rising pulse, narrow pulse pressure**, ejection click, quiet 2nd HS if severe (∵ difficult to close aortic valve)	3rd HS (∵ rapid ventricular filling), thrusting/displaced apex, **collapsing pulse, wide pulse pressure**, head bobbing (De Musset's sign), nailbed pulsation (Quincke's sign)
Mx	· AF – anticoagulation · Asymptomatic - monitor with regular echos · Symptomatic - percutaneous mitral balloon valvotomy - mitral valve surgery	· Medical: nitrates, diuretics, +ve inotropes, intra-aortic balloon pump to ↑cardiac output · HF: ACEI, β-blockers, spironolactone · Surgical: repair if damage is due to degeneration; otherwise, valve replacement is indicated	· Asmx but valvular gradient >40 mmHg + features of LV systolic dysfunction, consider surgery · Smx: ⚕ valve replacement ⚕ balloon – reserved for children (with no aortic valve calcification) and adults not fit for surgery ! Nitrates CI in aortic stenosis	· Medical Mx of HF · If smx or asmx with LV systolic dysfunction, surgery indicated

Murmurs

· **Pansystolic** ("holosystolic")
 - Mitral/tricuspid regurgitation
  ↳ TR louder during inspiration
 - Ventricular septal defect
  ↳ harsh murmur
· **Ejection systolic**
 - Aortic stenosis
 - HOCM
 - Pulmonary stenosis
 - Atrial septal defect
 - Tetralogy of Fallot
· **Late systolic**
 - Mitral valve prolapse
 - Coarctation of the aorta

· **Early diastolic**
 - Aortic regurgitation
 - Pulmonary regurgitation
  ↳ Graham-Steel murmur; similar to aortic regurgitation murmur
· **Mid-diastolic**
 - Mitral stenosis
 - Severe aortic regurgitation
  ↳ Austin-Flint murmur

· **Continuous machine-like**
 - Patent ductus arteriosus

Mnemonics
· RILE: right-sided murmurs best heard on inspiration; left-sided best heard on expiration
· ASMR: aortic stenosis & mitral regurg during **systole**
· ARMS: aortic regurg & mitral stenosis during **diastole**

Rheumatic fever

D: autoimmune disease usually following Strep pyogenes infxn

P: · type II hypersensitivity thought to be caused by molecular mimicry
· M protein on Strep pyogenes is structurally similar to myosin → cross-reactivity; autoimmune response against myosin on the heart walls and arterial smooth muscle

S/smx: "J♡NES" [major criteria]
· Joints: polyarthritis
· ♡: carditis and valvulitis
· Nodules (subcutaneous)
· Erythema marginatum
· Sydenham's chorea (late)

S/smx (continued):
· Minor criteria: ↑ESR/CRP, fever, athralgia, prolonged PR interval
· Dx confirmed if
 - evidence of recent strep infxn and
 - 2 major criteria, or
 - 1 major + 2 minor criteria

Ix: strep swabs, strep antibodies / antigen test, ECG

Mx: · oral penicillin V
 ↳ may prevent rheumatic fever
· NSAIDs
· Tx complications as they occur

P: 30-50% of pts with rheumatic fever will develop rheumatic heart disease - >70% if initial attack severe, or if ≥1 recurrence

Prosthetic heart valves
· Biological
 - usually bovine or porcine origin
 - structural deterioration and calcification over time
 - long term anticoagulation not needed
  ↳ aspirin long term
  ↳ ± warfarin for first 3mo
· Mechanical valves
 - bileaflet valve most common now
 - low failure rate
 - increased risk of thrombosis → requires long-term anticoagulation with warfarin
  ↳ target INR for aortic 3.0, mitral 3.5

Pulses
· Pulsus paradoxus
 - ≥10 mmHg fall in SBP during inspiration
 - seen in cardiac tamponade or severe asthma
· Slow-rising: aortic stenosis
· Collapsing: aortic regurg, patent ductus arteriosus, hyperkinetic states (eg anaemia, thyrotoxicosis)
· Pulsus alternans
 - arterial pulse with alternating strong and weak beats
 - seen in severe LV failure
· Bisferiens pulse ≈ double pulse with 2 systolic peaks
 - Seen in mixed aortic valve disease, sometimes in HOCM
· "Jerky" pulse – seen in HOCM

Heart sounds
· S1 ("lub") – closure of mitral and tricuspid valves
· S2 ("dub") – closure of aortic and pulmonary valves
 - splitting during inspiration is normal
· S3 – caused by rapid ventricular filling of the ventricle during diastole
 - normal if <30yo, may persist in some women ≤50yo
 - LV failure (eg dilated cardiomyopathy), constrictive pericarditis and mitral regurgitation
· S4 – caused by atrial contraction against a stiff ventricle
 - aortic stenosis, HTN, HOCM

© bjpm / pfsm

HOCM — Hypertrophic obstructive cardiomyopathy

D: AD genetic disorder characterised by LV hypertrophy without an identifiable cause. ~1:500

R: FHx of HOCM or sudden cardiac death. A/w Friedreich's ataxia, WFW

A/P: most common defect involve mutation in the gene encoding β-myosin heavy chain protein or myosin-binding protein C
- Results in predominantly **diastolic** dysfunction: left ventricular hypertrophy → ↓compliance → ↓cardiac output
- Myofibrillar hypertrophy with chaotic and disorganised fashion myocytes ('disarray') and fibrosis

S/smx: can be asmx
- Exertional dyspnea, angina, syncope (usually after exercise; 2/2 functional aortic stenosis)
- Sudden death (usually 2/2 ventricular arrhythmia), HF
- Jerky pulse, large 'a' waves, double apex beat
- Systolic murmurs
  - Ejection systolic murmur – ↑ with Valsava manouvre and ↓ with squatting
  - pansystolic murmur due to mitral regurgitation

Ix: ECG (LVH, deep Q waves, AFib, non-specific signs), echo ("MR SAM ASH" - mitral regurg, systolic anterior motion of the anterior mitral valve leaflet, asymmetric hypertrophy)

Mx: "ABCDE"
- Amiodarone
- β-blockers or verapamil
- Cardioverter defibrillator
- Dual chamber pacemaker
- ± Endocarditis prophylaxis

❗ Drugs to AVOID: nitrates, ACEIs, inotropes

Arrhythmogenic right ventricular cardiomyopathy

D: primary cardiomyopathy characterised by fibrofatty replacement of the right ventricular myocardium
- Autosomal dominant

R: FHx, usually presents in late 20s (second most common cause of sudden cardiac death in the young after HOCM), M>F (1.6x), intense exercise
- A/w Naxos disease (triad of ARVC, palmoplantar keratosis, woolly hair)

A: mutations in various genes; 50% pts have mutation of several genes which encode components of desmosome

S/smx: · palpitations
- syncope
- sudden cardiac death

Mx: ⟲ sotalol
- Catheter ablation or ICD to prevent ventricular tachycardia

diagram from Wikipedia

Takotsubo cardiomyopathy

= "octopus trap" – transient, apical ballooning of the myocardium brought about by stress
- S/smx: CP, features of HF
- Ix: ECG – ST elevation; normal coronary angiogram (ie no infarction)
- Mx: supportive; most pts improve with supportive tx

Dilated cardiomyopathy

D: disease of heart muscle characterised by enlargement and dilation of one or both of ventricles along with impaired contractility
↳ LVEF ≤40% and systolic dysfunction (by definition)

Causes
- Idiopathic
- Ischaemic heart disease & HTN
- Myocarditis, eg Coxsackie B virus, HIV, Chagas disease
- Peripartum
- Iatrogenic, eg doxorubicin
- Substance abuse, eg alcohol, cocaine
- Inherited, eg Duchenne muscular dystrophy
- Infiltrative, eg haemochromatosis, sarcoidosis
- Thiamine deficiency leading to wet beri beri

P: myocardial remodelling → eccentric hypertrophy of ventricles → ↓systolic dysfunction predominantly
- Can lead to significant tricuspid and mitral valve insufficiency → ↓ejection fraction

S/smx:
- Heart failure s/smx + S3
- Tricuspid and mitral valve regurgitation will cause pansystolic murmur

Ix: CXR – balloon appearance of heart on CXR. Others as per HF

Mx → as per HF

Chronic heart failure

D: dysfunction of the left ventricle, resulting in insufficient delivery of blood to vital organs. HFpEF (>50%) and HFrEF (<40%).

NYHA classification:
I. smx do not affect daily activities
II. smx occur at moderate effort, slightly restricting daily activities
III. smx occur at minimal effort, significantly restricting daily activities
IV. delibitating smx at rest

R: CAD, HTN, ↑chol, DM, smoking, radiation, some chemotherapy. FHx.

A/P: HTN, CAD, ↑chol → ↑peripheral vascular resistance → hypertrophy of heart to compensate → stressor (e.g. vol overload, arrhythmia, MI) may cause heart to decompensation
- Main issue is during **diastole** – impaired relaxation and/or ↑filling. Impaired elasticity or compliance of myocardium

systolic HF - impaired contraction
diastolic HF - impaired filling

S/smx: · dyspnea, cough (pink/frothy) ± cardiac wheeze, orthopnea, paroxysmal nocturnal dyspnea (pt wakes up at night struggling to breathe),
- wt loss (cardiac cachexia; may be masked by water gain)
- Peripheral oedema (sacral, pedal)
- Signs of right heart failure: ↑JVP, ankle oedema, hepatomegaly

Ix: ⟲ NTproBNP (≥400 ng/L = high)
⟲ **TTEcho w/in 2w** (+ estimating EF)
- Other Ix as appropriate, including bloods (eg FBC, U&Es), CXR, ECG, etc

CXR: bilat pleural effusions, fluid in interlobar fissures and fluid in septal lines (Kerley B lines)

Cor pulmonale

= Right heart failure arises from lung disease specifically – COPD, PE, interstitial lung disease, cystic fibrosis, pulmonary HTN

Mx:
- ACEI + β-blocker (eg bisoprolol)
- Start one drug at a time
- Aldosterone antag (eg eplenerone)
- Monitor renal function (drugs can cause hyperK)
- SGLT2 inhibitor
3rd line: (started by specialist)
- Ivabradine – use if sinus rhythm HR >75, LVEF <35%
- Sacubitril-valsartan (LVEF <35%, must have ACEI washout)
- Digoxin – can improve smx, esp useful if coexisting AF
- Hyradalzine and nitrate (esp in Afro-Caribbean pts)
- Cardiac resynchronisation therapy
- Others: annual influenza vaccine, one-off pneumococcal vaccine

Acute heart failure – Mx
"Pour SOD"
- **P**our away fluids – fluid restriction
- **S**it them upright
- **O**xygen – target 94-98% sats
  - CPAP if respiratory failure
- **D**iuretics, eg IV furosemide
- In patients with hypotension or cardiogenic shock
  - Ionotropic agents, eg dobutamine
  - Vasopressors, eg norepinephrine
  - Mechanical circulatory assistance, eg ventricular assist devices
- Other treatments
  - Vasodilators – consider in concomitant myocardial ischaemia, severe hypertension, aortic regurgitation or mitral regurgitation
  - Opiates – not routinely offered
- Continue regular medications for HF
  - β-blockers – stop only if HR <50, 2nd/3rd degree AV block, or shock

High output heart failure
= A normal heart is unable to pump enough blood to meet metabolic needs of the body
Eg severe anaemia, pregnancy, Paget's disease, thiamine deficiency

Deep vein thrombosis

D: blood clot in a major deep vein, classically in the lower limbs, impairing venous blood flow

R: ↑age, recent surgery, immobility >3d, previous VTE, cancer, pregnancy, COCP, HRT, trauma, clotting disorder

A/P: Virchow's triad (stasis, endothelial damage, **hypercoagulopathy**). Can lead to PE if clot embolises

S/Smx based on **Well's score**
· Risk factors (as above)
· Localised tenderness along distribution of venous system
· Entire leg swollen
· Calf swelling ≥3cm larger than other leg
· Pitting oedema of affected side
· Collateral superficial veins

Ix & Mx based on Well's score
Wells score ≥2 points
(1) proximal leg USS within 4h, *or*
(2) D-dimer + anticoagulate + scan w/in 24h
· If scan -ve: DVT + anticoagulate
· If scan -ve: D-dimer + anticoagulate
· If D-dimer +ve but scan -ve: stop anticoagulating, repeat scan in 1w
· If D-dimer -ve and scan -ve: stop anticoagulating – alternative Dx
· If 2nd scan +ve: DVT + anticoagulate
· If 2nd scan -ve: alternative Dx
Wells score ≤1 point
(1) D-dimer with result within 4h, *or*
(2) D-dimer + interim anticoagulation
· D-dimer -ve: stop anticoagulating, consider alternative Dx
· D-dimer +ve: treat as per Wells ≥2

Anticoagulation
· ⚡ DOAC (apixaban, rivaroxaban)
· ⚡ LMWH followed by dabigatran/edoxaban, *or* LWMH followed by warfarin
· Special situations
- Cancer: still use DOAC
- Renal impairment: LWMH → warfarin
- Antiphospholipid syndrome (esp triple +ve): LMWH → warfarin
· Length of anticoagulation
- If provoked, treat for 3mo
- If provoked by cancer, length depends on continued risk (3-6mo)
- If unprovoked, treat for 6mo + may need Ix to check for causes of DVT (eg CTTAP to look for cancer)

Pulmonary embolism

D: occlusion in pulmonary vasculature due to thrombus that arises in or travels to the lungs, most often originating from a deep vein.

R: as per DVT

A/P: most often, DVT that breaks off and gets stuck in the lungs

S/Smx based on **Well's score**
· Risk factors (as for DVT)
· Clinical s/smx of DVT
· HR >100   · Haemoptysis

Other s/smx: ↑RR (>20), crackles on chest, fever, pleuritic chest pain

Ix & Mx based on PERC & Wells score
· Pulmonary embolism rule-out criteria (PERC) – <2% probability of PE if *all* criteria ABSENT; if not, do Wells score
· Calculate Well's score
· Wells score ≥4 points
(1) Immediate CTPA, *or*
(2) Interim DOAC while awaiting CTPA
- CTPA +ve = PE + anticoagulate
- CTPA -ve → consider proximal leg vein USS if DVT suspected
- If CTPA contraindicated (eg pregnant, renal impairment), use V/Q scan
· Wells score <4 points
(1) D-dimer test
- If D-dimer +ve, treat as per Wells ≥4
- If D-dimer -ve, stop anticoagulation, consider alternative Dx

Other Ix while awaiting results:
· ECG - most commonly showing sinus tachy. S1Q3T3 only in 20%, RBBB and RAD may be a/w PE
· CXR - for all pts. Usually normal CXR unless large PE (wedge-shaped opacification)
· ABG, FBC (including clotting screen)

Mx: **anticoagulation**
· As per DVT
· If massive PE + circulatory failure (eg hypotension), ⚡ thrombolysis
· Pulmonary embolism severity index (PESI) used to determine who can be treated as outpatient
- Takes into account haemodynamic stability, comorbidities, etc
· Repeat PEs: consider IVC filter

Infective endocarditis

D: infection involving the endocardial surface of the heart, including valvular structures, etc.

R: prior hx of IE, prosthetic heart valves, congenital heart disease, heart transplant, sources of bacteraemia (vasc cath, recent dental work, IVDU), etc

A: *Strep. viridians, S. aureus, Strep. bovis., Enterococci.* Culture -ve HACEK
P: thrombi develop on valvular surfaces due to ↑endothelial damage, act as foci for bacteria to colonise and grow

Most common culture -ve causes incl fastidious organisms (zoonotic agents, fungi), **Strep** in pts who have received prior abx

HACEK: *Haemophilus, Aggregatibacter* (prev *Actinobacillus*), *Cardiobacterium, Eikenella, Kingella*

S/Smx: **fever**, murmur, constitutional smx, weakness, arthralgia, HA, dyspnea. Janeway lesions, Osler nodes, Roth spots, splinter haemorrhages

Ix: blood cultures (3x **10 mL** from different sites at 30-min intervals), echo, FBC, CRP, U&E, LFT, urinalysis, ECG

Mx: sepsis pathway if needed, broad spectrum then adjust according to culture results. May need urgent surgery

Indications for surgery for IE
· Severe valvular incompetence
· Aortic abscess (↑PR interval)
· Infxns resistant to abx (* fungal infxn)
· HF refractory to medical tx
· Recurrent emboli after abx

P: ↑mortality if elderly and resulting in HF. Possible cerebral comp. Surgery a/w ↓mortality.

Long-haul flights
· Slight ↑risk esp on long haul travel
· If no major risk factors for VTE, no special measures required
· If other risk factors,
- wear anti-embolism stockings
- ? seek medical advice about use of LMWH
· No role for aspirin

Pericarditis

D: inflammation of the pericardium.
> Acute: lasting ≤6w.
> Fibrinous vs effusive

R: M>F, 20-50yo, STEMI, cardiac surgery, cancer, infxn (esp viral), uraemia, dialysis, autoimmune.

A: 90% idiopathic or viral infxn; 10% other. Infxn, autoimmune, 2' immune, heart-related, metabolic, traumatic, neoplastic, drug-related, idiopathic.
P: Inflammation may lead to effusion or fibrosis

S/Smx: chest pain (acute, sharp, pleuritic/stabbing; relieved by sitting forward; may mimic MI but not relieved by GTN), pericardial rub (<33%), fever, myalgia

Clinical Dx confirmed by 2 of 4: **characteristic chest pain**, pericardial friction rub, ECG Δ, new/ worsening pericardial effusion. ❗ r/o PE.

Ix: ECG - ST elevation &/or PR depression. TTEcho. Bloods. Pericardiocentesis. CXR.

Mx: · suspected cardiac tamponade, urgent pericardiocentesis required
· **NSAID, PPI, colchicine**
· If present, treat underlying cause
- most 2/2 viral smx, no so specific tx
- if bacterial (purulent), IV abx
· Advice pt to avoid strenuous activity until smx resolve

P: poorer outcome if large effusion, high fever, subacute course, failure to respond

Constrictive pericarditis

D: A form of diastolic heart failure that arises because an inelastic pericardium inhibits cardiac filling

A: similar causes to pericarditis.
↳ most common cause is TB
· Can also occur following heart surgery or mediastinal radiation (M>F 3:1)

P: during healing, granulation tissue forms. This may contract over time ± calcify → constrictive picture

S/smx: · Dyspnoea
· Right heart failure: ↑JVP, ascites, oedema, hepatomegaly
· JVP: prominent x and y descent
· Pericardial knock (loud S3)
· Kussmaul's sign +ve
↳ paradoxical rise in JVP during inspiration

Ix: as per acute pericarditis
· CXR may show pericardial calcification

Mx: surgical pericardiectomy is the only effective tx for chronic constrictive pericarditis
· If inflammatory process still ongoing, pt may respond to NSAIDs or other anti-inflammatory agents

Pericardial rub - "**fresh snow**" sound best heard left sternal edge leaning forward, end-exp. Still heard when holding breath ∵ heart sound not respi-related. Likely need to examine repeatedly.

Uraemic pericarditis: tx intensive dialysis.

Dressler's syndrome: post-MI pericarditis (? inflammatory reaction). Usually 2-4w post MI Mx as per pericarditis.

PERC - must all be negative to r/o PE
· ≥50yo   · HR ≥100   · O2 sats ≤94%
· previous DVT/PE
· recent surgery/trauma in past 4w
· haemoptysis
· unilateral leg swelling   · oestrogen use

Cardiac tamponade

D: Accumulation of pericardial fluid, blood, pus or air within the pericardial space. ❗ Medical emergency.

R: malignancy (esp lung and breast), aortic dissection, purulent pericarditis, heart surgery, TB

A: iatrogenic (eg surgery), trauma, malignancy, idiopathic

P: ↑pericardial pressure 2/2 accumulation of fluid in pericardial space → if pericardial pressure is greater than intra-chamber pressures, heart will collapse

S/smx:
- Beck's triad – hypotension, ↑JVP, muffled heart sounds
- Dyspnea, ↑HR, pulsus paradoxus, ± Kussmaul's sign

Ix: ECG, TTE, CXR, bloods (FBC, cardiac enzymes)

- Pulsus paradoxus: ↑↑drop in BP during inspiration
- Kussmaul's sign: paradoxical rise in right atrial pressure during inspiration
- Electrical alternans: QRS complex amplitude changes in alternate cycles

Mx: urgent pericardiocentesis if pt is unstable (needle is inserted into the pericardial sac and allows drainage of fluid)

Antihypertensives

ACE inhibitors (-pril)
- Adverse effects
  - dry cough in 15%, 2/2 ↑bradykinin levels – may be intolerable for some
  - Angioedema (may occur up to a year after starting tx)
  - Hyperkalaemia
  - First dose orthostatic hypotension
- Contraindicated / caution in
  - pregnancy & bfding (teratogenic)
  - Renovascular disease
    ↳ think esp renal artery stenosis!
  - Aortic stenosis - may cause hypotension
  - Hereditary idiopathic angioedema
- Monitoring
  - U&Es – can cause transient ↑SCr up to 30% from baseline, transient ↑K up to 5.5mmol/L
  - Renal impairment – think about undiagnosed bilateral renal artery stenosis

Angiotensin II blockers (ARBs) (-sartan)
- Generally used where ACE inhibitors are not tolerated
- Similar contraindications and cautions with ACE inhibitors

β-blockers (-olol)
- Adverse effects:
  - bronchospasm   - cold peripheries
  - fatigue   - sleep disturbances
  - erectile dysfunction
- Contraindications / cautions
  - Uncontrolled HF
  - Asthma (∵ bronchospasm)
  - Sick sinus syndrome
  - Concurrent verapamil use – may precipitate severe bradycardia

α-blockers
- Not commonly used for HTN
- Eg doxazosin, tamsulosin
- Adverse effects: orthostatic hypotension drowsiness, dyspnea, cough
- Methyldopa – used to control BP in pregnancy

Calcium channel blockers
- *Non-dihydropyridine CCBs:* verapamil and diltiazem
- *Verapamil*
  - Adverse effects: HF, constipation, hypotension, bradycardia, flushing
  - DO NOT give with β-blockers
- *Diltiazem*
  - Adverse effects: HF, hypotension, bradycardia, ankle swelling
- *Dihydropiridine CCBs*
  - eg amlodipine, nifedipine
  - Affect the peripheral vascular smooth muscle more than heart; do not result in worsening of HF but can cause ↑ankle swelling
  - Adverse effects: flushing, HA, ankle swelling
  - Nifedipine can be used in pregnancy

Thiazide diuretics
- Eg indapamide, chlortalidone
- MOA: inhibit sodium reabsorption in kidneys (can result in ↑K loss)
- Adverse effects: dehydration, orthostatic hypotension, ↓K, ↓Na, ↑Ca (and also ↓Ca in urine = hypo-calciuria), gout, impaired glucose tolerance, impotence
- Rarely can also cause pancreatitis

Loop diuretics
- Eg furosemide, bumetanide
- MOA: inhibit NaCl reabsorption in kidneys by inhibiting Na-K-2Cl cotransporter
- Pts with poor renal function may require ↑↑dose to ensure sufficient concentration in renal tubules
- Adverse effects: hypotension, ↓Na, ↓K, ↓Mg, ↓Ca, hypochloraemic alkalosis, ototoxicity, renal impairment, hyperglycaemia, gout

Aldosterone antagonists
- Eg spironolactone, eplenerone
- Sometimes known as potassium-sparing diuretics
- MOA: ↓Na absorption in collecting ducts
- Adverse effects: ↑K, gynaecomastia (less common with eplenerone)

Adenosine

MOA: causes transient heart block in AV node
- α1 agonist at the AV node
- T1/2 of 8-10 s
- Used to terminate SVT

❗ Administer via large-bore cannulas due to short half life

- Avoid in asthmatics due to possible bronchospasm
- AE: CP, bronchospasm, transient flushing, ↑ventricular rate

Amiodarone

MOA: blocks K ± Na channels
- very long t1/2 (20-100d)

❗ Admin via central veins due to thrombophlebitis + loading dose

Monitoring:
- Prior to tx: TFT, LFT, CXR
- q6mo: TFT, LFT

Adverse effects
- thyroid dysfunction: both ↑ and ↓
- corneal deposits
- pulmonary fibrosis/pneumonitis
- liver fibrosis/hepatitis
- peripheral neuropathy
- myopathy
- photosensitivity
- 'slate-grey' appearance
- thrombophlebitis and injection site reactions
- bradycardia
- lengthens QT interval

Antiplatelets   LL = lifelong

	1st line	2nd line
ACS or PCI	aspirin (LL) ticagrelor (12mo)	clopidogrel (LL)
TIA or stroke	Clopidogrel (LL)	aspirin (LL) dipyridamole (LL)
PAD	Clopidogrel (LL)	aspirin (LL)

Aspirin - MOA: irreversible COX1,2 inhibitor
- Do not use in <16yo due to risk of Reye's syndrome (except in Kawasaki disease)
- British Society for Haematology recommends that aspirin monotherapy can be continued for most noncardiac procedures unless bleeding risk is high – in which case, omit 3d before until 7d after operation
- CABG – continue aspirin

Clopidogrel, ticagrelor, prasugrel
- MOA: P2Y12 adenosine diphosphate (ADP) receptor inhibitor
- May be less effective if used with PPIs
  - ?best PPI to use with is lansoprazole

DLVA cardiovascular disorders

- ACS: 4 weeks off driving
  ↳ 1 week if successfully treated by PCI
- Angina: driving must cease if smx occur at rest/at the wheel
- Aortic aneurysm ≥6 cm: notify DVLA
  ↳ Licensing will be permitted subject to annual review
- AA ≥ 6.5 cm: pt disqualified from driving
- CABG: 4 weeks off driving
- Catheter ablation for arrhythmia: 2d off
- Heart transplant: do not drive for 6 weeks, no need to notify DVLA
- HTN: can drive unless tx causes unacceptable AE, no need to notify DVLA
  ↳ for HGV: no driving if consistently SBP >180 and/or DBP >100
- ICD for sustained ventricular arrhythmia: cease driving for 6 months
- ICD for prophylaxis: 1 month off driving
  ↳ HGV: ICD placement – permanent ban
- Pacemaker insertion: 1 week off driving
- PCI (elective): 1 week off driving

Peripheral arterial disease

D: arterial disease caused by atherosclerotic obstruction of arteries *outside the heart and brain*
÷ intermittent claudication, critical limb ischaemia, & acute limb-threatening ischaemia

R: **smoking**, DM, HTN, ↑cholesterol, >40yo, Hx of CAD/stroke/TIA

A: atherosclerosis
P: fat deposits → clog peripheral arteries

S/smx:
Intermittent claudication
· Aching or burning in leg muscles during or after walking
· Predictable distance before smx start, relieved on stopping
· Pain not present at rest
Critical limb ischaemia
· **Rest pain** in foot for **≥2w**, ulceration and/or gangrene
Acute limb-threatening ischaemia
· ≥1'P's: pale, pulseless, painful, paralysed, paraesthetic (numb/sensory changes), perishingly cold

Ix: leg pulses ± hand-held Doppler exam, ankle-brachial pressure index (ABPI), duplex US, MRI angiography, ECG

Mx: · STOP SMOKING
· Mx comorbidities
· Statin (atorvastatin 80 mg)
  + clopidogrel for all pts + analgesia
· Exercise training
Severe PAD / Limb-threatening
· Acute Mx
  - ABCDE + analgesia (eg IV opioids)
  - IV UFH to prevent thrombus enlargement
  - Vascular review asap
· Definitive Mx options
  - Angioplasty ± stent
  - Endovascular interventions for short segment stenosis, aortic iliac disease, high-risk pts
  - Surgical revasc (open): long segment lesions (>10cm), multifocal lesions, lesions of common femoral artery and purely infrapopliteal disease
  - Amputation: worst-case option

Aortic aneurysm

D: permanent pathological dilation of the aorta. 1.5x expected AP diameter for segment, given pt's sex and body size. >3cm. 90% below renal arteries.

R: **!** **smoking**, FHx, ↑age, M>F incidence, F>M rupture, connective tissue disorders. ± hyperlipid, HTN, atherosclerosis, etc

A/P: degradation of aortic wall connective tissue by enzymes, inflam & immune response, wall stress and genetics

S/Smx: most asmx, picked up on screening. Palpable pulsatile mass. If rupture, shock, LOC, pain.

Ix: Aortic US, contrast CTA to plan for surgery, bloods (G&S, X-match, clotting, FBC, etc).

Mx: · stop smoking!!
· **Ruptured** - vascular surgical repair (lap repair or endovascular aneurysm repair using stent inserted via femoral arteries)
· If stable but **≥5.5cm, or >4cm and growing >1cm/year**, urgent ref to vascular surgery
· Surveillance for those not meeting criteria

> Screening offered to all men in England – one-off US at 65yo
> → CT yearly for 3-4.4cm
> → CT q3mo for 4.5-5.4 cm

P: high morbidity for rupture, ↑morbidity and mortality a/w surgical intervention. If pt survives intervention, low risk of complications

Leriche syndrome
· D: atheromatous disease of the iliac vessels → ↓blood flow to pelvic viscera
  ↳ ?subtype of peripheral arterial disease
· S/smx: (triad) buttock claudication, impotence and no femoral pulses
· Ix: angiography
· Mx: endovascular angioplasty and stent insertion

Aortic dissection

D: a separation occuring in aortic wall intima, causing blood flow into a new false channel composed of the inner and outer layers of the media

R: aneurysms, Marfan, Ehlers-Danlos, bicuspid aortic valve, coarctation, smoking, FHx, HTN

A/P: intimal tear that extends into the media of the aortic wall → blood passes through the media (antero or retrograde), creating a false lumen → can cause occlusion to branches of the aorta

Stanford classification
A: asc. aorta, prox to L subclavian a
B: distal to L subclavian a
DeBakey classification
I = A+B   II = A   II = B

S/Smx: ▶ abrupt severe chest pain, abd pain ("tearing") ± syncope. Pt can present with shock, HF, cardiac tamponade (Beck's triad: muffled heart sound, hypotension, ↑JVP)

Ix: ECG, CXR, bloods. **CT** for definitive Dx. TTE ideally

Mx: 1. **initial resus**: O2, fluids, inotropes, pain control
2. **monitor vitals**
   · HR <60, SBP ≤100-120
   · IV βB, verapamil or diltiazem
3. **definitive Mx**
   · A: emergency surgery
   · complicated B: urgent TEVAR or open surgery if TEVAR is CI
   · uncomplicated B: continue medical tx, TEVAR w/in 6w if ↑risk for comp
4. chronic aortic dissection (>90d after surgery)
   · Mx HR and BP carefully
   · Mx risk factors – smoking, chol

TEVAR = thoracic endovascular aortic repair

P: left untreated, up to 60% mortality in 24h in type A + rupture

Varicose veins

D: Subcutaneous, permanently dilated veins

R: ↑age, FHx, F>M, ↑number of pregnancies, DVT, obesity

S/smx: · Visibly bulging veins – usually more apparent when standing
· Aching, throbbing   · Itchy
· ± Other signs of chronic insufficiency

Ix: Venous duplex US (retrograde venous flow)

Mx: · Conservative, eg leg elevation, wt loss, regular exercise, graduated compression stockings
· Referral to vascular surgery if
  - Significant smx
  - Previous bleeding from varicose veins
  - Skin changes 2/2 chronic venous insufficiency
  - Superficial thrombophlebitis
  - Active or healed venous leg ulcer
  - Possible treatments
  ↳ currently under NICE tx can only be offered if significant smx
  - Endothermal ablation (using radio-frequency or endovenous laser tx)
  - Foam sclerotherapy
  - Surgery: ligation or stripping of veins

P: Even if treated, new varicosities likely will develop over time

Chronic insufficiency skin changes
· Telangiectasia
· Reticular veins (dilated, non-palpable, subdermal veins ≤3mm)
· Corona phlebectatica = malleolar flare or ankle flare (fan-shaped pattern of small veins on the ankle or foot)
· Varicose veins
· Atrophie blanche (localised, round areas of white, shiny, atrophic skin surrounded by small dilated capillaries)
· Lipodermatosclerosis (localised chronic inflammatory and fibrotic condition, esp in the malleolar region)
· Hyperpigmentation (reddish-brown discolouration = "brawny oedema")
  - due to deposition of haemosiderin
· Dry, scaling eczema – venous stasis dermatitis
· Venous ulcers in gaiter area

Lower leg ulcers

Venous leg ulcers
· Located above ankle
· Usually painless
· Shallow ulcer, undefined borders
· A/w - Previous DVT - Oedema
  - Chronic insufficiency skin changes
· Ix: Dopper US
· Mx: Compression banding after r/o arterial disease
  - If no healing in 12w or large ulcer, skin grafting may be needed

Marjolin's ulcer
· Squamous cell carcinoma
· Located at sites of chronic inflammation, eg burns

Arterial ulcers
· Located on toes and heels
· Painful, with deep punched appearance
· A/w gangrene, peripheral arterial disease
· Ix: low ABPI

Neuropathic ulcers
· Located on plantar surface of meta-tarsal head and plantar surface of hallux
· Esp in diabetics
· Ix: r/o other possible causes
· Mx: advice pts to wear cushioned shoes to reduce callus formation

Pyoderma gangrenosum
See 09.02

Ankle-brachial pressure index (ABPI)
= ratio of systolic BP in lower leg to that in the arms
↳ in diabetics, may need to do toe-brachial pressure index (TBPI)
· >1.2 – calcified, stiff arteries
· 0.9-1.2 – normal / acceptable
· <0.9 – likely peripheral arterial disease (do not do compression banding)
  - <0.5 – severe disease

Asthma

CRAB: **C**hronic, **R**eversible obstruction, **A**irway hypersensitivity, **B**ronchial inflammation

D: chronic inflammatory airway disease characterised by **intermittent reversible airway obstruction and hyperreactivity**

R: Fhx, allergens, atopic hx ± nasal polyposis, obesity, GORD, apnea

A/P: **(1) inflammation, (2) airway hyper-responsiveness (AHR).** The large airways and small airways <2µm are the sites of inflammation and airway obstruction.
(1) occurs due to inflammatory cells, mediators, etc. Initial trigger → Th2 response + other cells move to airway epithelium and cause Δ.
(2) smooth muscle contraction → AHR. Baseline fixed (∵ airway remodelling) + episodic variable element (∵ acute inflammation).

S/smx: recurrent dyspnea, chest tightness, wheezing, coughing. Allergens. Night time smx that wake pt from sleep in severe asthma.
In exacerbation, wheezing audible; chest may be silent if severe

Dx ≥17yo: spirometry & bronchodilator reversibility (BDR) + FeNO (>40 ppm)
Dx 5-16yo: spirometry & BDR + FeNO (if normal spirometry or obstructive smx and -ve BDR test)
Dx <5yo: Dx on clinical judgment
Reversibility testing: +ve if ↑FEV of ≥12% or ≥200 mL
Peak flow variability: ask pt if better on holidays/away from work

Mx: Step wise.
Monitoring: daily PEFR readings
1. SABA prn
2. + low dose ICS or cromolyn / montelukast
3. Δ medium dose ICS
4. + LABA or montelukast
5. Δ high dose ICS
6. + PO steroids

BTS classification of acute asthma

Moderate	Severe
PEFR 50-75%	PEFR 33-50%
Speech normal	Incomplete sentences
RR <25	RR >25
HR <110	HR >110

Life-threatening	PEFR <33%
O2 sats <92%	"Normal" PCO2

Silent chest, cyanosis or feeble respi effort
↑HR, ↓RR, dysrhythmia
Exhaustion, confusion, coma

Acute exacerbation (mod to severe)
S/Smx: SOB, cough, wheeze, ↑chest tightness, ↓PFT, ↑HR, ↑RR, accessory muscle use, sleep disturbance, **!** **silent chest [impending respi failure]**
Ix: ABG (repeat in 1h if continuing issues), peak flow (and 15-30 min after starting tx), O2 sats, CXR [not routine].
Mx: O2, SABA (inh / IV), steroid PO/IV, ipratropium bromide nebs ± MgSO4, aminophylline IV, intubate & ventilate + ITU if not responding

COPD

D: disease state characterised by **progressive airflow limitation** that is not fully reversible. Compasses both emphysema and chronic bronchitis.

R: **!** smoking, ↑age, genetics (AATD), childhood lung issues

A/P: chronic inflammation that affects central and peripheral airways, lung parenchyma and alveoli, and pulmonary vasculature. Repeated injury and repair → structure and physiologic Δ.
· Narrowing and remodelling of airways
· ↑ no of goblet cells
· ↑ size of mucus-secreting glands of central airways
· Alveolar loss
· Vascular bed changes → pul HTN
Emphysema ∵ elastin breakdown causing loss of alveolar integrity

Complications:
· Cor pulmonale (engorged neck veins, edema, hepatomegaly)
 - Tx with long term oxygen therapy (LTOT).
· ↑risk of recurrent pneumonia and depression.
· Variable course of disease - prognosis may be estimated using FEV1.

Respiratory failure
Type I: ↓O2 → CPAP
Type II: ↓O2 + ↑CO2 → BiPAP
Type III: peri-op / atelectasis
Type IV: septic shock / respi failure 2/2 ↑metabolic requirements

S/Smx: cough (morning cough, then becomes constant), SOB, sputum.
± barrel chest, hyper-resonance, wheezing ("continuous musical lung sound"), coarse crackles

Ix: spirometry (**FEV1/FVC<0.7**; FEV6 also acceptable), mMRC scale (see right) to Ax smx, O2 sats, ABG, CXR, FBC, ECG (Ax for comorbidities). ± α1-antitrypsin levels, exercise testing, sputum culture, etc

Mx of stable COPD
General advice
· Smoking cessation, incl nicotine replacement, varenicline, bupropion
· Annual flu jab
· One off pneumococcal vaccination
· Pulmonary rehab if functional disability

Bronchodilator
 SABA or SAMA eg ipratropium
 Asthmatic/steroid-responsive
· if prev Dx of asthma or atopy, diurnal variation in PEF (≥20%), variation in FEV1 (≥400 mL) over time, or ↑↑ eosinophil count
 - LABA + ICS
 - LAMA + ICS + LABA
  ↳ if pt on SAMA, switch to SABA
 No asthmatic features
· LABA + LAMA

Exacerbation of COPD
· Common infxns: **H. influenzae,** S pneumoniae, M. catarrhalis
· ABG should show compensated respiratory acidosis
· Ensure sats **88-92%** in known CO2 retainers
 - use Venturi mask to give specific %O2.
 - if bicarb is normal, aim for >94% (less risk of retaining CO2)
· **Mx**: prednisolone 30 mg OD for 5d, regular inhaler/ nebuliser
 - abx only if s/smx of pneumonia – amoxicillin, clarithromycin or doxycycline

Blue bloaters: chronic bronchitis. Productive cough, frequent RTI, progressive cardiorespi failure with edema and wt gain
 → obese, accessory muscles, coarse ronchi

Pink puffers: emphysema - long hx of progressive SOB, late onset of non-productive cough. Occasional RTI. Eventual cachexia and respi failure
 → thin and barrel shaped chest, pursed lips, tripod, hyper-resonant chest, distant heart sounds

MRC Dyspnea Scale
1 - SOB on strenuous exercise
2 - SOB walking up hill
3 - SOB that slows walking on flat ground
4 - SOB after 100m flat
5 - unable to leave house ∵ SOB

SABA · **salbutamol** (blue inhaler)
LABA · salmeterol · vilenterol
 · **formoterol**
SAMA · ipratropium
LAMA · tiotropium (Respimat)
 · glycopyrronium
 · umeclindinium (Ellipta)
ICS · beclometasone · fluticasone
 · budesonide

ICS = inhaled corticosteroid

· Fostair (LABA + ICS – beclometasone + formoterol) = "**pink inhaler**"
· Symbicort (LABA + ICS – budesonide + formoterol)
· Seretide (LABA + ICS – salmeterol + fluticasone)
· Trelegy Ellipta (LABA + LAMA + ICS – vilanterol + umeclidinium + fluticasone)
· **Blue inhaler** = salbutamol
· **Brown inhaler** = beclometasone

COPD rescue packs
· Prednisolone 30mg OD 7-14d
· Abx: amoxicillin (500 mg tds x 5d), doxycycline (200 mg first day, then 100 mg OD, total 5d) or clarithromycin (500 mg bds x 5d)
! ↑use of rescue packs indicates worsening COPD

Step down tx: trial ↓25-50% in dose of ICS

Tests

PEFR = peak expiratory flow rate	**Spirometry** is a test which measures the **volume** and **flow** of air during exhalation and inhalation.	**Methacholine challenge**	In asthma,	In COPD, **fixed ↓FEV1/FVC** ratio <70%

PEFR = peak expiratory flow rate
· PEFR test: hard, fast blow into peak flow meter; best of 3 tries

FeNO = fractional exhaled nitric oxide

Spirometry is a test which measures the **volume** and **flow** of air during exhalation and inhalation.

FEV1 = forced expiratory volume at the end of 1s of forced expiration
FVC = forced vital capacity; volume exhaled after maximal inspiration following full inspiration

Methacholine challenge
· Methacholine administered sequentially in ↑conc ranging from 0.016 to 16 mg/m via nebuliser
· FEV1 measured at 30s and 90s
· Dose/conc ↑ until FEV1 ↓ >20% and PD20/PC20 is determined
· +ve test if PD20 ≤200 mcg or **PC20 ≤8 mg/mL**

In asthma,
FEV1 – ↓↓↓
FVC – normal
FEV1/FVC <70%
! REVERSIBLE

In COPD, **fixed ↓FEV1/FVC** ratio <70%

Gold staging based on %FEV1 of predicted
>80% – Stage 1 (mild)
50-79% – Stage 2 (mod)
30-49% – Stage 3 (severe)
<30% – Stage 4 (v severe)

Small cell lung cancer SCLC

Non-small cell lung cancer NSCLC

Mesothelioma

Bronchiectasis

Idiopathic pulmonary fibrosis

Small cell lung cancer / Non-small cell lung cancer

D: aggressive malignant epithelial tumour of cells in the lower respiratory tract.

R: smoking, smoke exposure, radon

R: smoking, smoke exposure, COPD, FHx, radon, ↑age

P: usually arises from APUD cells, a/w ectopic ADH, ACTH secretion and Lambert Eaton (myasthenia-like)
Histology: small and densely packed, with scant cytoplasm, finely granular nuclear chromatin, and absence of nucleoli

APUD = Amine, Precursor Uptake, Decarboxylase

- Adenocarcinoma: located peripherally
- Large cell lung cancer: located peripherally, anaplastic/ poorly-differentiated, β-HCG secretion, a/w poor prog
- Squamous cell carcinoma: typically central, a/w PTHrp & hyperCa, clubbing, HPOA

S/Smx: cough, chest pain, haemoptysis, dyspnea, wt loss ± hoarseness, clubbing, smx also depending on metastasis, etc.

Ix: CXR, CTTAP, FBC (& other bloods), sputum cytology ± bronchoscopy, biopsy, thoracentesis, thoracoscopy, CT/MRI brain, bone scan, PET, etc

Mx: if limited disease, CT+RT. If extensive or mets, chemo only, RT for mets (palliative use). Consider prophylactic cranial irradiation.

Mx:
- I to IIIA curable
  - surgery (lobectomy) or SABR
  - adjuvant chemo
  - If not suitable for above, external beam RT + double plat chemo.
- IIIB to IV reverse, delay or palliate
- Some tumours can be treated with specific drugs, eg EGFR +ve, ALK rearrangement +ve tumours.
- Many complications of surgery, RT and chemo - weigh pros and cons :(

Complications: pneumonia, haematologic toxicity, radiation-induced esophageal injury, SVC syndrome, paraneoplastic syndromes, radiation-induced lung injury

Paraneoplastic syndromes
S - SIADH
C - Cushing's syndrome
L - Lambert-Eaton syndrome
C - Cerebellar syndrome

P: The 5-year survival rates are ~12% to 24% for limited stage and 1% to 5% for extensive stage

Complications: pneumonia, SVC syndrome, paraneoplastic syndromes
P: poor prognosis a/w poor performance status, pre-tx wt loss, mets, and ↑age.
- Prognosis depends more on pathological state (histological).
- Prognosis ↓ as stage ↑.

HPOA = hypertrophic pulmonary osteoarthropathy

CT = chemotherapy
RT = radiotherapy

Lung cancers :(

Small cell lung cancers (15%)

Non-small cell lung cancers (80%)

AC 40% SCC 20% LCC 10% Others 10%

AC = adenocarcinoma
SCC = squamous cell carcinoma
LCC = large cell cancer

Mesothelioma

D: aggressive epithelial neoplasm from lining of the lung (90%)
→ rarely can occur in peritoneum, pericardium, and tunica vaginalis.

R: asbestos (latency 30-40y; pts tend to present at 60-90yo), M>F 3:1.
Occupations – shipyard, construction, maintenance, mechanics, etc

A/P: asbestos taken up by alveolar macrophages and neutrophils → production of reactive oxygen & nitrogen species causes damage to DNA, Δ gene expression → cancer

S/smx:
- Dyspnea, dry cough, chest pain
- Non-specific smx: clubbing, wt loss
- Painless pleural effusion → ↓breath sounds, dullness to percussion, etc
- ! Check for occupational Hx + exposure to asbestos

Ix: CXR (pleural thickening), CT with contrast, thoracocentesis + cytology & biopsy, thoracoscopy
If considering surgical resection, lung function tests, echo, mediastinoscopy

Mx: extra-pleural pneumonectomy (EPP) and pleurectomy with decortication, but surgery alone rarely curative. Chemo (platinum based), adjvant RT. Palliative (eg talc pleurodesis)

P: high surgical morbidity, many side effects of RT/CT. Median survival is 10-15mo, 5y survival 5-10%.

Pleural plaques
- Develop 20-40y after exposure to asbestos that is most common
- Benign; do not undergo malignant change

Asbestosis
- Lower lobe fibrosis due exposure to asbestos (latency 15-30y, severity related to length of exposure)
- S/smx: dyspnea, clubbing, bilateral end-inspiratory crackles, restrictive pattern in lung function tests
- Ix as per mesothelioma (need to r/o malignancy)
- Mx: conservative; no benefit to treatment

Bronchiectasis

D: permanent dilation of bronchi ∵ destruction of the elastic and muscular components of the bronchial wall

R: CF, immunodeficiency, previous infxn, congenital disorders of bronchial airways (eg Young's), primary ciliary dyskinesia

A: Frequently 2/2 recurrent pul infxn, esp H influenzae → progressive bronchial damage. [various other causes]
P: persistent airway inflammation → bronchial wall edema, ↑mucus → damage, which may serve as foci for further colonisation & infxn

S/smx:
- Persistent productive cough ± large volume sputum
- Dyspnea • Haemoptysis • Clubbing
- Coarse crackles and wheezing

Brochiectasis severity index (BSI) - takes into account age, BMI, FEV1, hosp adm w/in 2y, MRC breathless score, microbiology, radiological severity.

Ix: FBC, sputum cultures. CXR. CT best for Dx (tree in bud pattern, signet ring sign). ± tests for aetiology (depending on RF). Spirometry, 6-min walk test, pH testing.

Mx:
- Physical training (eg inspiratory muscle training)
- Airway clearance - hydration, chest physio, nebulised saline ± mucolytic agents. 15-30min bds/tds
- Lifestyle modifications: ↑exercise, pulmonary rehabilitation
- Vaccinations & treatment of infxns
- If localised disease, consider surgery (eg lobectomy)

P: irreversible condition - waxing waning course.

Idiopathic pulmonary fibrosis

D: chronic, life-threatening disease characterised by formation of scar tissue w/in the lungs and ↑SOB

R: Fhx, smoking, ↑age (>50), M>F.

A/P: unknown. ?unidentified insult causes damage to alveolar epithelium, endothelium and BM → inflammatory cells damage the lung + dysregulation of normal repair process.

S/smx: • Progressive exertional dyspnea
- Bibasal fine end-inspiratory crepitations
- Dry cough • Clubbing

Ix: • Spirometry - restrictive picture (FEV1 -/↓, FVC ↓, FEV1/FVC ↑)
- Impaired gas exchange
- CXR, high res CT - "ground glass" pattern, "honeycombing"

Mx: • Pulmonary rehabilitation
- Some evidence for pirfenidone and nintedanib
- Lung transplant in long term

P: median survival of 2-5y at Dx.

Fibrosis in UPPER zones "CHARTS"
- Coal workers' pneumonitis
- Hypersensitivity
- Ankylosing spondylosis
- Radiation
- TB
- Silicosis – egg shell calcification
- Sarcoidosis

Fibrosis in LOWER zones
- Idiopathic pulmonary fibrosis
- Connective tissue disorders, eg SLE
- Drug induced (amiodarone, bleomycin, methotrexate)
- Asbestosis

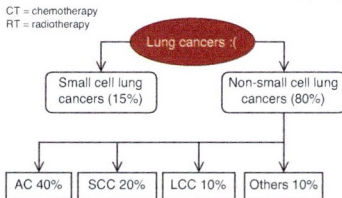

Pneumonia

D: **inflammation of the lungs** with consolidation or interstitial lung infiltrates, most often categorised according to the causative organism

Community acquired pneumonia

D: pneumonia acquired outside hospital or healthcare facilities

A: **50% Strep pneumoniae, 20% H. influenzae**. M. catarrhalis (in immunocomp or chronic lung disease), Ps. aeruginosa (CF or bronchiectasis), S. aureus (CF)

S/Smx: cough+sputum, SOB, pleuritic CP, fever/rigors, confusion, night sweats, confusion
► signs of sepsis: ↑HR, ↑RR, ↓O2, ↓BP, fever, confusion ►

! **CURB-65** (or CRB-65)
· **C**onfusion
· **U**rea > 7
· **R**R ≥30
· **B**P – SBP <90 or DBP <60
· **≥65**yo

Ix: obs, **CXR**, ABG, bloods (U&E, FBC, CRP, LFTs).
If sepsis suspected or severe disease, blood cultures, sputum culture

Mx based on CURB score:
· CURB 0-1 – at home
PO amoxicillin for 5d; clarithromycin or doxycycline if penicillin allergy
· CURB ≥2 – hospitalisation
PO amoxicillin + clarithromycin for 5d [or doxycycline if pen allergy]
· CURB ≥4 – consider ITU
IV co-amoxiclav + clarithromycin for 5d [or levofloxacin if pen allergy]

P: 30-day mortality based on CURB-65 score – <5% if 0-1; 15% if 3; >25% if 4-5
NICE's advice on resolution of smx:
· 1w: fever should resolve
· 4w: CP, sputum ↓↓
· 6w: cough, breathlessness ↓↓
  ↳ **follow-up CXR**
· 3mo: most smx ↓↓; fatigue may remain
· 6mo: most ppl back to normal

Hospital acquired pneumonia

D: acute LRTI acquired **after ≥48h of admission to hospital** and is not incubating at the time of admission

A: early onset (<5d after adm) – Strep pneumoniae. Late onset – **MRSA, Ps. aeruginosa, E. coli, Klebsiella pneumoniae**, Acinetobacter spp, etc

S/Smx & Ix – see CAP

Mx of non-severe smx
⚬ **co-amoxiclav** 500/125mg tds x 5d
⚬ doxycycline, cefalexin, co-trimoxazole, levofloxacin
Mx of severe smx (+sepsis)
→ review in 48h, consider switch to PO (see non-severe) for 5d
⚬ **tazocin** 4.5g tds-qds
⚬ ceftazidime, ceftriaxone, cefuroxime, meropenem, levofloxacin
Mx of MRSA (suspected or confirmed)
⚬ vancomycin
⚬ teicoplanin, linezolid

Atypical pneumonia is caused by organisms that cannot be cultured in the normal way or detected by Gram stains.

"Legions of psittaci MCQs"
· **Legionella**: infected water supplies or air conditioning, can cause hypoNa. typical pt "cheap hotel holiday, hypoNa"
· **Chlamydia psittaci**: infected birds. typical pt "parrot owner"
· **Mycoplasma pneumoniae**: milder pneumonia, erythema multiforme (target lesions), neurological smx, cold agglutinin disease
· **Chlamydophilia pneumoniae**: ?rare – moderate chronic pneumonia + wheeze
· **Q fever; Coxiella burnetti**: exposure to animals and their bodily fluids; typical pt "farmer with flu-like illness"

→ coverage by macrolides, fluroquinolones or tetracyclines

Pneumonia in immunocompromised pts

Pneumocystis jirovecii pneumonia
· D: fungal lung infection typically affecting HIV pts with CD4 <200
· S/Smx - may be first presentation of HIV
- Fever, dry cough, dyspnea
- May present with other s/smx of immuno-compromise, eg oesophageal candidiasis
- Pneumothorax (as a complication)
- Extrapulmonary: hepatosplenomegaly, lymphadenopathy, choroid lesions ("moles" on the posterior uvea)
· Ix: CXR (bilateral interstitial infiltrates, lobar consolidation, or just normal), exercise-induced desaturation, bronchoalveolar lavage (silver stain shows cysts)
· Mx: ⚬ Cotrimoxazole IV/PO x 21d
- If severe, IV or aerosolised pentamidine, consider ITU admission
- If hypoxic, steroids (reduces risk of respi failure and death)
· **Prophylaxis** for pts CD4 <200: Cotrimox – pts can be taken off prophylaxis when CD4 >200

Aspergillosis
· D: fungal lung infection typically affecting immunocomp pts, typically allogenic stem cell transplantation (25%), haematologic malignancy (28%), solid organ transplant, AIDS, etc
· A: Aspergillus spp. (~70% A. fumigatus)
· P: inhalation of spores + neutropenia and ↓CD4 (<100) or ↓macrophage → invasive disease
- dissemination via haematogenous or via the parasinus cavity may occur, affecting many organs
· S/Smx: cough (non-productive, mild-mod), HA, fever, congestion or sinus tenderness.
► pleuritic chest pain
► high suspicion for pts w/ prolonged neutropenia (>10d) + risk factors
· Ix: CXR, HRCT, other scans according to smx, sputum culture. Consider BAL
· Mx: amphotericin B, voriconazole, or other antifungals
- reverse underlying immunosuppression!
- Aspergilloma – ?surgical removal
· P: if immunosuppression can be reversed, pt usually recovers well

Tuberculosis

D: an infectious disease caused by Mycobacterium tuberculosis

R: prolonged exposure, birth in endemic country (Asia, Latin America, Africa), HIV and immunosupp [reactivation], silicosis apical fibrosis, etc

A/P: 1. Inhalation of TB
2. Engulfed by alveolar macrophages
3. Survive, multiply in macrophages
4. Kill macrophages → released
5. Migration to regional lymph nodes
- affected LN + lesion = Ghon complex
6. TH1 response → granuloma
- Type 4 hypersensitivity
- central caseous, necrotic material
- peripheral granulation tissue (macrophages, lymphocytes)
=> latent infxn, non-infectious, normal CXR, tuberculin skin +ve
7. Reactivation ∴ immunosuppression
  ↳ disseminated (miliary) TB

S/Smx: cough, fatigue, wt loss, night sweats, haemoptysis, clubbing, etc

Dx of latent TB – Mantoux test
· 0.1 ml of 1:1,000 purified protein derivative (PPD) injected intradermally
· result read 2-3d later

<6mm: -ve (no rxn), give BCG if unvaccinated
6-15mm: previous BCG or TB infxn; do not give BCG
>15mm: +ve; suggests TB infxn

False -ve: miliary TB, sarcoidosis, HIV, lymphoma, <6mo old

Dx of active TB
· CXR: upper lobe cavitation, bilateral hilar lymphadenopathy
· Sputum smear
- 3 samples, stained acid-fast
- sens 50-80%; ↓ in HIV (20-30%)
· Sputum culture [gold standard]
- 1-3w in liquid media, longer in solid
- can assess drug sens too
· NAAT
- rapid Dx (w/in 48h)
- more sens than smear, less sens than culture

Mx of active TB
RIPE 4 drugs for 2mo, 2 drugs for 4mo
· rifampin & isoniazid for 6mo
  - with pyridoxine (B6)
· pyrazinamide & ethambutol for 2mo

Mx of latent TB
· rifampicin + isoniazid for 3mo
· OR isoniazid for 6mo

Drugs adverse effects
Rifampicin
· Liver enzyme inducer
· Red pee   · Hepatotoxicity
Isoniazid
· Peripheral neuropathy (give B6!!)
· Agranulocytosis   · Hepatotoxicity
· Liver enzyme inhibitor
Pyrazinamide
· Hyperuricemia causing gout
· Athralgia, myalgia · Hepatotoxicity
Ethambutol
· Optic neuritis: check visual acuity before, during tx

Secondary / extra-pulmonary TB
· Tuberculous meningitis (CNS)
· Potts disease (vertebral bodies)
· Scrofuloderma (cervical LN)
· Renal · GI · anywhere
· Disseminated TB (multiple organs) – haematogenous spread
Higher mortality than pulmonary TB

Pedantic notes: "Pneumonia is a radiological diagnosis"; the right term is pneumonitis until confirmed by CXR

Sarcoidosis

D: **chronic granulomatous disorder** of unknown aetiology, commonly affecting the lungs, skin, and eyes
Characterised by accumulation of lymphocytes and macrophages and the formation of **non-caseating granulomas** in the lungs and other organs

R: age 20-40, FHx, Scandinavian origin, F>M, non-smokers

S/smx:
· Respi: dry cough, dyspnea
· Extrapulmonary: athralgia, lymphade-nopathy, eye smx (photophobia, red painful eye, blurred vision)
· **erythema nodosum** (painful lesions on shins of legs - good prognosis)
· **lupus pernio** - indurated plaques with discolouration on face; more common in black women - poor prognosis)

Ix: **CXR** - stage 0 = normal
1 = bilateral hilar lymphadenopathy
2 = BHL + interstitial infiltrates
3 = diffuse interstitial infiltrates only
4 = diffuse fibrosis
Spirometry (restrictive pattern), **tissue biopsy** (non-caseating granulomas), **bloods** (ACE ↑60%, ↑Ca, ↑ESR)

Mx: **Most pts get better with no tx**
Steroids - indications: CXR stage 2-3 + smx (if asmx, don't treat); hyperCa; eye, heart or neuro involvement

P: poor prognosis a/w insidious onset, smx >6mo, absence of erythema nodosum, extrapulmonary manifestations (e.g. lupus pernio, splenomegaly), CXR stage 3-4, black ethnicity

Pneumothorax   shorted to pnt in this section

D: air within the pleural space
– 1': occurs in people with no known respiratory illness
– 2': pre-existing respi illness
– tension: usually 2/2 trauma

R: smoking, pre-existing lung disease (COPD, asthma, CF, lung cancer, PJP), Marfan's (M>F, young), RA, ventilation (incl non-invasive)

A/P: spontaneous, trauma, iatrogenic, lung pathologies
· **catamenial pneumothorax** – 3-6% of spontaneous pnt in menstruating F; 2/2 endometriosis w/in the thorax

S/smx: SOB, chest pain (often pleuritic), sweating, ↑HR, ↑RR
· In tension pnt: ↓ breath sounds, tracheal tug (late/rare)

Ix: CXR. If tension pnt is suspected, go to Mx immediately!

Mx (see below)
· **Aspiration** = insertion of fine needle (14G) into 2nd intercostal space at mid-clavicular line
  - If no success, proceed to chest drain
· Chest drain = insertion of large drain into incision at the safe triangle
  - external end placed under water
  - air will exit and bubble through
  - swinging should be seen due to respiration
  - Complications: air leaks (persistent bubbling on coughing), surgical emphysema
· Surgical methods
  - Abrasive pleurodesis (using direct physical irritation of the pleura)
  - Chemical pleurodesis (chemicals, eg talc, used to irritate the pleura)
  - Pleurectomy (removal of the pleura)
· Discharge advice
  - stop smoking
  - only fly 2w after successful drainage or 1w post CXR clear
  - permanently avoid diving unless complete resolution

Mx of spontaneous pneumothorax

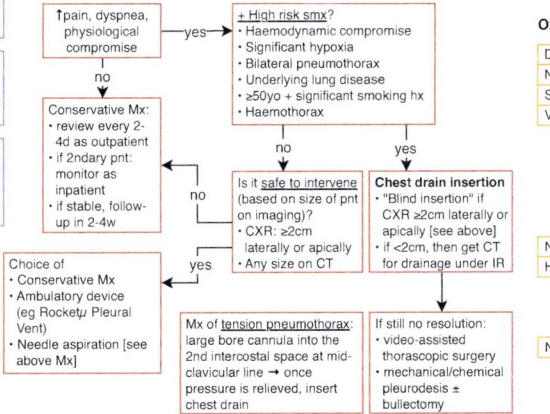

Choice of
· Conservative Mx
· Ambulatory device (eg Rocketₜ Pleural Vent)
· Needle aspiration [see above Mx]

IR = interventional radiology

Pleural effusions

Transudate <30 g/L
· Heart failure
· Hypoalbunaemia
· Hypothyroidism
· Meig's: benign ovarian tumour + ascites

Exudate >30 g/L
· Infection
· Connective tissue disease: RA, SLE
· Neoplasm
· Pancreatitis
· PE
· Dressler's syndrome
· Yellow nail syndrome

Acute respiratory distress syndrome
· D: non-cardiogenic pulmonary oedema and diffuse lung inflammation syndrome
· Conditions linked to development of ARDS: sepsis, pneumonia, acute pancreatitis, massive transfusions, smoke inhalation, cardio-pulmonary bypass
· S/smx: sudden onset of severe dyspnoea, ↑RR, bilateral lung crackles, low O2 sats
· Ix: CXR, ABG - repeated
· **Dx criteria**:
  - acute onset (<1w of known clinical insult)
  - pulmonary oedema on CXR
  - Respi failure not fully explained by HF or fluid overload
  - pO2 / FiO2 <40 kPa (300 mmHg)
· Mx: ITU + organ support, ↑O2 (including ventilation), prone positioning may help
· Prognosis is very poor; mortality 30-50%, death most often due to multiple organ failure

Oxygen delivery

Delivery	Flow (L/min)	FiO2 (%)
Nasal cannulae	1-6	0.24-0.40
Simple face mask	5-10	0.35-0.60
Venturi mask	2-5	0.24-0.56

	Flow	FiO2	
Blue	2L	24%	For high and fixed O2 requirements, eg COPD
White	4L	28%	
Orange	6L	31%	
Yellow	8L	35%	
Red	10L	40%	
Green	15L	60%	

Non-rebreather mask	10-15	0.60-0.90
High-flow NC	15-60	0.30-1.0

Good for pts with air hunger as it ↑work of breathing. Every 10L = 1 positive end expiratory pressure; helps to keep alveoli open

Non-invasive ventilation (NIV) ÷ BiPAP, CPAP, etc

Indicated for · cardiogenic pulmonary edema
· COPD exacerbation
· Extubation of COPD pts
· Immunocompromised hosts
NIV requires more monitoring!

Cystic fibrosis

D: autosomal recessive disorder, ~1:2500 incidence at birth, ~1:25 carriers. mutation on CFTR gene on chr7, coding a Cl channel

R: FHx, ethnicity (white)

A/P: mutation leads to abn salt transportation → thick secretion :(
· Pancreas – blockage of exocrine glands, eventual autodestruction of exocrine pancreas
· Intestines – bulky stools
· Respi: mucus retention, ↑infxns, inflammation, eventual destruction of lung tissue

Presenting features:
· neonatal period (20%)
  - meconium ileus
  - prolonged jaundice
· recurrent chest infxns (40%)
· malabsorption (30%): steatorrhea, failure to thrive
· others (10%): liver failure

Other s/smx:
· short stature   · DM
· delayed puberty · rectal prolapse
· nasal polyps   · in/subfertility

Screening in newborns:
· immunoreactive trypsinogen (IRT)
· ± 2-stage genetic testing (4±29 mutations) on the newborn blood spot test (Guthrie card)
Dx: sweat test +ve if Cl >60 mEq/L
· technically challenging

Mx: · regular (≥bds) chest physio and postural drainage
· high calorie diet (incl ↑fat)
· social distancing to ↓infxns
· vitamin supplementation
· pancreatic enzyme replacement therapy (PERT) with meals
· lung transplant
  - chronic infxn with *Burkholderia cepacia* is an impt CF-specific CI to lung transplant
· Orkambi: for pts homozygous for ΔF508 mutation

Acute cholecystitis

D: acute inflammation of the gall bladder ("cystitis")

R: gallstones, severe illness, TPN, DM

A: 90% gallstones
P: obstruction causes acute inflammation of the gallbladder
! jaundice does not normally occur ∴ bile can still pass into the cystic ducts
- only occurs in Mirizzi's syndrome where gallbladder inflammation ↑pressure on contiguous biliary ducts

S/Smx: RUQ pain and tenderness, Murphy's +ve, palpable mass (rare), s/smx of inflammation

Ix: labs - LFT usually normal
↙ US   MRCP ± ERCP

Mx: IV abx, then elective early lap chole (w/in 1w). If not fit for surgery, long-term ursodeoxycholic acid

Ascending cholangitis

D: acute, ascending inflammation of the biliary tree

R: >50yo, gallstones, benign or malignant stricture, post-procedure injury of bile ducts (eg ERCP), hx of 1' or 2' sclerosing cholangitis

A: gallstones stuck in the biliary tree, and biliary obstruction
P: then causes bacterial seeding in the gallbladder + sludge formation
→ haematogenous spread can lead to sepsis too

S/Smx: Charcot's triad – fever, RUQ pain, jaundice / Reynolds' pentad (+ shock, altered mental stasis)

Ix: labs – ↑ inflammation, Δ LFTs (stasis picture). ↙ US

Mx: IV abx, resus, then ERCP w/in 24-48h to relieve obstruction

Biliary colic: spasmodic pain that arises from contraction of the gallbladder or biliary ducts around gallstones
- "Fat, female, fertile and in their forties"
- Pt is systemically well, but this can progress to acute cholecystitis
- Eventually will require cholecystectomy to manage root cause

Primary sclerosing cholangitis

D: chronic, progressive, cholestatic liver disease. Characterised by inflammation and fibrosis of the bile ducts, causing multi-focal stricture formation.

R: male (2:1), IBD (75%, typically UC), genetics

A/P: likely immune related. Inflammation and injury of medium and large bile ducts → strictures → fibrosis → bile stasis → stones and liver damage

S/smx: abd pain, pruritus, fatigue, wt loss, fever, jaundice. Also steatorrhea, splenomegaly, ascites, encephalopathy

Ix: LFTs (ALP, GGT, AST, ALT, bilirubin, albumin), FBC, PT, antibodies, abd US, MRCP, ERCP, CT. **imaging is essential for Dx – strictures. ** p-ANCA

Mx of early disease
- Conservative: lifestyle Δ
  - Mx of pruritus
  - Mx of hepatic osteopenia – Cal+D, bisphosphonate, HRT
  - ERCP and balloon dilation of stricture
- End stage liver disease: liver transplant

Hepatic osteopenia arises due to impairment of bile function → ↓abs of fat soluble vitamins, incl Vit D

P: high risk of cirrhosis and attendant problems, cholangiocarcinoma, other cancers and osteoporosis. ↑morbidity - median survival from time of Dx to death or liver transplant is 7-14y. Can recur in 10-20% pts post-transplant.

Acalculous cholecystitis
- D: gallbladder inflam with no gallstones
- A/w ongoing illness (eg DM, organ failure)
- S/smx: pt is more unwell than in normal cholecystitis – high fever, shock
- Mx: cholecystectomy

Primary biliary cholangitis

D: chronic disease of the small intrahepatic bile ducts that is characterised by progressive bile duct damage (and eventual loss) occurring in the context of chronic portal tract inflammation

R: female (10:1), >45yo, PMH or FHx of autoimmune disorders

A/P: autoimmune disease – antimitochondrial abs (95%).
(1) biliary epithelial cells damaged and destroyed + (2) chronic portal tract inflammation → bile stasis, fibrosis, cirrhosis

S: abd pain, pruritis, fatigue, wt loss, fever, jaundice. Also steatorrhea, splenomegaly, ascites, encephalopathy

Ix: LFTs, FBC, PT, antibodies, MRCP, liver biopsy. antimitochondrial abs

Dx based on
(1) cholestatic LFTs
(2) auto-abs – antimitochondrial abs or PBC-characteristic ANA
(3) compatible or diagnostic liver histology on biopsy – +ve for classic bile duct lesions, portal tract inflammation, granuloma formation

Mx: ursodeoxycholic acid [bile acid analogue; ↓chol saturation of bile] &/or obeticholic acid. See also general Mx of PSC.

Mx of pruritus
↙ colestyramine [bile acid seques-trant, ↑excretion of bile] **bad taste
↙ naltrexone, rifampin
✗ avoid antihistamines ∴ no effect

P: ↑risk of mortality from liver and non-liver related causes (?linked to inflam). ↓QoL – itch and fatigue. Disease itself may progress slowly and pt may not suffer heavily from it

Hepatocellular carcinoma

D: aka hepatoma. Primary cancer arising from hepatocytes in predominantly cirrhotic liver
- 3rd most common cause of cancer worldwide

R: cirrhosis, chronic HBV (most common cause worldwide), HCV (most common in Europe), ↑alcohol use, DM, obesity, FHx

A/P: chronic inflammation and cirrhosis; any condition leading to cirrhosis is thus a risk factor

S/smx: tends to present late :(
- Cirrhosis: jaundice, ascites, RUQ pain, hepatomegaly, pruritus, splenomegaly
  - may present decompensated
- raised AFP

Ix: screening with US (± AFP) should be considered for high risk groups (pts with existing cirrhosis)

Mx:
- early disease: surgical resection
- liver transplantation
- radiofrequency ablation
- transarterial chemoembolisation
- sorafenib: multikinase inhibitor

P: 5y survival for symptomatic HCC is 0-10% - very aggressive tumour. For all, 5y survival is 20%

Cholangiocarcinoma

D: aka biliary tree cancer; cancer arising from the bile duct epithelium ÷ intrahepatic or extrahepatic

R: >50yo, cholangitis (esp primary sclerosing cholangitis), other bile duct problems

A/P: >95% are adenocarcinomas; most are infiltrating nodular or diffusely infiltrating

S/smx:
- Persistent biliary colic smx
- A/w anorexia, jaundice, wt loss
- Palpable mass in RUQ
- ± Sister Mary Joseph nodes (periumbili-cal lymph node) and Virchow nodes (left supra-clavicular node)
- Raised Ca19-9 levels - useful for detecting cholangiocarcinoma in pts with PSC

Ix: LFTs, Ca19-9, CEA, Ca-125, abdominal US, CT/MRI

Mx: • Surgery if resectable
- If unresectable, liver transplant ± chemo/radiotherapy if possible
- Palliation if extensive disease

Origins of secondary liver tumours
Common in men: stomach, lung, colon
Common in women:
  breast, colon, stomach, uterus
Less common in either: pancreas, leukemia, lymphoma, carcinoid tumours

Primary liver tumours

Malignant - regardless of type, prognosis is poor	Benign • Cysts
• HCC • Cholangiocarcinoma	• Haemangioma (common; F>M 5:1)
• Angiosarcoma	• Adenoma (common; tx only if smx or >5cm)
• Hepatoblastoma	• Focal nodular hyperplasia
• Fibrosarcoma	• Fibroma
• Hepatic GIST	• Benign GIST (=leiomyoma)

Alcohol-related liver disease

D: liver damage caused by chronic heavy alcohol intake. 3 stages: steatosis, alcoholic hepatitis (inflammation & necrosis), and alcoholic liver cirrhosis

R: ↑alc use, hep C, female (most cases are male, but F tolerance for alc is lower)

A/P: upregulation of **alcohol and acetal-aldehyde dehydrogenase** which reduce NAD to NADH → ↑NADH:NAD inhibits gluconeogenesis and ↑fatty acid oxidation → fatty infiltration in liver. upregulation of **CYP2E1** generates more free radicals.↑TNF-a and ↑ ROS in mitochondria of Kupffer cells. Inflamm rxn drives liver damage.

S/Smx: • May be asmx until decompensation (body cannot cope with liver damage anymore)
• Abdominal pain, hepatomegaly
• Decompensated liver disease
- haemetemesis   - melena
- venous collaterals (eg spider naevi)
- splenomegaly   - jaundice
- palmar erythema   - asterexis
- ascites   - hepatic encephalopathy

Ix: LFTs, FBC, U&Es (+Mg, PO4), clotting, hepatic US. Consider ammonia, folate, viral hep serology, liver biopsy.

• AST:ALT >2 in 70% of cases
• ↑ALP & GGT – a/w cholestasis
• ↓Na in advanced ALD; ↓K, ↓Mg – muscle weakness; ↓Mg can cause persistent hypoK, predisposing to seizures during alcohol withdrawal

Complications: hepatic encephalopathy, portal HTN (+esophageal varices), GI bleeds, coagulopathy, renal failure, hepatorenal syndrome, sepsis

Alcoholic hepatitis
= acute episodes of inflammation
• S/smx: rapid onset of jaundice, malaise, tender hepatomegaly, etc
• Ix: AST:ALT >2
• Mx: glucocorticoids
- Maddrey's discriminant function used to determine who will benefit
- ℞ Pentoxyphylline

Varices + bleeding
• 2/2 portal hypertension, causing distention of oesophageal veins, ↑bleeding, ↑risk of death

Mx • Prophylaxis: β-blocker, band ligation, TIPSS
• Acute: - ABCDE + resus
- Correct clotting (FFP, platelets, etc)
- Terlipressin (2nd line: octreotide)
- Prophylactic abx – quinolones
- Endoscopy ± band ligation, Sengstaken-Blakemore tube, TIPSS

Ascites
= abnormal collection of fluid in the abdomen
• in ArLD, this is 2/2 portal HTN

Mx • ↓dietary Na ± fluid restriction
• **Aldosterone antagonists**, eg spironolactone ± loop diuretics
• Drainage of tense ascites
- for large volume paracentesis, IV albumin required to prevent circulatory dysfunction and death
• Prophylactic PO ciprofloxacin to prevent spontaneous bacterial peritonitis (in some pts)
• Consider TIPSS

Hepatic encephalopathy
• neuropsychiatric syndrome caused by acute or chronic advanced hepatic insufficiency – likely due to excess ammonia & glutamine
• metabolic encephalopathy (↑NH4), brain atrophy and/or brain oedema

Grade 1 (early smx)
• Trivial lack of awareness
• Sleep rhythm alterations
• Shortened attention span
• Impaired addition/subtraction
• Euphoria or anxiety - ?irritable

G2 • Confusion and inappropriate behaviour
G3 • Incoherent and restless
G4 • Coma

Mx • Tx underlying cause (eg infxn)
• ℞ Lactulose (↑excretion of NH4) + rifaximin (↓NH4 production – 2ndary prophylaxis)

Alcohol withdrawal

Smx are brought on by abstinence from alcohol in a person with alcohol dependence. Characterised by **overactivity of the sympathetic nervous system**
• Chronic alcohol use → ↑regulation of NMDA receptors, ↓regulation of GABA receptors.
• ↓blood ethanol conc → imbalance between stimulatory NMDA and inhibitory GABA systems in the CNS
• Excessive stimulatory effect leads to development of clinical s/smx of alcohol withdrawal

Dx is usually clinical (Hx, O/E)
• Smx start at **6-12h**, usually autonomic smx eg tremor, sweating, ↑HR, anxiety
• Seizures – peak incidence at **36h**
• Delirium tremens
- peak incidence at **48-72h**
- coarse tremor, confusion, delusions, auditory and visual hallucinations, fever, ↑HR

Glasgow modified alcohol withdrawal scale (GMAWS) - 0, 1 or 2 pts for each
• Tremor   • Sweating
• Hallucinations • Orientation
• Agitation

Clinical institute withdrawal assessment of alcohol, revised (CIWA-Ar) scale is more detailed; max 67 points
• probably better for delirium tremens

Mx (if GMAWS ≥2 or CIWA-Ar ≥10)
• Admit under medics if complex withdrawals (DT, seizures, etc)
• ℞ chlordiazepoxide or diazepam (long-acting benzodiazepine)
- ℞ lorazepam if liver failure
- ℞ carbamazepine
• Thiamine (or Pabrinex) to prevent Wernicke's or Korsakoff

Hepatorenal syndrome: kidneys ↓↓blood flow distribution in response to the altered blood flow in the liver, which ↓MAP due to extreme vasodilation

---

Copper

D: autosomal recessive disorder of excessive copper deposition

R: ATP7B gene mutation, FHx

A/P: ATP7B encodes a metal P-type ATPase for trans-membrane transport of Cu within hepatocytes. No protein → ↓excretion from liver + copper overload in hepatocytes + overflow into circulation or organs

S/smx 2/2 Cu deposition in organs:
• onset 10-25yo – children usually liver disease, adolescents psychiatric
• Liver: hepatitis, cirrhosis
• **Neurological**
- basal ganglia degeneration
- speech, behavioural, psychiatric problems (eg depression, mania, etc)
- asterixis, chorea, dementia, parkinsonism
• Kayser-Fleischer rings (50% in all, 90% in those with neuro issues)
• Renal tubular acidosis (esp Fanconi syndrome)
• Haemolysis   • Blue nails

Ix: • Eyes: slit-lamp
• ↓ serum caeruloplasmin
• ↓ total serum copper
• ↑ 24h urinary Cu excretion
• Dx confirmed by genetic analysis

Mx: • ℞ penicillamine (chelates Cu)
• ℞ trientine hydrochloride
• ?? tetrathiomolybdate (new)

Spontaneous bacterial peritonitis
• D: peritonitis occuring in patients with ascites 2/2 liver cirrhosis
- Most commonly caused by **E. coli**
• S/smx: ascites, abdo pain, fever
• Dx/Ix: paracentesis (neutrophil count >250 cells/μL + culture)
• Mx: ℞ IV cefotaxime
• Prophylaxis with PO ciprofloxacin or norfloxacin if
- Previous episode of SBP
- Fluid protein <15 g/L and Child-Pugh score ≥9 or hepatorenal syndrome

---

Iron

D: autosomal recessive disorder. dysregulated dietary iron absorption and increased iron release from macrophages

R: middle age, M>F, Caucasian (1:10 carry mutation; 1:200 prevalence – more common than CF), FHx

A/P: HFE gene mutation (chr 6) → ↑absorption of Fe

S/smx:
• early smx: fatigue, erectile dysfunction and arthralgia (often of the hands)
• 'bronze' skin pigmentation
• diabetes mellitus
• liver: stigmata of chronic liver disease hepatomegaly, cirrhosis, hepatocellular deposition)
• cardiac failure (2/2 dilated cardiomyopathy)
• hypogonadism (2/2 cirrhosis and pituitary dysfunction – hypogonado-trophic hypogonadism)

Complications
• Reversible: cardiomyopathy, skin pigmentation
• Irreversible: cirrhosis, DM, hypogona-dism, arthropathy

Ix: • **Iron studies**
- ↑transferrin saturation >50-55%
- ↑ferritin (can be normal early on)
- ↓TIBC (∵ no more capacity)
• Genetic testing (for HFE mutation),
• Others: LFTs, biopsy

Mx: ℞ venesection – tailored to ↓transferrin <50%, ferritin <50μg/L
℞ desferrioxamine

Hepatitis A

D: liver infection caused by HBA. HBA is an RNA virus transmitted by the faecal-oral route.

R: travel to endemic areas, consumption of contaminated food/water, MSM, IVDU, childcare centre

A/P: virus replicates in hepatocytes, cellular damage may be mediated by Th1.

S/Smx: • onset ~2-4w after infxn
• Prodromal illness (fever, NV, bowel Δ, flu-like smx, etc) before jaundice
• Hepatomegaly & RUQ pain in 70-80% of symptomatic pts
• Clay coloured stools

Ix: LFTs (AST, ALT, bilirubin), U&E, PT, IgM anti-HAV. Consider PCR

Mx: • Confirmed infxn: supportive symptomatic care (eg paracetamol, metoclopramide, chlorpheniramine, etc)
• Avoid alcohol, avoid work/school until not infectious (~7d after smx onset)
• Ensure good hygiene to ↓spread
• Vaccination only for those at high risk (single dose + booster 6-12mo after)
  - Travel to endemic areas
  - Chronic liver disease (eg hep B/C)
  - Haemophiliacs receiving platelets
  - IVDU   - **MSM**   - (others)

P: 85% have full recovery w/in 3mo, nearly all recover w/in 6mo. In 10-20% of smx pts, prolonged course possible. Fulminant course very rare

Hepatitis E

Hep E - faecal-oral route, esp contaminated water. Usually self-limiting infxn, resolves w/in 2-6w. Flu-like smx, abd pain, jaundice, itching, rash, joint pain, slight hepatomegaly. Rarely fulminant hepatitis. Supportive care.

Hepatitis B

D: liver infection caused by HBV. HBV is a dsDNA virus transmitted by blood, sexual activity or vertically.

R: perinatal exposure, high risk sexual behaviours, IVDU, birth in endemic region, FHx, hx of incarceration

A/P: liver damage likely 2/2 host's immune response to viral antigens.

S/Smx: • Incubation 6-20w
• May be asymptomatic
• Acute episode: fever, jaundice, ↑LFTs
• Long-term complications
  - Chronic hepatitis (5-10%)
  - Fulminant liver failure (1%)
  - **HCC** - Glomerulonephritis
  - Polyarteritis nodosa
  - Cyroglobulinaemia

Ix: LFTs, FBC, U&Es, coag profile, HBV bloods. If more severe liver damage expected, US, CT and biopsy
• Chronic hepatitis: ground-glass hepatocytes on histology

Mx: pegylated interferon-α, antivirals, liver transplant. ! IMMUNISATION

C/P: 95% of immunocompetent pts with acute infxn will achieve seroconversion in absence of tx. Rarely, liver failure, cirrhosis. **Hepatocellular carcinoma** (HBV accounts for 50% of cases worldwide).

Hep B tests

HBs**Ag**: *acute infxn + infectious*

HBsAb/anti-HBs: protected against infxn [previous infxn or vaccinated]
→ HBs is given as vaccination, so if pt is +ve for *only HBsAb* = vaccination

HB**c**Ab: previous or current infxn

IgM anti-HBc: acute infxn
IgG anti-HBc: past infxn

Infxn with **Hep D** can only occur with current Hep B infxn.

Hepatitis C

D: liver infection caused by HBC. HCV is an RNA virus transmitted by blood, sexual activity or vertically. Chronic infxn ≥6mo of persistent serum HCV RNA.

R: needle stick injury (2% transmission), perinatal exposure (6%, ↑risk if +HIV), high risk sexual behaviours (~5%), IVDU, heavy alcohol use, HIV, incarceration

no vaccination available!!

A/P: majority of pts fail to clear virus, which may lead to progressive liver damage. Hepatic inflammation and fibrosis due to inflammatory reaction

S/Smx: Incubation 6-9w
• 30% develop symptoms in acute episode: flu-like illness, jaundice, ↑LFTs
• Fulminant hepatic failure very rare, but would present with decompensation
• Chronic hepatitis C (55-85%)
  - Arthralgia, arthritis   - Sjogren's
  - Cirrhosis (5-20%)   - **HCC**
  - Cryoglobulinaemia
  - Porphyria cutanea tarda
  - Glomerulonephritis

Ix: HCV antibody enzyme immunoassay, PCR, LFTs. Consider testing for co-infxns (HBV, HIV)

Mx: • acute & chronic infxn Mx same – start on antivirals asap
• Monitor bloods (FBC, metabolics, BCG) at 4w while on antivirals (esp rivabarin)
• Sustained virologic response = undetectable HCV RNA ≥12w after tx completion
• If ongoing infxn, monitor for progression of liver disease

P: 10y survival 79%. Among pts who develop cirrhosis, decompensation occurs in 30% at 10y. Higher morbidity than HIV, but possibly due to lifestyle issues rather than HCV infxn.

Child-Pugh scoring	MELD formula
• Bilirubin	• Bilirubiun
• **Albumin**	• Creatinine
• Prothrombin time	• INR
• Encephalopathy	
• Ascites	

Autoimmune hepatitis

D: Chronic inflammatory disease of the liver of unknown aetiology
• Type I: ANA &/or anti-smooth muscle abs – affects both adults & children
• Type II: Anti-liver/kidney microsomal type 1 antibodies – affects children only
• Type III: Soluble liver-kidney antigen – affects adults in middle-age

R: F>M, genetic pre-disposition (HLA B8, DR3), other autoimmune disorders

a/w: pernicious anaemia, UC, glomerulo-nephritis, autoimmune thyroiditis, autoimmune haemolysis, DM, PSC

S/smx:
• S/smx of chronic liver disease
• Acute hepatitis: fever, jaundice etc (only 25% present in this way)
• **Amenorrhoea** in F (common)

Ix: ANA/SMA/LKM1 antibodies, ↑IgG
• Liver biopsy: inflammation extending beyond limiting plate 'piecemeal necrosis', **bridging necrosis**

Mx: steroids, other immunosuppressants, liver transplantation

Non-alcoholic fatty liver disease (NAFLD)

D: spectrum of liver disease – macrovesicular hepatic steatosis with no excessive alcohol intake
• Steatosis = fat in the liver
• Steatohepatitis = fat + inflammation = non-alcoholic steatohepatitis (NASH)
• Fibrosis, cirrhosis

R: obesity, insulin resistance or T2DM, dyslipidaemia, HTN, metabolic syn, rapid wt loss, hepatotoxic meds, TPN

A/P: insulin resistance → ↑excessive triglyceride in liver → hepatic steatosis. 2nd hit or oxidative injury triggers inflammatory reaction and fibrosis.

S/Smx: • Usually asymptomatic
• Hepatomegaly ± ?non-specific smx
• If fibrosis/cirrhosis develops: jaundice, portal hypertension, etc

Ix: LFTs, FBC, metabolic panel, lipid panel, clotting, albumin, iron studies – mainly as baseline
• **Enhanced liver fibrosis** (ELF) blood test to check for advanced fibrosis
  - Hyaluronic acid, procollagen III, tissue inhibitor of metalloproteinase 1
• If ELF unavailable, FIB4 score or NAFLD fibrosis score may be used
• Fibroscan (transient elastography – how bouncy the liver is)

AST, ALT >1-4x ULN. ↑ALT more than AST. AST:ALT <1

Mx: • Lifestyle modification – **wt loss**
• Tx insulin resistance, hyperlipid.
• Vit E a/w improved clinical outcomes
• No evidence for ursodeoxycholic acid
• Severe disease may require TIPS and liver transplant

P: • "bland" steatosis – good prognosis, stable disease.
• NASH progressive, esp with comorbidities (DM, high BMI) – 9 to 20% progress to cirrhosis

Paracetamol overdose

1. Time of overdose
2. Amount ingested
3. Weigh pt → ≥40kg vs <40kg
   ↳ <40kg use Toxbase
4. Calculate mg/kg

Staggered OD (taken over ≥1h)
· start SNAP protocol stat
· send bloods 4h after last ingestion
0-4h
· If <1h, consider activated charcoal if pt has no acute smx
· Send bloods 4h after last ingestion
· If bloods ≥100 mg/L paracetamol at 4h, start SNAP
4-8h
· Send bloods stat
· Start SNAP stat if bloods not likely to return in 8h
· When bloods return, continue SNAP if above tx line
8-24h · Send bloods immediately
· Start SNAP immediately if >150mg/kg ingested
· When bloods return, continue SNAP if above tx line
>24h · Send bloods immediately
· Start SNAP if jaundice or hepatic tenderness +ve
· When bloods return, start SNAP if
  - INR >3   - ALT >3x ULN
· paracetamol detected

SNAP: 1st bag NAC 100 mg/kg over 2h, 2nd bag NAC 200 mg/kg over 10h → total 300 mg/kg over 12h
· N-acetylcysteine anaphylactoid rxn
  - pause infusion
  - antihistamine, eg chlorpheniramine
  - salbutamol nebs if bronchospasm
  - ondansetron 4 mg IV for N&V
  - restart tx when pt is settled

Risk factors for hepatotoxicity: pts taking enzyme-inducing drugs (rifampicin, phenytoin, carbamazepine, chronic alcohol excess, St John's wort), malnourished pts
** Acute alcohol intake ?protective

Liver transplantation
(King's College Criteria)
· Arterial pH <7.3, 24h after ingestion
· PT >100s + SrCr > 300 umol/L + grade III or IV encephalopathy

Acute pancreatitis

D: disorder of the exocrine pancreas, a/w acinar cell injury with local and systemic inflammatory responses.

R: middle-aged, gallstones, alcohol, hypertrigly, drugs (azathioprine, thiazides, furosemide), ERCP, trauma, SLE, Sjogren's.

A/P: [I GET SMASHED] - idiopathic, **gallstones**, **ethanol**, trauma, steroids, mumps, autoimmune, scorpion sting, hyperlipidaemia, **ERCP**, drugs (see below)

S/Smx: · severe epigastric pain radiating to back (stabbing pain, worsens on movement; pt may be in fetal position)
· A/w NV, abdo tenderness, systemically unwell (possible shock)

Haemorrhagic pancreatitis: ecchymotic bruising (1%) Cullen's (periumbilical), Grey-Turner's (flanks), Fox's (inguinal lig)

Dx confirmation (≥2 of 3):
· upper abdo pain
· ↑lipase or **amylase** 3x ULN
  - Amylase 90% sens for pancreatitis
  - Lipase more sens/spec but often less available; longer half-life – useful for late presentations
· characteristic imaging findings (CT, MRCP, **US** – but only request if doubt)
Other Ix: FBC+diff, CRP (>200 high risk of developing necrosis), U&Es (look for AKI and hypovolemia), O2 sats, LFTs (↑ALTs – ?gallstones as cause)

Mx: **!** aggressive IV fluids + analgesia
· Offer enteral nutrition (NGT) for pts with moderate to severe pancreatitis
  - NBM only for specific reasons (eg pt keeps vomiting)
· Do not offer routine / prophylactic abx
· Surgery or procedures (ERCP, cholecystectomy, drainage, etc) as indicated

Complications:
· Peripeancreatic fluid collections – aspirate and drain
· Pseudocysts (~4w) – observe for 12w; half resolve, other tx with cystectomy
· Pancreatic necrosis – conservative Mx
· Pancreatic abscess – requires drainage
· Haemorrhage   · ARDS

Glasgow score using PANCREAS mnemonic:
PaO2 <8 kPa
Age >55
Neutrophils (WBC >15)
Calcium <2 (hypoCa)
uRea >16
Enzymes (AST/ALT>200)
Albumin <32
Sugar (glucose >10)

Drugs a/w pancreatitis
· Azathioprine
· Mesalazine
· Bendroflumethiazide
· Furosemide
· Steroids
· Sodium valproate
· Didanosine
· Pentamidine

Chronic pancreatitis

D: Recurrent or persistent pancreatic inflammation, resulting in scarring and loss of function. ÷ 4 types: recurrent acute, idiopathic, chronic relapsing, or established chronic

R: >75% a/w chronic alcohol use. Others: smoking, FHx, coeliac

A/P: Alcohol, CF, haemochromatosis, or ductal obstruction (incl anatomical anomalies such as annular pancreas) repeated inflammation → collagen deposits, fibrosis, pain, etc

S/Smx: · abdo pain – epigastric, dull, radiates to back, ↓by sitting forwards, worsens ~30min after eating
· jaundice   · steatorrhea
· ± wt loss (∴ fear of food causing pain)
· malnutrition   · NV   · bloating
· **DM** (~20y after smx begin)

Ix: AXR (pancreatic calcification in 30%), **CT**, functional tests (faecal elastase to Ax exocrine function if inconclusive)

Mx: · Stop alcohol and smoking
· Ref to dietician (small meals, high protein), pancreatic enzyme replacement therapy (PERT).
· Pain Mx – step-wise analgesia
· Endoscopic procedures to dilate strictures, remove stones, drain cysts, etc. Surgical decompression or PPPD.

P: 20-30% lower survival than gen pop. Cardiovascular disease most common cause of death in alcoholic pancreatitis.

Pancreatic cancer

D: primary pancreatic ductal adeno-carcinoma (>90% of pancreatic cancers)

R: smoking, FHx, other hereditary cancer syndromes (eg Peutz-Jeghers, HNPCC, BRCA2, KRAS gene mutation), pancreatitis, DM

A/P: 65% head of pancreas, 15% body, 10% tail, 10% multifocal. LN mets common, also perineural and vascular invasion. Distant mets usually found in liver, lung, skin and brain

S/smx:
· classically, painless jaundice + pale stools, dark urine, pruritus
· Hepatomegaly, gb mass (Courvoisier's law = painless obstructive jaundice), epigastric mass
· Non-specific smx: anorexia, wt loss
· Loss of exocrine function eg steatorrhea
· Loss of endocrine function, eg DM
· Atypical back pain
· Migratory thrombophlebitis (Trousseau sign), which can lead to DVT/PE

Ix: US sens 60-90%, **high res CT** best if Dx suspected
  - double duct sign = simultaneous dilation of common bile and pancreatic ducts
· Ca19-9   · ↑ LFTs (cholestatic)

Mx:
· <20% suitable for surgery at Dx
· Whipple's resection (PD/PPPD) for resectable lesions at head of pancreas
  - SE: dumping syndrome, PUD
· Adjuvant chemo after surgery
· ERCP with stenting for palliation

P: mean survival <6mo. 5y survival 3%, 5-14% with Whipple's/PPPD.

Neuroendocrine tumours

Aka carcinoid tumours
· Secretory NETs that release serotonin, kinins, and other vasoactive peptides
· Carcinoid syndrome develops only in 40% pts with NETs
· If NETs metastasise to the liver, 95% of pts will have smx

R: MEN1, ~50yo   A/P: unknown

S/smx (Carcinoid syndrome):
· "B-FDR": bronchospasm, flushing, diarrhoea, right heart valvular stenosis
· Hypotension
· Other molecules such as ACTH and GHRH may also be secreted
  - Cushing's may develop
· Pellagra can rarely develop as dietary tryptophan is diverted to serotonin by the tumour

Ix: U&Es, VIP radioimmunoassay, LFTs, urinary 5-HIAA, plasma chromogranin A

Mx: somatostatin analogues (octreotide), cyproheptadine (for diarrhea), PERT, etc

Small bowel bacterial overgrowth syndrome

D: ↑↑ bacteria in small intestine causing dysfunction
RF: neonates with congenital GI abn, scleroderma, DM
S/smx: chronic diarrhoea, bloating, flatulence, abd pain
Dx: hydrogen breath test
Mx: correction of underlying disorder ± rifaximin, co-amoxiclav, or metronidazole

Crohn's disease

D: a type of IBD characterised by transmural inflammation of the GIT

R: white ethnicity and Ashkenazi Jewish ancestry, age 15-40yo or 50-60yo, FHx of CD

A/P: · unknown cause. ? genetics
· inflammation is transmural - all layers → ↑risk of strictures, fistulas and adhesions
· Mouth to anus, skip lesions!
· 80% involve small bowel, usually in the ileum; ~30% have ileitis exclusively

S/smx
· Non-specific, including wt loss, fatigue
· Diarrhoea ± bloody (colitis)
· Abdo pain, esp in children
· Perianal disease, eg skin tags
· Extra-intestinal features (esp in pts with colitis or perianal disease)

Ix: · Bloods (FBC – anaemia, ↑CRP/ESR, ↓vit B12, ↓vit D); stool (↑faecal calprotectin)
  - Can use CRP to track disease activity
· Colonoscopy: deep ulcers, skip lesions
· Histology: transmural inflammation, goblet cells, granulomas
· Small bowel enema:
  - high s/s for exam of terminal ileum
  - strictures: 'Kantor's string sign'
  - Proximal bowel dilation
  - 'Rose thorn' ulcers
  - Fistulae

Crohns disease activity index
· General wellbeing
· Abdominal pain
· Number of liquid stools/day
· Abdominal mass
· Complications
  – Arthralgia   – Uveitis
  – Erythema nodosum
  – Pyoderma gangrenosum
  – Aphthous ulcers
  – Anal fissure   – New fistula
  – Abscess

Mx
Inducing remission
· Glucocorticoids (topical, PO, IV) ± enteral feeding
  ↪ 5ASA, eg mesalazine
· Add-ons: azathioprine, mercapto-purine, methotrexate
· In refractory disease and fistulas: infliximab
· Isolated peri-anal disease: metronidazole

Maintaining remission
↪ Azathioprine, mercaptopurine
  - TPMT activity must be assessed
↪ Methotrexate

Surgery
· Stricturing ileal disease – ileocecal resection
· Segmental small bowel resection
· Strictuloplasty
· Mx of perianal fistulae
  - Ix: MRI
  - PO metronidazole, draining seton (↓risk abscess)
· Mx of perianal abscess: I&D + abx ± draining seton

Other notes
· Stop smoking
· ?? stop NSAIDs/COCP

C: small bowel cancer (40x risk), colorectal cancer (2x), osteoporosis

---

Extra-intestinal features of both CD and UC

Related to disease activity
· Arthritis: pauciarticular, asym
· Erythema nodosum
· Episcleritis
· Osteoporosis

Unrelated to disease activity
· Arthritis: polyarticular, sym
· Uveitis
· Pyoderma gangrenosum
· Clubbing
· PSC (more common in UC)

Ulcerative colitis

D: a type of IBD characteristically involving the rectum, extending proximally to affect a variable length of the colon

R: FHx of IBD, HLA B27, infection

A/P: · unknown cause. ? genetics
· inflammation limited to the submucosa (unless fulminant disease)
· inflammation limited to colon, unless incompetent ileocecal valve

S/smx:
· Bloody diarrhoea
· Urgency   · Tenesmus
· Abd pain, esp in LLQ
· Extra-intestinal features

Ix: · Colonoscopy
  - Avoid in severe colitis due to risk of perforation; *flexible sigmoidoscopy* preferred
  - No inflammation beyond submucosa, widespread ulceration with 'pseudopolyps',
· Histology: inflammatory cells within the lamina propria, crypt abscesses (·. neutrophils), depletion of goblet cells and mucin
· Barium enema: loss of haustrations, superficial ulceration, 'psuedopolyps', 'drain-pipe colon' (short and narrow colon)
· Stool sample: ↑faecal calprotectin

Toxic megacolon
· total or segmental *non-obstructive* colonic distension a/w systemic toxicity
· Complication of colitis ± C.diff infxn
· Diagnostic criteria (≥3 + XR)
  - Fever >38.6°C   - HR >120
  - WBC >10.5   - Anaemia
  - Radiographical evidence
· Mx: treat underlying cause
  - If C.diff +ve, IV abx
  - If severe colitis flare, IV steroids
  - If no improvement in 72h, surgery

Mx
Inducing remission in mild to mod UC
(1) Proctitis
  1. Rectal mesalazine
  2. PO mesalazine if remission not achieved w/in 4w ± topical/PO corticosteroids
(2) Proctosigmoiditis
  1. Rectal mesalazine
  2. PO mesalazine ± topical corticosteroids if remission not achieved w/in 4w
  3. stop topical, PO mesalazine and PO steroids
(3) Extensive disease
  1. PO mesalazine + PO steroids
  2. ↑mesalazine dose if remission not achieved w/in 4w
Inducing remission in severe UC
· Admit – IV steroids or ciclosporin
· After 72h, if no improvement, add ciclosporin or consider surgery

Maintaining remission
(1) Proctitis ± sigmoiditis
· topical mesalazine daily or as and when necessaryand/or PO mesalazine
(2) Extensive disease
· Low maintenance dose of PO mesalazine

Severe relapse or
≥2 exacerbations in past year
· PO azathioprine
· PO mercaptopurine

· PO methotrexate is not recommended
· ? probiotics may be useful

Mayo classification
· Stool frequency
· Rectal bleeding
· Findings on endoscopy
· Physician's global assessment

Truelove & Witts severity index
· Stool frequency (≥6 severe)
· Blood in stool
· T>37.8°C
· HR>90 (severe)
· Anaemia
· ESR (>30 severe)

Coeliac disease

D: a systemic autoimmune disease triggered by dietary gluten peptides found in wheat, rye, barley and related grains

R: FHx, IgA def, T1DM, autoimmune thyroid disease

A/P: gluten peptides trigger innate and adaptive immune reaction → **villous atrophy, hypertrophy of intestinal crypts,** ↑lymphocytes in epithelium and lamina propria → GI smx and malabsorption

S/Smx: · Diarrhoea: chronic or intermittent
· GI smx (persistent or unexplained) – nausea, vomiting, abdo pain, cramping, distention
  - Lactose intolerance may develop
· Wt loss (sudden or unexpected)
· Fatigue or failure to thrive
  - likely 2/2 iron-deficiency anaemia (or other anaemias), or vitamin deficiencies

Comnplications: · Hyposplenism
· Anaemia (2/2 iron, folate or B12 deficiency)
· Osteoporosis, osteomalacia
· Enteropathy-associated T-cell lymphoma of small intestine
· Subfertility   · Oesophageal cancer

Ix: ! Pts should be on gluten-*full* diet ≥6w
· Serology - < IgA-TTG
  + Endomyseal ab (IgA) to r/o IgA deficiency
· Endoscopic intestinal biopsy [gold standard]
  - duodenum usually, or jejunum
  - findings as above (under A/P)
· Other Ix to look for complications, eg FBC to look for anaemia

IgA-tTG = IgA tissue transglutaminase

Mx: · Gluten-free diet
· Immunisations: pneumococcal vaccine every 5y (due to hyposplenism – ↑susceptibility to encapsulated organisms) + influenza yearly

P: good - 90% complete, lasting resolution of smx on gluten-free diet. <1% refractory.

Dermatitis herpetiformis - intensely pruritic papulovesicular lesions that occur symmetrically over extensor surfaces of arms and legs, buttocks, trunk, neck and scalp. Almost always a/w coeliac disease.

Appendicitis

D: acute inflammation of the vermiform appendix

A: obstruction of the lumen of the appendix (eg by faecolith, normal stool or lymphoid hyperplasia)
P: obstruction + growth of bacteria → ↑pressure and distention

S/smx: Alvarado score
- Migration of abdominal pain =1
  - general at first as only visceral peritoneum is affected
  - localises to right iliac fossa (RIF) after 24-48h when parietal peritoneum is affected
  - worse on movement, eg coughing
    ↳ in children, ask them to hop on left to right leg to test ("hop test")
- Anorexia (no hunger) =1
- Nausea =1   ≥9 in males or
- Tenderness in RLQ =2   ≥10 females –
- Rebound pain =1   very likely
- Fever (>37.3°C) =1   appendicitis
- Leucocytosis =1
- Shift of WBC count to the left (neutrophil predominant) =1
- Others
  - Rovsing's sign: palpating LLQ causes pain in RLQ
  - Psoas sign: pain on extending hip if appendix is retrocaecal
  - Guarding and rigidity

Ix & Mx:
- bloods – CRP, ↑WCC (as above)
- urine dip – r/o pregnancy, UTI
- If Alvarado 4-6, CT scan; score ≥7, refer to surgeons
- Imaging
  - not generally indicated unless unsure about Dx; ↑CRP + clinical picture should be sufficient (esp in kids)
  - US not useful to visualise appendix, but can help look for gynaecological pathologies that may present similarly

If suspected appendicitis,
- Refer to surgeons + NBM
- Prophylactic IV abx, eg co-amoxiclav + metronidazole
- Appendicectomy (usually laparascopic)
- If pt is not fit for surgery, IV abx may be all that is needed (but risk of recurrence 12-24%)

Small bowel obstruction

D: mechanical disruption in the patency of the small intestines

R: previous abdominal surgery (causing adhesions), malrotation, Crohn's, hernia, appendicitis, intestinal malignancy, intussusception, volvulus

S/smx:
- Diffuse, central abdominal pain
- Nausea, vomiting
  - typically bilious (green) vomit
- Constipation with complete obstruction and lack of flatulence
- ± abdominal distention
- ± Tinkling bowel sounds

Ix: • CXR (to look for abdominal perforation – free air)
- abdominal XR (dilated small bowel >3cm thick + fluid levels)
- CT scan to confirm

Mx:
- NBM + IV fluids + Ryles tube
  - "drip and suck" – Ryles tube helps to relieve pressure
- ± Gastrografin (a contrast dye that is osmotic in nature)
- Surgery if not settled

Imaging (abdo XR)
- Small bowel: valvulae conniventes that extend all the way across
- Large bowel: haustra extend about 1/3 of the way across

Pilonidal disease

D: "ingrown hairs" in the skin of the natal cleft of the sacrococcygeal area → chronic inflammatory reaction

R: M>F, 16-40yo, FHx

A/P: ingrown hair → inflammation → sinus formation + discharge ± infection

Large bowel obstruction

D: mechanical disruption in the patency of the large intestines

R: colorectal cancer (and its risk factors), diverticular disease, current/previous hernia, gynaecological conditions, previous abdominal surgery, previous radiotherapy

A: • 60% colorectal cancer
- 20% diverticular strictures
- 5% volvulus (sigmoid in older, caecal in younger)
- Rarely, endometriosis

S/smx:
- Constipation ± absence of flatus
- Abdominal pain ± distention
- NV (late sign)
- ± Peritonism if perforated bowel

Ix: • CXR (to look for abdominal perforation – free air)
- abdominal XR
  - >6cm for colon is abnormal
  - >9cm for caecum is abnormal
  - if there is an incompetent ileocaecal valve, the small bowel may be distended too (>3cm)
- CT scan to confirm

Mx:
- NBM + IV fluids + Ryles tube
- Conservative Mx may be sufficient – trial for 72h if tolerated
- Surgery – urgent if perforated bowel + IV abx

S/smx: • Painful ± purulent discharge
- Fluctuant swelling at the sacrum-coccyx
- May be cyclical (comes and goes)

Mx: • Asymx: clean carefully + hygiene
- Symptomatic: I&D of sinuses, allow wound to close by secondary intention
  - Pain relief
  - Abx if infected / abscess
- If chronic or recurrent, excision of sinuses (including complete excision of cavities)

Hernias

D: the protrusion of viscera through the wall of a cavity in which its contents are contained

÷ congenital vs acquired
- Acquired hernias arise due to weakness of abdominal wall due to aging or previous surgery or ↑abdo pressure (eg heaving lifting, pregnancy)

÷ characteristics
- Reducible: the hernia can go away by manipulation (eg pressing down)
- Irreducible
- Incarcerated: irreducible + painful
- Strangulated: blood supply has been compromised, leading to ischaemia

S/smx: dependent on type of hernia and where it is located
- Hernias should have cough impulse (ie ask the pt to cough, and the hernia should expand)
  ↳ helps to differentiate between other swellings, eg hydrocele
- If strangulated: pain, fever, peritonism (eg abdo rigidity), bowel obstruction (eg NV, distention), bowel ischaemia (eg malaena)

Ix: clinical Dx ± CT to guide surgical management

Mx:
- Hernias should be treated even if asmx (prevents future problems)
- Most can be managed electively unless there is incarceration or strangulation → emergency
- Mesh repair – a mesh is placed to reinforce the abdominal wall
- Unilateral inguinal hernias: open approach
- Bilateral and recurrent inguinal hernias: laparoscopic approach
- If pt not fit for surgery, hernia support belts are the next best option

Inguinal hernias
- 75% of abdo wall hernias, M>>F
- Located above and medial to pubic tubercle
- Rarely strangulate
- ÷ direct and indirect hernias, but Mx is the same

Femoral hernias
- F>M, esp in multiparous women
- Located below and lateral to pubic tubercle
- High risk of incarceration and strangulation → must be repaired

Umbilical hernia
- Symmetrical bulge under umbilicus

Paraumbilical hernia
- Asymmetric bulge above/below the umbilicus

Epigastric hernia
- Lump in the midline between xiphisternum and umbilicus
- R: extensive physical training, chronic coughing, obesity

Incisional hernia
- up to 10% of abdominal operations

Spigelian hernia
- aka lateral ventral hernia
- hernia through the spigelian fascia
- Located roughly beside the rectus abdominis muscles anteriorly

Obturator hernia
- F>M
- Hernia passing through the obturator foramen
- Typically presents with bowel obstruction + strangulation

Richter hernia
- Herniation of only part of the bowel wall through a fascial defect
  - ie not the whole circumference of the bowel, but part of it
- Strangulation but no bowel obstruction

Anal fissures

D: a split in the skin of the distal anal canal.
· chronic: >6w, usually with features, eg indurated edges, skin tags, visible internal anal sphincter fibres

R: hard stool, pregnancy (3rd trim or post-partum), opiates (↑constipation), STIs (eg HIV, syphilis)

A/P: hard stools tear the anal skin from the pectin at the dentate line. Likely an ischaemic ulcer ∴ poor circulation and spasm of internal anal sphincter → ↓healing

S/Smx: · Pain on defecation ("passing broken glass") → ! DO NOT do a DRE
· Tearing or burning sensation
· Fresh blood on wiping (PR bleeding),
· Anal spasm · ± sentinel pile (20%)
· Visible fissure (40%)

Ix: clinical Dx, no tests at initial presentation. 2nd line: anal manometry and US in resistant fissures

Mx: Conservative for acute <1w – ↑fibre, fluids. Sitz bath, stool softeners and analgesics
· Medical for chronic >6w: topical GTN or CCBs – 6-8w even if smx resolve early (↑risk of recurrence)
· surgical tx ↑rate of healing but risk of incontinence
  - Lateral internal sphincterotomy (LIS) - a small portion of anal sphincter muscle is cut to ↓spasm and pain, promote healing

P: 60% achieve healing at 6-8w; further 20% heal after topic diltiazem. Some may relapse. Around 30% require surgery.

Anal fistulae

D: chronic manifestation of the acute perirectal process that forms an anal abscess. When the abscess is drained, an epithelialised track can form that connects the abscess in the anus/ rectum with the perirectal skin.

R: Crohn's, M>F (2:1), obstetric injury, pelvic radiation, rectal foreign bodies, infxn (eg chlamydia L, TB), malignancy

A/P: cryptoglandular fistulas originate from infected anal crypt glands. In Crohn's, penetrating inflammation causes these fistulae to form.

S/Smx: · Non-healing anorectal abscess following drainage or chronic pus/ pustule-like lesion in perianal area
· Intermittent rectal pain with defecation, sitting, activity.
· Others: pruritus, excoriation, induration.

Ix: Clinical Dx. Imaging for complex fistulae (esp in Crohn's) may be required – MRI, endosonography, fistulography (contrast + XR)

Mx: EUA, fistulotomy (cut open the tract, curette, marsupialisation, packing). Draining seton, etc, for complex fistulae

P: if non-complex fistula, low recurrence, but risk of incontinence

Low anterior resection (LAR) vs Abdomino-perineal resection (APR)
· APR removes tumour along with anal canal and sphincter complex
· LAR preserves remaining anorectum (& sphincter complex)

Hartmann's procedure
· sigmoid colectomy
· end colostomy + rectal pouch (Hartmann's pouch)
· reversal considered 3mo after initial surgery

Ileostomy – loop/end	Colostomy – loop/end
· Mid/distal small bowel	· Any part of large bowel
· Spouted	· Flush
· Prominent mucosal folds	· Flat mucosal folds
· Dark pink / red	· Light pink
· Most commonly on right side	· Most commonly on left side

Haemorrhoids

D: vascular-rich connective tissue cushions located within anal canal (3, 7 & 11 o'clock).
· Internal haemorrhoids lie proximal to dentate line, external haemorrhoids distal.

Classes of internal haemorrhoids
· Grade 1: protrusion w/in anal canal
· 2: beyond anal canal, but reduces spontaneously on cessation of straining
· 3: reduces on manual pressure
· 4: irreducible

R: 45-65yo, constipation, pregnancy, space-occupying pelvic lesion

A/P: straining → haemorrhoids are pulled lower and engorged → bleeding occurs when epithelial lining is torn

S/Smx: PR bleeding (fresh), perianal pain/discomfort ± pruritus, palpable lesion or mass

Ix: anoscopic exam, colonoscopy or flex sig ± FBC, stool for occult haem (if no significant tissue seen on exam)

Mx: conservative: ↑fibre, fluids ± topical steroids if pruritic
· Surgical: rubber band ligation.
  - Other options: sclerotherapy, photo-coagualtion, arterial ligation, staples.
  - Surgical haemorrhoidectomy for grade 4 or external haemorrhoids

P: recurrence likely if risk factors continue Surgical option best outcome, with <20% recurrence low re-treatment rates compared to rubber band ligation.

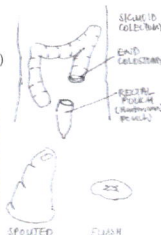

Colorectal cancer

D: cancers of the colon
· majority are adenocarcinomas
· 66% arise in the colon, 30% rectum
· others: carcinoid tumours, GI stromal cell tumours (GISTs), lymphomas

R: ↑age, FHx, genetic syndromes (eg Lynch), inflammatory bowel disease (esp pancolitis and left-sided colitis), obesity

S/smx:
· altered bowel habits ►
· rectal bleeding of any kind ►
· abdo pain and discomfort
· unexplained weight loss ►
· anaemia
  - any new iron deficiency anaemia in an elderly pt should be a red flag
· bowel obstruction ► ►

Screening: Home-based faecal immunochemical test (FIT)
· a type of faecal occult blood test
· uses antibodies that specifically recognise human Hb
· every 2y in 60-74yo in England
· every 2y in 50-74yo in Scotland
· pts ≥75yo can request screening
· pts are informed whether test was normal or abnormal – if abn, pts are offered a colonoscopy (1 in 10 will be found to have cancer)

Ix: · bloods (FBC – looking for iron deficiency anaemia)
· endoscopy + colonoscopy if source of occult blood cannot be established ("up and down")
· CTTAP for staging

Dukes' classification	5y survival
A: tumour confined to mucosa	95%
B: invading bowel wall	80%
C: lymph node mets	65%
D: distant mets	5%

Mx · Pts who meet any ► → 2ww referral
· Definitive Mx: resection
  - caecal, ascending or proximal transverse colon tumour: right hemicolectomy
  - distal transverse, descending colon tumour: left hemicolectomy
  - sigmoid colon: high anterior resection (preserves part of the rectum)
  - rectal tumours: anterior resection
  - anal verge tumours: abdomino-perineal excision of rectum
· Most pts will have an anastomosis where the proximal and distal segments of the colon are joined together
  - in emergency settings, end colostomies may be needed which can be reversed (ie anastomosed later on), eg Hartmann's pouch
· Chemotherapy or radiotherapy are likely indicated (before/after)

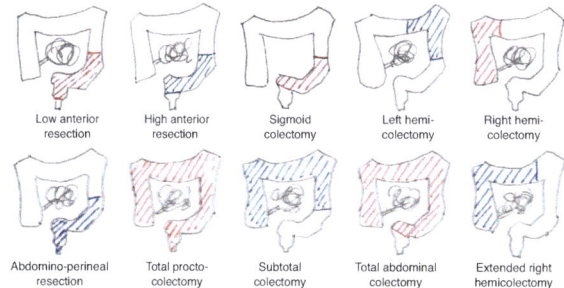

Low anterior resection · High anterior resection · Sigmoid colectomy · Left hemicolectomy · Right hemicolectomy

Abdomino-perineal resection · Total procto-colectomy · Subtotal colectomy · Total abdominal colectomy · Extended right hemicolectomy

GORD

D: smx/complications arising from reflux of gastric contents into the esophagus, oral cavity or lung

R: FHx, ↑age, hiatus hernia, obesity

A/P: ↑relaxation of lower oesophageal sphincter allows reflux of gastric contents
- Severity of damage depends on duration of contact with gastric contents, what contents, and resistance of epithelium to damage
- Acid in lower oesophagus → vagal stimulation → chronic coughing, throat clearing.

S/Smx: • Heartburn (esp after meals)
- Dyspepsia   • Regurgitation
- Cough (esp at night when lying down)
- Halitosis, globus, enamel erosion
- Bloating
► dysphagia, haemetemesis, melena, persistent vomiting, wt loss, anemia → 2ww URGENT REF ►

Ix: GORD is a clinical Dx; PPI trial first.
± pH monitoring, esophageal manometry, barium swallow, OGD.
Indications for UGI endoscope:
- >55yo   • smx >4w or despite tx
- Dysphagia   • Relapsing smx
- Wt loss

Mx: • Lifestyle Δ (wt loss, ↓triggers, stop smoking, avoid late night eating)
- If not endoscopically proven, treat as per dyspepsia
  - Review meds   - Full dose PPI
- Endoscopically proven
  - Full dose PPI 1-2mo
  - If response, then ↓dose, continue
  - If no response, then 2x dose
- Endoscopically -ve
  - Full dose PPI for 1mo
  - If response, then ↓dose prn (limit number of repeat prescription)
  - If no response, then Δ to H2RA or prokinetic for 1mo

P: most pts have smx control w/ PPIs – most pts relapse if PPI therapy is stopped.

Gastritis

D: histological presence of gastric mucosal inflammation

R: H. pylori infxn, NSAIDs, steroids, alc use, toxic ingestions, prev gastric surgery, critically ill pts, autoimmune disease

A/P: H. pylori induces severe inflam → gastric mucin degradation, ↑mucosal permeability → gastric epithelial cytotoxicity
NSAIDs and alcohol: ↓gastric mucosal blood flow, loss of mucosal protective barrier. NSAIDs ↓prostaglidins.
Autoimmune gastritis: antiparietal cell antibodies (abs) stimulate inflam → loss of parietal and chief cells
Gastric atrophy and acid blocking meds: ↑pH, disrupt acid barrier to bacterial overgrowth

S/Smx: • Epigastric discomfort ± NV
- ↓appetite.
- If severe: acute abd pain, ↑↑emesis, fever, altered reflexes and cognitive impairment (if 2/2 B12 deficiency), glossitis

Ix: H. pylori urea breath test, fecal antigen test, FBC ± histology, endoscopy, serum B12, cultures, parietal cell abs, intrinsic factor abs.

Mx of H. pylori infxn:
- ● triple tx (PPI + clarithromycin, amoxicillin or metronidazole) x14d
- ● quadruple tx (PPI, bismuth, tetracycline, metronidazole) x14d
Mx of non H. pylori induced gastritis:
- Stop offending drugs
- Autoimmune gastritis: B12 supplements

P: if H. pylori is untx, ↑risk of gastric cancers. Untx gastritis ↑risk of PUD. Generally good prognosis except for phlegmonous gastritis (rare disorder)

Stopping medications before OGD
1d: gaviscon
2w: PPI
3d: H2RA
4w: abx

For urea breath test: stop PPI and abx

Peptic ulcer disease

D: break in mucosal lining of stomach or duodenum >5mm in diameter, with depth to the submucosa.
→ ulcers smaller than this or without obvious depth = erosions

R: H. pylori infxn, NSAIDs, SSRIs, steroids, bisphosphonates, smoking, ↑age, personal hx of PUD, FHx, ITU pts

A/P: inbalance btwn factors that damage the gastroduodenal mucosal lining and defense mechanisms (mucus bicarb layer secreted by mucus cells).
- gastric ulcers: secretion of gastric acid low or normal
- duodenal ulcers: ↑↑gastric acid ∵ H. pylori impairs secretion of somatostatin
- Zollinger-Ellison: NET ↑gastric acid

S/Smx:
- Epigastric pain, "pointing sign" (pt can point to particular spot)
  - Gastric: pain on eating ± 1-2h after
  - Duodenal: pain several hours after eating
- Nausea, vomitting, diarrhoea
- Early satiety, wt loss
- Smx of anaemia (eg fatigue)
- If bleeding: haemetemesis, melaena, ↓BP, ↑HR
- If perforated: pain, shock, syncope

Ix in acute settings:
- Erect CXR (to check for free air under diaphragm → perforation).
- Bloods (incl G&S, cross match)
Other Ix: H. pylori testing, FBC, etc

Mx: • Bleeding or perforation: - ABCDE + resus, IV PPI
  - ● Endoscopic interventions
  - ● Interventional radiology or surgery
- Stable: tx underlying cause + PPI
  - H. pylori +ve: H. pylori eradication

P: With PPIs, duodenal ulcers heal w/in 4w, gastric ulcers w/in 8w. If H. pylori eradication, prognosis is good.
- NSAID-induced ulcers – low rate of recurrence if stopped.

Oesophageal cancer → see ENT 06.06, section under Dysphagia

Oesophageal conditions

Mallory-Weiss tear
- D: Superficial mucosal laceration of the oesophagus
- R: heavy alcohol use, bulimia nervosa, hyperemesis gravidarum, GORD
- S/smx: pt usually has Hx of retching or vomiting
  - streaks of fresh blood in vomit
  - no other systemic smx
- Mx: pt may need antiemetic to stop vomiting (and therefore stop the cause of the Mallory-Weiss tear)

Boerhaave syndrome
- D: spontaneous rupture of the oesophagus
- R: similar to Mallory-Weiss tear, essentially anything that ↑↑intra-abdominal pressure
- S/smx: triad of vomiting, lower thoracic pain, and subcutaneous emphysema
- Ix: CXR may show widened mediastinum + CT contrast swallow
- Mx: thoracotomy and lavage
  - <12h onset, primary repair
  - >12h, insertion of T tube to create a controlled fistula between the oesophagus and the skin (allows for drainage of blood out)
- P: up to 40% mortality, delays >24h a/w very high mortality
- Complications: severe sepsis 2/2 to mediastinitis (entry of gut contents into the thorax)

Hiatus hernia
- D: Protrusion of the stomach through the diaphragm into the thoracic cavity
- R: obesity, ↑abdominal pressure (eg multiparity, ascites)
- S/smx: heartburn, dysphagia, regurgitation, chest pain
- Ix: barium swallow, endoscopy
- Mx: weight loss, PPIs
  - Surgery only if refractory

Plummer-Vinson Syndrome
- D: rare condition characterised by classic triad
  - iron-deficiency anaemia
  - oesophageal webbing
  - dysphagia
- R: middle-aged women, coeliac, Crohn's, RA, thyroid disease
- A: unknown ?autoimmune
- S/smx: as above
  - glossitis (big tongue)
  - angular cheilitis (red, swollen patches at corners of the mouth)
- Ix: barium swallow ± videofluoroscopy, endoscopy (to look for oesophageal webs)
  - other tests as necessary to r/o malignant causes
- Mx: - iron supplementation
  - may require endoscopic dilation if severe
  - advise pt to eat slowly, chew thoroughly

See also 06.06 ENT – Dysphagia for Oesophageal carcinoma and Barrett's oesophagus

ERCP Endoscopic retrograde cholangiopancreatography

Indications:
- Extraction of biliary stones
- Relief of jaundice 2/2 benign or malignant strictures with stents
- Ampullary biopsy, biliary brushings

Consent: risks of pancreatitis, cholangitis, bleeding, perforation. 1/50.

1. Advance side-viewing endoscope to 2nd part of duodenum
2. Locate, cannulate ampulla
3. Sphincterectomy (knife/balloon) prn
4. Do definitive procedure

TIPS Transjugular intrahepatic portosystemic shunt

Indications:
- Oesophageal or gastric varices 2/2 portal hypertension
- Budd-Chiari syndrome

Interventional radiology procedure
- Right internal jugular vein cannulated
- Catheter advanced to hepatic vein
  ↳ usually the right HV
- Venogram (XR) obtained
- Direct needle towards right portal vein
- Dilate angioplasty balloon
- Deploy stent, widen to ~8mm
- Confirm placement with venogram

Upper GI bleed UGIB

D: GI blood loss whose origin is proximal to the ligament of Treitz at the duodenojejunal junction

S/smx
- Haemetemesis
  = blood in vomit
  - ranges from bright red to "cofffee ground" vomit
- Melaena
  = digested blood in poo
  - in contrast to fresh blood PR (aka haematochezia), melaena is black and tarry (sticky)
- ↑urea due to ↑digested protein

DDx (localising bleed)
Swallowed blood
- Epistaxis (nosebleed)
- Haemoptysis
Oesophagus
- Varices
  - large amount of fresh blood vommited ± melaena
  - may stop spontaneously, but rebleeds are common
- Mallory-Weiss tear
  - small to moderate amounts of fresh blood after vomiting and retching
- Reflux oesophagitis
  - small amount of fresh blood, like streaks in vomit
  - Hx of GORD
- Oesophageal carcinoma
  - variable amounts of blood
  - a/w s/smx of cancer – dysphagia, wt loss, etc
Stomach
- Peptic ulcer
  - Small bleeds
  - Presents more often as iron deficiency anaemia
  - Erosion into significant vessel may cause major haemorrhage
  - May have Hx of NSAID or steroid use without PPI cover
- Gastric cancer (carcinoma, GIST)
  - range of presentations

DDx (localising bleed)
Stomach (continued)
- Dieulafoy lesion (vascular malformation in the GI tract)
  - often no prodromal features prior to bleed, but can produce considerable haemorrhage
- Hereditary haemorrhagic telangiectasia
  - autosomal dominant disorder
  - bleeds tend to occur in mucosae, eg nasal bleeds, GI bleeds
Duodenum
- Duodenal ulcer
  - bleeds at **gastroduodenal artery** most common
  - pain occurs hours after eating
- Aorto-duodenal fistula
  - occurs in pts with abdominal aortic aneurysm surgery
- Duodenal diverticulae
  - 90% are asymptomatic
  - rarely can cause bleeding, obstruction, infxn, perforation
- Invasive pancreatic tumours
- Haemobilia
  = bleeding from and/or into the biliary tract
  - most of them are iatrogenic, 2/2 invasive procedures eg ERCP
  - classic triad of RUQ pain, jaundice, overt UGIB

DDx (underlying disorders)
- Bleeding disorders
  - liver disease associated
  - thrombocytopaenia
  - haemophilia
- Drugs
  - anticoagulation   - aspirin
  - NSAIDs   - steroids
- Others
  - uraemia
  - connective tissue disorders

Ix
- Glasgow-Blatchford score to determine whether pts need to be admitted
  - Composed of urea, Hb, SBP, HR, liver disease, heart disease, and whether pt presents with melaena and syncope
  - If score = 0, consider early discharge
- Rockall score, used AFTER endoscopy to determine risk of rebleeding and mortality
- Endoscopy
  - offered immediately after resus in pts with severe bleed
  - **ALL pts should have endoscopy within 24h**

Mx
- RESUS
  - ABC, 2x wide bore IV access
  - platelet transfusion if platelet <50
  - FFP if fibrinogen <1g/L or PT or APTT >1.5x normal
  - PCC + vitamin K if pts are on warfarin and actively bleeding
- Mx of non-variceal bleeds
  - DO NOT give PPIs before endoscopy; give *after*
  - if further bleeds, repeat endoscopy, ref to interventional radiology and upper GI surgery
- Mx of variceal bleeds
  - **terlipressin** and **prophylactic abx** at presentation
    ↳ give before endoscopy
  - **band ligation** for oesophageal varices; injections of cyanoacrylate for gastric varices
  - Sengstaken-Blakemore tube if uncontrolled bleeding
  - TIPS offered if bleeding cannot be controlled with above measures
- Prophylaxis of variceal bleeds
  - propranolol
  - endoscopic variceal band ligation

Lower GI bleed

D: GI blood loss whose origin is distal to the ligament of Treitz at the duodenojejunal junction

S/smx:
- Haematochezia = fresh blood PR
  - Bright red blood – may be mixed with stool or on toilet paper (when wiping after a poo)
- Melaena (as per UGIB)
- Occult bleeding – blood cannot be visibly seen, but is revealed on faecal occult blood test

DDx (localising bleed)
Small intestines
- Meckel's diverticulum
  - tends to occur in children and young adults
  - painless melaena or hematochezia; "currant jelly" bleeding
  - abdo mass may be palpated
- Intussusception
  - bloody stool occurs with abdo pain, vomiting and SBO
  - if occurring in adults, a lead point due to cancer is often present
- Mesenteric infarction
  - periumbilical pain that is sudden, severe – out of proportion to initial physical exam
- Aortoenteric fistula
  = wall of aorta erodes into adjacent GI system
  - usually occurs 2/2 endovascular surgical interventions
  - "herald" GI bleeds often occur, followed by catastrophic massive bleeds that are life-threatening

Colon and rectum
- Colorectal cancer
- Polyps
- Diverticular disease
- Inflammatory bowel disease
- Ischaemic colitis
- Rectal prolapse
- Angiodysplasia
  - typically >60yo
  - painless hematochezia
  - ± Hx of ESRD, von Willebrand disease, aortic stenosis or anticoagulant therapy

DDx (localising bleed)
Colon and rectum (continued)
- Irradiation colitis or proctitis
  - Hx of radiotherapy
  - Smx typically occur ~9w to 4mo after radiation injury
  - S/smx: diarrhea, rectal pain or urgency, faecal incontinence, obstructed defecation
- Solitary rectal ulcer
  - + passage of mucus, straining during defecation, tenesmus

Anus
- Haemorrhoids
- Fissure-in-ano
- Carcinoma
- Trauma

Others
- Endometriosis
  - Possible Hx of dysmenorrhea, pelvic pain, dyspareunia, infertility

See also underlying disorders in UGIB

Ix:
- DRE if pt is not in pain
  - if painless: diverticular disease more common in older adults
  - ‼ do not do DRE in anal fissure
- Faecal occult blood testing if micro-scopic blood is suspected, eg iron deficiency anaemia in older population
- Faecal calprotectin if suspecting IBD
- Colonoscopy for direct visualisation of lesions
- Barium enema
- Angiography (in acute bleeding phase)

Mx:
- Resus as per UGIB
- Deal with underlying condition

Irritable bowel syndrome

D: chronic condition characterised by abd pain assoc w/ bowel dysf. No structural abn. Multifactorial.

R: phy&sex abuse, PTSD, <50yo, F>M (2:1), previous enteric inxn, FHx, stress

A/P: Δ gastric motility, inflam or immune system involvement, microbiota Δ, bile acid malabsorption. Dysfunction in motor and sensory aspects of GIT.

Dx - consider if ≥6mo of **ABC**
· abdominal pain &/or
· bloating &/or · change in bowel habit
+ve diagnosis if ≥2 of 4 + pain relieved by defecation:
· altered stool passage
· abd bloating, distension, tension or hardness
· smx made worse by eating
· passage of mucus

Ix: FBC, ESR/CRP, coeliac disease screen (IgA TTG)
· Enquire for red flags: rectal bleeding, unexplained wt loss, FHx of bowel or ovarian cancer, >60yo

Mx:
 antispasmodic agents, laxatives (not lactulose), loperamide
  ↳ consider linaclotide if max loperamide or constip ≥12mo
 low dose TCAs (amitriptyline 5-10 mg preferred to SSRIs)
Others
· psychological: CBT, etc
· do not encourage use of acupuncture or reflexology
· general dietary advice
 - regular meals, eat slowly
 - limit tea/coffee intake, consider limiting intake of high fibre foods, limit fresh fruit to 3 portions
 - for wind and bloating consider ↑oat intake and linseeds

P: normal life expectancy, and no long-term complications, but ↓QoL.

Diverticular disease

D: clinical state caused by smx pertaining to colonic diverticula
· Colonic diverticul**osis** = herniation of mucosa and submucosa through muscular layer of the colonic wall.
· Diverticul**itis** = inflammation of diverticula, possibly ∴ infxn

R: >50yo, low dietary fibre ± ↑salt, meat, sugar intake, obesity, NSAID and opioid use

A/P: low fibre diet → ↑intestinal transit time → ↑stool vol → ↑intraluminal pressure and colonic segmentation → predisposes to diverticula formation

S/Smx:
· Generally diverticula are asmx → becomes symptomatic when there is inflammation (diverticul**itis**)
· LLQ abd pain, ↑WCC, fever ± PR bleeding, bloating, constipation, diarrhoea
· DRE: tenderness, palpable mass

Ix: FBC, U&Es, CRP.
· colonoscopy, CT cologram or barium enema
· if acutely unwell, CXR and AXR

Hinchey severity classification
I: para-colonic abscess
II: pelvic abscess
III: purulent peritonitis
IV: faecal peritonitis

Mx: ↑dietary fibre intake
· mild attacks: conservative - abx
· peri-colonic abscesses: drained surgically or radiologically
· recurrent episodes requiring admission: segmental resection
· Hinchey IV: resection + stoma; high risk of post-op complications

P: 1/3 pts have recurrent diverticular disease, mostly w/in 5y (↑risk in young pts, abscess formation at index Dx). A/w high mortality, ↓response to therapy. After surgery, 1/4 pts remain symptomatic.

Ischaemic bowel disease

D: umbrella term including
· Acute **mesenteric ischaemia**
  ↳ further ÷ into embolic, thrombotic or venous
· Chronic mesenteric ischaemia
· Colonic ischaemia

R: ↑age, smoking, hypercoagulable state (eg previous VTE), atrial fibrillation, MI, Hx of vasculitis

A: embolism (50%), thrombosis (15-20%), vasculitis, venous thrombosis (5%), hypoperfusion (eg shock, heart failure, recent surgery)
P: ischaemia 2/2 hypoperfusion of intestinal segment

S/smx:
· Abdominal pain severe, sudden-onset, out of keeping with physical findings
· PR bleeding – melaena

Ix: urgent CT scan with contrast or CT angiogram, erect CXR (will show free air if perforation present)

Mx:
· Resus + supportive
· Empirical IV abx
· Immediate laparotomy is usually required, esp if signs of advanced ischaemia
· Thereafter, Mx of risk factors - pt may need to be on LMWH

Abdominal pain DDx

Gastroduodenal
· GORD
· Peptic ulcer
· Gastritis
· Malignancy
· Gastric volvulus

Intestinal
· Appendicitis
· Obstruction
· Diverticulitis
· Gastroenteritis
· Mesenteric adenitis
· Strangulated hernia
· IBD + Celiac + lactose
· Intussusception
· Volvulus
· TB

Hepatobiliary
· Cholecystitis
· Cholangitis
· Hepatitis

Pancreatic
· Pancreatitis
· Malignancy

Splenic
· Infarction
· Spontaneous rupture

Urinary tract
· Cystitis
· Acute retention of urine
· Acute pyelonephritis
· Ureteric colic
· Hydronephrosis
· Tumour
· Pyonephrosis
· Polycystic kidney

Gynaecological
· Ruptured ectopic pregnancy
· Torsion of ovarian cyst
· Ruptured ovarian cyst
· Salpingitis
· Severe dysmenorrhoea
· Mittelschmerz
· Endometriosis
· Red degeneration of a fibroid

Vascular
· Aortic aneurysm
· Mesenteric embolus
· Mesenteric angina (claudication)
· Mesenteric venous thrombosis
· Ischaemic colitis
· Acute aortic dissection

Peritoneum
· Peritonitis

Abdominal wall
· Strangulated hernia
· Rectus sheath haematoma
· Cellulitis

Retroperitoneal
· Haemorrhage (eg anticoagulants)

Referred pain
· Myocardial infarction
· Pericarditis
· Testicular torsion
· Pleurisy
· Herpes zoster
· Lobar pneumonia
· Thoracic spine disease, e.g. disc, tumour

'Medical' causes
· Hypercalcaemia
· Uraemia
· Diabetic ketoacidosis
· Sickle cell disease
· Addison's disease
· Acute intermittent porphyria
· Henoch–Schönlein purpura
· Tabes dorsalis

Red flags
► severe pain
► signs of shock
► peritoneal signs (rebound tenderness, ↓bowel sounds, new or worsening ascites, fever/chills)
► abdo distension
► blood in stool / urine
► anorexia, wt loss
► abdo mass / organomegaly
► fever
► jaundice
► awakening pain / nocturnal pain

R hypochondrium	Epigastric	L hypochondrium
· Liver + GB · R kidney + adr · Small intestine · Ascending colon	· Stomach · Transverse colon · Liver, spleen, pancreas, SI	· Spleen · Pancreas · L kidney + adr · Descending colon
R flank	**Umbilical**	**L flank**
· Liver + GB · Ascending colon	· SI (incl duodenum)	· L kidney · Descending colon
RIF	**Hypogastric**	**LIF**
· Ileocecal junction · Appendix ± Ovaries, fallopian tube	· Bladder · Sigmoid colon ± Uterus ± Male repro	· Descending and sigmoid colon ± Ovaries, fallopian tube

General anaesthesia

D: inducing loss of consciousness in a controlled environment, to prevent response to noxious stimuli
- Triad of analgesia, amnesia/hypnosis, and muscle relaxation or paralysis

Pre-op checks
- Talking to pt – PMH, meds/**allergies**, discussing any concerns, consenting pt. to GA
  - Ask pt about previous anaesthetic use, or FHx of issues with anaesthesia
- Risks to discuss: dental damage, sore throat, post-op N&V, risks of MI & stroke
- Functional status (ASA grade):
  - 1 Normally fit and well
  - 2 Mild systemic disease, controlled
  - 3 Severe systemic disease
  - 4 Incapacitating disease, threat to life
  - 5 Moribund (won't survive >24h even with operation)
  - 6 Brain dead - for organ donation
- Airway Ax "LEMON"
  - Look externally, eg abnormal neck large tongue, dental issues, etc
  - Evaluate 332
    ◊ 3 fingers between teeth
    ◊ 2 btwn hyoid and mentum
    ◊ 2 btwn hyoid and thyroid
  - Mallampati score (look it up)
  - Obstruction / obesity
  - Neck mobility – ↓in trauma, elderly

Pre-op instructions
- Meds to stop (unless otherwise directed by surgeon/anaesthetist)
  - Anticoagulants (incl DOACs) usually stopped before op, and pt is usually on enoxaparin injections as inpt. Seek clear instruction from consultant
  - Antiplatelets: stop 5-7d before surgery
  - If pt on dual antiplatelet therapy to prevent stent thrombosis, ?delay surgery for 1y if possible. If not, seek cardiology advice
  - NSAIDs: stop
  - Insulin: **continue** basal insulin, but skip oral hypoglycaemics and fast-acting insulin when NBM
  - Contraceptive pill & HRT: stop 4w before major surgery, restart 2w after if pt mobile
- NBM 6h before surgery, clear fluids up till 2h before surgery

Induction of GA
Inhalation, eg sevoflurane, isoflurane
- A/w malignant hyperthermia
Intravenous
- Propofol – fast acting and good recovery characteristics
  - Can cause hypotension
- Thiopental – not used much nowadays
- Ketamine – usually in paeds
  - Can cause hypertension

Paralytic agents
- Used in operations where surgeons do not want change in abdominal pressure due to the diaphragm moving (eg laparoscopic procedures, major abdominal surgery)
- Agents include suxamethonium and rocuronium
- If used, will require intubation and ventilation until pt regains ability to maintain their own airway

Maintenance of GA
Maintenance of unconsciousness
- Inhalation, eg sevoflurane
- Intravenous, eg propofol
Maintenance of analgesia
- Impt to remember that pt can be unconscious but still experience pain – this may be reflected in ↑HR, ↑BP
- Opioids, eg remifentanil, alfentanil
- Local anaesthetics

Stopping/reversing GA
- Usually involves stopping the induction/maintenance agent while maintaining the analgesic component
- Neostigmine can be given to reverse residual muscle paralysis and ↓anti-cholinergic side effects (eg salivation) as pt wakes up
- More predictable in total intravenous anaesthesia (TIVA) than with inhaled agents
- Variable time as to when pts wake up
- Should only be extubated when they can obey commands and demonstrate muscle tone (eg "squeeze my hand")

Airway adjuncts

Most airway adjuncts help to open up the airway to promote air delivery, but *only* endotracheal intubation and tracheo-stomies properly protect the airway

Oropharyngeal / Guedal airway (OPA)
- Measure by putting tube on pt's cheek, with the wide part near the pt's front teeth; the smaller opening should sit on the angle of the jaw ("hard to hard")
- In adults, insert upside down, then twist 180° when getting to the back of the throat
- Poorly tolerated in conscious or semi-conscious individuals as they can cause gag reflex

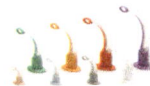

Nasopharyngeal airway (NPA)
- = tube that goes through nostril to the back of throat; helps bypass obstruct-ions in the mouth / base of tongue
- Measure by putting one end on tip of the nose, and the other end should sit at the tragus of the ear ("soft to soft")
- Insert as if inserting an NG tube – aim straight (not downwards)
- Contraindicated if suspected skull base fracture (might go into the brain)

Bag-valve-mask (BVM)
- Mask has to be placed over nose and mouth (usually with head tilt-chin lift manoeuvre + tight seal)
- Compression of the bag → ↑pressure → opening of valve → air passes through into the mask
- Can be hooked up to oxygen ± gas supply for pre-oxygenation
- Allows for manual ventilation just before intubation

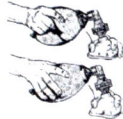

Supraglottic airway
÷ laryngeal mask airway (LMA) & iGel
- The end of these airways sit at the vocal cords and form a seal to block off the oesophagal opening, so they help to lower the risk of aspiration
- However, because they do not go completely into the trachea, there is still a risk of aspiration and thus cannot be properly said to fully protect the airway
- Useful in the cases of short or low risk procedures (eg incision and drainage of simple abscesses)

Laryngeal mask airway
- Reusable supraglottic device
- Some versions have seals that are inflatable (better seal) and also gastric ports to allow for drainage/suction of secretions

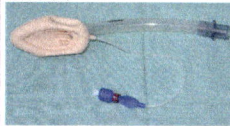

iGel
- Single use supraglottic device
- Seal at the end is activated by body temperature due to characteristics of the plastic used – no inflation required

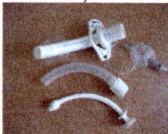

Tracheostomy tube

Endotracheal tube
- Tube inserted with the help of a laryngoscope or fibreoptic camera into the trachea
- Usually size 7 for women, size 8 for men – but may need to be resized based on weight if not standard
- Depth of tube needs to be marked – usually 20-24 cm at the teeth → then needs to be taped to secure
- Inflatable cuff helps to seal the trachea and prevent aspiration

Laryngoscope
- Consists of "blades" and a torchlight
- Used to lift the soft tissues and the epiglottis and directly visualise the larynx so that the tube can be inserted into the trachea past the vocal folds
- Pt needs to be able to bend their neck backwards so that laryngoscope can be inserted

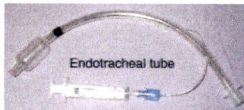

Endotracheal tube

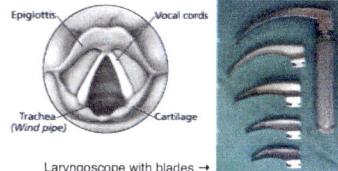

Laryngoscope with blades →

Tracheostomies
- Bypass upper airway, direct ventilation through trachea into lungs
- Cricothyroidectomy – done in emergencies; incision made through membrane between cricoid and thyroid cartilage, and tube is inserted through incision
- Surgical tracheostomy – incision made through trachea itself, and tracheostomy is inserted through this incision

Regional / local anaesthesia

- Divided into peripheral nerve blocks and neuraxial anaesthesia (further ÷ spinal & epidural)

Peripheral nerve blocks
- Using local anaesthetics (LA) such as lidocaine, bupivacaine and prilocaine
  - Long-acting: bupivacaine (also takes longer to work), levobupivacaine, ropivacaine
  - Middle-acting: lidocaine (esp good for mucous membranes), prilocaine, mepivacaine
  - Short-acting: procaine
- Adrenaline can be mixed in
  - Causes vasoconstriction so that the LA remain at the site of injection and is effective for longer
  - Also allows for higher doses of LA to be given since ↓risk of LA entering systemic distribution
- Can be used to block specific nerves (eg femoral nerve block for NOF#), or injected at incision sites during surgery

Risks of LA
- Systemic distribution (ie when LA is accidentally injected intravenously)
  - S/smx: perioral tingling, tongue numbness, lightheadedness, tinnitus. If severe, can result in seizures, apnoea, cardiac depression, coma
  - Mx: stop LA
    ◇ 20% lipid emulsion (Intralipid) – MOA: binds to LA in circulation
    ◇ Resuscitate as necessary (may require intubation, ventilation, etc)
    ◇ Seizure Mx
- Other risks: failure, nerve injury, bleeding

Neuraxial blocks
- Injection of anaesthetic (eg LA, opioids) into the epidural or the subarachoid space
  - Injection level should be around L3/L4. L4/L5 level can be estimated as the line between the iliac crests
  - Not higher as spinal cord ends ~L1; ↑risk of transecting spinal cord
- Needle passes through
  - Skin
  - Subcutaneous fat
  - Supraspinous ligament
  - Interspinous ligament
  - Ligamentum flavum
  - Epidural space   ← epidural needle
  - Dura mater   stops here
  - Arachnoid mater   spinal needle
  - Subarachnoid space ← stops here
- This is a sterile procedure (requires scrubbing in)
- Usually some local anaesthetic (to the skin and surrounding soft tissue) is given before the needle is advanced into the epidural or subarachnoid space
- Blocks are tested by using cold spray to determine dermatomal level at which the block ends

Absolute contraindications to neuraxial anaesthesia
- Anticoagulant states (due to ↑risk of bleeding at the cord)
- Local sepsis (risk of CSF infection)
- Shock or hypovolaemic states
- Raised ICP (risk of coning)
- Unwilling or uncooperative pt (risk to pt & risk to healthcare staff)
- Fixed output states (eg mitral and aortic stenosis)

Spinal anaesthetic
- Aims to anaesthetise the spinal roots passing through the space
- Single dose – only suitable for short procedures otherwise may wear out
- Risks
  - some degree of lightheadedness and ↓BP – conservative Mx
  - total spinal block (↓HR, ↓BP, anxiety, apnoea, loss of consciousness); requires resuscitation asap
  - HA (possibly due to dural puncture)
  - Urinary retention
  - Permanent neurological damage (rare)

Epidural anaesthetic
- Epidural space is larger than the subarachnoid space, and a larger volume of anaesthetic is needed
- Can be given as a single dose, or a catheter can stay in, hooked up to a continuous infusion or patient-controlled analgesia (PCA) machine
- Usually given in labour for pregnancy as catheter can sit in and allow for continuous anaesthesia
- Risk
  - Dural puncture leading to headache
    ◇ Mx with caffeine & oral fluids, bed rest, and analgesia.
    ◇ If headache > 24-48h, blood patch (introducing a small amount of pt's own blood into CSF space to patch the dural puncture)
  - Vessel puncture and inadvertent injection: Mx with resuscitation (symptomatic treatment)
  - Hypoventilation due to motor block of intercostal muscles – may require ventilation
  - Inadvertent spinal anaesthesia – large volume injected into CSF (≈total spinal block): resuscitation required
  - Epidural haematoma / abscess: requires referral to neuro asap

Post-op nausea & vomiting PONV

R: • Patient factors: F>M (3:1), previous Hx of PONV, obesity, motion sickness, pre-op anxiety
- Anaesthesia: opioids (esp morphine), nitrous oxide, etomidate, ketamine, volatile agents
  - TIVA with propofol ↓risk of PONV
- Surgery type: GI, GU, gynae, neuro-surgery, ENT (specifically middle ear), ophthalmic
- Post-op factors: dehydration, ↓BP, hypoxia, early oral intake

P: Common pathway is the stimulation of the vomiting centre in the medulla, which itself is stimulated by
- Higher centres (sensory input, personality, anxiety, etc)
- Chemoreceptor trigger zone (drugs)
- Somatic and visceral afferents
- Middle ear / labyrinth (eg motion)

Mx: • ↓anxiety before op
- ↓risk factors, eg hydration, oxygenation
- Good prevention of PONV esp in pts with known risk factors using anti-emetics (eg ondansetron, cyclizine)

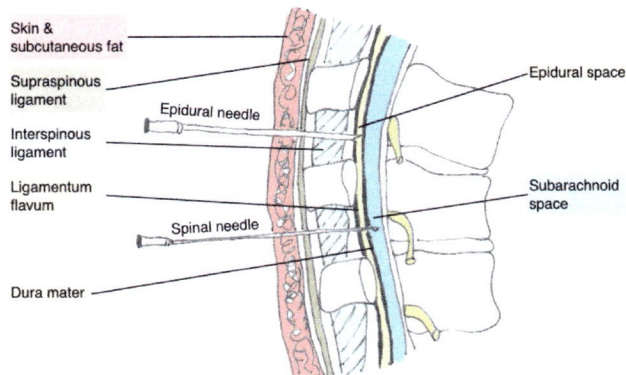

Skin & subcutaneous fat

Supraspinous ligament

Interspinous ligament

Ligamentum flavum

Dura mater

Epidural needle

Spinal needle

Epidural space

Subarachnoid space

Migraine

D: chronic, episodic neurological disorder characterised chiefly by severe headaches ± aura

Chronic = 8d/mo for ≥3mo

R: FHx, F>M (~3:1), young to middle age, obesity (BMI>30), stress, sleep disorder

A: uncertain; ?hyperexcitable brain. Strong genetic component

P: neurogenic inflammation of trigeminal sensory neurons →
vasodilation of blood vessels → HA
· Aura: neuronal dysfunction

S/smx: · HA 4-72h
· Unilateral location
· Pulsatile quality
· Mod-severe pain
· Aggravation by or causing avoidance of usual activity
· ± NV, photophobia, phonophobia
· ± in F, may be a/w menses
· ± Aura (25%): visual smx (eg scotoma)

Ix: clinical Dx; r/o red flag smx

Mx of acute migraines
· sumatriptan + NSAID/paracetamol
   ↳ in 12-17yo, consider nasal triptan instead of PO
· ☢ non-PO metoclopramide or prochlorperazine, consider non-PO NSAID or triptan

Prophylaxis of migraines
· propranolol
· topiramate (NOT in women of child-bearing age; teratogenic)
· amitriptyline
· for F with predictable menses-related migraines, frovatriptan or zolmitriptan may be given
   ↳ ± mefenamic acid, caffeine
· in pregnancy, paracetamol + NSAIDs (2nd line); avoid aspirin and opioids
· Migraines with aura are an absolute CI against COCP ∴ ↑↑risk of stroke
· HRT might worsen migraines

Cluster headache

D: a trigeminal autonomic cephal-algia causing HAs that occur in a cluster of weeks around once a year

R: M>F (3:1), FHx, head injury, smoking, alcohol use (can trigger)

A: unknown
P: trigeminal distribution, ipsilateral cranial autonomic smx, occuring a few weeks a year

S/smx: · HA 15min to 2h
· Clusters typically ~4-12w
· Intense, sharp stabbing pain around one eye (described as the one of the worst kinds of pain)
· a/w lacrimation, redness, lid swelling
· ± miosis, ptosis
· Pt is often *restless* during attacks (as opposed to migraines where pt often just wants to lie down)

Ix: MRI head with gadolinium

Mx: · ref to neurology
· 100% oxygen & subcut triptan
   ↳ 80% and 75% respond w/in 15min for each tx respectively
· Prophylaxis: verapamil
   ± tapering dose of prednisolone

Trigeminal autonomic cephalalgia

D: group of primary HA disorders characterized by
· unilateral head pain
· a/w generally prominent ipsilateral cranial autonomic features

Include   · cluster HA
· paroxysmal hemicrania
· short-lasting unilateral neuralgiform headache attacks with conjunctival injection and tearing (SUNCT)
· short-lasting unilateral neuralgiform headache attacks with cranial autonomic symptoms (SUNA)

Trigeminal neuralgia

D: facial pain syndrome in the distribution of ≥1 divisions of the trigeminal nerve (CN V)

R: ↑age, multiple sclerosis (20x), ?F>M (3:2), ?HTN

A: · focal compression of CN V root by aberrant vascular loop
· idiopathic / other causes

P: focal demyelination → conduction dysfunction → pain

S/smx: · brief (seconds) - sudden onset and sudden cessation
· electric shock-like pain
· limited to distribution of CN V
· triggered by any movement / sensation to the CN V distribution, eg touching the face, shaving, brushing teeth, etc

Ix: clinical Dx; r/o red flags

Mx: · carbamazepine
· if no response, ref to neurology

Tension headache   aka tension-type HA

D: HA characterised by generalised distribution like a "tight band around the head"

R: mental tension / stress, fatigue, missing meals, dehydration

A: unknown. ? muscle tension
P: release and activation of inflam-matory agents → pain

S/smx: · "tight band around head"
· can coexist with migraine HA, but does not have features of migraine

Mx: ☢ paracetamol, NSAIDs, aspirin
· Avoid known triggers

Medication overuse HA

D: chronic HA 2/2 overuse of analgesics; ≥15d/mo. Common.

A/P: not fully understood. ? overuse of analgesics leads to ↓sensitivity of receptors to analgesia → when analgesic is withdrawn, paradoxical pain ("rebound effect")

Dx: · pre-existing HA disorder resulting in the need for analgesia
· HA ≥15d/mo
· regular analgesic overuse for >3mo – people taking triptans or opioids at ↑risk
· not better accounted for by other HA syndromes

Mx: · if pt is on paracetamol, NSAID or triptan, withdraw abruptly
   ↳ warn pt that HA will get worse then better; persist!
· if pt is on opioids, gradual ↓
· Withdrawal smx: NV, hypotension, ↑HR, restlessness, anxiety, sleep disturbance, etc – persist!!

Temporal arteritis

for more info, see Giant Cell Arteritis under Rheumatology; this section only covers headache

D: aka giant cell arteritis
Vasculitis affecting medium and large arteries – in this case, temporal artery

R: >50-60yo, F>M, ?FHx

S/smx: · HA occurs in 85% of pts with GCA, with a tender, palpable temporal artery
· Rapid onset, Hx of <1mo, unilateral
· Jaw claudication in 65%
· ± ocular complications

Ix: ↑ESR. Temporal artery biopsy to confirm (may require >1 biopsy due to skip lesions)

Other causes of headaches

Acute, single episodes
· ▶ Subarachnoid haemorrhage
   ↳ occipital location
   ↳ "thunderclap" - sudden onset
   ↳ "worse headache of my life"
· ▶ Glaucoma (acute, closed-angle)
   ↳ severe pain; can be ocular or generalised HA
   ↳ + ↓visual acuity, hard red eye, semi-dilated non-reacting pupil
· ▶ Mengititis / encephalitis
   ↳ non-specific smx
· Head injury
· Sinusitis
   ↳ a/w rhinorrhea, allergic type smx
· Tropical illness, eg malaria

Chronic
· **Idiopathic intracranial hypertension**
   - R: obesity, F>M, pregnancy, drugs (COCP, steroids, tetracyclines, retinoids, lithium)
   - Smx: + blurred vision, papilloedema, enlarged blind spot + CN VI palsy (see section ICP →04.12)
· Chronically raised ICP
· Paget's disease of the bone
   - 2/2 mechanical compression or ↓blood flow to neural tissue
   - occipital HA, worse on coughing
· Psychological

Headache red flags

"SNOOP4"
· Systemic smx, incl fever
· Neoplasm in PMH, FHx
· Neurologic deficit or Δ
· Onset – sudden/abrupt
· Older age >50yo
· Pattern Δ or recent onset
· Positional HA
· Precipitated by sneezing, coughing, exercise
· Papilloedema
· Progressive HA + atypical smx
· Pregnancy or puerperium
· Painful eye with autonomic features
· Post-traumatic HA
· Pathology of immune system eg HIV
· Painkiller overuse or new drug at onset of HA

Vascular dementia shortened to VD in Neuro

D: chronic progressive cerebrovascular disease of the brain bringing about cognitive impairment. 2nd most common dementia after AD.

R: >60yo, obesity, HTN, smoking, risk factors for stroke (eg AF)

A/P: **infarction** (2/2 emboli, thrombi, lacunar infarction, hypoxia, etc), **leukoaraiosis** (subcortical leuko-encephalopathy), **haemorrhage**
Vascular changes exhaust the brain's compensatory mechanisms and lead to dementia

S/Smx: • **Stroke Hx** strongly suggestive.
• <u>Frontal cognitive syndrome</u>: difficulty solving problems, apathy, disinhibition, slowed processing, poor attention, retrieval memory deficit, frontal release reflexes (grasp, glabella tap, jaw jerk).
• ± focal neurological signs, impaired gait and balance

Dx/Ix: • Cognitive testing (eg MMSE)
• Imaging: MRI (best) or CT
• Bloods (baseline, eg FBC, vit B12, etc), consider syphilis serology (possibility of neurosyphilis)

NINDS-AIREN criteria for Dx of VD
(1) Dementia - impairment in memory + ≥2 other domains (eg orientation, attention, language, executive function)
(2) Cerebrovascular disease - focal signs on neuro exam (eg hemiparesis)
(3) Time relationship - step-wise decline or dementia w/in 3mo after stroke
(4) Clinical s/smx consistent, eg gait disturbance, urinary incontinence, etc

Mx: • Consider referral to specialist dementia clinic or neuro services
• 2ndary prevention of stroke (eg antiplatelets, antihypertensives)
• No specific drugs for VD
• Non-pharm: cognitive stimulation programmes, music & art therapy, etc
• Ensure social support for family / carers

Organic vs psychiatric causes of memory loss – serial 7s (psych usually intact)

Alzheimer's disease AD

D: chronic neurodegenerative disease with insidious onset and progressive but slow decline (generally)

R: ↑age, FHx, genetics, **Down's** (early onset), CVD, smoking, midlife obesity, ↑saturated fats (linked to apoprotein E allele E4), alcohol >14U/w or 0/w

A/P: ↑interneuronal amyloid peptides ∵ ↓clearance of β-amyloid → **amyloid plaques & neurofibrillary tangles** → microglial activation, cytokine and complement activation → neuritic plaques → synaptic and neuritic injury and cell death.
• Presenilin 1 and 2 genes - missense mutations → early onset AD
• Cerebral cortical & hippocampal atrophy

S/Smx: cognitive deficits (loss of recent memory, then ↓executive function, nominal dysphasia). Insidious onset, gradual progression of smx.
Early signs:
1. memory loss that disrupts daily life
2. challenges in planning or solving problems
3. difficulty completing familiar tasks
4. confusion with time or place
5. trouble understanding visual images and spatial relationships
6. new problems with words in speaking or writing
7. misplacing things and losing ability to retrace steps
8. judgment
9. withdrawal from work/social activities
10. change in mood and personality

Ix: • Cognitive testing (eg MMSE)
• Bloods as baseline

Mx: • Non-pharmacological (eg reminiscence therapy, cognitive rehab)
• 💊 Acetylcholinesterase inhibitors
  - eg donepezil, galantamine, rivastigmine
  - for mild to moderate AD
• 💊 Memantine (NMDA receptor antagonist) - add on or monotherapy
• Antipsychotics ONLY for pts at risk of self-harm or severe distress from smx
  - a/w ↑mortality in dementia

P: 8-10y deterioration

Lewy body dementia LBD

D: A neurodegenerative disorder with parkinsonism, progressive cognitive decline, prominent executive dysfunction, and visuospatial impairment.

R: ↑ age

A: unknown
P: accumulation of Lewy bodies in vulnerable sites. Course mimics idiopathic Parkinson's disease.
• Lewy bodies: α-synuclein (a cytoplasmic protein a/w synaptic vesicles), **neurofilament, ubiquitin**
• ↓↓ ACh, dopamine

S/Smx: cognitive **fluctuations**, visual hallucinations (80%), parkinsonian features, REM sleep disturbance.
• Autonomic dysfunction (falls, syncope, urinary incontinence, constip, etc), delusions, ↑/↓sleep

In LBD, neuropsych smx and motor smx w/in 1y. Dementia can also develop in PD (but occurs >1y *after* motor smx).

Ix: • Clinical Dx
• Imaging: SPECT

Mx: • As per AD - use of cholinesterase inhibitors and memantine
• Avoid use of antipsychotics (esp first generation) due to risk of EPSE that can worsen parkinsonian smx
• Non-pharmacological interventions as per VD and AD

P: avg survival of 5-7y upon smx onset

Cholinesterase inhibitors (ChEI)
eg rivastigmine, donepezil, galantamine
→ for mild to mod AD
→ MOA: ↑cholinergic activity
→ SE: GI upset, GU Δ, sleep disorders
Note: rivastigmine relatively CI in pts with bradycardia

NMDA receptor antagonists
eg memantine
→ for severe AD; better tolerated
→ SE: GI upset, balance

Frontotemporal lobar degeneration FTLD

D: spectrum of primary neurodegenerative brain diseases affecting the frontal and/or temporal lobes
• Behavioural variant ≈ Pick's disease
• Progressive nonfluent aphasia ≈ chronic progressive aphasia (CPA)
• Semantic dementia

R: mutations in some genes, ?TBI

A: genetics (~30%), traumatic brain injury
P: neuronal loss, gliosis, microvascular Δ of frontotemporal cortex. Neuronal and glial abnormal inclusions: FTLD-tau (hyperphosphorylated tau), TDP, FET

S/smx:
• For all variants: onset ≤65yo, insidious onset, relatively preserved memory, and changes in personality / social conduct problems
• Behavioural variant: disinhibition, apathy/inertia, ↑appetite, perseveration
• CPA: effortful language output, loss of grammar, motor speech deficits
• Semantic dementia: progressive loss of knowledge about words and objects

Ix: MMSE, MRI (atrophy of frontal and temporal lobes; behavioural variant will show focal gyral atrophy)
• Post mortem biopsy - histology may show Pick bodies (tau protein bodies on silver staining), gliosis, neuro-fibrillary tangles and senile plaques

Mx: • Supportive care
• ChEIs and memantine not rec

P: median survival from Dx 7-13y. Generally shorter survival and faster decline than in AD.

Normal pressure hydrocephalus
• D: Condition characterised by clinical features of hydrocephalus but with no significant ↑CSF pressure
• R: >65yo, vascular disease
• A/P: not well understood: ? ↓blood flow to basal ganglia
• S/smx: "wet, wobbly, whacky"
  - Gait apraxia not responding to levodopa
  - Cognitive impairment
  - Urinary incontinence

Delirium

D: acute, fluctuating changes in mental status - inattention, disorganised thinking, altered level of consciousness
÷ Hyperactive, hypoactive, mixed

R: >65yo, past/present cognitive impairment or dementia, current hip fracture, severe illness

A/P: reduced functional reserve + precipitating insult = delirium
Insults - drugs and withdrawal, primary neurological injury, acute illness (infxn, hypoxia, shock, dehydration, fever, constipation), metabolic abn, surgery, pain, sleep deprivation, environmental factors (use of physical restraints, catheters, ITU stay)

S/Smx: • Acute onset (hours to days)
• Decreased cognition (often fluctuating)
• Impairment of consciousness (more drowsy than normal)
• Agitation, fear, delusions
• Abnormal perceptions, eg hallucinating
• Smx usually worse at night interspersed with periods of normality

Ix: Cognitive testing (eg MMSE), look for source of delirium (eg U&Es to look for AKI, FBC to look for ↑WCC)

Prevention: Ax for risk factors, familiarity
Mx: remove precipitating insult, Mx risk factors (eg med review). Give clear instructions, signage, visits, etc
• If pt gets aggressive,
  💊 haloperidol 0.5 mg PO bds →
  increase to 2.5 mg PO if no effect
  💊 IM haloperidol if no choice
  - If 2/2 alcohol withdrawal, give chlordiazepoxide or diazepam

• Ix: CTH or MRI head, levodopa challenge, LP
• Imaging will show hydrocephalus with ventriculomegaly out of proportion to sulcal enlargement
• Mx: 💊 ventriculoperitoneal shunting
  - Complications: seizures, infxn, bleeding (ICH), stroke
• P: shunting is lifelong

Parkinson's disease PD

D: chronic progressive neurological disorder characterised by **motor symptoms of resting tremor, rigidity, bradykinesia, and postural instability**

R: ↑age, M>F, FHx, genetics, MPTP exposure

RF for faster progression: older age at smx onset, rigidity/bradykinesia as presenting smx, assoc comorbidities, ↓ response to dopaminergic meds

A: considered a sporadic disorder, with some genetic forms. Environmental factors, oxidative stress, etc.

P: Selective **loss of nigrostriatal dopaminergic neurons in the substantia nigra pars compacta** + Lewy bodies and neurites (composed of synuclein)

S/Smx: "TRAP"
• **Tremor** (resting) • **Rigidity** (cogwheel)
• **Akinesia / bradykinesia** • **Postural instability**
• Others: mask-like facies, micrographia, depression (40%), sleep disorder, etc
• Drug-induced parkinsonism tends to be more symmetrical than idiopathic PD

Ix: clinical Dx based on Hx and exam

Mx: • Referral to specialist
• Motor smx affecting QoL 👍 levodopa
• Motor smx not affecting QoL: dopamine agonist, levodopa, or monoamine oxidase B (MAO-B) inhibitor
• Risk of impulse control disorders with these meds - ensure pts know warning signs
• Med review to remove drug-drug interactions

Levodopa
• MOA: precursor to dopamine
• Usually combined with decarboxylase inhibitor (eg carbidopa) to ↓ peripheral metabolism of levodopa → ↓SE
• SE of levodopa: (see mnemonic)
  - End-of-dose wearing off
  - On-off phenomenon (large variations in motor performance)
  - Dyskinesias at peak dose: dystonia, chorea and athetosis
• Counselling: ❗ do NOT abruptly stop levodopa. If pt cannot take PO medications, dopamine agonist (eg cabergoline) can be given as rescue medication

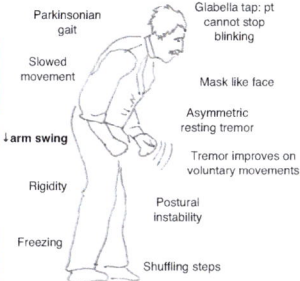

Glabella tap: pt cannot stop blinking

Parkinsonian gait

Slowed movement

↓arm swing

Rigidity

Freezing

Mask like face

Asymmetric resting tremor

Tremor improves on voluntary movements

Postural instability

Shuffling steps

Dopamine agonists
• Eg ropinirole, apomorphine, cabergoline, bromocriptine
• MOA: active dopamine receptors
• SE: ↑risk of impulse control disorders
  - Excessive daytime somnolence - do not drive or operate machinery!
  - Hallucinations in older pts
  - ↑risk of pulmonary, retroperitoneal and cardiac fibrosis a/w cabergoline & bromo
    ↳ Baseline echo, CXR, ESR & creatinine
    ↳ Closely monitor pts

MAO-B inhibitors
• Eg selegiline. Not often used first line.
• MOA: Inhibits breakdown of dopamine
• SE: arrhythmias, anticholinergic effects, can potential effects of levodopa (may need to reduce levodopa dosage 10-30%)
• Don't take with cheese (tyramine thingy)

COMT inhibitors
• Eg entacapone, tolcapone
• MOA: inhibits breakdown of dopamine; often used as adjunct to levodopa

Antimuscarinics
• Eg procyclidine, benzotropine, etc
• MOA: blocks cholinergic receptors - often used to treat drug-induced parkinsonism

P: after 5y of levodopa tx, **motor complications** develop, and eventually smx such as freezing, falling, dementia develop. Cognitive dysfunction and non-dopaminergic smx main determinants of ↑disability in first 5y of disease

---

Parkinson-plus syndromes

D: disorders that have classic features of PD, plus features that distinguish them from PD.

Progressive Supranuclear Palsy (PSP)

The supranuclear gaze palsy from which PSP is named causes restriction of voluntary eye movements in the vertical plane (up/down/both)

• **Rigidity and frequent falls**
• Problems with balance and mobility
• **Difficulty looking up/down & blinking**
  → staring expression & double vision
• Change in behaviour (eg, apathy, impulsivity)
• Dysarthria and dysphagia
  - "chaotic dysarthrophonia", less spontaneous speech
• Slowness of thought, irritability, mood changes

Corticobasal degeneration (CBD)

• Limb rigidity or akinesia
• Limb dystonia
• Limb myoclonus   *** Cortical signs!**
• Orobuccal or limb apraxia
• Cortical sensory deficit
• Alien limb phenomena
  → usually asymmetrical

Multiple system atrophy (MSA)

• **Autonomic failure** involving
  - urinary incontinence or
  - BP↓ (orthostatic hypotensio) w/in 3min of standing by SBP ≥30 or DBP ≥15 mmHg
  - Parkinsonian smx not responsive to levodopa
• **Cerebellar syndrome** (gait ± limb ataxia, dysarthria, oculomotor dysf)

Dopamine adverse effects
Dyskinesia
On-off phenomenon
Psychosis
Arterial BP ↓
Mouth dryness
Insomnia
Nausea, vomiting
Excessive daytime sleepiness

Motor neuron disease MND

D: group of rare neurodegenerative disorders that selectively affect motor neurons. ÷ 4 subtypes
• ALS – 50% (as below)
• Primary lateral sclerosis: only UMN signs first. Slower progress than ALS
• Progressive muscular atrophy: only LMN signs first. Best prognosis.
• Progressive bulbar palsy - worst prog.

Amyotrophic lateral sclerosis ALS

D: progressive disease characterised by degeneration of the motor neurons with cortical, brainstem, and ventral cord locations.

R: genetics (≤7%), >40yo
A: unknown; various theories

P: progressive loss of cortical (fronto-temporal), bulbar (pons, medulla), and ventral cord MNs → retrograde axonal degeneration → denervation and reinnervation in affected muscles

S/Smx: **UMN+LMN** signs; clinical Dx
• Asymmetrical limb involvement (70%), then spreads to contiguous segment of motor neuron (e.g. cervical → thoracic motor neuron)
• **UMN signs**: weakness, **spasticity**, ↑reflexes (and Babinski's, jaw jerk)
• **LMN signs**: weakness, atrophy, fasciculations. Tongue fasciculations – bulbar onset MND
• No remissions; progressive disease

Ix: nerve conduction (normal motor conduction), MRI (r/o cord compression or myelopathy) ± LP (r/o infxn)

Mx: • Riluzole - ↓stimulation of glutamate receptors. Prolongs life ~3mo
• BiPAP at night - survival benefit ~7mo
• Nutrition via PEG

P: mean survival 3-5y. Prolonged survival with NIV (BiPAP), enteral nutrition, younger age at Dx, limb onset, baseline FVC >75%. -ve prog: older, bulbar onset, +frontotemoral dementia, FVC <75%

Huntington disease

D: slowly progressive neurodegenerative disorder with specific smx

R: expansion of the CAG repeat length at the N-terminal end of the huntingtin gene (≥40 copies), FHx

A: **autosomal dominant**, trinucleotide repeat disorder.
P: expanded CAG repeat generates an elongated polyglutamine tail on the huntingtin protein, which leads to cleavage and the generation of toxic fragments of this abnormal protein
→ primarily affects the striatum

S/Smx: earliest smx relate to loss of executive function (eg
↓concentration,
↑errors in complex tasks, slips, misjudgments, needing more help).
• **Behavioural** smx (irritability, impulsivity, personality changes).
• **Motor** smx (chorea, twitching, rigidity, bradykinesia, saccadic eye movements)
• "Anticipation" - disease presents earlier in successive generations

Ix: Clinical Dx, CAG testing, MRI/CT

Mx: • Counselling & supportive care
  - Ensure good support system
• Behavioural smx: SSRIs, CBT, etc
• Motor smx (specialist Mx):
  - tetrabenazine, antipsychotics, benzodiazepines, etc

P: ~20y from Dx to death.
Stage I: disability
Stage II: managing behaviour
Stage III: dependence
Stage IV: placement, end of life

See also 04.14 for section on abnormal involuntary movements.

Bacterial meningitis

D: inflammation of the meninges by various microbes

R: ↑age, crowding, exposure hx, ↓immunity, brain defects (eg AV defects), cochlear implants, sickle cell disease

A: ÷ according to age groups
0-3mo I GBS, E. coli, L. monocytogenes
3mo - 6y I N. meningitidis,
S. pneumoniae, H. influenzae
6-60y I N. meningitidis, S. pneumoniae
> 60y I S. pneumoniae, N.
meningitidis, L. monocytogenes
Immunosuppressed I L. monocytogenes

P: haematological spread or direct contiguous spread → multiple quickly in the subarachnoid space → bacterial components in the CSF trigger inflammation → influx of WCC → cerebral edema, ↑ICP → damage, death

S/Smx: • Early signs – HA, neck stiffness, fever, ↓ consciousness
• Late signs ► shock, sepsis/rash, respi or cardiac compromise, bleeding, ↑ICP (focal neuro signs, papilloedema, seizures, ↓GCS)►

Ix + Mx pathway
• If pt presents at GP, send to hospital asap. Give IM benzylpenicillin if this does not result in delay
• ABCDE + senior review if red flags (eg GCS <12, RR <8 or >30)
• Decide whether to do LP
 - Delay if pt is in rapid deterioration, pt is very unstable (eg severe sepsis), or signs of raised ICP (eg papilloedema, GCS ≤12, focal neuro signs, seizures)
 - If LP cannot be done w/in first hour, give IV abx after blood cultures
• Abx + IV dexamethasone + fluids
 - For 3mo - 50yo, give IV cefotaxime or ceftriaxone
 - Add amoxicillin if <3mo or >50yo
• Mx of exposed contacts within 7d before onset of smx: PO ciprofloxacin
 - Alternative: rifampicin
 - Offer meningococcal vaccination if confirmed
 - No prophylaxis for pneumococcal meningitis unless cluster of cases

Viral meningitis

D: inflammation of the meninges by a virus

R: very young or old, immunocomp, summer and autumn, unvaccinated for mumps, IVDU

A: non-polio enteroviruses (eg coxsackie virus, echovirus), mumps, HSV, CMV, HZV/VZV, HIV, measles

P: see bacterial

S/Smx: presents similarly to bacterial meningitis, but possibly less severe

Ix: r/o bacterial meningitis – LP, PCR

Mx: • Supportive Mx generally
• If HSV meningitis suspected, consider using aciclovir
• If bacterial meningitis or encephalitis suspected, tx until otherwise proven
 - IV ceftriaxone and aciclovir

P: generally good, but post-viral syndrome (HA, malaise) may persist for weeks. May recur.

Cryptococcus neoformans – stains with India ink

Complications of bacterial meningitis:
• Sensorineural hearing loss (25-35% after pneumococcal meningitis, 5-10% after HiB)
• Seizures (Mx with benzos, may require long-term anticonvulsants)
• Focal neurological deficit, cognitive or behavioural problems
• Infection: sepsis, abscess
• ↑Pressure: herniation, hydrocephalus
• Waterhouse-Friderichsen syndrome (adrenal insufficiency 2/2 adrenal haemorrhage) esp a/w meningococcal meningitis

Kernig's sign (11%): Pain in the lower back or back of thigh on extension of knee when hip is flexed to a 90° right angle
Brudzinski's sign (9%): Forced flexion of the neck elicits a reflex flexion of the hips

Encephalitis

D: inflammation of the brain parenchyma a/w neuro dysfunction

R: <1yo or >65yo, immunocomp, post-infxn, blood/fluids exposure, organ transplant, animal/insect bites, location, season, swimming in certain places

A: causative agent found in only 50%. Viruses, bacterial, immune-mediated, etc
P: similar to meningitis but involving the brain parenchyma

Dx criteria (1 + ≥3 minor criteria for probable encephalitis)
(1) Δ mental status lasting ≥24h with no alternative cause identified
(2) fever ≥38˚C w/in 72h before/after presentation
(3) partial/general seizures
(4) new onset focal neurological findings
(5) CSF WCC ≥5
(6) +ve neuroimaging findings
(7) +ve EEG findings

Ix: • LP (CSF – ↑WCC, ↑protein + PCR for HSV, VZV and enteroviruses)
• Neuroimaging - MRI better
 - Normal in 1/3 pts
 - May show medial temporal and inferior frontal changes
• EEG: lateralised periodic discharges at 2Hz
• Bloods + blood cultures

Mx: • Hospitalisation + isolation.
• IV aciclovir if suspected encephalitis
• Supportive care (airway, fluids, analgesia, etc)

P: depends on aetiology. 12% mortality for infectious aetiology in England

Herpes simplex encephalitis
• D: encephalitis 2/2 herpes simplex infection – characteristically affects temporal & inferior frontal lobes
 - HSV-1 causes 95% cases
• S/smx: - As above
 - Focal features of temporal lobe infxn, eg aphasia
• Ix: CT may show bilateral temporal lobe changes

Brain abscess

D: suppurative collection of microbes w/in a gliotic capsule occurring within brain parenchyma – single/multiple

R: infxn elsewhere (esp sinusitis, otitis, dental procedure/infxn, endocarditis), brain op, AVM, immunocomp, DM

A: infxn w/ bacterial, fungal, or parasitic organisms. Possibly polymicrobial.
P: organisms enter into brain via haem spread or direct innoculation. Most often originates in ischaemic white matter adjacent to the cortex
(1) early cerebritis: ~3d, local inflam, necrosis, neutrophilic infiltration, activation of microglia and astrocytes
(2) late cerebritis: day 4-9, lymphocytic and microglial infiltration
(3) frank abscess formation: after day 10 – encapsulation and suppuration

Dx relies on identifying risk factors
S/Smx: HA, signs of ↑ICP, CN palsy, fever, focal neuro deficit

Ix: bloods (FBC, CRP/ESR), blood cultures, neuroimaging (MRI better) → ↑CRP/ESR favours Dx of abscess over tumours

Mx: • Initially, IV abx (ceftriaxone and metronidazole) asap
• If needed, anticonvulsants, steroids (only if pt is unstable)
• Confirmed Dx, surgical drainage

P: permanent hemiparesis and long-term seizures <50%, mortality <13%. main prognostic factor is pt's neurological status upon presentation

Spinal epidural abscess

D: inflammation with pus within the epidural space

R: IVDU, recent surgery/trauma, indwelling catheter, immunocomp, DM, concomitant bacteremia or endocarditis

A: infxn – haem spread in up to 50% cases, contiguous spread (30%), direct inoculation 2/2 surgery, trauma

P: epidural venous plexus (valveless veins running from foramen magnum to sacrum) + lymphatics allow for spread of bacteria. Neurological impairment 2/2 vascular compromise of spinal cord or roots and direct pressure on tissue.
Clinical stages: (1) localised muscle, bone pain (2) radicular pain and paraesthesias (3) muscle weakness, sensory loss, sphincter dysfunction (4) paralysis

S/Smx: classic triad of focal back pain, fever and neurological deficit present in only 10%.

Ix: bloods (FBC, CRP/ESR), blood cultures, MRI spine

Mx: empirical → culture-directed abx ± surgical mx. Supportive therapy – hypotension, DVT prevention

P: ~5% mortality, most impt prognostic factor is pt's neurological status upon presentation. morbidity can be significant – paralysis lasting ≥24-36h is likely to last

Toxoplasmosis

D: infxn by the protozoan parasite *Toxoplasma gondii*, usually smx only in immunocomp pts

R: immunocompromise (HIV, etc), exposure during pregnancy (risk for child), ingestion of raw/undercooked meat, exposure to cat faeces

A: *Toxoplasma gondii* found in cat faeces → ingested, spread haem from GIT throughout the human body
P: 90% asmx if immunocompetent. In immunocomp pts, ↑dissemination (esp in neural and muscular tissues) → inflammation → smx

S/Smx:
• In immunocompetent pts, s/smx resemble infectious mononucleosis
  - Fever, malaise, lymphadenopathy
  - Rarely, meningoencephalitis and myocarditis
• In immunocompromised pts: HA, confusion, drowsiness, vision issues
• Toxoplasmic chorioretinitis: blurry vision. Fundoscopy may show lesions
• Congenital: cerebral calcification, hydrocephalus, chorioretinitis, retinopathy, cataracts

Ix: serology, CT (single or multiple ring-enhancing brain lesions, often involving basal ganglia ± mass effect)

Mx: • Not needed in immunocompetent
• In immunosuppressed & congenital:
  - Pyrimethamine + sulphadiazine + calcium folinate – ≥6w course
  - Treat until CD4 >200 for ≥6mo
• Eye disease – steroids to ↓inflam
• Prophylaxis for HIV pts with CD4+ count <100: cotrimoxazole

P: in immunocompromised, infxn is lifelong. Chronic suppressive therapy unless CD4+ >200

Primary CNS lymphoma

D: extranodal non-Hodgkin lymphoma that is confined to the brain, eyes, and cerebrospinal fluid without evidence of systemic spread

R: HIV + EBV. usually >60yo

A/P: various mutations. Usually has diffuse large B-cell lymphoma histology.

S/Smx: focal neurologic deficits, Δ mental status, behavioural Δ, ↑ICP (HA, NV, papilloedema), seizures

Ix: CT/MRI – homogenously enhancing mass lesion, most commonly in the brain, less frequently in the eyes/spine. PET scan for non-CNS disease.
Dx procedure: stereotactic biopsy or vitrectomy or CSF cytology

Mx: high dose MTX + rituximab ± other chemo ± radiation. Surgery limited use.

P: 10-15% primary refractory, 50% pts relapse → poor prognosis, median survival of 2mo w/o added tx. Median time to relapse is 10-18mo, most relapses occur w/in 2y of initial dx.

Cryptococcosis

D: opportunistic fungal infection caused by *Cryptococcus* species

R: HIV (80% cases; CD4 <100), immunosupp, comorbs and smoking

A/P: in immunosuppressed pts, majority of infxns are caused by *Cryptococcus neoformans*. Usually starts in lungs.
(1) Lungs – dry yeast cells are inhaled and deposited
(2) Alveolar macrophages release cytokines, chemokines to recruit other inflammatory cells
(3) Th1 → **granulomatous inflam**
There is haematogenous dissemination in multiple organs

S/Smx: • Smx onset 1-2w in HIV
• Pulmonary infxn: fever, productive cough, dyspnea, CP, wt loss
• CNS involvement: HA, fever, cranial nerve palsies, change in mental status over days

Ix: cryptococcal polysaccharide antigen in serum, CSF and pleural fluid, cultures, HIV abs, CXR, LP

Mx: • antifungal therapy (fluconazole)
  - If relapse or refractory, amphotericin B
• If HIV +ve, start ART.
• Other supportive tx as needed
• Mx other smx (↑ICP)

P: 70% fatal if untx, 20-30% fatal in high-income countries

Progressive multifocal leukoencephalopathy (PML)

D: devastating CNS infection caused by JC virus (JCV)

R: immunocomp (esp HIV, but also drug-induced)

A/P: JCV establishes asmx, lifelong persistent or latent infxn in the general population.
• In immunocompromise, JCV can reactivate, and cause lytic infxn of CNS glial cells (! demyelination) → PML
• "classic PML": triad of multifocal demyelination, oligodendroglia with enlarged hyperchromatic nuclei, and enlarged, bizarre astrocytes with irregularly lobulated nuclei

S/Smx: multifocal neurological smx, Δ mental status, blindness, aphasia, progressive CN ↓, motor ↓ or sensory ↓ and ultimately coma. Rarely, seizures.

Dx: brain biopsy is definitive. PCR from CSF or other sources possible, but not sensitive

Mx: direct antiviral therapies or ↑antiviral immune response.

P: if ART is started early in disease course, there is better chance at some improvement, but 70% have residual neurological disability. JCV persists in the host

Glasgow Coma Scale (GCS)

Eyes
4 spontaneously
3 opens to voice
2 opens to pain
1 no opening

Verbal
5 oriented
4 confusion
3 inappropriate words
2 sounds
1 none

Motor
6 obeys commands
5 localises to pain
4 withdraws from pain
3 abnormal flexion to pain
2 extends to pain
1 none

! If GCS <8, requires intubation (pt may not be able to secure their own airway). Minimum score of GCS is 3.

	Normal	Bacterial	Viral	TB	Fungal
Opening pressure	12-20	↑	normal, mildly ↑	↑	↑
Appearance	Clear	Turbid, cloudy, purulent	Clear	Clear or cloudy	Clear or cloudy
WCC	<5	↑, typically >100	↑, 5-1000	↑, 5-500	↑, 5-500
Predominant cell type	n/a	Neutrophils	Lymphocytes	Lymphocytes	Lymphocytes
Protein (g/L)	<0.4	↑	mildly ↑	↑↑	↑
Glucose (mmol)	2.6 to 4.5	↓↓	normal, slightly ↓	↓↓	↓
CSF/plasma glucose ratio	>0.66	↓↓	normal, slightly ↓	↓↓	↓

Seizures & Epilepsy

Seizure: a transient occurrence of s/smx ÷ abnormal excessive or synchronous neuronal activity in the brain

Epilepsy - must fulfil any of the criteria
1. ≥2 unprovoked seizures occurring >24h apart
2. 1 unprovoked seizure and probability of further seizures after 2 unprovoked seizures occurring over 10y
3. Dx of an epilepsy syndrome

Classified based on
1. **Where** seizure began in the brain
2. **Level of awareness** during seizure
3. Other **features** of the seizure

Focal seizures

• Start in a specific area of the brain, typically the temporal lobe
  + further ÷ by awareness
  + further ÷ by motor vs non-motor
• Temporal lobe seizures
  - Usually has aura, eg rising epigastric sensation, experiential phenomena (eg deja vu or jamais vu), rarely hallucinations
  - Seizures are typically automatisms ~1min (eg lip smacking, grabbing, plucking)
• Frontal lobe seizures
  - Motor seizures – eg Jacksonian march (twitching starts in one side of body and spreads proximally)
  - Post-ictal weakness (Todd's paresis = focal *uni*lateral weakness usually of the limbs)
• Parietal lobe: sensory seizures
• Occipital lobe: visual seizures (eg flashers)

Mx: • **lamotrigine or levetiracetam**
  ⚕ carbamazepine, oxcarbazepine, zonisamide

Generalised seizure

Subtypes: tonic-clonic (=grand mal), tonic, clonic, typical absence (=petit mal), myoclonic (brief, rapid jerks), atonic (drop)

Generalised tonic clonic seizures (GTCS)
(1) Loss of consciousness (LOC)
(2) Phasic tonic stiffening
(3) Repetitive tonic jerking
Other smx: tongue biting, incontinence, irregular breathing + post-ictal confusion

Mx: [M] **sodium valproate**
  [F] **lamotrigine** or levetiracetam

Absence seizures involve LOC + pt stares into space (10-20s) and abruptly returns to normal

Mx: ⚕ ethosuximide
  ⚕ carbamazepine, oxcarbazepine, zonisamide

Atonic seizures involve LOC + brief lapses in muscle tone (≤3min) = pt drops to the ground

Mx: [M] sodium valproate [F] lamotrigine

Other causes of recurrent seizures

Febrile convulsions
• children 6mo to 5yo, ~3% of children
• occurs early in viral infxn when temp ↑ rapidly
• brief, generalised tonic-clonic or tonic

Psychogenic non-epileptic seizures
• Aka "pseudoseizures" (don't say to pt)
• Seizure-like, but no EEG Δ
  - May have gradual onset
• Ix: normal serum prolactin

Alcohol withdrawal seizures
• Peak incidence ~36h after last drink
• Mx: ⚕ chlordiazepoxide, diazepam

Psychogenic non-epileptic seizures PNES

D: episodic events that appear similar to epileptic seizures but *without* abnormal EEG findings
• Do not refer to as "pseudoseizures"

R: trauma (incl PTSD), acute stressors, mood and personality disorders
• Can occur together with epilepsy

A/P: poorly understood; previously thought of as a conversion disorder (see 14.05). Pts have actual structural neuro-logical changes. Pts should not be thought of as "making up" their seizures

S/smx: PNES appears similar to epileptic seizures, but some factors point towards PNES
  - Pelvic thrusting
  - Family member with epilepsy
  - Occurring only with others around
  - Gradual onset, prolonged event (>10 min)
  - Forced eye closure during seizure
  - Crying during/after seizure
  - Remembering events during seizure
  - Lack of post-ictal confusion
• PNES can have features that resemble epileptic seizures, including urinary incontinence and tongue biting

Ix: EEG, video telemetry, serum prolactin (↑prolactin favours epileptic seizures)

Mx: • Explain diagnosis empathetically
• No consensus on best treatment; CBT + treat co-morbid psychiatric conditions

Anticonvulsants / Antiepileptics

Sodium valproate
⚒ modulates voltage gated Na channels
 - bind to inactivated Na channel
 - use-dependent blocking action

AE: • CYP450 inhibitor
• **teratogenic** (neural tube defects)
• **liver damage**
• pancreatitis • GI: wt gain
• hair loss (regrowth curly??)
• tremor   • ataxia
• thrombocytopaenia
• hyponatraemia

• To stop, reduce dose over 4w
• Monitoring: LFT and FBC (baseline and during first 6mo)
• Pregnancy: if females are on sodium valproate, they should be on **contraceptives**

Carbamazepine
⚒ binds to voltage gated Na channels, ↑refractory period

AE: • P450 enzyme inducer
 - Carbamazepine is an auto-inducer, ie may ↑CYP450 and result in ↑clearance of itself
 - Seizures may return in 3-4w of starting or increasing dose
 - Need to titrate until this stops
• dizziness   • ataxia
• drowsiness   • HA
• visual disturbances (esp diplopia)
• SJS
• **leukopenia, agranulocytosis**,
• **hypoNa** (2/2 SIADH)

Monitoring: LFT and FBC (no clear guidance on this)

Lamotrigine
⚒ Na channel blocker

AE: SJS

Monitoring: no specific requirements

Levetiracetam
⚒ ? Ca channel blocker

AE: Blood dyscrasias, QT prolongation

Monitoring: no specific requirements

Phenytoin
⚒ MOA ≈ carbamazepine

AE: • dizziness   • ataxia
• diplopia, nystagmus, slurred speech, dyskinesia
• gingival hyperplasia, hirsutism, coarsening of facial features
• megaloblastic anaemia (2/2 folate metabolism dysfunction)
• peripheral neuropathy
• **toxic epidermal necrolysis**
• hepatitis / liver failure
• ! teratogenic: cleft palate and congenital heart disease
• CYP450 inducer

Monitoring
• check if starting or adjusting dose, suspected toxicity, suspected non-adherence to meds
• Measure trough (lowest) levels immediately before dose

→ **04.14** for DVLA rules
→ **15.12** for epilepsy in children

Status epilepticus

D: (1) single seizure >5min, or
(2) ≥2 seizures within a 5min period without the individual returning to baseline in between the seizures
! medical emergency

Mx: • Airway: secure airway
• Breathing: high-flow oxygen
• Circulation: IV access if possible
• Disability: check blood glucose

⚕ Benzos • No IV access: PR diazepam or buccal midazolam
• IV access: IV lorazepam
• Repeat once after 5-10 min

• If >5-10min, start second line agent eg IV levetiracetam, phenytoin infusion or sodium valproate
• If >45 min (refractory), general anaesthesia or phenobarbital

Seizures	Syncope
Rhythmic jerking (tonic-clonic)	Twitching, jerking
Incontinence more common	Incontinence rare
Post-ictal confusion	More rapid recovery
Aura	Prodromal smx
Unconscious >5min	Unconcious <1min

Syncope

D: sudden and transient loss of consciousness a/w loss of postural tone, and resolves spontaneously and completely without intervention

A: ÷ cardiac & non-cardiac causes
P: the common end-point in syncopal syndromes is transient insufficiency of cerebral blood flow

Ix: • Cardiovascular examination
• Postural blood pressure measurement (aka lying-standing BP / LSBP)
  - ↓SBP >20 or ↓DBP >10 is diagnostic of orthostatic hypotension
• ECG for all pts
• Other tests depend on clinical features

Mx of reflex syncope
• Pt education usually sufficient
  - prevent known triggers
    ↳ eg ensure good hydration
  - know prodromal smx
  - respond and try to abort
    ↳ physical counter-pressure manouvers, eg squatting, arm tensing, leg crossing
  - standing training – standing for progressively longer periods of time
• Fludrocortisone (volume expansion), midodrine (α1-agonist)

Cardiac syncope
• Arrythmias
  - bradycardias (AV conduction eg heart block ≈ Stokes-Adam attack, sinus node dysfunction, etc)
  - Tachycardias (supraventricular or ventricular)
• Structural
  - valvular heart disease
  - MI
  - HOCM
• Others: pulmonary embolism

Stokes-Adam = transient LOC 2/2 AV block causing ↓cardiac output
Cataplexy = sudden muscle weakness triggered by strong emotions (eg laughter)

→ 04.14 for DVLA rules

Non-cardiac syncope

Reflex syncope
(neurally-mediated reflex syncope)
• D: a group of related conditions in which symptomatic hypotension occurs as a result of neural reflex vasodilation and/or bradycardia
• Vasovagal syncope: stimuli (varied; emotional, pain, etc) → vagal nerve stimulation → vasodilation & ↓ BP → ↓perfusion of brain → syncope
• Carotid sinus syndrome: pressure on carotid sinus → ↓HR, vasodilation, ↓BP
• Situational: cough, micturition, GI stimulation (eg swallowing, defecation)
• Reflex anoxic seizures
  - (not a true seizure)
  - syncope in response to pain or emotional stimuli
  - ? neurally-mediated transient asystole in children (6mo - 3yo)
  - child goes very pale → drops to floor → rapid recovery
  - no long term sequelae

Orthostatic syncope
• Dysautonomia (eg in Parkinson's Disease, diabetic neuropathy)
• Hypovolaemia
• Drug-induced (eg β-blockers)

Syncope 2/2 anatomical problems
• Subclavian steal syndrome (subclavian artery steals blood from the vertebrobasilar artery circulation, causing ↓blood flow to brain)

Neurological causes
• SAH
• Traumatic brain injury
• Migraine (uncommon)

Metabolic
• Hypoglycaemia
• Hypoxia
• Hyperventilation + hypocapnia

Presyncope – feeling of almost passing out but without loss of consciousness
↳ same causes as syncope

Brain tumours

Metastases
• Most common type of brain tumour, most commonly from lungs, breast, bowel, skin (melanoma) and renal cancers
• Mx: radiotherapy, chemotherapy, palliation. Surgery rarely an option

Glioblastoma multiforme
• 45% of primary brain/CNS tumours; 5y survival of only 5.5%
• CT/MRI: lesions with central necrosis + vasogenic oedema
• Histology: pleomorphic tumour cells around necrotic centre
• Mx: surgery + chemo ± RT
  ↳ dexamethasone for swelling

Meningioma
• Tumour originating from meningeal layer of the brain or spinal cord
• Majority of them are benign, but can undergo malignant transformation (32-64% 5y survival)
• 37% of primary brain/CNS tumours
• R: neurofibromatosis type 2, radiation, hormonal therapy, FHx
• CT/MRI - 65% show dural tail
• Histology: spindle cells in concentric whorls ("onions") and calcified psammoma bodies
• Mx: surgery + chemo ± RT
  ↳ if no smx, ?watch and wait

Vestibular schwannoma
• See entry under ENT

Ependymoma
• Malignancy of the cells lining the ventricular system; commonly in the 4th ventricle. Rare (1.7%)
• Histology: perivascular pseudo-rosettes (rose-like pattern)

Oligodendroglioma
• Malignancy of the gray matter, commonly in the frontal lobes
• Usually benign & slow-growing
• Histology: "fried egg"-like microscopic calcifications

Pilocytic astrocytoma
• Malignancy of the astrocytes
  ↳ pilocytic = hair-like
• Most common brain cancer in children, usually slow growing. Good prognosis
• Histology: Rosenthal fibres (corkscrew eosinophilic bundle)
• Mx: resection is usually curative

Medulloblastoma
• Most common *malignant* brain tumour in children; very aggressive
• Arises and spreads from fourth ventricle; can spread to whole CNS
• Histology: small round cells with high nuclear to cytoplasm ratio. Very invasive :(

Craniopharyngioma
• Most common supratentorial brain tumour in children
• Malignancy from the remnants of Rathke's pouch (located near the pituitary gland)
• S/smx: can cause bitemporal hemianopia (∵ location)

Haemangioblastoma
• Vascular tumour that can occur in the brain, spinal cord and retina
• a/w Hippel-Lindau syndrome
  ↳ multiple tumours over lifetime
• Histology: foam cells, high vascularity

Pituitary adenoma
• Benign tumours of the pituitary gland
  ÷ secretory or non-secretory, also ÷ into micro (<1cm) or macro (>1cm) adenomas
• Secretory cause s/smx of hormone excess, eg Cushing's due to ↑ACTH, acromegaly due to ↑GH
• Bitemporal hemianopia classically ∵ compression of optic chiasm
• Mx: hormonal ± surgical (trans-sphenoidal approach)

Unless otherwise noted, most brain tumours are treated with a combination of surgery, radiotherapy ± chemo.

Bitemporal hemianopia
• Lower = craniopharyngioma
• Upper = pituitary adenoma

Brain lesion localisation

Parietal lobe lesions
• Sensory inattention
• Apraxia = pt can understand but cannot perform commands
• Asterognosis = inability to discriminate shape & size by touch, inability to recognise objects by touch
• Inferior homonymous quadrantopia
• Gerstmann's syndrome

Occipital lobe lesions
• Homonymous hemianopia with macula sparing
• Cortical blindness = eyes are ok but person cannot see
• Visual agnosia = cannot recognise objections despite seeing them

Temporal lobe lesions
• Wernicke's aphasia (fluent speech but unrelated with word substitutions, neologisms)
• Superior homonymous quadrantopia
• Auditory agonisa = inability to recognise words heard
• Prosopagnosia = difficulty recognising faces

Frontal lobe lesions
• Broca (expressive)'s aphasia = pt knows what to say but cannot convey it; causes non-fluent, laboured and slow speech
• Disinhibition
• Perseveration = insistent repetition
• Anosmia = cannot smell
• Inability to generate a list

Cerebellar lesions "DANISH"
• Dysdochokinesia (pt cannot alternate between actions rapidly)
• Ataxia = inability to coordinate + Gait is unstable
• Nystagmus
• Intention tremor + past pointing
• Speech changes (dysarthria)
• Hypotonia + heel-shin test fail

See also →04.14 Aphasia

Transient ischaemic attack — TIA

D: transient episode of neurologic dysfunction caused by focal brain, spinal cord, or retinal ischaemia, without acute infarction ± smx last <24h

Mx

1. Aspirin 300 mg STAT unless CI
· CI in pts already on anticoag (CTH to r/o haemorrhage), pt alr on aspirin, etc

2. Arrange for specialist review w/in 24h
· If >1 TIA ("crescendo TIA") – admit
· Advise not to drive for ≥4w

At specialist review,
· **MRI brain** - more sensitive for small infarcts
· Urgent **carotid doppler** unless not candidate for endarterectomy

3. Secondary prevention
· Antiplatelet: **Clopidogrel**
  ↳ If CI, then aspirin + dipyridamole
· **Atorvastatin** 20-80 mg
· **BP** control - anti hypertensives

If pt also has AF (paroxysmal, persistent or permanent) and haemorrhage r/o,
· **Anticoagulation**: warfarin, dabigatran, apixaban, edoxaban, or rivaroxaban

Haemorrhagic stroke — specifically referring to intracerebral haemorrhage (ICH)

R: HTN, ↑age, M>F, heavy alcohol use, illicit drug use, FHx, blood/ clotting disorders, sickle cell disease, anticoagulation, pregnancy, etc

A: cerebral amyloid angiopathy and HTN can directly cause ICH
· 2ndary ICH: cerebral infarction or tumour, drug misuse (eg cocaine, meth), AVMs

P: vascular rupture → bleeding into brain parenchyma → direct damage to brain tissue
± expanding haematoma may cause mass effect

Ischaemic stroke

Ix: non-contrast CT head
  ↳ r/o haemorrhagic stroke

Acute Mx
All pts: Give **300 mg aspirin** if no bleed

IV thrombolysis with alteplase
· within 4.5h of onset of smx
  - if haemorrhage definitively r/o + no CI
· within 9h if CT/MRI evidence of potential to salvage brain tissue
  - within 9h of known onset, or
  - within 9h of midpoint of sleep if they awoke with smx
· lower BP to ≤185/110 before thrombolysis

Thrombectomy within 6h
· + IV thrombolysis (if within 4.5h)
· for confirmed occlusion of **proximal anterior circulation** (seen on CTA or MRA)

Thrombectomy within 24h
· for **proximal anterior circulation** occlusion and potential to salvage brain tissue (seen on CT/MRI – limited infarct core volume)
· consider for **proximal posterior circulation** (ie basilar or PCA) occlusion and potential to salvage brain tissue

Rosier score for stroke
-1 LOC/syncope or seizure
+1 asym facial weakness
+1 asym arm weakness
+1 asym leg weakness
+1 speech disturbance
+1 visual field defect
Stroke likely if **Rosier >0**

Absolute CI to thrombolysis
- Previous ICH
- Seizure at onset of stroke
- Intracranial neoplasm
- Suspected SAH
- Stroke or TBI in preceding 3mo
- LP in preceding 7d
- GI haemorrhage in preceding 3w
- Active bleeding
- Pregnancy
- Oesophageal varices
- Uncontrolled HTN >200/120

Relative CI
- Concurrent anticoag (INR >1.7)
- Haemorrhagic diathesis
- Active diabetic haemorrhagic retinopathy
- Suspected intracardiac thrombus
- Major surgery / trauma in the preceding 2w

Young <55yo: screen for thrombophilia and autoimmune disorders or cardiac disorders (eg ASD)

→ 04.14 for DVLA rules

S/smx: similar to ischaemic stroke (clinically indistinguishable)

Ix: non-contrast CT head
· Once ICH is confirmed, CT angiogram

Mx
· Stabilise pt (ABCDE)
  - consider endotracheal intubation
· Refer immediately to neuro and neurosurgeons
· Rapid control of SBP if >150-220
  - aim for SBP ≤140 ensuring drop does not exceed 60 mmHg within 1h
· Urgent reversal of anticoagulation
· Supportive care as necessary
· Definitive Mx if undertaken is coiling or craniotomy and clipping

Secondary prevention
· Antiplatelet: clopidogrel
  - aspirin + modified-release dipyridamole
· Statin: if cholesterol >3.5mmol/L
  - usually started >48h after due to risk of haemorrhagic transformation
· Carotid artery endarterectomy only if carotid stenosis >50-70%
  - performed within 7d
· If 2/2 to AF: start DOAC or warfarin 14d after ischaemic stroke

According to arterial distribution

Anterior cerebral artery	Medial and superolateral cerebral hemispheres (except occipital lobe)	CL hemiparesis – L>U CL sensory loss – L>U
Middle cerebral artery	Lateral aspect of cerebral hemispheres	CL hemiparesis – U>L CL sensory loss – U>L CL homonymous hemianopia Aphasia
Posterior cerebral artery	Inferior cerebellar and occipital lobe	CL homonymous hemianopia with macular sparing Visual agnosia
Branches of PCA supplying midbrain	= Weber's Midbrain	CL weakness of U&L limbs IL CN III palsy
Posterior inferior cerebellar artery	= Lat med = Wallenburg Posteroinferior cerebellum	Ataxia, nystagmus IL facial pain, temp loss CL limb/torso pain, temp loss
Anterior inferior cerebellar artery	Inferior cerebellum	Ataxia, nystagmus IL facial paralysis, deafness CL limb/torso pain, temp loss

CL = contralateral (opposite side)
IL = ipsilateral (same side)
L = lower / U = upper

Bamford-Oxford classification

TACS 1+2+3	1. Unilat weakness ± sensory deficit 2. Homonymous hemianopia 3. Higher cerebral dysf (e.g. dysphasia, visuospatial disorder)
PACS 2 of 3	
POCS Any 1	· CN palsy + CL motor/sensory deficit · Bilat motor/sensory deficit · Conjugate eye movement disorder · Cerebellar dysfunction (e.g. vertigo, nystagmus, ataxia) · Isolated homonymous hemianopia
Lacunar Any 1	· Pure sensory stroke · Pure motor stroke · Sensori-motor stroke · Ataxic hemiparesis

TACS = total anterior circulation stroke
PACS = partial anterior circulation stroke
POCS = posterior circulation stroke

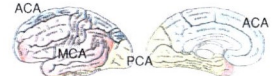

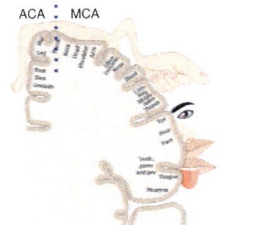

diagrams from Wikipedia

Subarachnoid haemorrhage — SAH

D: intracranial haemorrhage into the subarachnoid space ("on the surface of the brain")

÷ traumatic and spontaneous

R: HTN, smoking, FHx, autosomal dominant polycystic kidney disease

A: intracranial aneurysm (berry aneurysms) – 85%, a/w ADPKD, Ehlers-Danlos, coarctation of the aorta; AVMs; pituitary apoplexy, infective aneurysms

S/smx:
- HA: sudden onset "thunderclap" – peak intensity within 1min of onset - occipital location. "Worst HA I've ever had" ± Hx of less severe 'sentinel' HA in weeks prior to presentation
- Nausea & vomiting
- Meningism (photophobia, neck stiffness)
- Seizures, coma
- ECG Δ if big bleed – ST elevation

Ix: ⚡ non-contrast CT head
- SAH shows up as bright white (=blood) signal typically in the basal cisterns and sulci
- Ideally done within 6h of onset
- If CTH within 6h + normal, do not do LP
- If CTH >6h + normal, do LP
  - LP should be done ≥12h after smx onset to allow development of xanthochromia
  - normal or raised opening pressure
- If CTH confirms SAH, refer asap to neurosurgery
  → order CT angiogram to guide neurosurgical Mx
  → order bloods, G+S & cross match to to prep for surgery

Mx
- Stabilise pt (ABCDE)
- **Nimodipine** to prevent vasospasm
- Supportive: bed rest, analgesia, VTE prophylaxis
- Reversal of anticoagulation
- Definitive Mx if undertaken should be within 24h: coiling, or craniotomy and clipping by neurosurgeons

Complications
- Rebleeding
  - in 10% of pts, most common in first 12h of initial SAH
  - if suspected, repeat CTH
  - a/w high mortality :(
- Hydrocephalus
  - bleep neurosurgeons
  - temporarily treated with external ventricular drain
  - may need long term ventriculoperitoneal (VP) shunt
- Vasospasm
  - aka delayed cerebral ischaemia
  - usually 7-14d after SAH
  - prevent with euvolaemia (normal blood count)
  - may require tx with vasopressor
- Hyponatraemia
  - usually 2/2 SIADH
- Seizures (due to damage to brain parenchyma)

Prognosis: factors a/w with poorer prog – ↓consciousness on admission, ↑age, ↑amount of blood visible on CTH

Subdural haematoma

D: collection of blood between dura and arachnoid layer of meninges

÷ acute, subacute, chronic

R: trauma, coagulopathy / anti-coagulant use, >65yo (esp chronic), ± alcoholic

A: Trauma most common (eg falls, shaken baby syndrome)
P: tortional forces disrupt the bridging cortical veins → bleed into the dural venous sinuses
  ↳ elderly people & alcoholics ↑risk due to brain atrophy

S/smx: wide range depending on how the trauma was sustained
- Can be asmx
- Confusion, ↓consciousness, neurological deficit
- Acute: can present with other associated injuries or picked up on CT scan ordered for head injury
- Chronic: present for weeks to months, slowly developing confusion, ↓consciousness, neuro deficit

Ix: CTH
- Sickle ("C") shaped collection not limited by suture lines
  - acute: bright white signal (=blood)
  - chronic: hypodense (dark) compared to brain tissue
  ± mass effect (eg midline shift)

Mx: • Conservative: watch and wait
- Surgical
  - monitor intracranial pressure
  - Burr hole drainage
  - Decompressive craniectomy

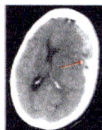

Subdural = SICKLE

Extradural haematoma

aka epidural haematoma
D: collection of blood above the dural meninges - blood collects between the dura and skull

A: trauma - typically a low impact hit to the head or a fall
- Collection tends to be at the pterion (confluence of 4 skull bones) where skull is thin and the **middle meningeal artery** sits under the pterion

S/smx:
- Classically "talk and die"
  - Pt initially loses consciousness
  - Then they regain consciousness ("lucid interval") where they appear to improve
  - Then they lose consciousness again due to expanding haematoma and brain herniation
- If severe, can cause brain herniation → blown out pupil due to compression of CN III

Ix: CTH
- Egg-shaped bright white lesion
  - blood movement is limited by suture lines of the skull
  (also described as biconvex or lentiform shaped lesion)

Mx:
- Conservative if pt is asymptomatic – requires careful monitoring as pts may present in the lucid interval
- Definitive Mx: craniotomy and evacuation of haematoma

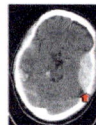

Epidural or extradural = EGG

Cerebral aneurysm

D: focal abnormal dilation of the wall of an artery in the brain

R: smoking (formation, growth, rupture), mod to high alcohol con-sumption (rupture), FHx (esp in siblings; ? autosomal dominant), previous SAH, heritable connective tissue disease (eg ADPKD, Ehlers Danlos)

A: haemodynamically induced injury to the vascular wall

S/smx: can be asmx, picked up incidentally on imaging
- HA (variable character)
- Uncommon (? 2/2 mass effect of aneurysm): seizures, nuchal rigidity, ↓consciousness, focal neuro deficit

Ix: CTH + catheter-based angiogram or CT angiogram

Mx:
- Unruptured: case by case
  - Choice for observation vs treatment has to be undertaken by neuro-surgeons and pt
  - If smx present, generally treated
  - If enlarging (>1mm), treat
  - Small aneurysms (<7mm) can generally be observed
- Ruptured: see ICH [→04.10] or SAH
  - Coiling or clipping

Monroe Kellie doctrine: what makes up the brain - parenchyma 80%, CSF 10%, blood 10%

CT scans from Wikipedia

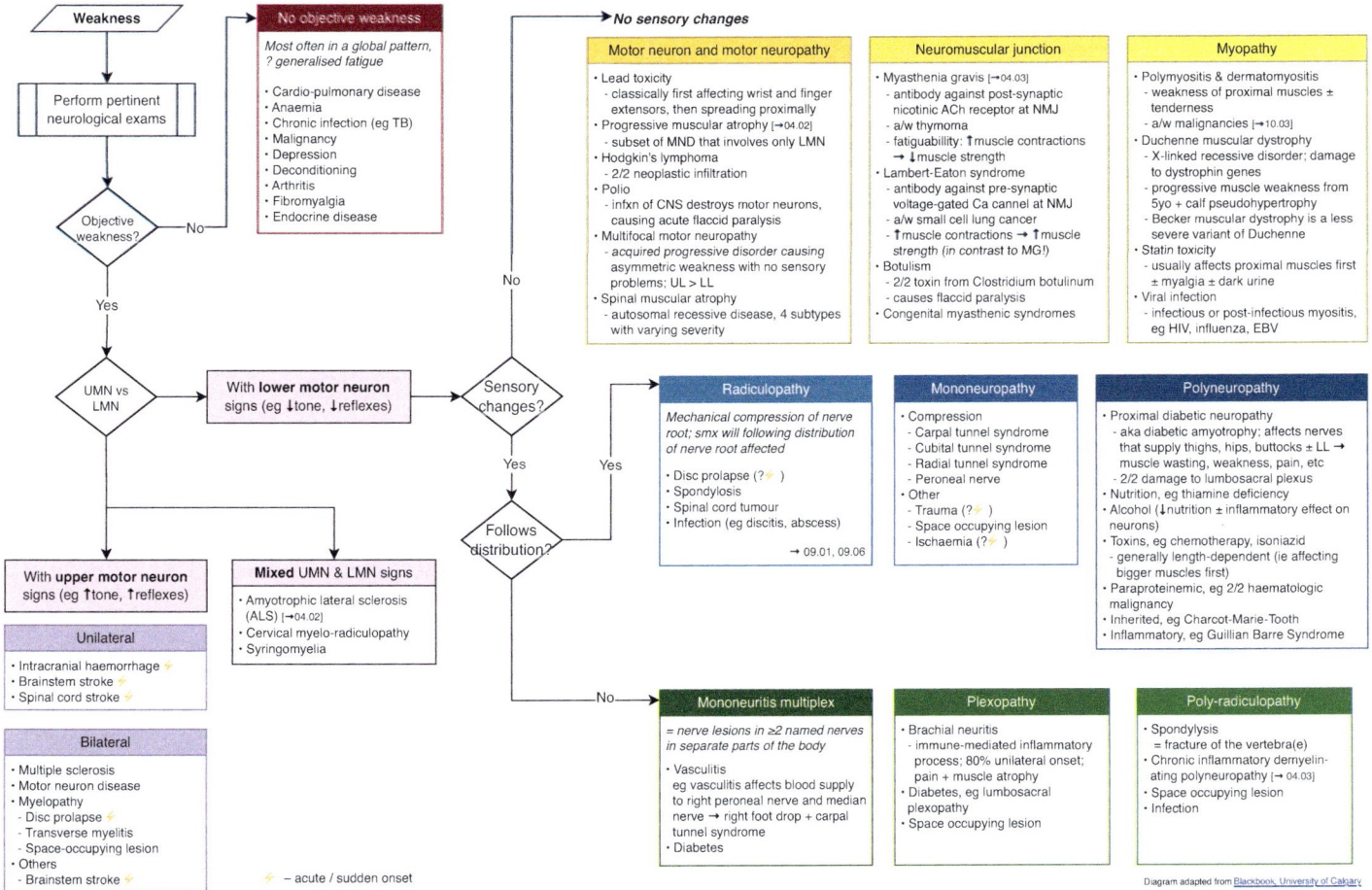

Weakness

↓

Perform pertinent neurological exams

↓

Objective weakness? —No→

No objective weakness

Most often in a global pattern, ? generalised fatigue

- Cardio-pulmonary disease
- Anaemia
- Chronic infection (eg TB)
- Malignancy
- Depression
- Deconditioning
- Arthritis
- Fibromyalgia
- Endocrine disease

Yes ↓

UMN vs LMN →

With lower motor neuron signs (eg ↓tone, ↓reflexes)

→ **Sensory changes?**

No sensory changes

Motor neuron and motor neuropathy

- Lead toxicity
  - classically first affecting wrist and finger extensors, then spreading proximally
- Progressive muscular atrophy [→04.02]
  - subset of MND that involves only LMN
- Hodgkin's lymphoma
  - 2/2 neoplastic infiltration
- Polio
  - infxn of CNS destroys motor neurons, causing acute flaccid paralysis
- Multifocal motor neuropathy
  - acquired progressive disorder causing asymmetric weakness with no sensory problems; UL > LL
- Spinal muscular atrophy
  - autosomal recessive disease, 4 subtypes with varying severity

Neuromuscular junction

- Myasthenia gravis [→04.03]
  - antibody against post-synaptic nicotinic ACh receptor at NMJ
  - a/w thymoma
  - fatiguability: ↑muscle contractions → ↓muscle strength
- Lambert-Eaton syndrome
  - antibody against pre-synaptic voltage-gated Ca cannel in NMJ
  - a/w small cell lung cancer
  - ↑muscle contractions → ↑muscle strength (in contrast to MG!)
- Botulism
  - 2/2 toxin from Clostridium botulinum
  - causes flaccid paralysis
- Congenital myasthenic syndromes

Myopathy

- Polymyositis & dermatomyositis
  - weakness of proximal muscles ± tenderness
  - a/w malignancies [→10.03]
- Duchenne muscular dystrophy
  - X-linked recessive disorder; damage to dystrophin genes
  - progressive muscle weakness from 5yo + calf pseudohypertrophy
  - Becker muscular dystrophy is a less severe variant of Duchenne
- Statin toxicity
  - usually affects proximal muscles first ± myalgia ± dark urine
- Viral infection
  - infectious or post-infectious myositis, eg HIV, influenza, EBV

Sensory changes? —No→ (to Motor neuron box)

Yes ↓

Follows distribution?

Yes →

Radiculopathy

Mechanical compression of nerve root; smx will following distribution of nerve root affected

- Disc prolapse (?⚡)
- Spondylosis
- Spinal cord tumour
- Infection (eg discitis, abscess)

→ 09.01, 09.06

Mononeuropathy

- Compression
  - Carpal tunnel syndrome
  - Cubital tunnel syndrome
  - Radial tunnel syndrome
  - Peroneal nerve
- Other
  - Trauma (?⚡)
  - Space occupying lesion
  - Ischaemia (?⚡)

Polyneuropathy

- Proximal diabetic neuropathy
  - aka diabetic amyotrophy; affects nerves that supply thighs, hips, buttocks ± LL → muscle wasting, weakness, pain, etc
  - 2/2 damage to lumbosacral plexus
- Nutrition, eg thiamine deficiency
- Alcohol (↓nutrition ± inflammatory effect on neurons)
- Toxins, eg chemotherapy, isoniazid
  - generally length-dependent (ie affecting bigger muscles first)
- Paraproteinemic, eg 2/2 haematologic malignancy
- Inherited, eg Charcot-Marie-Tooth
- Inflammatory, eg Guillian Barre Syndrome

No ↓

Mononeuritis multiplex

= nerve lesions in ≥2 named nerves in separate parts of the body

- Vasculitis
  eg vasculitis affects blood supply to right peroneal nerve and median nerve → right foot drop + carpal tunnel syndrome
- Diabetes

Plexopathy

- Brachial neuritis
  - immune-mediated inflammatory process; 80% unilateral onset; pain + muscle atrophy
- Diabetes, eg lumbosacral plexopathy
- Space occupying lesion

Poly-radiculopathy

- Spondylysis
  = fracture of the vertebra(e)
- Chronic inflammatory demyelinating polyneuropathy [→ 04.03]
- Space occupying lesion
- Infection

With upper motor neuron signs (eg ↑tone, ↑reflexes)

Mixed UMN & LMN signs

- Amyotrophic lateral sclerosis (ALS) [→04.02]
- Cervical myelo-radiculopathy
- Syringomyelia

Unilateral

- Intracranial haemorrhage ⚡
- Brainstem stroke ⚡
- Spinal cord stroke ⚡

Bilateral

- Multiple sclerosis
- Motor neuron disease
- Myelopathy
  - Disc prolapse ⚡
  - Transverse myelitis
  - Space-occupying lesion
- Others
  - Brainstem stroke ⚡

⚡ – acute / sudden onset

Diagram adapted from Blackbook, University of Calgary

Multiple sclerosis

D: demyelinating CNS condition clinically defined by ≥2 episodes of neurological dysf (brain, spinal cord, or optic nerves) separated in space and time.

R: F>M 3:1, FHx, northern latitude, autoimmune disorders
↳ "typical pt" - 20-40yo white female

A: genetics + environment
P: activated T cells against an unknown antigen → cascade of inflammation, demyelination and axonal loss.
! multifocal areas of demyelination, ↓oligodendrocytes, loss of axons in the white matter of the CNS
· if episode/s not disseminated in time and space, considered clinically isolated syndrome (CIS)
· relapsing remitting MS (RRMS) 85%
  - acute attacks (1-2mo) followed by periods of remission
· secondary progressive
  - 65% of RRMS go on to this, generally within 15y of diagnosis
· primary progressive - no period of RRMS, just deterioration

S/Smx: · Significant lethargy
· Visual: ! optic neuritis, optic atrophy, Uhtoff's phenomenon (worsening of vision with rise in body temp), internuclear ophthalmoplegia
· Sensory: pins & needles, numbness, trigeminal neuralgia, Lhermitte's syndrome (paresthesiae in limbs on neck flexion)
· Motor: spastic weakness, esp in legs
· Cerebellar: ataxia, tremor
· Others: urinary incontinence, sexual dysfunction, intellectual deterioration

Ix: MRI (brain and spinal cord), LP, visual evoked potentials

P: variable prognosis. -ve prognosis a/w frequent relapses, motor or cerebellar onset, ↑MRI lesion burden

---

Mx of relapses:
· High dose steroids (eg IV methylpred) for 5d – shortens duration of smx but does not influence degree of recovery
· DMARDs
  - ↘ natalizumab IV, ocrelizumab IV
    ↳ best evidence for this
  - others: finoglimod PO, β-interferon SC/IM, glatiramer acetate SC
· Fatigue: r/o other causes (eg anaemia), trial of amantadine, CBT
· Spasticity: ↘ baclofen & gabapentin
  - Others: diazepam, dantrolene
· Urinary incontinence
  - Bladder US to Ax bladder emptying
  - If significant residual volume, intermittent self-catheterisation
  - If not, anticholinergics may help

Neuromyelitis optica
aka Devic disease
· D: chronic disorder of the brain and spinal cord dominated by optic neuritis and myelitis
· R: autoimmune disorders (PMH or FHx), non-white predominance relative to MS
· A/P: similar to MS; antibody-mediated disease
· S/smx: - may be preceded by viral infxn
  - optic neuritis
  - transverse myelitis: motor, sensory and autonomic dysfunction below a certain spinal level, may be unilateral
· Ix: as per MS + labs
  - ! test for anti-aquaporin 4 and anti-myelin oligodendrocyte glycoprotein abs → AQP4-IgG is highly specific, moderately sensitive for NSOMD
· Mx: - high dose IV methylprednisolone
  - plasmapheresis
  - long-term immunosuppression
· P: in most cases, there is a partial recovery. Permanent loss of function can occur in recurring episodes

---

Guillain Barre syndrome

D: acute inflammatory polyneuro-pathy ÷ into axonal and demyelinating forms

R: preceding infxn (viral, bacterial, mosquito-borne, hep E) ~6w before, esp a/w Campylobacter jejuni and CMV

A/P: immune-mediated attack on the myelin sheath or Schwann cells of sensory and motor nerves; ∴ cellular and humoral immune mechanisms
· Cross-reaction of abs to gangliosides

S/Smx:
· Progressive symmetrical muscle weakness of all limbs
  - Legs first then arms (ascending)
  - Flaccid paralysis - Areflexia
  - Paraesthesia in feet and hands
· Acute development over 2-4w, then plateau of smx
· Mild dysautonomia (2/3 pts): urinary retention, ileus, respiratory failure (20-30% require mechanical ventilation)
· Cranial nerve involvement: diplopia, bilateral facial nerve palsy, oropharyngeal weakness
· Rarely, papilloedema

Ix: LP (↑protein with normal WBC), nerve conduction studies (↓motor conduction)

Mx: · ↘ IVIG or plasma exchange
· Supportive Mx, including VTE prophylaxis, mechanical ventilation prn, rehab

P: 85% good functional recovery. -ve prognosis a/w severe weakness, rapid onset, ↑age, muscle wasting, electrical inexcitable nerves, preceding diarrheal illness

---

Miller-Fisher syndrome

· Subset of GBS
· S/smx: ophthalmoplegia, ataxia, and areflexia
  - Usually descending paralysis

Chronic inflammatory demyelinating (poly)neuropathy

D: acquired demyelinating peripheral neuropathy of presumed autoimmune aetiology

R: M>F, autoimmune, DM, infxn, monoclonal gammopathy of undetermined significance (MGUS)

A: unclear. 20-30% preceded by infxn, immunisation or surgical procedure.
P: autoimmune disease against myelin – cell-mediated

S/Smx of typical CIDP:
· Condition is chronically progressive, step-wise, or recurrent
· Symmetrical proximal and distal weakness and sensory dysfunction of all extremities
· Develops over ≥2mo
· ↓ or absent tendon reflexes in all extremities
There are many variants of CIDP

Ix: nerve conduction studies (slow conduction, ↑latency, block), LP (WCC <10, protein >45 mg/dL)

Mx: · IVIG, corticosteroids, or plasma exchange
· Analgesia for neuropathic pain
· Rehabilitation

P: 80% respond to tx w/in first few months. 50% go into remission, 10% poor outcomes (severe disability or death)
-ve prognosis a/w age, progressive, CNS involvementt, axonal loss on biopsy

No cross over between the demyelinating syndromes due to differing underlying pathology
· MS affects the oligodendrocytes in CNS
· GBS and CIDP affect the Schwann cells in the PNS

Drugs that worsen MG: β-blockers, lithium, abx (gentamicin, macrolides, quinolones, tetracyclines), phenytoin, quinidine, procainamide, penicillamine

---

Myasthenia gravis

D: chronic autoimmune disorder of the post-synaptic membrane at the NMJ in skeletal muscle

Epidimiology: in females, <40yo; in males, >60yo. Link with thymoma (20-40% pts with thymoma develop MG). A/w autoimmune disorders

A/P: abs against nicotinic AChR on post-synaptic membrane at the NMJ (90%) → complement-mediated destruction of the post-synaptic membrane → ↓action potential in skeletal muscle → weakness
Also, anti-muscle-specific tyrosine kinase abs (10-40%)

S/Smx: · Muscle fatiguability
  - pts usually complain that they get weaker at the end of day
· Ptosis, diplopia   · Dysphagia
· Dysarthria   · Facial paresis
· Proximal limb weakness
Classification
Class I: any eye weakness ± ptosis
II: mild weakness of other muscles
III: moderate weakness
IV: severe weakness
V: intubation to maintain airway
* classes II to IV split into a and b
  ↳ a – predominantly limb/axial/both
  ↳ b – oropharyngeal/respi/both

Myasthenic crisis: acute worsening of smx, often triggered by stressors – can lead to respiratory failure

Ix: single fibre electromyography (high sensitivity; >92%), CT thorax to r/o thymoma, CK (normal), autoantibodies to AChR. In crises, use forced vital capactiv to monitor lung function

Mx of class I to III
    pyridostigmine
    corticosteroids, immunosupp (eg azathioprine, rituzimab), thymectomy
Mx of class IV to V ↘ + ↘
Mx of myasthenic crisis
(1) serial FVC ± mechanical ventilation
(2) plasmapheresis or IVIG
(3) supportive care, remove trigger
Mx of MG in pregnancy
PO pyridostigmine (not IV),
prednisolone, azathioprine, tacrolimus, ciclosporin, IVIG, plasmapheresis

---

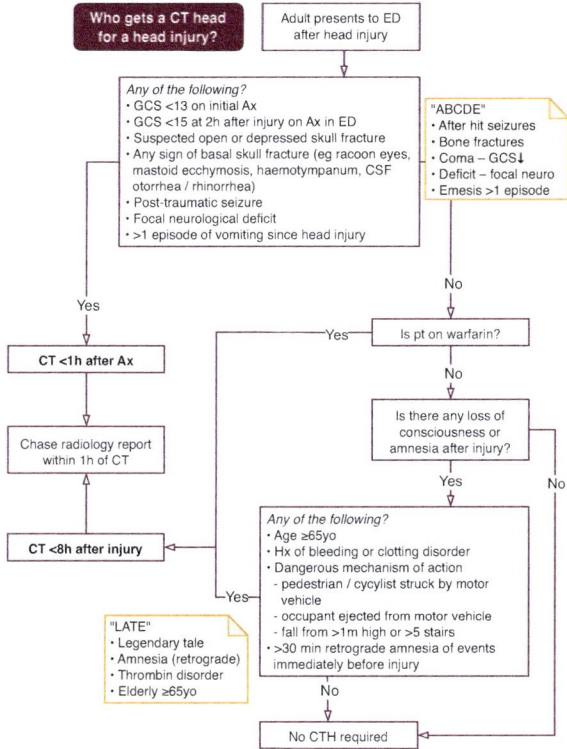

Who gets a CT head for a head injury?

Adult presents to ED after head injury

Any of the following?
- GCS <13 on initial Ax
- GCS <15 at 2h after injury on Ax in ED
- Suspected open or depressed skull fracture
- Any sign of basal skull fracture (eg racoon eyes, mastoid ecchymosis, haemotympanum, CSF otorrhea / rhinorrhea)
- Post-traumatic seizure
- Focal neurological deficit
- >1 episode of vomiting since head injury

"ABCDE"
- After hit seizures
- Bone fractures
- Coma – GCS↓
- Deficit – focal neuro
- Emesis >1 episode

Yes → **CT <1h after Ax**

No → Is pt on warfarin?

Yes → **Chase radiology report within 1h of CT**

No → Is there any loss of consciousness or amnesia after injury?

Yes →

Any of the following?
- Age ≥65yo
- Hx of bleeding or clotting disorder
- Dangerous mechanism of action
  - pedestrian / cyclist struck by motor vehicle
  - occupant ejected from motor vehicle
  - fall from >1m high or >5 stairs
- >30 min retrograde amnesia of events immediately before injury

"LATE"
- Legendary tale
- Amnesia (retrograde)
- Thrombin disorder
- Elderly ≥65yo

Yes → **CT <8h after injury**

No → **No CTH required**

Head injury

TBI = traumatic brain injury

- Primary injuries ÷ focal or diffuse
- Focal
  - Contusion (bruising)
  - Haematoma – collection of blood
    ↳ see also 04.09 for haematomas
- Diffuse axonal injury
  - Occurs as a result of mechanical shearing after deceleration, causing disruption and tearing of axons
  - 90% end up in coma, very very poor prognosis

- Secondary brain injuries occur due to
  (1) the body's response to the primary injury, and
  (2) loss of autoregulatory mechanisms due to the primary injury
- Eg cerebral oedema, ischaemia, infection, tonsillar or tentorial herniation
- Cushing's reflex (see raised ICP) occurs as a preterminal event

Ix: • CTH (see algorithm)
- Full body survey
- ICP monitoring
  - mandatory if GCS 3-8 + abn CTH
  - consider if GCS 3-8 + normal CTH
- U&Es - may pick up hypoNa if SIADH develops due to brain injury

Mx:
- ABCDE + resuscitate
  - C-spine collar may be needed
  - Intubate & ventilate if GCS <8
- ICP monitoring as above
- If ↑↑ICP, decompressive craniotomy may need to be done
- Depressed skull fractures: surgical reduction and debridement
- Maintain cerebral perfusion pressure ≥70 mmHg in adults, 40-70 mmHg in children

Intracranial pressure

Normal: 7-15 mmHg; higher in adults than children
- Cerebral perfusion pressure = mean arterial pressure - intracranial pressure

Raised ICP — LP opening pressure >20 is suggestive

Causes
- traumatic head injuries (2/2 bleeding, haematomas)
- infections, eg meningitis, TB
- tumours
- hydrocephalus
- idiopathic intracranial HTN (a Dx of exclusion)

S/smx:
- HA: typically worse in morning or on lying down (due to ↑ICP)
- vomiting • ↓consciousness
- papilloedema
- Cushing's triad (late stage)
  - widening pulse pressure
  - bradycardia
  - irregular breathing

Ix: • CT/MRI
- If suspecting ↑ICP due to mass effect (eg in haematoma, tumours), **DO NOT** perform LP due to risk of herniation
  ↳ the mass has to be dealt with first to relieve pressure
- Invasive ICP monitoring
  - catheter is placed into the lateral ventricles of the brain to monitor ICP ± collect samples / drain small amounts

Mx
- Treat underlying cause if possible
  - Dexamethasone can help ↓swelling in brain tumours → ↓ICP
- Head elevation to 30°
- IV mannitol (osmotic diuretic)
- Controlled hyperventilation
  - ↓pCO2 = vasoconstriction of cerebral arteries → ↓ICP
  - temporary solution
- Removal of CSF
  - ventricular drain
  - repeated LPs (eg in IIH)
  - ventriculoperitoneal shunt (for hydrocephalus)

Idiopathic intracranial hypertension aka pseudotumour cerebri
- unknown cause
- R: F>M (~6:1), obesity & wt gain, some drugs (including COCP, steroids, lithium, tetracyclines, isotretinoin)
- S/smx: HA (typically worse on waking up or when lying down)
  - Papilloedema
  - Blurred vision, enlarged blind spot
  - ± CN VI palsy (pt cannot look laterally)
- Ix: as per ↑ICP; ! IIH is a Dx of exclusion
- Mx
  - repeated LP to ↓ICP temporarily
  - carbonic anhydrase inhibitors, eg acetazolamide, topiramate (not in pregnancy; teratogenic)
    ↳ MOA: ↓CSF production
  - long term: wt loss
  - surgery

Low ICP — LP opening pressure <4-5 mmHg

Causes
- Iatrogenic, eg lumbar punctuyre headache, post-epidural
- Spontaneous

Ix: MRI may show thickened meninges

Mx
- Bed rest, fluids, caffeine
  - after LP, pts should be advised to lie flat for ≥1h
  - In consenting for spinal epidural, pts should be warned about risk of low pressure HA
- Epidural blood patching:
  - pt's own blood is injected into the epidural space
  - blood acts as a tamponade and clots over the epidural leak
  - usually works very well

Brown-Sequard syndrome

D: hemisection of the spinal cord (incomplete transverse injury)

Tracts affected
- Lateral corticospinal tract
  - Ipsilateral weakness below lesion
- Dorsal columns
  - Ipsilateral loss of proprioception and vibration sensation
- Lateral spinothalamic tract
  - Contralateral loss of pain and temperature sensation

Subacute combined degeneration of the spinal cord

D: demyelination of the lateral and posterior columns of the spinal cord

A: vitamin B12 deficiency, recreational nitrous oxide inhalation (deactivates B12 from its active form)

Tracts affected + S/smx
- Dorsal columns
  - Tingling, burning or sensory loss
    ↳ symmetrical, LL>UL
  - Impaired proprioception and vibration sense
- Lateral corticospinal tracts
  - Muscle weakness, hyperreflexia and spasticity
  - UMN signs LL first then UL
    ↳ Brisk knee reflexes
    ↳ Absence ankle jerks
    ↳ Extensor plantars
- Spinocerebellar tracts
  - sensory ataxia & gait changes
  - +ve Romberg's sign

Mx: stop trigger, B12 replacement

Friedrich's ataxia

D: autosomal recessive trinucleotide repeat disorder

S/smx
- Onset 10-15yo
- Cerebellar ataxia & spinocerebellar tract degeneration
  - sensory ataxia & gait changes
  - +ve Romberg's sign
- Optic atrophy
- Hyporeflexia – absent ankle jerks and extensor plantar reflexes
- Other s/smx: cardiomyopathy (90% pts, most common cause of death), DM, kyphoscoliosis, foot deformities, high-arched palate

Anterior spinal artery occlusion

D: ischemic infarction of the anterior spinal artery (artery of Adamkiewicz) or generalised hypoperfusion
- The artery of Adamkiewicz is the only major arterial supply to the anterior spinal artery along the lower 2/3 of the spine

A: (many causes) aortic surgery, atherosclerotic disease, emboli, vasculitis, etc

Tracts affected + S/smx
- Lateral corticospinal tracts
  - Bilateral spastic paresis
- Lateral spinothalamic tracts
  - Bilateral loss of pain and temperature sensation
- Other s/smx: acutely can cause spinal shock; later findings include neurogenic bladder/bowel, sexual dysfunction

Syringomyelia

D: collection of CSF within the spinal cord (= syrinx)
- Syringobulbia = fluid-filled cavity within the medulla of the brainstem

A: Chiari malformation (type 1), trauma, tumours, idiopathic

Tracts affected + s/smx
- Ventral horns
  - flaccid paresis (usually starting with intrinsic hand muscles)
- Lateral spinothalamic tract
  - Loss of pain and temperature sensation, classically in a 'cape-like' pattern – neck, shoulders and arms
- Other s/smx: spastic weakness of the lower limbs, neuropathic pain, upgoing plantars, autonomic features (eg neurogenic bowel/bladder), scoliosis in the long term

Ix: full spine MRI + brain MRI (to look for Chiari malformation)

Mx: treat underlying cause
- If persistent or symptomatic, shunt into syrinx to drain

Tabes dorsalis

aka tabes dorsalis
D: syndrome 2/2 CNS infection by *Treponema pallidum*

Tracts affected + s/smx
- Dorsal columns and roots
  - Loss of propioception and vibratory sense
  - ataxia, lancinating pains, bladder dysfunction, paraesthesias
- Other neuro s/smx: pupillary abnormalities (Argyll Robertson pupils), ocular palsies, ↓reflexes, Charcot joints
- ! classically known as "the great imitator" – requires a degree of suspicion

Neurofibromatosis

D: Neurocutaneous genetic disorder autosomal dominantly inherited disorders - NF1 (more common), and NF2

R: FHx

A: genetic mutation
- NF1: mutation on gene encoding neurofibromin located on chr 17
- NF2: mutation on chr 22

P: ↓neurofibromin in Schwann cells, glia, melanocytes, mast cells, vascular endothelial and smooth cells, etc → dysplasias and neoplasias

S/smx of NF1
- Cafe au lait spots (≥6 spots) - flat light brown birthmarks
- Axilary/groin freckles
- Peripheral neurofibromas - tumours that hang off the skin
- Iris Lisch nodules (tiny tumours of the iris of the eye)
- Scoliosis
- Pheochromocytomas
S/smx of NF2
- Bilateral vestibular schwannomas
- Multiple intracranial schwannomas, meningiomas and ependymomas

Ix: MRI/CT scans, genetic testing to confirm NF1

Mx: symptomatic (as and when features of NF give problems)
- Neurofibromas need to be under surveillance and removed if assessed to be malignant

Tuberous sclerosis

D: Neurocutaneous and multi-systemic genetic disorder autosomal dominantly inherited disorders

R: FHx

A/P: mutations of TSC1 and TSC2 genes → cellular hyperplasia, tissue dysplasia and multi-organ hamartomas

S/smx:
- Hypopigmened "ash-leaf" spots which fluoresce under UV light
- Roughened patches of skin over lumbar spine (Shagreen patches)
- Adenoma sebaceum (angiofibromas) distributed over nose
- Fibromata beneath nails
- Cafe au lait spots
- Neuro problems
  - Developmental delay
  - Epilepsy (infantile spasms)
  - Intellectual impairment
- Retinal hamartomas
- Rhabdomyomas of the heart
- Gliomatous changes of the brain
- Polycystic kidneys, renal angiomyo-lipomata
- Lymphangio-leiomyomatosis (multiple lung cysts)

Ix: as per NF

Mx: As per NF
- mTOR inhibitors everolimus and sirolimus are approved for some indications under tuberous sclerosis

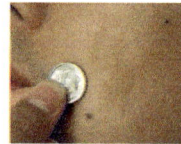

Cafe au lait spot

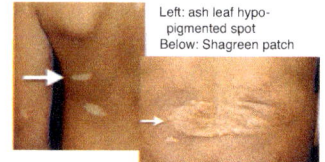

Left: ash leaf hypo-pigmented spot
Below: Shagreen patch

Restless legs syndrome

D: compulsive urge to move the legs

R: conditions a/w iron deficiency (eg ESRD); pregnancy; FHx (50%); use of antidepressants, antihistamines, metoclopramide; uraemia; DM

A/P: not fully understood; a/w iron and dopamine dysfunction?

S/smx:
· Akathisia: uncontrollable urge to move legs
· Usually occurs at night, but as condition progresses, some comes during the day
· May be a/w paraesthesias – crawling or throbbing sensations
· Movement during sleep may be noted by partner (period limb movements of sleep)

Ix: FBC & iron studies (esp ferritin) to r/o iron deficiency

Mx · Treat any iron deficiency
· Remove any potentially offending drugs
· Lifestyle modifications
  - Walking, stretching, massaging may help affected limbs
  - Stop smoking if relevant
  - Trial of cutting out caffeine and alcohol to see if smx improve
· 🔹 Dopamine agonist such as ropinirole or pramipexole
· Others: benzodiazepines, gabapentin may help

Essential tremor

Aka benign essential tremor
· D: progressive, mainly symmetrical, rhythmic, involuntary oscillatory movement disorder of the hands and forearms
  - Autosomal dominant
  - Usually absent at rest, present during intentional movements (eg asking pts to do finger-to-nose test)
  - Improves with alcohol & rest
    ↳ as opposed to Parkinson's
· A/w titbuation (head tremor)
· Mx: 🔹 propranolol   - ?? primidone

Abnormal involuntary movements

Chorea
· D: sudden, rapid, involuntary, rapid, and purposeless movements
  - Greek for dance / choreography
· Results from damage to basal ganglia
· Important causes
  - Neuro: Huntington's disease, Wilson's disease, ataxic telangiectasia, stroke/ TIA (affecting basal ganglia)
  - Rheumatic / autoimmune: SLE, anti-phospholipid syndrome, rheumatic fever (Sydenham's chorea)
  - Drugs: COCP, L-dopa, antipsychotics
  - Haem: polycythaemia rubra vera, neuroacanthocytosis
  - Pregnancy (chorea gravidarum)
  - Thyrotoxicosis
  - Carbon monoxide poisoning

Athetosis
· D: slower form of chorea that has a writhing snake-like quality
· Often accompanies chorea

Dystonia
· D: slow, prolonged contraction of trunk and limb muscles

Oculogyric crisis
· D: subtype of dystonia characterised by restlessness, agitation, and involuntary upward deviation of eyes
· Causes: antipsychotics (esp 1st gen), metoclopramide, postencephalitic PD
· Mx: stop offending drugs, IV antimuscarinics (eg benztropine, procyclidine)

Ballism & hemiballism
· D: severe form of chorea involving proximal muscles, characterised by violent flinging movements
· Hemiballism: only affects one side of the body
· Results from damage to subthalamic nucleus
· Mx: antidopaminergics (eg haloperidol)

Tics
· D: intermittent, stereotypical, repetitive, involuntary movements
· Tourette syndrome: multiple motor and vocal tics beginning in childhood ± comorbid neuropsychiatric disorders
· Eg blinking, shrugging
· Mx: clonidine, atypical antipsychotics

DVLA rules

Epilepsy / seizures
· First unprovoked & isolated seizure
  - If no structural abn on brain imaging + no definite epileptiform activity on EEG: no driving for 6mo
  - If structural abn or epileptiform activity on EEG: no driving for 12mo
· Established epilepsy or multiple unprovoked seizures
  - If seizure free for ≥12mo: ok
  - If no seizures ≥5y (± medication): ok
· If stopping antiepileptics: no driving while tapering down, and for 6mo after last dose

Syncope
· Simple fainting: no restrictions
· Single episode, explained & treated: no driving for 4w
· Single episode, unexplained: no driving for 6mo
· ≥2 episodes: no driving for 12mo

Stroke / TIA
· Single stroke / TIA: no driving for 1mo
  - If residual neuro deficit, inform DLVA
· Multiple TIAs over short period of time: no driving for 3mo + inform DLVA

Neurosurgery
· Craniotomy: no driving for 12mo
· Benign meningioma + no seizure Hx: license can be reconsidered for 6mo after surgery if no seizures
· Pituitary tumour
  - Craniotomy: no driving for 6mo
  - Transphenoidal surgery: if safe to drive, ok

Narcolepsy / Cataplexy
· On case by case basis, depending on control of smx

Chronic neurological disorders
(eg MS, MND)
· Inform DLVA + complete PK1 form
· On case by case basis

Aphasia

Wernicke's (receptive) aphasia
· 🔹 Superior temporal gyrus
· 🔹 inferior division of left MCA
· Comprehension impaired
· Speech fluent, but make no sense; word substitutions & neologisms. Repetition impaired.

Broca's (expressive) aphasia
· 🔹 Inferior frontal gyrus
· 🔹 superior division of left MCA
· Comprehension normal
· Speech non-fluent, laboured, halting. Repetition impaired.

Conduction aphasia
· 🔹 Arcuate fasciculus (connection between Wernicke's & Broca's areas)
· Comprehension normal
· Speech fluent.
  Repetition impaired.
  Pt is aware of errors they're making.

Global aphasia
· 🔹 Wernicke's area, Broca's area, and arcuate fasciculus
· Comprehension impaired
· Speech non-fluent.
  Repetition impaired.
· May still be able to communicate with gestures

Wernicke's encephalopathy
· D: Neuropsychiatric disorder caused by thiamine (B1) deficiency
· R: alcoholism, AIDS, tx with chemo-therapy (due to ↑vomiting), GI surgery, malnutrition
· P: ↓activity of thiamine dependent enzymes → neuronal death
· S/smx:
  - Oculomotor dysfunction: nystagmus, ophthalmoplegia (lateral rectus palsy)
  - Gait ataxia
  - Encephalopathy: confusion, disorienta-tion, indifference, inattentiveness
  - Peripheral sensory neuropathy
· Ix: MRI
· Mx: urgent replacement of thiamine
· P: if untx, Korsakoff's syndrome can develop (→ antero/retrograde amnesia and confabulation)
  - Confabulation = making up memories

Charcot-Marie-Tooth disease
· D: a hereditary motor and sensory neuropathy
· Different inheritance patterns. Can affect Schwann cells and myelin (CMT1), axons (CMT2). Look for FHx.
· S/smx:
  - Distal muscle weakness & atrophy
  - Hyporeflexia
  - High stepping gait / foot drop
    ↳ Hx of frequently sprained ankles
  - High-arched feet (pes cavus)
  - Hammer toes
  - Stork leg deformity
· Ix: nerve conduction studies, genetic testing
· Mx: supportive – physical and occupational therapy

Other random notes
· Local anaesthetic toxicity: Mx with 20% lipid emulsion IV
· Brain pathology causing NV: Mx with cyclizine

Retinal detachment

D: detachment of the neuroretina from the underlying epithelial pigment layer

R: DM (2/2 traction by the vitreous humour causing breaks in retina), myopia (> -8), ↑age, previous surgery for cataracts (accelerates posterior vitreous detachment), eye trauma

S/smx
- new onset **floaters or flashes**
  - pigment cells enter the vitreous space (floaters) or traction on the retina (flashes)
  - sudden onset, painless and progressive **visual field loss**
  - "curtain falling"; also, shadow progressing to the centre of the visual field from the periphery
- if the *macula* is involved, central visual acuity and visual outcomes become much worse
- peripheral visual fields ↓
- central acuity ↓ to hand movements if the macula is detached
- RAPD if the optic nerve is involved
- On fundoscopy
  - **red reflex lost**
  - retinal folds - pale, opaque or wrinkled
  - if break is small, may appear normal

Ix: visual acuity, slit-lamp exam
+ US of the eye if media opacity prevents visualisation of fundus
+ CT/MRI if injury suspected

Mx: same-day ref to eye A&E
- posterior vitreous detachment without break/tear: laser tx to ↓risk of retinal detachment
  - PVD = vitreous detaches from retina
  - if separates incompletely, can cause traction and pull on retina → ↑risk of retina detachment
- pneumatic retinopexy (surgeon positions an air bubble to push the retina back into place, then freezes it there)
- vitrectomy — for significant vitreous traction

Causes of sudden, sustained vision loss

Painless	Painful
- Anterior ischaemic optic neuropathy	- Acute glaucoma
- Retinal artery occlusion	- Severe corneal pathology
- Retinal vein occlusion	- Severe uveitis (anterior, panuveitis)
- Macular degeneration (wet)	- Endophthalmitis
- Retinal detachment	- Optic neuritis
- Vitreous detachment	
- Severe uveitis	

Anterior ischaemic optic neuropathy (AION)

90-95% non-arteritic

Retinal artery occlusion

- D: an interruption of the normal arterial supply to the retinal tissue = stroke 2/2 **thromboembolism** from atherosclerosis or **arteritis** (eg GCA)
- S/smx
  - sudden, painless unilateral visual loss
  - relative afferent pupillary defect
  - 'cherry red' spot on a pale retina
- Mx: tx underlying conditions
  - possible to attempt intra-arterial thrombolysis but mixed results
- Poor prognosis :(

5% arteritic

Giant cell arteritis

- AION from GCA is primarily due to occlusion of the **posterior ciliary artery** (branch of ophth artery)
- temp visual loss = **amaurosis fugax**
- permanent visual loss is the most feared complication of temporal arteritis and may develop suddenly
- diplopia may also result from the involvement of any part of the oculomotor system (e.g. CN)

- + HA (85%), jaw claudication (65%), temporal artery tenderness, PMR features (50%), systemic smx

See also 11.09 for Ocular trauma

Transient vision loss

- Amaurosis fugax / TIA
- Migraine
- Papilloedema causing transient visual obscuration
  ↳ 2/2 ↑ICP

Retinal vein occlusion

D: an interruption of the normal venous drainage from the retinal tissue
- central vein (= CRVO)
- one of the vein branches (= BRVO)

R: ↑age (>65), HTN, cardiovascular disease, glaucoma, polycythemia, DM, hyperlipidaemia, smoking, ↑BMI

S/smx:
- sudden, painless, ↓visual acuity, usually unilaterally
- On fundoscopy
  - widespread **hyperaemia**
  ↳ in the retina proximal to the occlusion, the affected venous system is tortuous and dilated
  - severe retinal haemorrhages – '**stormy sunset**'
  - retinal oedema

Mx:
- conservative tx (watch and wait)
  - manage co-morbidities, ↓risk
  - monitor for complications
- macular oedema: anti-VEGF injections
- retinal neovascularisation: laser photocoagulation

Retinal migraine

D: transient monocular scotoma or loss of vision that is accompanied or followed by a headache within 60 minutes of visual symptoms onset

S/smx:
- flashing lights
- scintillating scotoma with fortification spectrum (expanding zigzag lines)

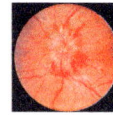

Papilloedema

D: optic disc swelling that is caused by increased intracranial pressure

A:
- space-occupying lesions: neoplastic, vascular
- malignant hypertension
- idiopathic intracranial hypertension
- hydrocephalus   · hypercapnia
- hypoparathyroidism, hypocalcaemia
- vitamin A toxicity

S/smx
- almost always bilateral
- venous engorgement (usually 1st sign)
- loss of venous pulsation (although many normal patients do not have normal pulsation)
- blurring of the optic disc margin
- elevation of optic disc
- loss of the optic cup
- Paton's lines: concentric/radial retinal lines cascading from the optic disc

---

Optic neuritis

D: inflammation of the optic nerve → most commonly idiopathic, a primary demyelinating disease in isolation or 2/2 multiple sclerosis

S/smx
- unilat ↓ in visual acuity over h-d
- poor discrimination of colours, 'red desaturation'
- pain worse on eye movement
- RAPD   · central scotoma

Ix: MRI brain, orbits with contrast

Mx: high dose steroids, taper in 4-6w

P: if > 3 white-matter lesions, 5-year risk of developing multiple sclerosis is ~50%

Vitreous haemorrhage

- 2/2 proliferative **diabetic retinopathy** >50% (→ 04.03), posterior vitreous detachment or ocular trauma
- S/smx: acute/subacute course
  - painless vision loss / haze
  - ± visual field defects if severe haemorrhage
  - red hue in vision
  - floaters, dark spots
- Ix: fundoscopy (haemorrhage), slit-lamp exam (RBC in anterior vitreous), US (to r/o retinal tear or detachment), fluorescein angiography (to look for neovascularisation), orbital CT (if open globe injury)

DDx of loss of colour vision (non-congenital)
- Optic neuritis / MS
- Optic nerve ischaemia
- Glaucoma
- ARMD
- Retina pigmentosa
- Thyroid eye disease
- DM (diabetic retinopathy)
- Drugs (chloroquine, hydroxychloro-quine, phenytoin, sildenafil, digoxin)

DDx of blurred vision
- Refractive error (eg myopia)
- Cataracts
- Retinal detachment
- ARMD
- Acute angle closure glaucoma
- Optic neuritis
- Amaurosis fugax

Ax:
- Snellen chart
  - Use pinhole occluders (if blurring improves, then likely cause is refractive error)
- Visual fields   · Fundoscopy

photo from Wikipedia

Red eye

Glaucoma = group of conditions causing optic nerve damage and vision loss

Angle-closure glaucoma

D: condition resulting from closure of the anterior-chamber angle resulting in elevation of the intra-ocular pressure
Acute ACG – relatively sudden blockage of the trabecular meshwork by the iris, via the pupillary block mechanism (iris is pushed upward, blocking outflow)
Chronic ACG – adhesional blockage
For open-angle glaucoma, see 05.04

R: hypermetropia (far-sighted), pupillary dilatation, lens growth a/w age, F>M, previous ACG

S/smx
· **severe** pain: may be ocular or HA
· ↓**visual acuity**
· Smx worse with mydriasis (e.g. watching TV in a dark room)
· **hard, red-eye**
· haloes around lights
· semi-dilated **non-reacting pupil**
· corneal oedema → dull/hazy cornea
· ± systemic upset, eg NV, abdo pain

Dx is clinical, immediate referral for same-day appt with ophthalmology
Ix: gonioscopy (examine the anterior chamber; unable to see trabecular meshwork), slit-lamp exam, automatic static perimetry

Mx – medical:
· Combination of eye drops
  - pilocarpine + timolol + apraclonidine
· IV acetazolamide 500 mg IV stat, then 250 mg/8h PO/IV
· ± topical steroids

Mx – surgical (definitive):
· laser peripheral iridotomy – tiny hole in iris to allow aq humour to flow out
· unaffected eye treated also

Anterior uveitis

D: irritation of the anterior uvea (**iris and ciliary body**)

R: other inflammatory diseases, HLA-B27 +ve, ocular trauma

A/w: · ankylosing spondylitis, reactive arthritis, IBD (UC, CD)
· Behcet's disease, sarcoidosis
· Juvenile idiopathic arthritis
· HSV, VZV, TB, syphilis, HIV
· Tarantular hairs (literally)

S/smx · **acute** onset (h-d) **red eye**
· ocular **discomfort & pain**
· pupil may be small ± oval/irregular (due to sphincter muscle contraction)
· **photophobia** (often intense)
· blurred vision · lacrimation
· **ciliary flush**: a ring of red spreading outwards
· **hypopyon** – pus and inflammatory cells in the anterior chamber → visible fluid level
· visual acuity initially normal, then **impaired**
Hx · ask about systemic disease

Dx is clinical
Ix: use slit lamp exam to monitor inflam-mation. Can recur, so f/u is critical.

Mx: · **urgent review** by ophth
· cycloplegics (dilates the pupil which helps to relieve pain and photophobia), eg atropine, cyclopentolate
· steroid eye drops

Other types of uveitis
· Intermediate: vitreous chamber
· Posterior: choroid ± retina
· Panuveitis – all
· S/smx: painless, blurry vision/floaters, eye *not red*
· Ix: fundus fluorescein, indocyanine green-angiography
· Mx: systemic or intraocular therapies, eg adalimumab, steroid implants
· Complications: vision loss :(

Episcleritis + Scleritis

D: inflammation of the epi/sclera

A/w: IBD (UC, Crohns), RA. F>M

S/smx
· red eye ~30-50% bilateral
· Pain
  - Episcleritis – not as painful
  - Scleritis – constant, severe dull ache that 'bores' into their eye, can wake pt up at night. Eye movements are painful ± HA
· ± watering and photophobia
· Scleritis: gradual ↓vision
· On exam,
  - Episcleritis – the injected vessels are mobile when gentle pressure is applied on the sclera
· DDx between episcleritis and scleritis:
  - **phenylephrine** blanches the conjunctival and episcleral vessels but not the scleral vessels
  - if the eye redness *improves after phenylephrine* → episcleritis

Mx of scleritis
· Urgent referral to A&E eye unit
· Non-necrotising anterior scleritis: PO NSAIDs ± PO high-dose prednisolone
· Posterior / necrotising scleritis: systemic immunosuppression (cyclophosphamide or rituximab)
· Recalcitrant disease: infliximab
· Globe perforation: emergency surgery

Mx of episcleritis
· conservative ± artificial tears

P: vision loss highly likely in necrotising scleritis / perforation of globe

Contact lens care
· Don't reuse daily disposable CL
· Do not swim or shower wearing CL
· Follow manufacturer's instructions on how to clean lenses
  - avoid tap water → acanthamoeba
· Wash hands before handling CL
· Replace container every 3mo

Keratitis

D: inflammation of the cornea.
Infectious keratitis refers to microbial invasion of the cornea causing inflammation and damage to the corneal epithelium, stroma, or endothelium

R: contact lenses, corneal trauma, abrasion/erosion (+ recurrent), PMH of autoimmune disease, immunosupp

Aetiology – *infectious*
· bacterial – typically **S. aureus**
  - *P. aeruginosa* in contact lenses
· Fungal
· Amoebic (acanthamoebic keratitis) – 5% of cases, ↑risk if exposure to soil or contaminated water
  - pain out of proportion to findings
· Parasitic: onchocercal keratitis ('river blindness')
· Viral – herpes simplex keratitis (HSV1)

Aetiology – *others* (rare)
· Environmental: photokeratitis (welder's arc eye), exposure keratitis, contact lens acute red eye (CLARE)

hypopyon: white area on the cornea indicating a collection of white cells in corneal tissue

S/smx:
· red eye: pain and erythema
· photophobia · ± hypopyon
· foreign body, gritty sensation

Ix: corneal scraping – microscope slide, MC&S. For contact lens wearers, slit lamp may be required

Mx: · same-day ref to eye specialist
· stop wearing contact lenses
· Topical abx (typically quinolones)
· Cycloplegic for pain relief (e.g. cyclopentate)

P: corneal scarring, perforation, endophthalmitis, visual loss

Medication	MOA	Notes
Prostaglandin analogues (PGA) · Latanoprost	↑uveoscleral outflow	· OD administration · AE: brown pigmentation of iris, ↑eyelash length
ββ · Timolol · Betaxolol	↓aq humour production	· Avoid in asthma, heart block
Sympathomimetics · Brimonidine (α2 agonist)	↓aq humour production ↑outflow	· Avoid in MAOI, TCA · AE: hyperaemia
Carbonic anhydrase inhibitors · Acetazolamide	↓aq humour production	· Systemic absorption may cause sulphonamide-like reactions
Miotics · Pilocarpine (M3 receptor agonist)	↑uveoscleral outflow	· contraction of ciliary muscle · AE: myosis, HA, blurred vision

photo from Wikipedia

···· Red eye ····

Conjunctivitis

D: inflammation of the lining of the eyelids and eyeball

Aetiology · Allergic
· Infectious – bacterial or viral

R: exposure to infected person (or public areas with ↑risk), environmental irritants or allergen exposure, other infection (+ prior infxn with HSV1), atopy, contact lens use, trauma, oculogenital spread, vaginal delivery in neonates

S/smx of infectious conjunctivitis
· Bacterial – purulent discharge, eyes stuck together
· Viral – serous discharge, recent URTI, preauricular LN

S/smx of allergic conjunctivitis
· Bilateral symptoms conjunctival erythema, chemosis and itch!!
· ± swollen eyelids
· Generally in PMH of atopy, spring/ summer, or due to environmental exposure

Ix: cultures only needed if gonorrhoea or chlamydia suspected, neonatal, or recurrent / refractory

Mx of infectious conjunctivitis
· conservative – ww 1-2w
· offer topical abx (eg chloramphenicol eye drops q2-3h; ointment qds)
  - alt in pregnant women: fusidic acid
· for CL users: do not wear CL; topical fluoresceins to identify corneal staining
· advice all pts do not share towels, wash hands properly
· school exclusion not necessary

Mx of allergic conjunctivitis
· ▪ topical or PO antihistamines
· ▪ topical mast-cell stabilisers, e.g. sodium cromoglicate and nedocromil
· Advice to pts
  - remove allergens
  - cold compresses, artificial tears, PO antihistamines, nasal steroid sprays

···· External eye problems ····

Blepharitis

D: inflammation of the eyelid margin
· Posterior blepharitis: meibomian gland dysfunction (common)
· Anterior: seborrhoeic dermatitis or staphylococcal infection

S/smx · typically bilateral
· **grittiness and discomfort** esp around eyelid margins
· ± sticky in the morning
· ± red and swollen eyelid margins (esp in Staph infxn)
· styes and chalazions common
· secondary conjunctivitis may occur

Mx · hot compresses 10min bds
· lid hygiene – cotton wool buds dipped in boiled water + baby shampoo
  - or tsp of sodium bicarb in cup of cooled water
· ± artificial tears if dry eye or abn tear film

Blepharospasm

· D: dystonia of the upper eyelids; involuntary contraction of the orbicularis oculi, often in response to ocular pain
  - Focal dystonia = repetitive blepharospasm
· A: idiopathic, drugs (neuroleptics, PD, progressive supranuclear palsy, paraneoplastic)
· S/smx: - F>M (3:1)
  - Often preceded by exaggerated blinking ± other dystonias
  - Starts unilat → then bilateral
  - Pt may develop mechanisms to manage, eg pulling eyelids
· Mx: medical
· Botulinum neurotoxin inj q3mo.
  - MOA: flaccid paralysis by inhibiting release of ACh
· Anticholinergics, eg trihexyphenidyl
· Dopamine agonists, eg levodopa
· Supportive tx: wearing goggles

Entropion

= in-turning of (usually lower) eyelid → eyelashes irritate the cornea. >40yo
· Mx: taping eyelid, botulinum toxin injury, surgery

Ectropion

= out-turning of (lower) eyelid → watering ± exposure keratitis
· a/w old age, facial palsy
· Mx: plastic surgery, surgical correction with implant

Pinguecula

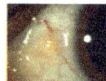

· D: degenerative vascular yellow-gray nodules on the conjunctiva on either side of the cornea (esp nasal side)
· A/w: M>F, ↑hair and skin pigment, sun-related skin damage
· Mx: - Pingueculitis: topical steroids
  - Corneal invasion ("pterygium"): surgery

Hordeolum (stye)

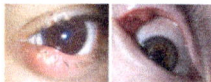

H externum   Chalazion
(points out)   (points inside)

Hordeolum **externum** – abscess or infxn in a lash follicle
  - glands of Moll (sweat gland)
  - glands of Zeis (sebum-producing; attached directly to follicles)
· They point outwards ("externum")
· Mx: warm compress 5-10 min a few times a day until it resolves

Hordeolum **internum** – abscess or infxn in a Meibomian gland
· Leaves a residual swelling called a **chalazion** (= Meibomian cyst)
· firm, painless lump in eyelid
· They point inward and open to the conjunctiva. Less local reaction.
· Mx: chalazion needs incision and curettage under local anaesthesia

Ophthalmic shingles

= Herpes zoster ophthalmicus (HZO)
· VZV usually affects children (chickenpox), then lays dormant. Usually reactivated >60yo
· Most common in thoracic nerves 50%, then CN V1 (20%)

S/smx: · pain and neuralgia in V1 distribution
· vesicular rash (blistering, inflamed) around eye ± involvement of eye
· Hutchinson's sign: rash on tip or side of nose
  - strong RF for ocular involvement
· Ocular involvement: corneal signs ± iritis

Ix / referral
· Normal visual acuity and corneal appearance is assuring
· Refer same-day if pain, redness, Δ vision or Hutchinson's sign

Mx
· antiviral **PO** for 7-10d
  - eg famciclovir, aciclovir
  - start w/in 72h
  - IV if severe infxn or immunosupp
  - ↓complications but will not prevent post-herpetic neuralgia
· steroid eye drops for secondary inflammation
· pregnant women with no immunity to VZV – isolate until vesicles dry up

Complications:
· conjunctivitis, keratitis, episcleritis, anterior uveitis, ptosis
· post-herpetic neuralgia – up to 45%, months to years; a/w ↑age, ocular involvement, severe rashes
  - Mx: TCAs, gabanergics
  - cited as commonest cause of suicide in pts with chronic pain >70yo :(
· Ramsay Hunt syndrome

See also Shingles 09.07

Other issues with external eye

Ptosis = abnormally low upper lid when pt looks forward
· A: congenital (absent nerve to levator muscle or poorly developed levator), myogenic, CNS
· Mx: surgical if (pupil) is covered in congenital ptosis
Pseudoptosis – due to abn position or size of globe

Dermatochalasis = excess eyelid skin hanging over eye; may obstruct sight

Lagophthalmos = inability to close eyelids
· A: exophthalmos (eg thyroid eye), mechanical impairment of lid movement (eg injury, leprosy, CN VII palsy)
→ Exposure keratopathy and corneal ulcers may follow
· Mx: lubricate eyes regular, tape eyes shut at night ± tarsorrhaphy (stitching eyelids together)

Xanthelasma = cholesterol deposit around the eye

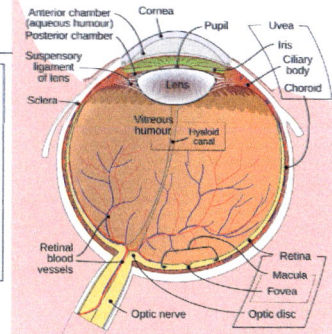

Anterior chamber (aqueous humour) · Cornea · Pupil · Uvea · Iris · Ciliary body · Choroid · Posterior chamber · Suspensory ligament of lens · Lens · Sclera · Vitreous humour · Hyaloid canal · Retinal blood vessels · Optic nerve · Retina · Macula · Fovea · Optic disc

Open-closure glaucoma

D: condition resulting from anatomically open angle but **obstructed and slowed drainage system outflow**. The trabecular network functionally causes ↑resistance to aqh outflow → ↑IOP

R: IOP >23, >50yo, FHx, Afro-Carribean, myopia, HTN, DM, steroid use

S/smx:
· *peripheral* visual field loss: nasal scotomas progressing to tunnel vision
· ↓visual acuity

Fundoscopy signs
· **Optic disc cupping** – cup-to-disc ratio >0.7; loss of disc substance makes optic cup widen and deepen
· **Optic disc pallor**; 2/2 retinal atrophy
· **Bayonetting** of vessels – vessels have breaks as they disappear into the deep cup and re-appear at the base
· Cup notching, usually inferior where vessels enter disc
· Disc haemorrhages

Dx: usually found via screening in pts with risk factors
Ix: · automated perimetry (Ax visual fields)
· slit lamp examination with pupil dilatation (Ax optic nerve and fundus as baseline)
· applanation tonometry (measure IOP)
· central corneal thickness measurement
· gonioscopy (Ax peripheral anterior chamber configuration and depth)
· Ax risk of future visual impairment
  - RF: ↑IOP, central corneal thickness, FHx, life expectancy

Mx: · PGA eye drops (eg. latanoprost)
· βB, acetazolamide, sympathomimetic eye drops
· + surgical/laser (trabeculectomy)
· regular reAx to check progression

Age-related macular degeneration

D: a potentially progressive maculopathy
Dry macular degeneration (90%)
· drusen – yellow round spots in Bruch's membrane

Wet macular degeneration (10%)
= exudative or neovascular macular degeneration; 'late' AMD
· choroidal neovascularisation
· leakage of serous fluid and blood can result in a rapid loss of vision
· worst prognosis

R: ↑age, smoking, FHx

S/smx:
· subacute reduction in visual acuity, esp for near field objects
· difficulties in **dark adaptation** with an overall deterioration in vision at night
· *fluctuations* in visual disturbance which may vary significantly from day to day
· **photopsia** (perception of flickering or flashing lights) + glare around objects
· distortion of line perception on Amsler grid testing
· fundoscopy: drusen, macular scar, well-demarcated red patches (intra-retinal or sub-retinal fluid leakage or haemorrhage)

Ix: · OCT to visualise macula
· slit-lamp microscopy
  - looking for pigmentary, exudative or haemorrhagic changes of the retina
· + colour fundus photography (baseline)
· fluorescein angiography if neovascular ARMD is suspected
  - guide intervention with anti-VEGF therapy
  - indocyanine green angiography to visualise any changes in the choroidal circulation
· ocular coherence tomography
  - to visualise the retina in 3D (to see areas that microscope cannot)

Mx: · Zinc + multivit – ↓progression
· anti-VEGF; start w/in 2mo of Dx of wet ARMD, e.g. bevacizumab. Admin q 4w via infusion
· laser photocoagulation
· ! warn pt can cause acute visual loss

Cataracts

D: opacification of the crystalline lens that results from normal ageing process
· leading cause of blindness worldwide
· can be due to normal ageing, but can also be due to other reasons

Classification
· Nuclear: change in lens refractive index (='2nd sight'; pt becomes more myopic and regains reading vision). Common in ↑age
· Cortical: wedge-shaped opacities
· Posterior subcapsular: progress faster, cause the classic glare from bright sunlight and lights while driving at night

S/smx: · clouded, blurred vision (painless)
· ↓distance judgment (↓stereopsis)
· ± dazzle, ± monocular diplopia
· in adults, ↑difficulty driving
· in children, squinting, white pupil, nystagmus, amblyopia

Ix: slit lamp exam (↓red reflex, cataract visible), normal IOP

Mx: · Glasses, brighter lights
· Surgical if severe visual impairment, ↓QoL, pt choice
  - Lens removal by phacoemulsification (US to break up cataract, then aspirated), then artificial lens inserted into empty capsule
  - Usually day procedure under LA
  - 90-95% successful, 2% serious risks
· Complications of surgery
  - Posterior capsule opacification: tx with YAG laser capsulotomy
  - Retinal detachment
  - Posterior capsule rupture
  - Endophthalmitis (inflm of aq &/or vitreous humour, can cause blindness)
· Astigmatism: toric lens
  - Eyes may not be completely normal after (glare often remains)
Prevention: · sunglasses
· ↓oxidative stress · stop smoking!!

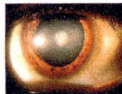

Diabetic retinopathy

D: chronic, progressive retinal disease 2/2 hyperglycaemic microvascular damage and neurodegenerative changes
· Most common cause of blindness in 35-65yo pts

R: longer duration of DM, poor glycaemic control, ↑lipids, HTN
· Proliferative: more common in T1DM

A/P: hyperglycaemia → ↑retinal blood flow and abnormal metabolism in retinal vessel walls → damage to endothelium and pericytes
· Endothelial damage → ↑vascular permeability → microaneurysms
· Pericyte damage → microaneurysms
· Retinal ischaemia → ↑growth factors → neovascularisation

S/smx: · Asmx initially
· Maculopathy – ↓visual acuity
· If/when proliferative retinopathy develops, blindness can come rapidly (50% blind in 5y)

Ix: fundoscopy
Non-proliferative (NPDR)
· Mild: ≥1 microaneurysm
· Mod: + blot haemorrhages
  + hard exudates (≈ maculopathy)
  + cotton wool spots (= retinal infarcts)
· Severe: above in all 4 quadrants
  + venous beading in >2 quadrants
  + intraretinal microvascular abn (IRMA)
Proliferative
· Retinal neovascularisation (can lead to vitreous haemorrhage)
· Fibrous tissues anterior to retinal discs

Mx:
· All: optimise glycaemic control, BP and lipids + regular review by ophthal
· Maculopathy (manifests as ↓visual acuity): intravitreal VEGF inhibitors
· NPDR: if severe, consider panretinal laser photocoagulation
· Proliferative retinopathy:
  - Panretinal laser photocoagulopathy
    ↳ warn pt 50% experience ↓visual fields due to scarring, ↓night vision
  - Intravitreal VEGF inhibitors
  - If severe, vitreoretinal surgery

Orbital & peri-orbital cellulitis

D: infection within the orbital soft tissues with associated ocular dysfunction
· Peri-orbital cellulitis (aka preseptal): inflammation & infection of the superficial eyelid

R: sinusitis, young (7-12yo), M>F, lack of Hib vaccination in children, facial infxn

Orbital – local spread of URTI, usually sinusitis, less often due to injury / fracture, dental infxns
Peri-orbital – superficial spread from inoculated site, eg insect bite
· Bony orbit is thin + many nerves & vessels + valveless veins → makes it easier for spread of infection

S/smx of orbital cellulitis:
· Redness, swelling around eye
· Severe ocular pain
· Visual disturbances   · Proptosis
· Ophthalmoplegia or pain with eye movements
· Eyelid oedema and ptosis
· Meningeal involvement (rare): drowsiness ± N&V

S/smx of peri-orbital cellulitis:
· Redness, swelling around eye only
· ± Fever

Ix: · FBC (↑WCC, ↑CRP)
· CT with contrast – helps differentiate between orbital & peri-orbital cellulitis
· Blood cultures & swabs

Mx: · Ophthalmology review asap
· Admit for IV abx if orbital cellulitis
· Peri-orbital cellulitis can be managed with PO abx

Thyroid eye disease

D: eye condition resulting from Grave's disease. Affects 20-30%.

A/P: autoimmune response to TSH receptor, causing retro-orbital inflammation → glycosaminogen and collagen deposition in muscles

S/smx: • Exophthalmos
• Conjunctival oedema
• Optic disc swelling
• Ophthalmoplegia
• Sore, dry eyes (2/2 inability to close eyelids) → can lead to exposure keratopathy
• Smx have no relation to thyroid status

Mx: ✎ topical lubricants
• Prevention
  - ❗ Stop smoking
  - ? Radioiodine tx, prednisolone
• Ophthal review if ▶
  - Unexplained ↓vision
  - Change in colour vision
  - Eye suddenly pops out (globe subluxation) – or Hx of this
  - Obvious corneal opacity
  - Cornea still visible when eyes closed
  - Disc swelling
• Definitive Mx involves treating Grave's disease, eg radiotherapy or surgery
• Advice pts about ▶ signs

Complications
• Exposure keratopathy – foreign body sensation, pain, photophobia. Can cause corneal scarring and blindness
• Optic neuropathy
  - Due to compression of optic nerve by extraocular muscles
  - Manifests as ↓acuity, colour vision deficits, visual field defects
  - Requires urgent medical attention
• Strabismus and diplopia
  - Due to enlargement of extraocular muscles → restriction of movement

Strabismus   aka squint

D: misalignment of the eyes
÷ concomitant and paralytic

R: FHx, prematurity, low birth wt, maternal smoking during pregnancy

A/P: poorly understood.
• Concomitant strabismus arises due to imbalance in extraocular muscles
  ↳ ÷ convergent and divergent
• Paralytic strabismus (rare) due to paralysis of extraocular muscles

S/smx:
• Convergent squint (esotropia) – one or both eyes turn inward
• Divergent (extropia) – one eye is turned out ± intermittent

Ix (screening)
• Corneal reflection: bright light will not fall symmetrically on each cornea due to misalignment
• Cover test
  - ask child to focus on an object
  - cover one eye, and observe movement of uncovered eye
  - cover other eye and repeat test
  - if neither eye moves, this indicates both eyes are fixating normally
  - if either eye moves, there is a squint present. When the fixating eye is covered, the non-fixating (squinting) eye moves to fixate on the object

Mx: • Optical: spectacles
• Orthoptic: patching the good eye can help encourage use of the squinting eye
• Operation: resection and recession of rectus muscles - helps alignment and can give good cosmetic results
  - botulinum toxin in some pts
• Best results if
  - early detection
  - conscientious and compliant tx
  - optimal glasses

C: if untreated, can lead to permanently damaged vision

Paralytic squint

D: paralysis of extraocular muscles resulting in diplopia

Causes of CN palsies
• all: trauma, stroke (ischaemic or haemorrhagic), tumour, congenital, DM
• CN III: cavernous sinus lesions, superior orbital fissure syndrome, posterior communicating artery syndrome
• CN VI: ↑ICP, trauma to skull base, multiple sclerosis

S/smx depends on which CN is affected:
• CN III, IV and VI palsies cause diplopia, esp on looking at the direction that the muscle would have been pulling at
• CN III palsy
  - ptosis (upper eyelid droops)
  - proptosis (protrusion of eye)
  - fixed pupil dilation
  - eye looks down and out
• CN IV palsy
  [superior oblique paralysed]
  - ocular torticollis (pt holds their head tilted to correct for diplopia)
  - slight upward deviation of eye
  - difficulty looking down and in
    ↳ difficulty walking down stairs
• CN VI palsy
  [lateral rectus paralysed]
  - diplopia in horizontal plane
  - eye is medially deviated, pt cannot look sideways on affected side

Anisocoria = unequal pupils

Causes
• Physiological (20% population)
• ▶ Horner's syndrome (see right)
• ▶ CN III palsy
• Migraine headache
• Drugs: cholinergics, cycloplegics, sympathomimetics
• Adie Tonic pupil
• ▶ Trauma

Pupil problems

÷ afferent or efferent or both
• Afferent (light go in): CN II problem
• Efferent (eye reacts): CN III

Afferent pupil problems
• No direct response to affected eye, but consensual response intact
  ↳ swinging flashlight test
• **Relative afferent pupillary defect**
  = when the light swings to affected eye, the pupil dilates slightly
• Compression of optic nerve can also cause ↓colour vision
  - test with Ishihara plates
• Causes: optic neuritis, optic atrophy, retinal disease

Efferent pupil problems (CN III)
• With complete palsy, there is complete ptosis, fixed dilated pupil, eye looks down and out
  - see left for CN III palsy causes
• Other causes of fixed dilated pupil
  - acute glaucoma
  - coning (uncal herniation)

Tonic (Adie) pupil
• D: parasympathetic denervation → poor constriction to light
• 2:1000 prevalence, F>M, mid-30s
• S/smx: blurry vision, difficulty reading up close
• Ix: slit lamp exam may show wormy movements ("iris streaming")

Argyll Robertson pupil
• Bilateral miosis, poor pupilary dilation, pupil irregularity
• Light-near dissociation where pupil does not respond to light but can still accommodate to near objects
• Causes: neurosyphilis, diabetes

Horner syndrome
• D: partial ptosis + miosis + facial anhidrosis due to disruption of sympathetic fibres in CN III
• Many causes (see left) including pancoast tumour, cervical adenopathy, mediastinal mass, etc
  ↳ sympathetic fibres emerge from T1 and below, so masses in the thorax can cause Horner's
• Congenital Horner's includes iris heterochromia

Tropical eye diseases

Xerophthalmia
• D: dry eyes a/w deficient vitamin A
  ↳ affects 40mil children worldwide
• S/smx: night blindness (nyctalopia), tunnel vision, poor acuity, dry eyes.
• Progression:
  - Cornea is unwettable
  - Cornea loses transparency
  - Small foamy plaques occur
  - Keratomalacia: cornea softens, thins and eventually ulcerates
  - Can lead to blindness :(
• Mx: improve nutrition, vitamin A (can reverse some changes), address associated causes (eg alcoholism)

Trachoma
• D: blindness 2/2 Chlamydia trachomatis (serotypes A B C)
  ↳ spread by flies in hot and dry places where people live near cattle
• Causes scarring on inner eye lids which damages cornea → causes eyelid to roll inwards, so that lashes rub directly on cornea, exacerbating damage → corneal scarring and ulceration
• Mx: "SAFE strategy" by WHO
  - Surgery, abx, facial cleanliness and environmental improvement
  - Abx: azithromycie, tetracycline 1% eye ointment
    ↳ mass tx if >10% population affected due to ↑risk of reinfection

Onchocerciasis (river blindness)
• D: blindness 2/2 Onchocerca volvulus (nematode parasite), transmitted btwn humans by black flies
  ↳ infxn causes blindness in 40%
• Parasite infects (or travels to) eye where they cause inflammation → fibrosis + corneal opacities
• Chronic iritis causes adhesions (synechiae) ± cataracts and fixed pupil
• Also causes skin smx where the parasite lodges in the subcutaneous tissue
• Mx: ivermectin + steroids

This page has been left blank intentionally.

Hypothyroidism

D: clinical disorder 2/2 ↓T3 and T4

Causes of primary hypothyroidism
- **Hashimoto's** (autoimmune)
  - anti-thyroid peroxidase and anti-thyroglobulin antibodies
  - a/w other autoimmune disorders
- Subacute thyroiditis (de Quervain's)
  - thought to occur after viral infxns
  - 4 phases: 1st phase (3-6w) with ↑T, painful goitre and ↑ESR; 2nd phase euthyroid; 3rd phase ↓T; 4th phase normal
  - scan will show ↓uptake of iodine-131
  - usually self-limiting
- Riedel thyroiditis
  - chronic inflammation and fibrosis of thyroid gland
- Post-thyroidectomy or post-radioiodine treatment
- Post-partum thyroiditis
- Drug therapy (eg lithium, amiodarone, and anti-thyroid drugs)
- Iodine deficiency (diet)

Causes of 2ndary hypothyroidism
- ↳ causes that don't directly affect the thyroid gland
- Down's syndrome
- Turn's syndrome
- Coeliac disease

S/smx: [body slows down]
- General: wt gain, lethargy, cold intolerance
- Skin: dry, cold skin; non-pitting oedema (on hands/face - can show up as peri-orbital oedema); dry, coarse scalp hair, loss of lateral aspect of eyebrows
- GI: constipation
- Gynae: menorrhagia (↑bleeding)
- Neuro: carpal tunnel syndrome

Ix: TFTs

Mx: levothyroxine 50-100 mcgod
- ↳ if >50yo, with IHD, start with 25 mcg od and slowly titrate up
- With dose ↑ or ↓, check TFTs after 8-12w

Note: amiodarone can cause both hyper and hypothyroidism

Mx (cont)
- Goal is to normalise TSH level – aim for 0.5-2.5 mU/L
- In pregnancy, increase dose by ≥25-50 mcg, monitor TSH
- Levothyroxine SE
  - hyperthyroidism
  - ↓bone mineral density: may need supplementing with calcium + D
  - worsening of angina   - AF
- In amiodarone-induced ↓T, continue amiodarone + give levothyroxine
- ❗ Interactions with levothyroxine
  - iron and calcium carbonate will ↓ absorption of levothyroxine – give ≥4h apart
- Levothyroxine is safe in bfding

Subclinical hypothyroidism
= ↑TSH but normal T3, T4 + no obvious smx
- Possible in pts who are non-compliant with levothyroxine

Mx
- If TSH >10 mU/L on 2 separate occasions 3mo apart (and T3 T4 normal range), consider offering levoT
- If TSH 5.5-10 mU/L on 2 separate occasions 3mo apart (and T3 T4 normal range + smx of hypothyroidism <65yo
  → consider 6mo trial of levothyroxine
- If TSH 5.5-10 mU/L in older people, watch and wait
- If TSH 5.5-10 mU/L + asmx, observe and repeat TFT in 6mo

Sick euthyroid syndrome
= non-thyroidal illness where ↓TSH, ↓T3, ↓T4
- Most of the time TSH is roughly in normal range
  - ↳ "inappropriate" since TSH should be high if T3 and T4 are low
- Usually result of systemic illness
- No tx needed if it reverses upon recovery

Myxoedema coma
= extremely decompensate hypoT
- S/smx: confusion, hypothermia
- Mx: - IV thyroid replacement
  - IV corticosteroids (due to possibility of coexisting adrenal insufficiency)
  - IV fluids   - correct electrolytes

Hyperthyroidism

D: clinical state 2/2 ↑T3 and ↑T4
- Thyrotoxicosis is an interchangeable term

Causes
- Graves' disease (most common)
- Toxic nodular goitre
- Postpartum thyroiditis
- Gestational hyperthyroidism
- TSH-producing pituitary adenoma
- Thyroid cancers (don't usually cause hyper or hypothyroidism)
- Iodine-induced ↑T (2/2 diet, contrast, drugs eg amiodarone)

S/smx of hyperthyroidism
- General: wt loss, sweating, heat intolerance, tremor, irritability
- Palpitations ± AF
- GI: diarrhoea
- Gynae: oligomenorrhoea
- See below for features specific to Graves'

Graves' disease
= autoimmune thyroid condition a/w hyperthyroidism
- ↳ abs to TSH receptor (90%) and abs to anti-thyroid peroxidase (75%)
- R: FHx, F>M (6:1), tobacco use
- Features specific to Graves'
  - Eyes (30%): exophthalmos & ophthalmoplegia [→05.05]
    - ↳ smoking ↑risk for eye disease
  - Pretibial myxoedema (scaly and lumpy skin on shins; non-pitting)
  - Thyroid acropachy
    - ◊ Digital clubbing
    - ◊ Soft tissue swelling of hands and feet
    - ◊ Periosteal new bone formation
- Ix: thyroid scintigraphy scan – diffuse, homogenous,↑uptake of iodine 131
- Mx
  - ⚡ Propranolol for smx control
  - Ref to endocrine
  - Will likely start carbimazole if smx not controlled with propranolol
  - If still refractory, radioiodine therapy may be considered
    - ↳ CI if pregnant, <16yo
  - →_____ for hyperthyroidism in pregnancy

Toxic multinodular goitre
= multiple autonomously functioning thyroid nodules
- Scan: patchy uptake
- Mx: radioiodine therapy

Thyroid storm
aka thyrotoxic crisis, life-threatening hyperthyroidism
- Precipitated by surgery, trauma, infxn or acute illness, acute iodine overload (eg contrast)
- S/smx:
  - Fever (>38.5℃)
  - CNS dysfunction (agitation, delirium, psychosis, lethargy++, seizure, coma)
  - ↑HR ± AF   - HF
  - GI dysfunction (NVD, abd pain, unexplained jaundice)
- Mx
  - ⚡ β-blockers: IV propranolol
  - Antithyroid drugs, eg propylthiouracil or methimazole
  - Dexamethasone ❗ blocks the conversion of T4 to T3
  - Lugol's iodine
  - Other smx treatment
  - Treat precipitating event

Anti-thyroid drugs, eg carbimazole
- MOA: inhibits thyroid peroxidase
- ❗ SE: agranulocytosis - need to warn pt to watch for infxns

---

Thyroid cancers

Papillary carcinoma (70%)
- F>M (3:1), young, good prognosis
- cancer of epithelial follicular cells, seldom encapsulated
- mets: usually via LN, rare haematologically

Follicular adenoma
- benign encapsulated tumour of the thyroid gland; usually presents as solitary thyroid nodule
- Requires histology to r/o malignancy

Follicular carcinoma (20%)
- malignant transformation of follicular adenoma; capsular invasion of tumour
  - ↳ vascular invasion usually
  - ↳ multifocal disease rare

Medullary carcinoma (5%)
- malignancy of the parafollicular C cells derived from neural crest
- secretes calcitonin
- a/w MEN2 (familial genetic disease accounts for ~20%)
- nodal disease a/w very poor prognosis

Anaplastic carcinoma (1%)
- aka undifferentiated thyroid carcinoma
- highly aggressive; very poor prognosis
- most common in elderly females
- Mx: resection where possible, palliation via isthmusectomy and radiotherapy
  - ↳ chemo not effective

Thyroid lymphoma (rare)
- a/w Hashimoto's
- Primary thyroid lymphoma – lymphoma affects thyroid first → LN → other organs
  - ↳ B-cell lymphoma most common
- 2ndary thyroid lymphoma – lymphoma affects LN → other organs → thyroid

---

Goitre
= neck swelling ∴ thyroid issue
- 5-12% malignant. Usually benign and asmx.
- Both hyper and hypothyroidism can cause goitre.

Dx - establish whether mass is intra or extra thyroidal - US + exam. Evaluate LN also. Thyroid will move with swallowing.

Cushing's

- Cushing's syndrome = clinical state 2/2 ↑cortisol from any cause
- Cushing's disease = 2/2 ACTH-secreting pituitary tumour

A: exogenous (eg steroid exposure), ACTH-secreting pituitary tumours, ectopic ACTH production (eg SCLC), adrenal adenoma/carcinoma, micro-nodular adrenal dysplasia [very rare], Carney complex

P: ↑cortisol → smx

S/smx: • facial plethora (moon face)
- central obesity & violaceous straie
- buffalo hump - enlarged fat pad on upper back
- proximal limb muscle wasting (causing proximal limb myopathy)
- menstrual irregularities + hirsutism
- thin skin → easy bruising, poor healing
- Mood changes, eg irritability
- In Cushing's disease: hyperpigmentation of skin
- Medical conditions 2/2 Cushing's
  - HTN   - Cardiac hypertrophy
  - T2DM / hyperglycaemia
  - Dyslipidaemia   - Osteoporosis

Ix
- VBG/ABG: metabolic alkalosis + ↓K ± hyperglycaemia
  ↳ ectopic ACTH → ↓↓K
- Low dose dexamethasone suppression test
  - in normal pts, dexa will suppress cortisol spike in the morning
  - in pts with Cushing's, no suppression ie, cortisol spike present
- 9 am & midnight ACTH + cortisol
  - ACTH-dependent cause will show suppressed cortisol
- High dose dexamethasone suppression test
  - Cortisol and ACTH suppressed = Cushing's disease
  - Cortisol and ACTH not suppressed = Ectopic ACTH syndrome
  - Cortisol not suppressed - Cushing's syndrome due to other causes (eg adrenal adenoma)

Mx:
- Resection of tumour wherever or taper down exogenous steroids
- Medical Mx
  - somatostatin analogue (pasireotide)
  - dopamine agonist (cabergoline)
  - steroidogenesis inhibitor (eg osilodrostat, ketoconazole)
  - glucocorticoid receptor antagonist (mifepristone)
- Pt may require post-surgical corticosteroid ± pituitary hormone replacement therapy
  - Clinically guided: monitor BP, check for orthostatic smx, etc

Note: Cushing's disease is usually 2/2 pituitary adenoma; carcinomas are rare

Non-functioning pituitary adenoma → ↑prolactin, 2ndary hypothyroidism, hypogonadism

Prolactinoma: HA, amenorrhea, visual field defects (bitemporal hemianopia most common) – see next pg

Ix (other tests)
- 24h urinary free cortisol
  - requires 2 measurements
- Bedtime salivary cortisol
  - requires 2 measurements
- CRH stimulation
  - CRH → ACTH → cortisol
  - if pituitary source, CRH will cause cortisol rise
  - if ectopic/adrenal source, no cortisol rise
- Petrosal sinus sampling
  - May be needed to differentiate between pituitary and ectopic ACTH secretion
- Insulin stress test: to r/o pseudo-Cushing's
- Imaging: MRI (for pituitary tumours), CTTAP (for adrenals or ectopic source)

Addison's disease

aka primary adrenal insufficiency
D: ↓cortisol, ↓aldosterone, ↓DHEA (adrenal androgen) due to disease affecting the adrenal cortex

A: autoimmune (majority), infxns (eg TB), metastases, infiltrative disease (eg amyloidosis), haemorrhagic infarction of adrenal glands (Waterhouse-Friderich-sen syndrome), adrenalectomy
- 2ndary Addison's (↓ACTH): pituitary disorders

R: F>>M, thrombembolic or hyper-coagulable states (eg anti-phospho-lipid syndrome), other autoimmune disease (esp coeliac disease)

S/smx: can be quite nonspecific
- lethargy, weakness, ↓appetite, NV, wt loss, 'salt-craving'
- vitiligo, loss of pubic hair in women, hypotension, hypoglycaemia
- hyperpigmentation (only in primary)
- ± ↓Na, ↑K
- Addison's crisis (see right)

Ix: ACTH stimulation test (short synacthen test)
  - plasma cortisol measured 30 min before and after giving synacthen 150 μg IM
- Alternatively, 9am cortisol
  - >500 nmol/L: Addison's unlikely
  - <100 nmol/L: Addison's likely
  - 100-500 nmol/L: ref for synacthen test
- U&Es: ↑K, ↓Na, ↓glucose, met acidosis

Mx: replace adrenal hormones
- Hydrocortisone ÷ 2-3 doses/day
  ↳ majority given in first half of day
- Fludrocortisone
- Sick day rules:
  - double hydrocortisone dose, fludrocortisone remains the same
  - drink lots of fluids
! DO NOT MISS DOSES
- Pts may need hydrocortisone for injection for adrenal crisis

Addisonian crisis
= acute exacerbation of adrenal insufficiency
- Usually a result of stress on the body (eg infxn) where the body requires but does not have sufficient cortisol ± aldosterone
- Can also be due to abrupt steroid withdrawal after long term therapy
- S/smx: shock, collapse, fever
- Mx:
  - Hydrocortisone 100 mg IM/IV stat
  - Then hydrocortisone 50 mg qds or 200 mg/24h IV until pt is stable
  - 0.9NaCl infusion
    ↳ continuous, monitor BP, UO
  - Monitor and treat hypoglycaemia
    ↳ dextrose IV if needed
  - PO hydrocortisone replacement 24h after, and taper down to maintenance dose over 3-4d
- Prevention: carry steroid card, ensure Drs/nurses know pt is on steroids and need for replacement if sick

Hyperaldosteronism

A: • bilateral idiopathic aldrenal hyperplasia 60-70% cases
- Conn syndrome (adrenal adenoma)
- Unilateral hyperplasia
- Familial hyperaldosteronism
- Adrenal carcinoma (rare)

P: ↑aldosterone → ↑Na reabsorption via kidneys, ↓K and ↓H

S/smx:
- treatment-resistant HTN
- ↓K ± metabolic alkalosis
  ↳ muscle weakness, ECG Δ etc
  ↳ more common with Conn's

Ix: • plasma aldosterone-renin ratio is the first line Ix
  ↳ ↑aldosterone + ↓renin
- CT abdo + adrenal vein sampling to identify cause of ↑aldosterone
  ↳ also helps show whether it is unilateral or bilateral

Mx: • tumour: adrenalectomy
- hyperplasia: aldosterone antagonist (eg spironolactone)

Acromegaly

D: disease resulting from excess growth hormone
- Gigantism = disease onset in childhood (prior to epiphyseal closure)

A: pituitary somatotroph adenoma (95%), with ↑prolactin in 25%. a/w MEN-1 in 6% pts

S/smx: "ABCDEFGHIJ"
- Arthropathy (painful joints)
- Big spade-like hands
- Coarse features & carpal tunnel syndrome
- Diabetes
- Enlarged tongue, heart, throat
- Field defects (bitemporal hemianopia)
- Gynaecomastia, galactorrhea (2/2 ↑prolactin) & greasy skin
- Hypertension
- Increasing size - shoes, hat, etc
- Jaw enlargement ± prognathism

Ix: • Serum IGF-1 levels (1st line)
- OGTT to confirm Dx if ↑IGF-1
  - in normal pts, OGTT will suppress GH (<2 mU/L)
  - in pts with acromegaly, no suppression of GH
  - ± impaired glucose tolerance
- MRI brain - ? pituitary tumour

Mx: • tumour resection (trans-sphenoidal surgery)
- if tumour is inoperable or surgery CI, then medical therapy
  - somatostatin analogue (↓GH), eg octreotide
  - GH receptor antagonist, eg pegvisomant subcut
  - dopamine agonists, eg bromocriptine; not particularly effective
- rarely, external irradiation

Prolactinoma

D: benign pituitary adenoma of prolactin-secreting cells

÷ into size
- Microadenoma <1cm
- Macroadenoma >1cm
÷ by hormonal status
- Secreting/functioning adenoma – ↑prolactin
- Non-secreting / non-functioning

S/smx:
- In females: amenorrhea, infertility, galactorrhea, osteoporosis
- In males: impotence, galactorrhea, loss of libido
- S/smx due to mass effect: HA, visual disturbances (bitemporal hemianopia)
- Hypopituitarism

Ix: MRI brain

Mx: ◄ medical - dopamine agonists (eg cabergoline, bromocriptine)
↳ MOA: inhibit release of prolactin from pituitary gland
◄ surgery (transsphenoidal)

Hyperparathyroidism

D: ↑PTH. ÷ into primary, secondary and tertiary hyperparathyroidism

Primary hyperparathyroidism
- Main problem is ↑PTH
- ↑PTH → ↑Ca, ↓PO4
- Causes: 80% solitary adenoma; 4% multifocal disease; 10% hyperplasia, ≤1% PTH carcinoma
- S/smx: asmx if mild
  - recurrent abdo pain
  - Δ emotional, cognitive state
  - XR: pepperpot skull, osteitis fibrosa cystica (OFC)
  ↳ OFC refers to bone disease specifically 2/2 ↑PTH; shows up as subperiosteal bone resorption

Secondary hyperparathyroidism
- Main problem is ↓Ca
- ↓Ca ± ↓Vit D → ↑PTH, ↑PO4
- Causes: usually 2/2 chronic renal failure (↓Vit D conversion → ↓Ca absorption)
- S/smx: few smx
  - eventually can develop bone disease, OFC, and soft tissue calcification

Tertiary hyperparathyroidism
- Main problem is ↑PTH that persists despite correction of Ca levels
- parathyroid hyperplasia → ↑PTH
  - labs: ↑PTH, -/↑Ca, ↓/- PO4, ↓/- vit D, ↑ALP
- Causes: parathyroid hyperplasia 2/2 chronic renal disease - non-responsive to correction of Ca levels
- S/smx: metastatic calcification, bone pain ± fractures, renal stones, pancreatitis

Ix: PTH, bone profile (Ca, PO4, etc), XR, CT/MRI neck

Mx: treat underlying cause
- 1' hyperparathyroidism
  - Surgical resection of tumours
  - Medical: calcimimetic eg cinacalcet
- 2' hyperparathyroidism
  - correct renal failure, supplement vitamin D and calcium
  - may require surgery
- 3' hyperparathyroidism
  - if it develops post-renal transplant, wait for 12mo as ↑PTH may resolve on its own
  - may require surgery

Hypoparathyroidism

D: ↓PTH → ↓Ca, ↑PO4

A: post-surgery (75% cases), genetics (eg DiGeorge), ↑or↓ Mg

S/smx: hypocalcaemia
- Tetany: muscle twitching, cramps, spasm
- Trousseau's sign: carpal spasm
- Chvostek's sign: tapping on facial nerve causes muscles to spasm
- ECG: prolonged QT interval

Mx: alfacalcidol (vitamin D analogue)

Pseudohypoparathyroidism
- Normal PTH levels, but target cells do not respond to PTH
↳ ↑PTH, ↓Ca, ↑PO4
- Genetic problem a/w low IQ, short stature, shortened fingers

Pseudopseudohypoparathyroidism
- Similar to pseudohypoPTH, but normal biochemistry

Multiple endocrine neoplasia

- Autosomal dominant disorder affecting various endocrine organs

MEN-1 (3Ps)
2/2 MEN1 gene mutation
- Hyperparathyroidism (90% cases)
- Pancreatic neuroendocrine tumour
  ↳ insulinoma, gastrinoma, etc
- Pituitary adenoma [anterior]
- Others: other NETs, adrenal cortical tumours, CNS tumours, thyroid tumours, etc
! Most likely to present with hyperCa

MEN-2A (2Ps)
2/2 RET oncogene mutation
- Hyperparathyroidism
- Phaeochromocytoma
- Medullary thyroid cancer
- a/w Hirschsprung disease, cutaneous lichen amyloidosis

MEN-2B (1P)
2/2 RET oncogene mutation
- Phaeochromocytoma
- Medullary thyroid cancer
- Marfinoid body habitus
- Mucosal intestinal ganglioneuromatosis

Other MEN
- MEN3: aka familial medullary thyroid cancer
- MEN4 (rare): parathyroid adenomas, pituitary adenomas, tumours affecting adrenal, renal and reproductive organs, GI NETs

HbA1c may be inaccurate in
- Haemoglobinopathies (eg sickle cell)
- Haemolytic anaemia
- Untreated iron deficiency anaemia
- Suspected GDM
- Children   • HIV   • CKD
- People taking medications causing hyperglycaemia (eg steroids)

Diabetes mellitus

Dx criteria for diabetes mellitus
In smx pts, random plasma glucose >11 1
Fasting plasma glucose ≥7.0
Plasma glucose ≥11.1 2h after 75 OGTT
HbA1c ≥48 mM (≥6.5%)

HbA1c	mmol/mol	%
Normal	<42	<6
pre-DM	42-47	6-6.4
DM	≥48	≥6.5
Goal for DM	58	7.5

Impaired fasting glucose 6.1-6.9

MODY 1/2/3 are autosomal dominant inherited forms of DM with onset btwn 2nd to 5th decade
· MODY 1&3 respond well to PO hypoglycaemic agents   See 15.16 for more

T1DM

D: metabolic disorder characterised by hyperglycemia ∴ **absolute insulin deficiency**.

A/P: autoimmune or idiopathic destruction of pancreatic β cells

S/S/mx: • peak Dx at 10-14
· Hyperglycemia, polyuria, polydipsia, wt loss and ↑fatigue
· In adults, hyperglycemia, ketosis, rapid wt loss, BMI<25. Often FHx.
! some present with DKA (next pg)

Ix: Glucose levels, plasma or urine ketones, C-peptide (low), diabetes-specific autoantibodies

Mx: basal-bolus insulin (long-acting insulin for basal, rapid-acting for bolus) in multiple daily injections regimen
· Metformin if BMI ≥25
· Monitor glucose before each meal and before bed (≥4x a day); more frequent monitoring if unwell, ↑exercising, pregnancy
! pregnant women with T1DM - aspirin 75 mg from 12w to birth of baby

T2DM

D: progressive disorder defined by **deficits in insulin secretion** and **increased insulin resistance** that lead to abn glucose metabolism and related metabolic derangements.

R: ↑age, obesity, PMH of GDM, prediabetes, FHx of T2DM, non-white ancestry, PCOS, HTN, dyslipid, CVD and stress

A/P: relative deficiency of insulin due to excess of adipose tissue - not enough insulin to "go around" all the excess fatty tissue

S/smx: polyuria, polydipsia ± wt loss, paraesthesias, acanthosis nigricans. Usually picked up incidentally

Ix: fasting lipid profile, urine ketones, ACR, eGFR, ECG, ABPI, LFT as baseline tests

Mx: lifestyle mod (diet, exercise, stop smoking), Mx of comorbidities. Pharmacological agents (see →)

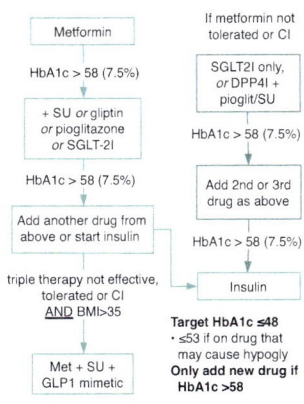

Metformin

HbA1c > 58 (7.5%)

+ SU or gliptin or pioglitazone or SGLT-2I

HbA1c > 58 (7.5%)

Add another drug from above or start insulin

triple therapy not effective, tolerated or CI AND BMI>35

Met + SU + GLP1 mimetic

If metformin not tolerated or CI

SGLT2I only, or DPP4I + pioglit/SU

HbA1c > 58 (7.5%)

Add 2nd or 3rd drug as above

HbA1c > 58 (7.5%)

Insulin

Target HbA1c ≤48
· ≤53 if on drug that may cause hypogly
Only add new drug if HbA1c >58

HTN + T2DM: BP target <140/90
· + ACEI (ARBs in African-Carribean pts)
· Avoid β-blockers
Lipids: offer statin if QRISK >10%

Drugs for DM

Metformin PO
· MOA: ↑ insulin sensitivity, ↓hep gluconeogenesis
· AE: GI upset, lactic acidosis
· CI: GFR<30   (see below also)

Sulfonylureas PO, eg glicazide
· MOA: ↑insulin secretion
· AE: hypogly, wt gain, hypoNa

Thiazolidinediones PO, eg pioglitazone
· MOA: activate PPAR-γ receptor in adipocytes to ↑adipogenesis and fatty acid uptake
· AE: wt gain, fluid retention

SGLT-2 inhibitors PO, eg capagli*flozin*, empagli*flozin*
· MOA: inhibits reabsorption of glucose in kidneys
· Start at any point if pt develops cardiovascular disease, QRISK ≥10% or chronic heart failure
· AE: **UTI**   · Good for wt loss

DPP4-inhibitors PO, eg sitagliptin
· MOA: ↑incretin by decreasing peripheral breakdown → inhibits glucagon secretion
· AE: ↑risk of pancreatitis

GLP-1 agonists SQ, eg liraglutide
· MOA: mimics incretin which inhibits glucagon secretion
· AE: NV, pancreatitis
· Note: good for wt loss

Insulin

Rapid acting
· Onset 5min   · Peak 1h
· Duration 3-5h
· Often used as bolus doses before meals
· Eg NovoRapid, Humalog

Short-acting
· Onset 30min   · Peak 3h
· Duration 6-8h
· Can be used as bolus dose (needs to be taken earlier)
· Eg Actrapid, Humulin S

Intermediate acting
· Onset 2h   · Peak 5-8h
· Duration 12-18h
· Can be used as basal dose given bds
· Eg isophane insulin

Long acting
· Onset 1-2h   · No peak!!
· Duration - up to 24h
· Used as basal dose
· Eg Levemir (od/bds dosing), Lantus (od)

Premixed preps
· Many different kinds

Administration
· Subcutaneous: rotate sites!
· Continuous SQ infusion (pumps)
· IV - only in hospital

Adjustments day before surgery
· OD insulin ↓20%

Day of surgery
· No adj: metformin, DPP4i, GLP-1
· Omit morning dose: SU, SGLT2
· BD insulin: morning dose ↓50%

Metformin: If pt requires procedure with contrast dye,
- GFR ≥60 (or SrCr normal range), metformin as per usual
- GFR <60 or ↑Cr, skip metformin on day of contrast and for 48h following contrast

→ 16.04 for Gestational diabetes mellitus

DLVA rules for DM

For general (group 1) license
· If diet-controlled, no need to inform DLVA
· If pt is on meds that can cause hypoglycaemia (eg SU)
  - ≤1 episode of hypoglycaemia requiring assistance of another person within preceding 12mo - ok to drive
  - if ≥2 such episodes, inform DLVA
· If pt is on insulin,
  - ≤1 episode of hypoglycaemia requiring assistance of another episode within preceding 12mo - ok to drive
  - pts are normally contacted by DLVA

For heavy goods vehicles drivers (group 2)
· Can drive only if
  - no severe hypoglycaemic event in previous 12mo
  - driver has full hypoglycaemic awareness
  - driver must regularly monitor BMs (≥ bds and at times relevant to driving)
  - driver must understand risks of hypoglycaemia
  - no other debarring complications of DM

Complications of DM

Macrovascular
Brain - stroke/TIA, cognitive impairment
Heart - HTN, atherosclerosis, CHD, MI
Extremities - peripheral vascular disease, ↑risk of ulcers, gangrene, amputation

Microvascular
Eye - diabetic retinopathy, cataracts, glaucoma
Kidney - diabetic nephropathy → CKD
Neuropathy - peripheral neuropathy (glove and stocking pattern), contributes to issues with extremities

DM sick day rules
· *DO NOT* stop insulin – risk of DKA
· ↑ monitoring ± check ketones
· consume 3L of fluids / 24h
· ± sugary drinks
· Drug management
  - Metformin: stop if risk of dehydration due to risk of lactic acidosis
  - SUs: caution due to ↑risk of hypoglycaemia
  - SGLT2i: check ketones, stop if acutely unwell + risk of dehydration (risk of euglycaemic DKA)
  - GLP1 receptor agonists: stop if risk of dehydration (risk of AKI)

Diabetic ketoacidosis

D: acute metabolic complication of diabetes, characterised by absolute or relative insulin deficiency

R: inadequate or inappropriate insulin therapy, **infection**, MI

A/P: **uncontrolled lipolysis** → ↑free fatty acids converted to ketone bodies

S/smx: **abd pain**, polyuria, polydipsia, dehydration, deep hyperventilation (Kussmaul), "pear drops" breath

Ix: blood glucose, ABG/VBG, urine dipstick, bloods, etc

Dx: • **D** - BGC >11 or Hx of DM
• Ketones >3mmol or urine ketones 2+
• **A** – pH <7.3 or bicarbs <15

Mx (general principles)
(1) **isotonic saline** (for all pts)
→ start D5 inf when BGC <15
(2) **insulin IV at 0.1 U/kg/h**
→ stop short-acting insulin
→ continue long-acting insulin
(3) monitor and correct **electrolyte abnormalities**, esp K
→ may require cardiac monitoring

DKA resolution – should be w/in 24h
• pH > 7.3
• Blood ketones <0.6 mmol/L
• Bicarbonate >15 mmol/L

Continued mx: E&D as tolerated, switch to SQ insulin, review by diabetes nurse

Complications   • ARDS   • AKI
• gastric stasis   • VTE
• arrhythmias 2/2 hyper/hypo K
• cerebral edema and hypoglycemia (iatrogenic)
- children/ young adults esp vulnerable to cerebral edema after fluid resus – 1:1 monitoring

Insulin infusion: using an insulin syringe, draw up 50U of Actrapid insulin. Add to 49.5mL 0.9NaCl in a 50 mL syringe → 1U insulin per 1mL solution

---

Mx (UHB guidelines)
• Consider ITU referral if
- young, elderly or pregnant
- heart, liver or kidney failure
- severe DKA - blood ketones >6, bicarb <5, pH <7.1, K<3.5, GCS <12, persistent hypoxia or persistent ↓/↑HR or anion gap >16

0-60 min
• Restore circulatory volume
- 500 mL of 0.9NaCl stat doses until BP>90
- Then 1L 0.9NaCl over 1h
• Start insulin therapy
- Fixed rate insulin infusion 0.1 mL/kg/h
- Continue pt's long acting insulin
• Senior review

60min to 6h
• 1L of 0.9NaCl with K over 2h
• Then, 1L of 0.9NaCl + K over 2h
• Then, 1L of 0.9NaCl + K over 4h
• Notes on K replacement
- <3.5: senior review
- 3.5-5.5: 40 mmol/L
- >5.5: no replacement

6-12h
• 1L of 0.9NaCl + K over 4h
• 1L of 0.9NaCl + K over 6h
• Senior review if DKA >12h
• Monitor for hypoglycemia
- start 500 mL 10% glucose at 125mL/h and reduce infusion rate by 50% (i.e. 0.05 mL/kg/h) when glucose ≤14

Monitoring
• Glucose & ketones qhly
• ABG for bicarb and K at 1h, 2h, and then q2hly thereafter
• Check infusion rate if
- ketones not ↓ by 0.5mmol/h
- bicarb not ↑ by 3 mmol/h
- glucose not ↓ by 3mmol/h

Hypoglycaemia
• If glu ≤4, follow hypoglycaemia guidelines, ensure fixed rate insulin infusion running at 0.05 mL/kg/h if DKA still persisting

Stopping tx
• When DKA is resolved, switch to VRIII insulin infusion if pt cannot E+D
• If pt can E+D, give SQ insulin dose, then stop infusion 0.5h later

---

Hyperosmotic hyperglycemic state

D: acute metabolic complication of DM, characterised by profound hyperglycaemia, hyperosmolarity, and volume depletion in the *absence* of ketoacidosis

R: infection, inadequate insulin or oral antidiabetic therapy, acute illness in a known patient with diabetes, nursing home residents (or just elderly pts)

A/P: • **Hyperglycaemia → osmotic diuresis** a/w loss of Na and K
• Severe **volume depletion** → significant raised serum osmolality (> 320 mOsm/kg) → hyperviscosity
• The typical patient with HHS may not look as dehydrated as they are as hypertonicity leads to preservation of intravascular volume

S/smx: fatigue, lethargy, N&V
• Neuro: altered consciousness, HA, papilloedema, weakness
• Haematological: hyperviscosity → MI, stroke and peripheral arterial thrombosis
• CVS: hypotension, tachycardia

Dx: 1. Hypovolaemia
2. BGC >30 mmol/L without significant ketonaemia or acidosis
3. Significantly raised serum osmolality (> 320 mosmol/kg)

Mx: 1. Gradually normalise the osmolality
- monitor serum osm, or infer from Na, glucose and urea
2. Replace fluid and electrolyte losses
- isotonic 0.9NaCl first, may need to switch to 0.45NaCl
- aim for +ve fluid balance 3-6L by 12h, and replace remaining fluid in next 12h
- monitor K levels – may need cautious K replacement
3. Gradually normalise blood glucose
- fluid resus will lower BGC
- insulin only needed if ketosis is significant, otherwise monitor

---

Hypoglycaemia

D: ↓blood glucose <3.3 mmol/L

A: • insulinoma
• drugs: insulin, sulphonylureas
• liver failure
• Addison's disease (↓↓cortisol)
• Alcohol – causes ↑↑insulin secretion

S/smx: • can be asmx early on (∴ pts need to monitor BMs!)
• Early on: sweating, shaking, hunger, anxiety, nausea
• Later on: weakness, vision Δ, confusion, dizziness
• Severe hypo: seizures, coma

Mx:
• In the community + pt is alert
- oral glucose 10-20g in any form
↳ ≈ 4 jelly babies, 200 mL of pure fruit juice, 200 mL sugary Coke
- or quick-acting carb eg Glucogel
- some pts may have Hypokit
• In hospital + pt is alert
- quick-carb eg Glucogel
• In hospital + pt is unable to swallow or unconscious: SQ/IM glucagon or IV 20% dextrose
• *Prevention*
- Pt education on s/smx
- Encourage frequent monitoring esp in T1DM where s/smx may not be as clear cut
- Give Hypokit (with glucagon)
• Note: β-blockers ↓hypoglycaemic awareness

Water deprivation test
• Method: pt stops drinking water + empty their bladder, then hourly urine and plasma osmolalities
• PP = psychogenic polydipsia
• DDAVP = desmopressin (synthetic ADH)

	Normal	PP	CDI	NDI
Starting plasma osm	Normal	Low	High	High
Final urine osm	>600	>400	<300	<300
Post DDAVP urine osm	>600	>400	**>600**	**<300**

Diabetes insipidus

D: metabolic disorder characterised by absolute or relative inability to concentrate urine, resulting in production of large quantities of dilute urine

Cranial DI: ↓production of antidiuretic hormone (ADH)
Nephrogenic DI: ↓sensitivity to ADH

Causes of cranial DI
• Idiopathic   • Post head injury / TBI
• Pituitary surgery   • Craniopharyngioma
• Infiltrative: histiocytosis X, sarcoidosis
• DI, DM, Optic Atrophy and Deafness (DIDMOAD, aka Wolfram syndrome)
• Haemochromatosis

Causes of nephrogenic DI
• Genetic (affecting the ADH receptor or aquaporin 2 channel)
• Electrolytes: hyperCa, hypoK
• Lithium (desensitises kidney to ADH)
• Demeclocycline
• Tubulo-interstitial disease: obstruction, sickle cell, pyelonephritis

S/smx: Polyuria, polydipsia, nocturia
• May have other signs depending on causative factor (eg visual field defects if 2/2 craniopharyngioma)

Ix: • high plasma osmolality, low urine osmolality (very diluted pee)
- Urine osmolality >700 mOsm/kg excludes DI
• Water deprivation test

Mx: • Nephrogenic DI: thiazides, low salt/protein diet
• Central DI: desmopressin

Acid-base imbalance

D: acidosis (pH <7.35), alkalosis (pH >7.45). Further ÷ metabolic and respiratory components.

Metabolic acidosis

↓pH, ↓HCO3 [↓PCO2 if compensated]
→ check anion gap: Na - (Cl + HCO3)

Normal anion gap metabolic acidosis
- Anion gap 6-12
- aka hyperchloremic MA
- GI or renal causes common
[HARDASS] Hyperalimentation, Addison, Renal tubular acidosis, Diarrhea, Acetazolamide, Spironolactone, Saline infusion

Anion gap metabolic acidosis
- Anion gap >12
[MUDPILES] Methanol, Uraemia, Diabetic ketoacidosis (also alcoholic ketones), Propylene glycol, Iron tabs, Isoniazid, Lactate (shock, sepsis, hypoxia, burns), Ethylene glycol, Salicylates (late)

Mx: sodium bicarbonate (IV/PO), ?HD

Renal tubular acidosis

→ Hyperchloraemic met acidosis + normal Sr anion gap and hypokalaemia (except IV)

Type I (distal): cannot excrete H+, often genetic • ↑urine pH

Type II (proximal): cannot reabs HCO3, often genetic or Faconi syndrome
→ ∴ ↓H+ secretion by NH3 or H-ATPase, or ↓NaHCO3 cotransporter, or ↓activity of carbonic anhydrase
• ↓urine pH
• Fanconi: urine glu, PO4 wasting

Congenital RTA - growth retardation & muscle weakness, failure to thrive, fructose intolerance (hypogly after fructose ingestion), rickets, renal stones. Fanconi a/w Balkan ethnicity.

Substances that can be cleared by HD:
[SLIME] Salicylates, lithium, isopropanol, methanol and ethylene glycol

Metabolic alkalosis

↑pH, ↑HCO3 (or ↓H)
[↑PCO2 if compensated]

[HALVE] Hyperaldosteronism, Antacids, Loop diuretics, Vomiting, Extremely low circulating volume (↑conc of HCO3)
→ may also be compensatory mechanism for pts w/ chronic respiratory acidosis (eg COPD)

S/Smx: tingling, muscle cramps, weakness, cardiac arrhythmias, seizures

Mx: [severe >7.6] controlled hypoventilation, using sedation and mechanical ventilation, correct volume depletion w/ NaCl, Mx of e- abn. If hypervolaemia, acetazolamide. If ↓renal function, HD.

Causes of ↑aldosterone: Conn's, cirrhosis, HF, loops, thiazides

Type III (mixed): any condition causing carbonic anhydrase deficiency, incl acetazolamide
• ↑urine pH, ↑fractional excretion of HCO3

Type IV (hyperkalaemic distal):
aldosterone deficiency or resistance
Inhib of Na reabs in distal nephron →
↓excretion of K (∴↑K) → ↓ammonia production → ↓buffering capacity of urine. Also ↓function of HATPase in distal nephron → ↑H.
• ↓urine pH + +ve urine anion gap

Ix: 1st line - Sr HCO3, Cl, Na, K, pH, anion gap, urine pH. Others - use for cause, eg Sr aldosterone, US, CT

Mx: alkali replacement (NaHCO3 or Shohl's solution), K replacement in Types I, II, III.

Respiratory acidosis

↓pH, ↑PCO2 (>6kPa)
[↑HCO3 (>24) if compensated]

[AACOW] Airway obstruction, acute lung disease, chronic lung disease (eg COPD), opioids/sedatives, weakening of lung muscles (eg myasthenia gravis)

S/Smx: hypoventilation, obtundation, haemodynamic instability, respiratory muscle fatigue (accessory muscle use, SOB, ↑RR)

Mx: O2 venturi mask or CPAP (sats 88-92% for COPD, others >94%).

Respiratory alkalosis

↑pH, ↓PCO2 (<4.7kPa)
[↓HCO3 (<24) if compensated]

[HAPPENS] Hyperventilation, ARDS, pneumonia, PE, Neoplasm, Sepsis

→ salicylates cause early RAlk followed by metabolic acidosis

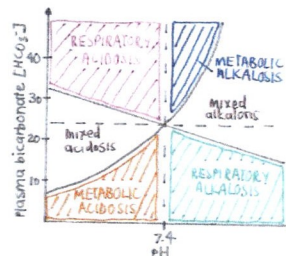

Arterial Blood Gas

pH: 7.35-7.45	pCO2: 4.7-6 kPa
	Respi failure
pO2: 10-14 kPa	→ I: ↑CO2 only
→ Hypoxia <8	→ II: ↑CO2, ↓O2

Base excess: -2 to 2 mmol/L
>2 - met alkalosis or respi acidosis
<2 - met acidosis or respi alkalosis

HCO3: 22-26 mmol/L

Lactate: <1 mmol/L. Raised in ↑ anaerobic respi; poor tissue perfusion

Anion gap raised >14

Hypercholesterolaemia

D: ↑total cholesterol (TC) and/or low-density lipoprotein cholesterol (LDL-C) or non-high-density lipoprotein cholesterol (HDL-C) ± ↑triglycerides, ↑apolipoprotein B, ↑lipoprotein(a)

R: insulin resistance, T2DM, BMI > 25, hypothyroidism, cholestatic liver disease

S/Smx: RF, Fhx, Hx of CVD, poor diet, ↑BMI (esp abd obesity), xanthelasma ± corneal arcus.

Mx: lifestyle advice (diet, smoking, exercise, wt loss, etc)
· no evidence for omega-3 fatty acids
■ Statins - HMG-CoA reductase inhibitors: ↓LDL 20-55% (↓1mM = ↓10% risk of mortality, ↓20% death due to heart disease, ↓27% MI, ↓21% stroke).
· If QRISK2>10%, ≥85yo, DM, CKD, atorvastatin 20 mg.
· If ACS/stroke, atorvastatin 80 mg
· Main SE: myositis, Δ LFTs.
■ (a) ezetimibe - inhibits absorption of cholesterol in the GIT. SE: HA
(b) fibrates (eg fenofibrate) - agonist of PPAR-α = ↑lipoprotein lipase.
· SE: myositis, pruritis, cholestasis
(c) nicotinic acid - ↓hepatic VLDL secretion. SE: flushing, myositis
(d) PCSK9 inhibitors - inhibits degradation of LDLR responsible for removing LDL. SE: athralgia, back pain, nausea, infxns
(e) bile acid sequestrants, eg cholestyramine - ↓bile reabsorption in SI, ↑cholesterol converted to bile.
· SE: GI side effects

Monitor:
· bloods every 6w until target LDL is achieved, then q6-12mo when stable
· ! Baseline LFTs before starting statin; no need to check regularly unless myositis

C: IHD/ACS, stroke, PVD, erectile dysfunction
P: overall good prognosis, esp with statins. Monitor for other comorbidities (eg HTN, DM) to improve outcomes.

Dx criteria:
· TC > 5.18 mmol/L
· LDL-C >2.6 [↑↑>4.9]
· Non-HDL <3.4
· HDL <1.04 (M), <1.29 (F)
· TG >1.7
· ± lipoprotein >50 mg/dL

Optimal levels:
· TC < 4.4-5.2
· LDL-C <1.8-2.6
· TG < 1.1-1.7

When to step up
■ at Dx
■ if statin not tolerated, or very high risk, or LDLC ≥1.8 despite statin

Scores - QRISK2/3. Framingham??

Hyperkalaemia

D: ERC classification - mild 5.5-5.9; mod 6-6.4; severe ≥ 6.5mmol/L

Causes
- AKI • Rhabdomyolysis
- Drugs: ACEI, ARBs, K-sparing eg spironolactone, ciclosporin, heparin (incl LMWH)
- Metabolic acidosis
- Addison's disease
- Massive blood transfusion

S/smx:
- muscle weakness, palpitations, paraesthesias
- ECG: - tall tented T waves
  - loss of P waves
  - broad QRS complexes
  - sinusoidal wave pattern
  - ventricular fibrillation

Ix: ECG, VBG (K+, HCO3, pH)

Mx: Stop offending drugs!
[C BIG K DROP]
- Calcium gluconate: 30 mL of CaGlu 10% IV over 5 min; repeat q10min until ECG normalises
- β-agonists: 10 mg neb salbutamol
- Insulin & glucose: 10 U Actrapid insulin using insulin syringe + 50 mL glucose 50% (25 g glucose) over 15-30 min into large vein
  - if pt is hyperglycaemic, do not give 50% glucose
  → monitor VBG q2hly
  → monitor BCG 0 min, 15, 30, 60, 90, 2h, 3, 4, 6, 8 and 12h, as delayed hypos reported frequently
- If pt is volume deplete
  - IV 0.9 NaCl 500-1000mL
- If pt is volume overloaded, give IV furosemide 50 mg
- If pH <7.3, bicarb <20, give 500 mL 1.26% sodium bicarb over 1h
- Monitor UO
- Ref urgently to renal team
  - consider HD ± K-sequestering agents

Hypokalaemia

D: mild 3-3.5 / mod 2.5-3 / severe ≤2.5 mmol/L

Causes
- ↓K with alkalosis
  - Vomiting - Thiazides, loops
  - Cushing's - Conn's
- ↓K with acidosis
  - Diarrhoea - Acetazolamide
  - Renal tubular acidosis
  - Partially treated DKA
- Others: ↓Mg!

S/smx: muscle weakness, hypotonia, digoxin toxicity
- ECG: - U waves
  - small or absent T waves
  - prolonged PR
  - prolonged QT
  - ST depression

Ix/Dx: FBC, glucose, U&Es (incl Mg), ECG

Mx: • Stop offending drugs
- Correct hypoMg first
- IV or PO replacement (eg SandoK)

K 3.0-3.5 mmol/L
- SandoK 2 tab 8hly, or
- If ECG Δ or taking digoxin, give 0.9 NaCl 1L with KCl 40 mmol/L as commercially premixed bag over 4h with continuous ECG monitoring

K 2.5-3.0 mmol/L
- SandoK 2 tabs 6hly, or
- If ECG Δ or taking digoxin, give 0.9 NaCl 1L with KCl 40 mmol/L as commercially premixed bag over 4h with continuous ECG monitoring

K <2.5 mmol/L
- Inform senior Dr
- Give 0.9 NaCl 1L with KCl 40 mmol/L as commercially premixed bag over 4h with continuous ECG monitoring

Note: do not replace K at rate >10 mmol/L

Hypercalcemia

D: normal Ca levels - 2.1-2.6 mmol/L
Mild: 2.6-2.9 / Mod: 3.0-3.4
Severe > 3.4 mmol/L

S/smx: unusual until Ca >3.0
- "moans stones bones groans"
- GI: NV, constipation, abd pain
- Renal: polyuria, polydipsia
- CVS: HTN, ECG (↑QT, ↑PR, wide QRS, arrythmias)
- CNS: depression, alt mental status, HA, ↓GCS, psychosis

Ix: U&Es, bone profile, CXR, ECG, PTH (purple top), FBC, ESR, myeloma screen, 25OH-VitD

Mx: • Ca 2.6-2.9: stop thiazides, Ca supplements, vitamin A/D + keep hydrated
- Ca 3.0-3.4 but asmx: 2-3L of water per day, or 2-3L IV 0.9 NaCl.
- Ca 3.0-3.4 + smx OR >3.4 mmol/L
  - Admit + fluids: IV 0.9NaCl 4-6L over 24h as tolerated
  - Monitor fluid balance
  - Measure U&Es and Ca 12hly
  - IV zolendronic acid 4mg over 15min if hyperCa persists after hydration
    ↳ ↓dose if eGFR <60
  - Consider HD if Ca >4.5
  - Ref to endocrinology

CHIMPANZEES
[causes of hyperCa]
C alcium supplementation
H yperparathyroidism
I atrogentic (thiazides)
M ilk Alkali syndrome
P aget disease of the bone
A cromegaly & Addison's
N eoplasia
Z olinger-Ellison Syndrome (MEN Type I)
E xcessive Vitamin D
E xcessive Vitamin A
S arcoidosis

Hypocalcaemia

D: corrected Ca < 2.10 mmol/L; smx typically arise when <1.9

Causes
- ↓PTH 2/2 surgery, ↓Mg (a/w PPI, diuretics, diarrhoea, malnutrition, alcoholism, renal loss), autoimmune disease, genetics
- Failure of release of calcium from bone
  - Osteomalacia (Vit D def, ESRD)
  - Drugs, eg cisplastin, calcitonin, PO phosphates
  - Osteoblastic metastases
- Failure of 1,25 OH D levels
  - Drugs, eg ketoconazole, PPI
  - Acute pancreatitis
- Complexing of calcium from circulation
  - Alkalosis: ↑albumin binding
  - Acute pancreatitis
  - Multiple blood transfusions

S/smx:
- Tingling, numbness, cramps, carpopedal spasm, stridor (2/2 laryngospasm), seizures
- Chvostek's sign, Trousseau's sign
- ECG: prolonged QT

Ix/Dx: ECG, bloods - CCa, PO4, PTH (purple top), U&E, 25OH-D, Mg

Mx of <1.9 + smx
- 10-20ml 10% calcium gluconate in 50-100ml of 5% dextrose IV over 10 minutes
- Repeat up to 3x until asmx
- Cardiac monitoring
- Anything more: refer to Trust guidelines & ALERT SENIOR

Mx of >1.9 / asmx
- PO calcium supp: eg SandoCal 1000 2 tab BD or equiv

Mx of underlying condition
- VitD or Mg def - supplementation
- Stop offending drugs
- Ref to ENT (if post-surgery) or endocrinology

Hypomagnesaemia

D: <0.9mmol/L; usually smx only if (0.4-0.5mmol/L)

Causes
- Drugs: diuretics, PPIs, TPN
- Diarrhoea - acute/chronic
- Alcohol >:(
- HypoK, hyperCa
- Metabolic disorders, eg Gitleman's and Bartter's

S/smx similar to hypoCa
- Paraesthesia • Tetany
- Seizures • Arrythmias
- Exacerbates digoxin toxicity
- ECG: prolonged QT

Mx in symptomatic pts
- IV Mg sulphate 50%, 20 mmol in 10mL, made up in 240 mL 0.9 NaCl at 50 ml/h (i.e. over 5h)
  - if faster rates, cardiac monitoring required
- While infusing, monitor obs, UO, and check for s/smx of toxicity
- May require up to 160 mmol to correct over 3-5d
- Measure Mg daily until normal
- In renal pts, lower replacement doses should be given (↓25-50%)
- NB: PO Mg poorly absorbed

↓Na
SrNa < 135

→ 🔲 Measure *serum* osmolarity

↑Na
(SrNa >145)
∴ net water loss or excess Na intake

→ **Unreplaced water losses**
- Diabetes insipidus [→06.08]
- Others: skin losses, GI losses, osmotic diuresis

→ **Water loss into cells**
Transient hyperNa due to severe exercise or electroshock-induced seizures. Usually returns to normal 5 to 15 min post event

→ **Sodium overload**
Accidental (eg NaHCO3 in tx of metabolic acidosis) or deliberate [idk how]

Syndrome of inappropriate antidiuretic hormone (SIADH)
- D: condition characterised by hypotonic hyponatraemia, concentrated urine, and a euvolaemic state
- Causes:
  - Malignancy: SCLC, pancreas, prostate
  - Neuro: stroke, SAH, subdural haematoma, meningitis, encephalitis, abscess
  - Infxns: TB, pneumonia
  - Drugs: sulfonylureas, SSRIs, TCAs, carbamazepine, vincristine, cyclophosphamide
  - Others: positive end-expiratory pressure, porphyrias
- Ix: ↑urine osmolality (concentrated urine),↑urine sodium concentration
- Mx: 💧 fluid restriction
  - Slow correction of Na to avoid precipitating central pontine myelinolysis
  - Others: demeclocycline, ADH receptor antagonists

Hypertonic ↓Na SrOs >295 mmol/kg
- Hyperglycemia
  - HHS [→04.05]
- Hypertonic fluid admin

Hypotonic ↓Na SrOs <275 mmol/kg
→ 🔲 Assess volume status
BP, HR, RR

Isotonic ↓Na SrOs 275-295 mmol/kg
Pseudohyponatremia

Most often due to ↑↑ serum chol. May be due to ↑in other blood components eg proteins

Hypervolemic hypotonic ↓Na

Euvolemic hypotonic ↓Na

Hypovolemic hypotonic ↓Na

→ 🔲 Measure *urine* sodium

Urine Na ≤20 mmol/L
- HF
- Cirrhosis
- Nephrotic syndrome

Urine Na >20 mmol/L
- Chronic renal failure

Urine Na >20 mmol/L
→ 🔲 Measure *urine* osmolality

Urine Na ≤20 mmol/L
Non-renal Na losses

Urine Na >20 mmol/L
Renal Na losses

Addison's or adrenal insufficiency: ↓cortisol & ↓aldosterone. ↑loss of Na (→↑loss of water), ↓BP

High urine osmolality
- SIADH (←)
- Medications

Variable urine osmolality
- Prolonged exercise
- High fluid intake

Low urine osmolality
- Potomania
- 1' polydipsia

- GI (vomiting, diarrhea)
- Urinary (diuretics, ↓aldosterone)
- Skin (burns, exudative lesions)
- Sequestration into third space (severe pancreatitis, crush injuries)
- Bleeding

Hypervolemic hypotonic hyponatraemia with normal urine Na
- ∴ fluid overload state eg HF, cirrhosis
- generally kidney function is preserved, therefore normal urine Na

Hypervolemic hypotonic hyponatraemia with ↑ urine Na
- fluid overload state with loss of kidney function (CKD)

Beer drinker's potomania arises from drinking >6L beer/d w/ poor dietary intake (usually s/smx ALD) → fluid overload, ↓renal function and no electrolytes to pee out

1' polydipsia: ↑fluid intake → dilutional hypoNa and dilution of urine. ?↑urine Na ∴ body is trying to excrete fluid.

Urgent considerations

Rapid Na decrease can lead to **cerebral edema**, CNS smx (HA, cramps, ataxia, psychosis, lethargy, apathy, anorexia, agitation) → ❗ can progress to coma, brainstem herniation, respi arrest, death.
Mx: Hypertonic saline (3%) 1-2 mL/kg/h, aim to ↑Na > 120 mM. If more aggressive replc needed, 4-6 mL/kg/h.
- Furosemide also given to prevent volume overload and ↑BP

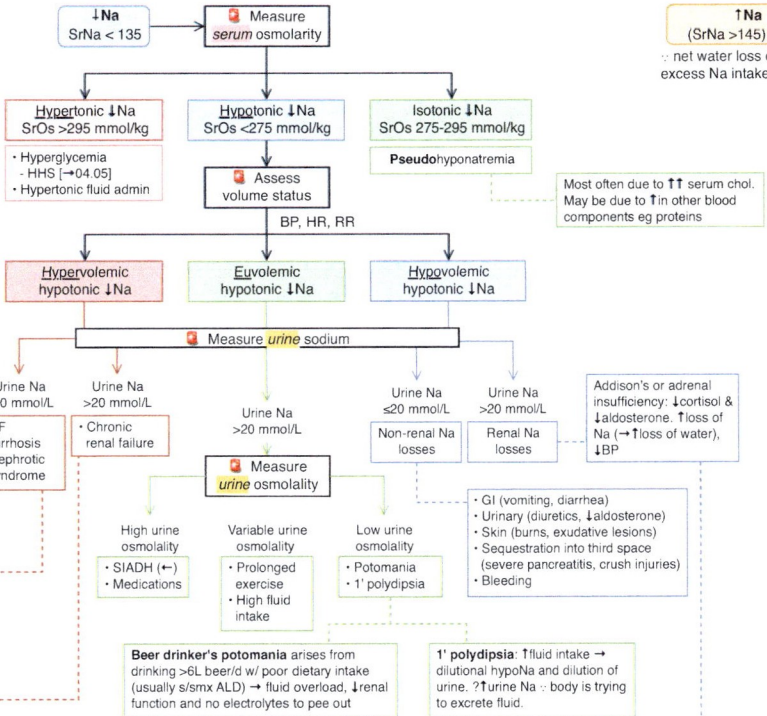

Adrenal crisis presents with weakness, postural hypotension, fatigue, ± hypovolemic shock.
Mx: IVF, glucocorticoid replacement
DO NOT delay treatment

Cerebral salt-wasting syndrome & SIADH (2/2 head injury, intracranial surgery, SAH, stroke, tumours).
If asmx, water restriction.
Smx, Na replacement.

From high to low, your brains will blow (cerebral edema)
From low to high, your pons will die (central pontine myelinosis)

Urine Na - tests for renal function
- ≤20 mmol/L indicates that kidneys kidneys are able to retain Na 💧
- >20 mmol/L may indicate acute tubular necrosis

Rapid Na increase can lead to **central pontine myelinolysis** (aka osmotic demyelination syndrome)
- In hypotonicity, astrocytes lose intra-cellular solutes to shed excess water and maintain isotonicity with plasma
- This causes the brain to "shrink" in size
- Rapid correction of hypoNa can cause the brain to shrink even further as water is given up to maintain isotonicity
  → This causes demyelination.
- Smx and +ve MRI scan may not be seen for as long as 4w after disease onset, therefore high degree of suspicion needed

Acute kidney injury AKI

D: acute decline in kidney function
According to KDIGO, defined as
- ↑SCr ≥26.5 μmol/L in 48h, or
- ↑SCr ≥1.5x baseline in last 7d
- UO <0.5 mL/kg/h for 6h

Further ÷ according to stages
1. ↑SCr ≥26.5 μmol/L, or
   ↑SCr 1.5-1.9x baseline, or
   UO <0.5 mL/kg/h for 6-12h
2. ↑SCr 2.0-2.9x baseline, or
   UO <0.5 mL/kg/h for ≥12h
3. ↑SCr ≥3x baseline, or
   ↑SCr ≥353.6 μmol/L, or
   UO <0.3 mL/kg/h for ≥24h, or
   UO = 0 (anuria) for ≥12h, or
   Initiation of RRT, or
   In pts <18yo, eGFR <35 mL/min

SCr = serum creatinine

A ÷ pre, intrinsic, post renal causes
- Pre-renal causes
  - ❗ hypovolaemia (eg dehydration,
    shock, diarrhoea)
  - renal artery stenosis
- Intrinsic renal disorders
  - glomerulonephritis
  - acute tubular necrosis →next pg
    ↳ 45% cases (eg 2/2 sepsis)
  - acute interstitial nephritis →next pg
  - rhabdomyolysis (eg fall + long lie)
  - tumour lysis syndrome
- Post-renal causes
  - kidney stones in ureter/bladder
  - benign prostatic hyperplasia
  - external compression of ureter

R: ↑age, underlying kidney disease (eg
diabetic nephropathy), hospitalisation for
various causes (15% inpatients develop
AKI), drugs (eg NSAIDs, amino-
glycosides, ACEIs, ARBs, diuretics)

S/smx: · may be asmx until late
- Usually picked up on routine bloods or
  when ↓UO
- Pulmonary & peripheral oedema
- Arrythmias 2/2 electrolyte disturbances
- Features of uraemia, eg encepha-
  lopathy, pericarditis

Ix:
- Bloods: U&Es
- Urinalysis (consider intrinsic cause if
  +ve blood & protein; consider infxn if
  +ve nitites, leukocytes)
- UO (?pts ideally on catheter to ensure
  accurate measurements)
- Imaging: renal US if no identifiable
  cause or if judged to be at risk of
  urinary tract obstruction

Mx: "STOP AKI"
Sepsis - screen & treat
Toxins - identify and stop
- Stop as the worsen renal function:
  NSAIDs (except baby aspirin), amino-
  glycosides, ACEI, ARBs, diuretics
- Stop as AKI ↑risk of toxicity: metformin,
  lithium, digoxin
Optimise vol status and BP
- IV crystalloid 500 mL bolus over 15 min
  (caution in HF, cirrhosis, etc)
- Withhold antihypertensives
- Pt may require inotropes
Prevent harm
- Tx reversible causes (eg obstruction)
- Tx life-threatening complications
- Modify doses of meds

Renal replacement therapy (RRT)
"AEIOU" indications
- Acidosis (pH <7.1)
- Electrolyte imbalance, eg K>6.5
- Intoxication ("SLIME" - salicylates,
  lithium, isopropanol, methanol,
  ethylene glycol) ± drug overdose
- Overload ± pulmonary oedema
- Uraemia (pericarditis, encephalopathy,
  end organ failure)

Mx of hyperkalaemia
- Cardiac protection with IV calcium
  chloride or calcium gluconate + ECG
- IV insulin/glucose + salbutamol neb
- (see notes on hyperkalaemia)

Chronic kidney disease CKD

D: abnormal kidney structure or function
≥3mo

By definition this includes pts who only have
one kidney (eg kidney donors)

A: · diabetic nephropathy
- hypertension
- chronic glomerulonephritis
- chronic pyelonephritis
- adult polycystic kidney disease
- (others)

÷ into 6 grades by GFR
G1. GFR >90 mL/min with evidence of
    kidney damage (eg histopathology,
    on imaging, on lab findings)
G2. 60-89 mL/min
G3a. 45-59 mL/min
G3b. 30-44 mL/min
G4. 15-29 mL/min
G5 (end stage). GFR <15

÷ by albumin to creatinine ratio (ACR)
↳ albumin and creatinine measured in
  urine. Albumin is not normally excreted
  in urine (∴ ↑ACR indicates severity)
A1. ACR <3 mg/mmol
= normal or mildly increased
A2. ACR 3-30 mg/mmol
= moderately increased
A3. >30 mg/mmol = severe

Note: protein:creatinine ratio is also used to
monitor kidney function, but ACR is preferred
in diabetics

S/smx: · asmx early on, picked up on
         routine bloods
- unspecific s/smx - lethargy, anorexia
  (wt loss), insomnia, NV
- in later stage kidney failure, pts can
  develop anaemia, pruritus (2/2 uraemia)

Ix: · bloods (U&Es)
- Urinalysis + ACR/PCR
- Imaging ± biopsy

Mx:
1. Slow progression
- Optimise DM control
- Optimise HTN control
  - ACEI or ARB
    ↳ can cause small ↓GFR (≤↓25% ok)
  - SGLT2 inhibitors - evidence of benefit
    in reducing progression; dapaglifozin
    only for now
    ↳ furosemide (esp when GFR ≤45
      mL/min; also helps ↓K)
- Tx glomerulonephritis

2. ↓risk of complications
- Exercise, wt loss, stop smoking
- Dietary advice
  - control dietary sodium intake esp
- Atorvastatin 20 mg for 1' prevention of
  cardiovascular disease

3. Treat complications
- Mineral bone disease Mx
- Anaemia Mx

4. End stage renal disease
- Renal replacement therapy
- Renal transplant
- At ESRD, if pt does not receive RRT,
  their average life expectancy is ~6mo

Mineral bone disease
- Pathophysiology
  - CKD → ↓vit D activation → ↓Ca
  - CKD → ↓excretion of PO4
  - ↑PO4 also causes bone degradation
    (osteomalacia)
  - 2ndary hyperparathyroidism [→06.03]
- Normalise PO4 levels
  - ↓PO4 in diet
  - PO4 binders (eg sevelamer)
    ↳ avoid calcium based binders as
      they can cause hyperCa and
      vascular calcification
- Normalise vit D levels
  - Supplementation: alfacalcidol
- Normalise PTH levels
  - parathyroidectomy if severe

CKD-related anaemia
- Pathophysiology
  - CKD → ↓erythropoietin → ↓RBC
    production ∴ anaemia
  - CKD → ↓absorption of iron
  - Causes a normochromic normocytic
    anaemia (normal Hb, just fewer RBC)
  - Can lead to left ventricular
    hypertrophy
- Mx: target Hb 10-12 g/dL
  - ❖ iron supplementation to optimise
    iron levels
  - if no improvement, offer EPO-
    analogues (eg darbepoietin)
  - pts may need blood transfusions

Renal replacement therapy (RRT)

Haemodialysis
- Pt is hooked up to machine which
  "cleans" the blood
- Usually required 3x/week, each
  session lasts 3-5h
- Access routes: arteriovenous fistula,
  graft or central venous catheter

Peritoneal dialysis
- Filtration occurs in pt's abdomen
- Requires insertion of PD catheter
  (surgically), via which pt can insert
  and drain PD fluid
- Continuous ambulatory PD - each
  exchange lasts 30-40 min, and the
  dwell time of fluid is 4-8h. It can go
  about normal activities while the
  dialysis solution is in their abdomen
- Automated PD - pt is hooked up to
  machine that fills and drains
  abdomen overnight

Renal transplant
- Kidney from live or deceased donor –
  usually placed in the right or left iliac
  fossa and attached to external iliac
  vessels
  ↳ native kidneys remain
- Requires life long immunosuppression to prevent rejection
- Lifespan of donor kidney is ~10-15y

Acute tubular necrosis

D: necrosis of the renal tubular epithelial cells resulting in AKI – usually reversible if identified and treated early on

Causes ÷ ischaemia & nephrotoxins
- Ischaemic: shock, sepsis
- Toxins: aminoglycosides, myoglobin 2/2 rhabdomyolysis, contrast dyes, lead

Injury to epithelial cells causes detachment of the basement membrane and tubular dysfunction.

S/smx: • Oliguria / anuria
- Hypotension   • ↑HR
- Other non-specific smx, eg thirst, malaise, anorexia, etc

Ix: U&Es (deranged), urine dip – muddy brown casts

Mx: • Treat underlying cause
- IV fluid boluses
- 3 phases: oliguric phase, polyuric phase, recovery phase

Acute interstitial nephritis

D: a pattern of AKI, localised to the kidney tubulo-interstitial space and usually triggered by medications

A: drugs - esp abx (penicillin, rifampicin), NSAIDs, allopurinol, furosemide
Systemic disease - SLE, sarcoidosis, Sjogren's syndrome
Infxns: Hanta virus, Staphylococci

P: histology: marked interstitial oedema and interstitial infiltrate in the connective tissue between renal tubules

S/Smx: • fever, rash, arthralgia, HTN
- FBC: eosinophilia
- mild renal impairment

Ix: monitor SrCr regularly, find underlying cause

Mx
- Accurate fluid balance monitoring (eg daily weights, UO chart)
- Monitor U&Es daily
- Review medications
- Ix and treat underlying cause
- Supportive therapy - O2, fluids, etc
- Uro referral if required

Diabetic nephropathy

D: • albuminuria (↑urinary excretion of albumin ≥30mg/g)
- progressive ↓eGFR
- against background of DM (T1/2)
- usually with retinopathy

A/P: • metabolic Δ (↑glucose, ↑lipids)
- haemodynamic Δ (HTN)
- → both promote ↑inflammation, endothelial dysf, oxidative stress, fibrosis, glomerular hyperfiltration
- Glomerular mesangium expansion due to ↑glucose, ↑glomerular pressure
- Glomerular sclerosis and fibrosis

R: sustained ↑BGC, HTN, FHx of HTN & CKD, obesity, smoking

Screening: all pts should be screened annually using urinary albumin:creatinine ratio (ACR)
- early morning specimen
- ACR > 2.5 = microalbuminuria

S/smx like oedema and retinopathy will show only when kidney disease becomes severe.

Mx: • dietary protein restriction
- tight glycaemic control
- BP control: aim for <140/90 mmHg
- ACEI or ARB
  ↳ start when urinary ACR ≥3
- control dyslipidaemia (statins, etc)

P: DKD a/w worsening of proteinuria, earlier complications, worse performance on dialysis. Other complications a/w DM

Lupus nephritis

D: severe manifestation of systemic lupus erythematosus (SLE)

A/P: type III hypersensitivity (immune complex formation 2/2 IgG abs to dsDNA and nuclear proteins)
In LN, immune complexes are deposited in the kidneys and cause inflammation

S/smx: fever, oedema, HTN, athralgia, myalgia, malar rash, frothy urine

Ix: bloods (FBC, UEs, ESR, ANA, anti-Smith, anti-dsDNA, complement levels), biopsy + histology

WHO classification
class I: normal kidney
class II: mesangial GN
class III: focal/segmental proliferative GN
class IV: diffuse proliferative GN
class V: diffuse membranous GN
class VI: sclerosing GN

Class IV (diffuse proliferative GN)
- Most common, most severe
- Microscopy
  ↳ glomeruli shows endothelial and mesangial proliferation, 'wire-loop' appearance
  ↳ capillary wall may be thickened 2/2 immune complex deposition
- Electron microscopy: subendothelial immune complex deposits
- Immunofluorescence: granular

Mx: • control HTN
- glucocorticoids + mycophenolate or cyclophosphamide
- Then, mycophenolate > azathioprine
  ↳ less risk of developing ESRD

ANCA glomerulonephritis

GN a/w
- granulomatosis with polyangiitis (Wegener's)
- eosinophilic granulomatosis with polyangiitis (Churg-Strauss)
- microscopic polyangiitis
- renal-limited vasculitis
→ immune complex deposition

A/P: (1) Neutrophil priming
(2) Neutrophil activation
(3) Acute inflammation, necrosis
(4) Chronic inflammation, scarring

S/Smx of renal disease: haematuria and proteinuria

Ix: AKI (↑SrCr), ANCA testing, biopsy + histology

Mx: steroids, immunosuppresant (eg MTX), supportive care. ± IVIG

→ ___ rheum

Myeloma kidney

- 50% of MM pts will have kidney disease, a/w poorer prognosis
- monoclonal production of Igs → light chain deposition within the renal tubules
- ∴ renal damage: presents as dehydration and increasing thirst
- other causes of renal impairment in myeloma: amyloidosis, nephro-calcinosis, nephrolithiasis
- Bence Jones proteins in urine

Mx: treat underlying cancer, renal replacement therapy

	A/P	Presentation	Examples
Nephritic syndrome	Glomerular inflm → GBM damage → loss of RBCs into urine → dysmorphic RBCs, haematuria	• Haematuria • RBC casts in urine • ↓GFR → oliguria, azotemia • Proteinuria (<3.5g/d usually, may be higher if severe)	• GN a/w infections • Goodpasture • IgA nephropathy • Alport syndrome • Membrano-proliferative GN
Nephrotic syndrome	Podocyte damage → impaired charge barrier → proteinuria	• Proteinuria (>3.5g/d) • Oedema, hypoalbunaemia • ↑hepatic lipogenesis • Hypercholesterol • Frothy urine with fatty casts • A/w hypercoagulable state	1' or 2' • Focal segmental GN • Minimal change [→15.10] • Membranous nephropathy • Amyloidosis • Diabetic GN
Mixed	Severe GBM damage → loss of RBCs and proteins into urine	• Proteinuria (>3.5g/d) • Haematuria • Mixed features	Most common a/w • Diffuse proliferative GN • Membrano-proliferative GN

Urinary tract infection: infection of the kidneys, bladder or urethra

Infectious cystitis

D: Infxn of the bladder
- Complicated: UTIs in pts with functional or structural impairments that reduce efficacy of abx therapy, or involvement of kidneys, ≥2 occurring during pregnancy
- Recurrent: ≥2 separate culture-proven episodes of acute UTIs and a/w smx within 6mo, or >3 UTIs in 12mo

R: F>M. Hx of UTI, urinary catheter, anatomical or functional abn in UTI, frequent sexual intercourse, DM, spinal cord injuries, pregnancy, immunosupp

A: 80% E.coli. Others - *Staph. saprophyticus, Kleb. pneumoniae*, etc

P: Bacteria usually ascends the UTI ± stasis of bladder urine impairs defence

S/Smx:
- **<65yo: dysuria, new nocturia, cloudy-looking urine**
- **≥65yo:** new onset of dysuria with ≥2 of the following
  - fever within last 12h
  - new frequency / urgency
  - new incontinence
  - new or worsening delirium
  - new suprapubic pain
  - new haematuria
  - **!** think SEPSIS
- ► fever, loin/back pain, N/V, renal angle tenderness on exam

Ix: ⚡ urine dipstick +ve for leukocytes and nitrites
- *DO NOT* routinely urine dip for ≥65yo or those with catheters (almost always positive anyway)
  - Dip is for elderly (to get sensitivities guiding treatment)
- Urine MC&S (for complicated or recurrent UTI, or haematuria)
- Imaging (US or CT) to look for structural abnormalities

Mx:
- **Non-complicated**
  - ⚡ Nitrofurantoin / trimethoprim 3d
  - Symptomatic Mx (eg paracetamol)
  - Pt education - Drink lots of water
    - Pee after sex
- **In pregnant women**
  - ⚡ Nitrofurantoin (except in near term) x 7d course
  - Amoxicillin or cefalexin
  - **!** Trimethoprim CI (teratogenic)
  - Requires test of cure
- **In males**
  - ⚡ Nitrofurantoin / trimethoprim 7d
  - Do not routinely refer to urology
- **≥65yo and those with catheters**
  - Urine dip does not guide tx
  - ***Tx only if symptomatic***
  - Remove/replace catheter
  - Abx for 7d

Pyelonephritis

D: severe infectious inflammatory disease of the renal parenchyma, calices, and pelvis

R: UTI, DM, stress incontinence, foreign body, anatomical abn, frequent sex, immunosuppression, pregnancy

A/P: causative agents similar to UTIs. Acute uncomp pyelonephritis usually 2/2 ascending UTI. Haematological seeding of kidneys in pts with bacteraemia.

S/Smx: flank pain, tenderness at costovertebral angle, flu-like smx, fever, N/V. Rapid development of smx (within 1d).

Ix: urine dipstick, urine C&S (≥100k CFU/mL), FBC, ESR/CRP, U&Es, blood culture (15-30% bacteraemic)

Mx:
- Uncomplicated: cefalexin 7-10d, adjust based on MC&S
- Analgesia as needed
- Pt education: drink lots of water
- Complicated: consider admitting; may need IV abx ± ↑support

Chronic pyelonephritis
- Definitive dx based on histology, but biopsies are rare
- Presumptive clinical dx: vesicoureteral reflux or prior surgery for obstruction or recurrent UTIs + imaging studies
- Tx underlying cause; may require nephrectomy ± abx

Epididymitis

D: inflammation of the epididymis. Acute ≤6w. Referred to as epididymo-orchitis if concurrent inflammation of testis.

R: unprotected sex, bladder outflow obstruction, catheter, etc

A/P: depends on risk factors. MSM usually STI; older males usually UTI. Retrograde infection from urethra and bladder likely.

S/Smx:
- unilateral scrotal pain
- swelling of gradual onset
- tenderness, hot, erythematous swollen hemiscrotum

Ix: urethral swab, urine dipstick, urine microscopy, C&S, NAAT for *Chlamydia* and *Neisseria*

Mx: Abx depending on suspected causative agent
- ?STI: ceftriaxone 500 mg IM (one dose) + doxycycline 100 mg bds for 10-14d
- ?UTI: empirical tx with PO fluoro-quinolone (eg ofloxacin)
- Supportive measures as needed

Prostatitis

D: inflammation of the prostate, usually a/w recent/ongoing bacterial infection

R: UTI, BPH, catheter, procedure

A/P: usually ascending infection, similar causative agents as cystitis (*E. coli*)

S/Smx:
- Lower urinary tract smx (LUTS)
- ± systemic signs, eg fever, malaise
- ± referred pain to genitalia, perineum, lower back, suprapubis
- ? more common <50 yo
- DRE: tender, boggy prostate gland

LUTS

Storage smx: frequency, urgency, nocturia, incontinence	
Voiding smx: weak stream, dribbling, dysuria, straining	

Ix: **!** urine dipstick - +ve for leuks & nitrites. urine C&S. blood culture (required for pts who are febrile)

Mx: PO quinolone (eg ciproflox) x14d, NSAIDs, relief of obstruction ± sepsis 6

Balanoposthitis

D: inflammation of the glans penis and prepuce. Balantitis = inflammation of the glans penis

R: congenital or acq dysfunctional foreskin, uncircumcised state, poor hygiene, over-washing, HPV

S/smx: broadly ÷ inflammatory, infective and pre-cancerous
- **Candidiasis:** after sex, a/w itching, white, non-urethral discharge
- Contact or allergic **dermatitis** - itchy ± painful ± a/w clear non-urethral discharge
- **Eczema or psoriasis** - very itchy, hx of inflammatory skin conditions elsewhere
- **Bacterial** (*Staph*) - painful ± itch, yellow non-urethral discharge
- **Anaerobic** - ± itchy, a/w very offensive yellow non-urethral discharge
- **Lichen planus** - ± itchy. Wickham's striae, violaceous papules
- **Circinate balanitis** - not itchy, not a/w discharge. Painless erosions, a/w reactive arthritis
- **Lichen sclerosus** - ± itchy, a/w white plaques, scarring
- Plasma cell **balanitis of Zoon** - not itchy, clearly circumscribed areas of inflammation

Not itchy: circinate balanitis, Zoon balanitis
Discharge - white: candidiasis
- Clear: contact/allergic dermatitis
- Yellow: bacterial, anaerobic (smelly)

Ix: Swab for MCS, virology

Mx: gentle saline washes, wash under foreskin; 1% hydrocortisone for itch
- Candidiasis: topical clotrimazole for 2w
- Bacterial: PO flucox / clarithromycin
- Anaerobic - top / PO metronidazole
- Dermatitis, circinate balanitis: low potency topical steroid (hydrocort)
- Lichen sclerosus, Zoon balanitis: high potency topical steroid (clobetasol) ± circumcision

Urinary tract stones

D: presence of crystalline stones (calculi) within the urinary system (kidneys and ureter)

R: dehydration, medullary sponge kidney, polycystic kidney disease, beryllium or cadmium exposure
Drugs that ↑risk of Ca stones: loop diuretics, steroids, acetazolamide, theophylline

S/smx:
· ureteric/renal colic – **severe, intermittent, stabbing pain** radiating from **loin to groin**
  ↳ pt is unable to keep still due to pain
· **haematuria** (usually microscopic)
· systemic smx, eg NV, ↑HR, fever
· loin/renal angle tenderness
· iliac fossa tenderness

Ix: urine dip + culture, bloods (U&Es, FBC, CRP), Ca and urate levels.
Imaging: <mark>non-contrast CT KUB</mark> in all pts within 14h of admission

Mx: · Analgesia (diclofenac PR/IM)
· Antiemetic (metoclopramide)
· IV fluid resus
· Mx of stones ≤5mm: watchful waiting (usually pass within 4w of smx onset)
· Mx of more severe stones:
  - shock wave lithotripsy
  - percutaneous nephrolithotomy
  - uretoscopy   - open surgery
· Mx of ureteric obstruction:
  ! Emergency – nephrostomy tube, ureteric catheters or stents

Shock wave lithotripsy
· Shock wave is generated outside
· Internally, cavitation bubbles and mechanical stress → fragmentation
· Risks – solid organ injury, ureteric obstruction
· Requires analgesia during and after
· For most pts with stone burden of <2 cm in aggregate

Ureteroscopy
· For pts in whom above is CI (eg pregnancy)
· Usually a stent is left for 4w post-procedure

Calcium oxalate 85%		R: Hypercalciuria, hyperoxaluria, hypocitraturia (∵ citrate forms complexes with Ca making it more soluble)
	Variable	· radio-opaque stones · Hyperuricosuria may cause uric acid stones to which calcium oxalate binds
Cystine 1%		Inherited recessive disorder of transmembrane cystine transport leading to ↓absorption of cystine from intestine and renal tubule
	Acidic to normal	· Multiple stones may form · Relatively radiodense (∵ may contain sulphur)
Uric acid 5-10%		R: gout, ↑purine diet (∵ purine metabolism → precipitate at low urinary pH); high cell turnover rate (malignancy); ileostomy (∵ urine becomes more acidic) inborn errors of metabolism
	Acidic	· Radiolucent
Calcium phosphate 10%		R: RTA types 1 and 3 (↑urinary pH → supersat of urine w Ca, PO4) · Radio-opaque stones (≈ bone) Urine pH: normal - alkaline
Struvite 2-20%		= Mg, ammonium and PO4 → made and ppt under alkaline conditions ∵ a/w urease-producing
	Alkaline	bacteria (∵ a/w chronic infections) · Slightly radio-opaque · Staghorn calculi: renal pelvis + ≥2 calyces. 2/2 Ureaplasma urealyticum and Proteus infxns

· **Prevention of Ca stones:** ↑water intake, ↓animal protein, ↓salt, ± thiazide diuretics
· Prevention of **oxalate stones**
  - Cholestyramine & pyridoxine
· Prevention of **uric acid stones**
  - Allopurinol
  - Urinary alkalinisation - bicarb

Percutaneous nephrolithotomy
· Access to renal collecting system
· Intra-corporeal lithotripsy or stone fragmentation is performed
· Stone fragments removed
· Reserved for complex renal calculi and staghorn calculi

Benign prostatic hyperplasia BPH

D: lower urinary tract smx (**LUTS**) caused by bladder obstruction due to prostate enlargemt (transitional zone). | R: >50yo |

A: hyperplasia of epithelial and stromal compartments.
P: · Static component: ↑tissue causes narrowing of urethral lumen
· Dynamic component: ↑prostatic smooth muscle tone mediated by α-receptors

LUTS

Storage smx: frequency, urgency, nocturia, incontinence

Voiding smx: weak stream, dribbling, dysuria, straining

▶ ref to urology: · Haematuria
· Neurological disease (?neurogenic bladder)
· Hx of prior urological surgeries and urethral stricture
· Recurrent or persistent UTI,
· Retention / palpable bladder
· Renal impairment 2/2 BPH,
· Abnormal DRE   · abn PSA levels

Ix: · urine dipstick (normal)
· PSA (check limits according to age)
· International Prostate Symptom Score
· Voiding diary - volume and frequency
· ± US, CT/MRI, cystoscopy

PSA - serine protease enzyme produced by normal and malignant prostate epithelial cells
· Refer to urology if
  - 50-69yo: PSA ≥3 or abnormal DRE
  - >70yo: PSA ≥5 or abnormal DRE
· Raised PSA seen in BPH, prostatitis and UTIs (wait 1mo), ejaculation (48h), vigorous exercise (48h), urinary retention, instrumentation (catheters)
· **!** Poor sensitivity and specificity

IPSS: 7 Qs, scale 0 to 5. Incomplete emptying, frequency, intermittency, urgency, weak stream, straining, nocturia. ± QoL 0-6. Mild 0-7, mod 8-19, severe 20-35

Mx:
· Conservative: watchful waiting
  - lifestyle mods, eg ↓fluids at night, ↓caffeine & alc, Δ diuretics timing,
· Medical
  - α-blockers (doxazosin, tamsulosin)
  - 5α-reductase inhibitors (finasteride) esp for pts at risk of progression,
  - PDE-5 inhibitors (sildenafil) to improve LUTS, ED and QoL
  - anticholinergics (tolterodine)
· Surgical - ref to urologists if complications 2/2 BPH (renal insufficiency, recurrent bladder stones, etc), &/or refractory response to meds → transurethral resection of prostate (TURP)

TURP syndrome
· life-threatening complication of TURP
· 2/2 large volumes of glycine used as irrigation fluid, which are absorbed systemically when prostatic venous sinuses are opened during prostate resection
  - hyponatraemia
  - breakdown of glycine causing hyperammonia and visual changes
· S/smx
  - appear 15 min to 24h post-op
  - Respi: distress, hypoxia, pulmonary oedema
  - GI: NV
  - Visual disturbances, eg blindness
  - Neuro: confusion, seizures, coma
  - AKI
  - Reflex bradycardia
· Mx: treat underlying cause (eg stop surgery). Other Mx is symptomatic
  - resus (ABC)
  - fluid overload: furosemide
  - seizures: benzodiazepines
  - hyponatraemia: if severe, use hypertonic saline

Cryptorchidism

→ 15.11

Erectile dysfunction ED

D: inability to achieve or maintain an erection satisfactory for sexual intercourse

· **Psychogenic:** Anxiety, depression.
· **Drugs:** SSRIs, β-blockers, recreational drugs, tobacco, alcohol
· Vascular: Hyperchol, atheroma, DM
· Metabolic/endrocine: Azotaemia, hypogonadism, hyperthyroidism, hyperprolactinaemia
· Neurological: Parkinson's disease, stroke/TIA, spinal injury, neurological damage following pelvic surgery, pelvic fracture, autonomic neuropathies
· Penile: Cavernositis, Peyronie's disease, previous priapism

S/smx
· Presence of morning erections strongly suggests psychogenic cause
· Small testicles, lack of sexual 2ndary characteristics - endocrine cause
· Lack of LL pulses - vascular cause
· Neuro deficits in S2-4 - neuro cause

Ix: bloods (glucose, lipids, U&Es, **free testosterone**, FSH/LH, prolactin, thyroid) Dynamic cavernosometry to look for venous/arterial cause ± angiography

Free testosterone - measure btwn 9 to 11 am. Measure for all men w/ ED.

Mx:
· Psychotherapy or specialist sexual counselling for psychogenic causes
· PO PDE5 inhibitors: -afils, eg sildenafil (Viagra, "little blue pill")
· Apomorphine sublingual
· Intracavernosal—prostaglandins, α-blockers, papaverine
· ?? people with ED who cycle for >3h/w should be advised to stop
· Refer young men who have always had difficulty achieving an erection to urology

Peyronie's disease: fibrous tissue in the penis leading to curvature during erection. A/w Duputyren's contracture

Renal cell carcinoma

D: renal malignancy arising from the renal parenchyma/cortex - 90% of kidney cancers, 2% of all cancers

R: smoking, M>F (3:1), >55yo, black/ American-Indian, obesity, HTN, FHx, Hx of hereditary syndromes (VHL, tuberous sclerosis) and acq renal cystic disease

VHL = von Hippel-Lindau syndrome

S/smx
- **Haematuria, loin pain, abd mass**
- Fever of unknown origin
- Endocrine: ↑EPO, PTH, renin, ACTH
- Paraneoplastic hepatic dysfunction syndrome
- Varicocele - L sided, nutcracker syndrome (compression of L renal vein)
- Stauffer syndrome
  - cholestasis / hepatosplenomegaly
  - paraneoplastic syndrome 2/2 ↑IL6

Ix: • Bloods (FBC, U&Es, etc)
- CTTAP pre- and post-IV contrast – enhanced CT → to see size, local extent, invasion, mets
- If evidence of bony mets, isotope bone scan

TMN staging
T1 = tumour ≤ 7cm, confined
T2 = tumour >7cm, confined to kidney
T3 = extends into major veins, invades adrenal gland or perinephric tissue.
T4 = extends beyond Gerota fascia or distant mets

Mx: surgery - partial if T1 tumour, otherwise total nephrectomy
- trials – α-interferon and IL2, receptor tyrosine kinase inhibitors
- Need to manage **anaemia** also

P: adverse risk factors - extracapsular spread, invasion of renal vein, LN involvement. Periodic radiological follow up recommended in most cases.

Bladder cancers

Urothelial carcinoma = transitional cell carcinoma → 90% of cases
SCC → 1-7% cases
Adenocarcinoma → 2% cases

D: malignancy of the urinary bladder

R: **smoking**, exposure to **aromatic amines** in rubber and dye, arsenic (esp in painters and hairdressers), >65yo, pelvic radiation, systemic chemo, **schistosoma** infxn (esp in Arabic population; ↑risk of SCC), M>F (3:1), chronic bladder inflammation, FHx

S/smx: 85% **painless, frank haematuria**

Transitional cell carcinoma
- Solitary or multifocal
- 70% papillary growth pattern; superficial in location, better prognosis
- 30% mixed papillary and solid growth or pure solid growth; more prone to local invasion, worse prognosis

TMN staging
Ta = non-invasive papillary carcinoma
T1 = invades sub-epithelial connective tissue
T2a = invades superficial muscularis propia
T2b = invades deep muscularis propia
T3 = extends to perivesical fat
T4a = invades uterus, prostate or bowel
T4b = invades pelvic sidewall, abd wall

N1 = single regional LN in true pelvis
N2 = multiple regional LNs in true pelvis
N3 = met to common iliac LN

Ix: urinalysis (haematuria), staging - **cystoscopy**, biopsy, pelvic MRI, CTTAP, PET-CT for mets

Mx: trans-urethral resection of bladder tumour (TURBT) may be sufficient for superficial lesions
- + intravesical chemo.
- May require radical cystectomy and ileal conduit or radical radiotherapy

P: LN involvement ↓survival a lot. 5y survival: T3 ≈35%, T4a ≤25%.

Prostate cancer

D: malignancy of the glandular prostate

High-grade prostatic intraepithelial neoplasia → 95% adenocarcinomas
- 70% multifocal, in peripheral zone
- graded using **Gleason** grading system
- LN spread - obturator LN first

R: >50yo, ? black ethnicity, FHx

S/smx: • most often **asmx**
- ↑tumour size: LUTS, **haematuria**, **haematospermia**, pain (back, perineal, testicular)
- DRE - asymmetrical, hard, nodular enlargement with loss of median sulcus
- Mets - usually bony mets causing bone pain

Ix: 🔍 **multiparametric MRI**
- Results reported using 5-point **Likert scale**
  - ≥3 - offer prostate biopsy
  - 1-2 - consider (discuss with pt)
- Complications of transrectal US guided (TRUS) biopsy: sepsis 1%, pain (≥2w in 15%, severe in 7%), fever 5%, haematuria, rectal bleeding

PSA - needs cautious interpretation
- Can be raised by
  - BPH   - urinary retention
  - Prostatitis & UTI (4w)
  - Ejaculation (48h)
  - Vigorous exercise (48h)
  - Instrumentation of urinary tract eg catheters
  - DRE
- Poor sensitivity and specificity for prostate cancer

Mx of **localised cancer** (T1/T2): watchful waiting, radical prostectomy, RT

Mx of **localised advanced cancer** (T3/T4): hormonal therapy (anti-androgens), radical prostatectomy, RT

Mx of **metastatic cancer**: anti-androgen therapy
- Synthetic GnRH agonists, eg **goserelin** (↓LH, ↓testosterone)
  ↳ must be covered with anti-androgen initially to prevent tumour-flare
- Bicalutamide = non-steroidal anti-androgen - blocks androgen receptor
- Cyproterone acetate = steroidal anti-androgen; prevents DHT binding
- Abiraterone = androgen synthesis inhibitor; 2nd line

Other Mx options
- Bilateral orchidectomy
- Chemo with docetaxel

Other urological topics

	Inguinal hernia	Hydrocele	Varicocele	Epididymal cyst	Epididymo-orchitis	Testicular torsion	Testicular tumour
Definition	Protrusion of abdominal or pelvic contents through internal or external inguinal ring	Collection of serous fluid between layers of membrane that surrounds testis or along spermatic cord	Abnormal enlargement of internal spermatic veins and pampiniform plexus	Collection of fluid that develops within the lining (contained in its own sac)	Infxn of epididymis ± testes "male equivalent of pelvic inflammatory disease"	Urological emergency caused by twisting of the testicle on the spermatic cord. Can result in constriction of vascular supply, ischaemia and necrosis ! Surgical emergency	Malignancy of the testes – most common malignancy in males 20-34yo
A/P	· Indirect: persistent processus vaginalis · Direct: acquired weakness of abdo wall	· Communicating hydrocele – see indirect inguinal hernia · Simple: imbalance between secretion and reabsorption of fluid	? ↑temp, incompetent valves, ↑hydrostatic pressure, nutcracker phenomenon	?? mountain bikers	Local spread of infxn from GUT – *C. trachomatis* & *N gonorrhoea* (in younger pts), *E. coli* (in older pts)		Starts with carcinoma in situ – growth beyond basement membrane. Seminoma vs non-seminoma
Risk factors	M>F, ↑age, FHx, prematurity, anatomical defects, ↑abdo pressure (eg pregnancy)	Prematurity, low birth wt, ↑abdominal pressure, inflammation or injury to scrotum, cancer, etc	?? taller + thinner, FHx	A/w polycystic kidney disease, cystic fibrosis, VHL syndrome	Unprotected sex, bladder outflow obstruction, catheters	<25yo (peak 13-15yo), neonates, bell clapper deformity	Infertility (3x risk), crypt-orchidism, FHx, mumps, gonadal dysgenesis / atrophy, white ethnicity, HIV
Key features on O/E	· Usually painless unless strangulated/incarcerated · ❌ Cannot get above it · ± Cough impulse · ± Reducible · Located superior, medial to pubic tubercle · Disappears on pressure on when pt lies down	· Painless · ✅ Can get above it · Soft, fluctuant · Transilluminates	· Painless · Usually on left side · "Bag of worms" feeling · Sub/infertility	· Painless · ✅ Can get above it · Clear / opalescent fluid · Located above and behind testes – separate from body of testicle	· May be tender · Pain eased by elevating testes ! R/o testicular torsion	· Painful – sudden, severe onset, not eased by elevating testes (Prehn's sign) · Pain may be referred to lower abdo, a/w N&V · "High riding testicle" · Absent cremasteric reflex	· Painless · Discrete lesion(s) · Craggy and hard · ± Hydrocele · Gynaecomastia (due to ↑oestrogen:androgen ratio)
Ix	Clinical Dx	Clinical Dx ± US	Clinical Dx Consider semen analysis – infertility	Dx confirmed by US	· STI workup · Midstream urine MC&S	Clinical Dx + US ("whirlpool sign")	Doppler US, CXR, CTTAP, **β-HCG, AFP**, LDH, histology post-op
Mx	· Tx even if no smx · ✂ Mesh repair - unilateral hernia repaired with open approach - bilateral or recurrent – laparoscopy · ✂ Hernia truss (eg if pt cannot undergo surgery)	· If no smx, watchful waiting · If smx – surgery	· Reassurance + observation · Surgery for grade II or III varicocele (asymmetrical, >2cm3 or >20% difference)	· If no smx, watchful waiting · If smx – surgery	· Ceftriaxone 500 mg IM single dose + doxycycline 100 mg PO bds for 10-14d	· Analgesia, antiemetics, IVF · Urgent surgical exploration · Orchidopexy for both sides	· ✂ Inguinal (radical) orchidectomy + chemo + radiotherapy · ✂ Testis sparing surgery – only if limited disease
Prognosis	· Pts can return to light work after 2-3w · Bruising, wound infxn, chronic pain, recurrence	· Majority of simple hydroceles resolve within first 2y of life · Low rate of recurrence	Comp of surgery: testicular atrophy, hydrocele 50-80% chance of catch-up growth of affected testis	(no info)	Rapidly resolves with abx. Can cause infertility if not adequately tx (eg pt stops tx early)	· "Time is testicle" · Can recur if not fixed (therefore preemptively fix the other side)	· Main complication is infertility · Excellent 5y survival if in early stages

Investigate testicular lumps with ULTRASOUND

Anthrax

- 🦠 Gram +ve Bacillus anthracis
- 📧 From animals – usually infected carcasses (sheep)
- 👤 Farmers, abattoirs

Toxins: • protective antigen
- Oedema factor: ↑cAMP
- Lethal factor: toxic to macrophages

S/smx: • painless black eschar
- typically painless and non-tender
- ± marked oedema ± GI bleeding

Mx: 💊 ciprofloxacin
- Further tx – expert advice

Bacillus cereus

- 🦠 Gram +ve rod Bacillus cereus
- 📧 From food (classically reheated rice), soil, water
- 👤 ?immunocompromised

Food poisoning syndromes
- Emetic syndrome: ∴ heat-stable exotoxin cereulide. Onset 0.5-6h of ingestion ± diarrhoea
- Diarrhoeal syndrome: ∴ exotoxin haemolysin. Onset 8-16h. Crampy abdo pain and diarrhoea
- Smx resolve w/in 24h for both
Other issues in immunosupp pts:
- Bacteraemia   • Endocarditis
- MSK and CNS infections

Mx of food poisoning: w&w
Others: β-lactamase + vancomycin

Campylobacter

- 🦠 Gram-ve rod Campylobacter jejuni
- 📧 faecal-oral route – incubate 1-6d

S/smx: prodromal HA and malaise
- Diarrhoea – bloody :(
- Abdo pain mimicking appendicitis

Mx: • self-limiting w&w
- Tx if immunocompromised or severe
- 💊 **clarithromycin** 💊 ciprofloxacin

Comp: a/w GBS classically, reactive arthritis, septicaemia, endocarditis

Botulism

- 🦠 Gram +ve anaerobic Clostridium botulinum (serotypes A-G)
- 📧 contaminated food (tinned food, honey), IVDU

MOA: botulinum toxin is a neurotoxin which irreversibly blocks the release of ACh – affects bulbar muscles and ANS

S/smx: **flaccid** paralysis (floppy), diplopia, ataxia, bulbar palsy
** pt is usually fully conscious, no sensory disturbance

Mx: botulism antitox, supportive care
- Antitoxin is only useful if given early, once toxin binds to AChR it cannot be reversed

Cat scratch disease

- 🦠 Gram -ve Bartonella henselae
- 📧 cat   👤 homeless :(

S/smx: fever, regional lymphadeno-pathy, HA, malaise, ±abd pain

Mx of mild infxn: analgesia, w&w
Infxns requiring abx: erythromycin, doxycycline, azithromycin

Cholera

- 🦠 Gram -ve Vibrio cholerae
- 📧 Contaminated water, badly cooked seafood

S/smx: profuse "rice-water" diarrhea, dehdyration, hypoglycemia

Mx: ORS, doxycycline or ciprofloxacin

Clostridioides difficile *C. diff*

- 🦠 Gram +ve rod anaerobic, spore-forming, toxin-producing
- 📧 Hospitalisation / nursing home
- R: abx exposure (esp clindamycin, cephalosporins), PPI use

S/smx:
- diarrhoea – classically very smelly (if you know you know)
- abdominal pain
- if severe, toxic megacolon may develop

Dx/Ix: • WCC
- Stool sample: C. difficile toxin – diagnostic
- Blood culture not very useful – C. diff antigen only shows *exposure*

Public Health England severity scale
- Mild: normal WCC
- Moderate: ↑WCC (10-15 x10⁹)
   - typically 3-5 loose stools per day
- Severe: ↑WCC (>15 x10⁹)
   - acute ↑creatinine (>1.5x baseline)
   - temp >38.5°C
   - evidence of severe colitis (abdominal or radiological signs)
- Life-threatening: hypotension
   - Partial or complete ileus
   - Toxic megacolon
   - CT evidence of severe disease

Mx: • Review medicines used
- First episode
   - 💊 PO vancomycin x10d
   - 💊 PO fidaxomicin
   - 3rd-line: PO vanco ± IV metronidazole
- Recurrent episode
   - Within 12w of smx resolution: PO fidaxomicin
   - After 12w: PO vanco or fidaxomicin
- Life-threatening infxn
   - PO vancomycin and IV metronidazole
   - Specialist advice: surgery
- Other meds: bezlotoxumab, faecal microbiota transplant (consider if ≥2 previous episodes)
- Prevention: isolation in side room until no more episodes of diarrhoea for ≥48h + PPE + hand wash with soap (alcohol rub not useful)

Diphtheria

- 🦠 Gram+ve Corynebacterium diphtheriae
- 📧 Contaminated water
- 👤 Visitors to Eastern Europe, Russia, Asia
MOA: exotoxin inhibits protein synthesis

S/smx:
- Sore throat with 'diphtheric membrane' (grey, pseudomembrane on posterior pharyngeal wall)
- Bulky cervical lymphadenopathy
   ↳ "bull neck"
- Neuritis   • Heart block

Ix: culture of throat swab (Loeffler's media)

Mx: IM penicillin, diphtheria antitoxin

Escherichia coli

- 🦠 facultative anaerobic, lactose-fermenting, Gram-ve rod
- 📧 normal gut commensal

Antigen-O (lipopolysaccharide)
K (capsule): neonatal meningitis
H (flagellin)
E. coli O157:H7 – found in contaminated ground beef.
- Severe, haemorrhagic watery diarrhoea → haemolytic uraemic syndrome

Klebsiella

- 🦠 Gram -ve; part of normal gut flora

Klebsiella pneumonia
- aspiration, alcoholics, DM
- "red-currant" sputum
- often affects upper lobe

Prognosis:
- Commonly causes lung abscess formation and empyema
- Mortality 30-50%

Enteric fever (typhoid / paratyphoid)

- 🦠 aerobic G-ve Salmonella typhi and paratyphi (types A, B, C)
- 📧 Faecal-oral route (contaminated food and water). Check travel Hx.

S/smx: systemic (HA, fever, athralgia), abdo pain, distention
- Relative bradycardia
- Constipation: more common than diarrhoea in typhoid
- Rose spots on trunk in 40%, more common in paratyphoid (tends to be a late sign)

Complications:
- Osteomyelitis (esp in sickle cell)
- GI bleeding
- Meningitis   • Cholecystitis
- Chronic carriage (1%, F>M)

Haemophilus influenzae

- 🦠 Gram-ve cocci   📧 respi droplets

- CAP
- Most common cause of bronchiectasis exacerbations
- Acute epiglottitis (type B) →15.04
   - rapid onset, high fever
   - stridor, drooling + tripod position (leaning forward)
   - Dx: direct visualisation
      ↳ CXR lat view – thumb sign
   - Mx: immediate senior help ± endotracheal intubation
      • do NOT examine throat
      • supplemental O2   • IV abx

Legionella

- 🦠 intracellular Legionella pneumophilia
- 📧 AC systems, contaminated water

S/smx: flu-like smx (>95%), dry cough, relative bradycardia, confusion, lymphopaenia, **hypoNa**, deranged LFTs, pleural effusion (30%)

Ix: urinary antigen, CXR (mid/lower zone patchy consolidation, pleural effusion)

Mx: erythromycin or clarithromycin

Leptospirosis

aka Legionnaire's disease
- *Leptospira interrogans*
- Rat urine
- Sewage workers, farmers, vets, abattoir + travellers going to tropics

Early phase 2/2 bacteraemia
- Last around 1w
- Fever, flu-like smx
- Subconjunctival suffusion (redness), haemorrhage
Second phase 2/2 immune rxn
= Weil's disease
- AKI 50%
- Hepatitis: jaundice, hepatomegaly
- Aseptic meningitis

Ix: serology (antibodies develop in 7d), PCR, culture (less useful)

Mx: high-dose benzylpenicillin or doxycycline

Leprosy

- *Mycobacterium leprae*
- Person to person

Degree of cell-mediated immunity determines type of leprosy developed

↓ Lepromatous leprosy ("multibaciliary")
- Extensive skin involvement
  - butt, face, limb extensors
- Symmetric nerve involvement

↑ Tuberculoid leprosy ("paucibaciliary")
- Limited skin disease
- Hair loss
- Asym nerve involevment → hyperesthesia

Mx: rifampicin, dapsone, clofazimine

See 16.06 for **Listeria**

Lyme disease

- spirochaete *Borrelia burgdoferi*
- ticks

Early features
- erythema migrans (80%)
  - target / bullseye rash at site of tick bite
  - 1-4w after initial bite
  - usually painless, >5cm, slowly ↑size
- systemic features: HA, lethargy, fever arthralgia

Late features (>30d)
- CVS: heart block, peri/myocarditis
- Neurological: CN VII palsy, radicular pain, meningitis

Ix: clinically if +ve rash
  ELISA antibodies to *Borrelia burgdoferi*
- Repeat in 4-6 w and 12w
- Immunoblot test to confirm

Mx of asmx tick bites
- Remove tick with fine-tipped tweezers, grasping tick as close to skin as possible + wash
- Abx not recommended
Mx of confirmed Lyme
- Doxycycline   Amoxicillin
- If disseminated: ceftriaxone
- Jarisch-Herxheimer seen sometimes – fever, rash, tachycardia

Pseudomonas aeruginosa

- Gram-ve rod
MOA: endotoxin (fever, shock)
Exotoxin A (↓protein synthesis)

S/smx:
- Chest infxns esp in CF
- Skin: burns, wound infxns, 'hot tub' folliculitis
- Otitis externa, esp in diabetics
- UTIs

Mycoplasma pneumoniae

- younger pts

S/smx: gradual onset, prolonged
- Flu-like smx → dry cough
- Bilat consolidation

Complications
- Haemolytic anaemia 2/2 cold agglutinins (IgM)
- Thrombocytopaenia
- Erythema multiforme, erythema nodosum
- meningoencephalitis
- GBS and other immune-mediated neurological diseases
- bullous myringitis: painful vesicles on the tympanic membrane
- pericarditis/myocarditis
- GI: hepatitis, pancreatitis
- renal: acute glomerulonephritis

Ix: Mycoplasma serology, +ve cold agglutination test

Mx: doxycycline or macrolide (erythromycin, clarithromycin)

Q fever

- *Coxiella burnetii*
- cattle – abattoir, infected dust

S/smx:
- Prodrome: fever, malaise
- Transaminitis
- Atypical pneumonia
- Culture -ve endocarditis

Mx: doxycycline

Staphylococci

- Gram+ve cocci
  Facultative anaerobe
S. aureus
- Catalse +ve, coagulase +ve
- Skin infxns, abscesses, osteomyelitis, toxic shock syndrome
- S. aureus pneumonia tends to follow influenza (2ndary bacterial pneumonia)
S. epidermidis
- Coagulase -ve
- Central line infxns, IE

MRSA

- Screen all admitted pts – elective and emergency
- Swab: nasal, axilla, groin

Suppression from carrier
- Nose: mupirocin 2% in white soft paraffin, tds for 5d
- Skin: chlorhexidine gluconate, daily for 5d – apply all over, but esp to axillae, groin, perineum

Mx: vancomycin, teicoplanin, linezolid
Avoid ∴ resistance: rifampicin, macrolides, tetracyclines, aminoglycosides, clindamycin

Toxic shock syndrome

- S. aureus producing TSST-1 superantigen toxin

CDC Dx criteria
- T ≥ 39°C   · SBP <90 mmHg
- Diffuse erythematous rash
- Desquamation of rash, esp palms and soles
- Involvement of ≥3 organ systems, eg GI (diarrhoea), mucous membrane erythema, renal failure, hepatitis, thrombocytopaenia, CNS involvement (confusion)

Mx: · remove infection focus (eg retained tampon)
- IV fluids   · IV abx

Tetanus

- *Clostridium tetani* producing exotoxin tetanospasmin
- spores in soil → wound/ IVDU
MOA: tetanospasmin prevents release of GABA

S/smx:
- Prodrome: fever, lethargy, HA
- Trismus (lockjaw)
- Risus sardonicus: facial spasms
- Opisthotonus (arched back, hyperextended neck)
- Spasms (e.g. dysphagia)

Mx: supportive (incl ventilatory, muscle relaxants)
- IM human tetanus immunoglobulin (IG) for high-risk wounds
- Metronidazole
Vaccination
- Complete = 5 doses
- last dose <10y ago: no vaccine or IG required
- last dose >10y ago: booster
  ↳ high-risk: + immunoglobulin
- Hx incomplete or unknown
  - booster + IG

Other *Clostridia*

- *Clostridium perfringens*
- MOA: produces α-toxin (lecithinase)
- Causes gas gangrene and haemolysis
- S/smx: - tender, oedematous skin
  - haemorrhagic blebs and bullae
  - crepitus on palpation

- *Clostridium botulinum* [→08.01]
- MOA: prevents acetylcholine release, leading to flaccid paralysis

- *Clostridium difficile* [→08.01]
- (old name, now Clostridioides)
- MOA: produces exotoxin & cytotoxin, causing pseudomembranous colitis

Streptococcus

Strep pneumoniae 🦠 α-haemolytic (partial haemolysis)
· Causes pneumonia, meningitis, otitis media

🦠 β-haemolytic (full haemolysis)

Scarlet fever

🦠 *Strep. pyogenes* (GAS)
✉ Respi droplets, or direct contact with
  nose and throat discharge
⏱ 2-6yo, peak at 4y
MOA: erythrogenic toxin

S/smx: · incubates 2-4d
· Fever: 24-48h
· Malaise, HA, vomiting
· Sore throat
· Strawberry tongue
· Rash – "pinhead" rash esp seen in
  flexures
  - flushed appearance
  - "sandpaper" texture

Dx: clinical + throat swab

Mx: · PO penicillin V x 10d
· azithromycin or clarithromycin
· Children can go back to school 24h
  after starting abx
· ! notifiable !

Complications
· Otitis media
· Rheumatic fever: ~20d after infxn (type
  II HS) [→01.05]
· Acute glomerulonephritis: ~10d after
  infxn (type III HS)
· Invasive comp rare (bacteraemia),
  meningitis, necrotising fasciitis)

Centor criteria for sore throat
· **C**ervical lymphadenopathy
· **E**xudate (tonsillar)
· **N**o cough
· **T**emperature (fever)

Treat if 3-4 criteria met (32-56% of
isolating Strep)

see also Sore throat 13.05

Group B Strep

= *Streptococcus agalactiae*

📧 Mother to child
  - 20-40% mothers have GBS in their
    bowel flora
Risk factors for transmission
· Premature birth
· Prolonged rupture of membrane
· Previous sibling GBS infxn
· Maternal pyrexia

Mx: benzylpenicillin
· universal screening for all females
· GBS +ve in previous pregnancy:
  - risk of carriage in this pregnancy is
    50%
  - offer intrapartum abx prophylaxis (IAP)
  - *or* testing in late pregnancy
    ◊ test at 35-37w or 3-5w before
      anticipated delivery
    ◊ if +ve, abx
· Previous baby with early or late-onset
  GBS disease: offer IAP
· Preterm labour: offer IAP regardless of
  GBS status
· Pyrexia during labour: IAP

Notifiable diseases

1. Acute encephalitis
2. Acute infectious hepatitis
3. Acute meningitis
4. Acute poliomyelitis
5. Anthrax
6. Botulism
7. Brucellosis
8. Chikungunya virus
9. Cholera
10. COVID-19
11. Diphtheria
12. Enteric fever
13. Food poisoning
14. HUS
15. Infectious bloody diarrhoea
16. Invasive GAS
17. Legionnaires disease
18. Leprosy
19. Malaria
20. Measles
21. Meningococcal septicaemia
22. Mumps
23. Plague
24. Rabies
25. Rubella
26. SARS
27. Scarlet fever
28. Smallpox
29. Tetanus
30. Tuberculosis
31. Typhus
32. Viral haemorrhagic fever
33. Whooping cough
34. Yellow fever

Influenza vaccination

Children
· **Intranasal** vaccine
  - More effective than injectable vaccine
· First dose at 2-3yo, then annually
· Live vaccine

· Contraindications
  - Immunocompromised
  - <2yo - Current febrile illness
  - Current wheeze / Hx of severe asthma
  - Egg allergy
  - Child is taking aspirin

· Side effects
  - Blocked nose / rhinorrhea
  - HA   - Anorexia

Adults & at-risk groups
· Inactivated vaccine
  - 75% effective (less in elderly)
  - Effective 10-14d post-immunisation
· Trivalent – consists of 2 subtypes of
  influenza A and 1 subtype of flu B
· Store between 2-8°C, shield from light

· Recommended yearly for all >65yo and
  those >6mo if
  - Chronic respi disease (incl asthma)
  - Chronic heart disease (eg HF, HTN)
  - Chronic kidney disease
  - Chronic liver disease
  - Chronic neurological disease
  - DM   - Immunosuppression
  - Asplenia / splenic dysfunction
  - Pregnant women
  - Adults BMI ≥40
  - Health & social care staff + carers
  - Long-stay in residential care homes

· Side effects: fever, malaise ~1-2d

Vaccination schedule

Age	Vaccine	Dose
8w	Diphtheria	1/5
	Poliomyelitis	1/5
	Tetanus	1/5
	HiB	1/4
	Pertussis	1/4
	Hep B	1/3
	MenB	1/3
	Rotavirus	1/2
12w	Diphtheria	2/5
	Poliomyelitis	2/5
	Tetanus	2/5
	HiB	2/4
	Pertussis	2/4
	Hep B	2/3
	Pneumococcal conjugate	1/2
	Rotavirus	2/2
16w	Diphtheria	3/5
	Poliomyelitis	3/5
	Tetanus	3/5
	HiB	3/4
	Pertussis	3/4
	Hep B	3/3
	MenB	2/3
1y	MMR	1/2
	MenB	3/3
	Pneumococcal conjugate	2/2
	HiB	4/4
2-3y	Influenza	
40mo	Diphtheria	4/5
	Poliomyelitis	4/5
	Tetanus	4/5
	Pertussis	4/4
	MMR	2/2
11y	HPV	
13y	MenA, MenC	
	Diphtheria	5/5
	Poliomyelitis	5/5
	Tetanus	5/5
65y	Pneumococcal polysaccharide	
70-79y	Herpes zoster (live or recomb)	

GRAM POSITIVE [purple] | **GRAM NEGATIVE [pink]**

Cocci | Anaerobes | Cocci/coccobacilli | Bacilli

Columns:
- MRSA
- S. epidermidis (coag -ve Staph)
- MSSA
- Enterococcus
- Streptococcus
- Clostridium Peptostrep
- Bacteriodes Fusobacterium
- N. meningitidis
- H. influenzae
- Moraxella
- E.coli
- Klebsiella
- Proteus mirabilis
- Pseudomonas
- Eschappm organisms
- Legionella

Drug coverage bands:

- Penicillin (MSSA–Streptococcus)
- Penicillin (N. meningitidis)
- Amoxicillin (MSSA–Clostridium Peptostrep)
- Amoxicillin (H. influenzae)
- Flucloxacillin (S. epidermidis–MSSA)
- Flucloxacillin (Streptococcus)
- Macrolides (Legionella)
- Ticarcillin-clavulanate (MSSA–Pseudomonas area)
- Piperacillin-tazobactam
- Clindamycin (MRSA)
- Clindamycin (MSSA–Enterococcus)
- Clindamycin (Streptococcus–Clostridium)
- Rifampicin/Fusidic acid (MRSA–MSSA)
- Metronidazole (Clostridium–Bacteriodes)
- Rifampicin/FA (N. meningitidis)
- Rifampicin (H. influenzae)
- Vancomycin / Teicoplanin, Linezolid, Daptomycin (MRSA–Streptococcus)
- Vanco, Teico (Clostridium)
- Co-trimoxazole (MRSA–Pseudomonas)
- Cotrim (Legionella)
- Trimethoprim (MSSA–Enterococcus)
- Trim (Eschappm organisms)
- Trim (Legionella)
- Gentamicin (MRSA)
- Genta / Tobramycin (S. epidermidis–Streptococcus)
- Gentamicin / Tobramycin (H. influenzae–Eschappm)
- Ciprofloxacin, Aztreonan (N. meningitidis–Eschappm)
- Cipro (Legionella)
- Moxifloxacin (S. epidermidis–Bacteriodes)
- Moxifloxacin (Eschappm–Legionella)
- Cephazolin (S. epidermidis)
- Cephazolin (MSSA)
- Cephazolin (N. meningitidis–Moraxella)
- Cephaz (Klebsiella)
- Cefu, ceftri (S. epidermidis)
- Cefuroxime, ceftriaxone (MSSA–Streptococcus)
- Cefuroxime, ceftriaxone (N. meningitidis–Proteus)
- Ceftazidime (Pseudomonas area)
- Cefepime (S. epidermidis)
- Cefepime (Streptococcus–Eschappm)
- Mero, imi, ertapenem (S. epidermidis–MSSA)
- Imipenem (Enterococcus)
- Meropenem, imipenem (Streptococcus–Eschappm)
- Ertapenem (Clostridium–Eschappm)
- Ertapenem (Eschappm)
- Tigecycline (MRSA–Bacteriodes)
- Tigecycline (H. influenzae–Proteus)
- Tigecycline (Eschappm)

Adapted from Intensive Care Drug Manual: Wellington ICU. Appendix 5 as seen on FOAMid.

Cytomegalovirus CMV

- CMV (subtype of *Herpes*)
- 50% people have been exposed, but only disease-causing in immunocompromised

- Congenital CMV
  - growth retardation
  - pinpoint petechial 'blueberry muffin' skin lesions
  - microcephaly
  - sensorineural deafness
  - encephalitis (seizures)
  - hepatosplenomegaly
- CMV mononucleosis
  - flu-like smx
  - can develop in healthy pts
- CMV retinitis
  - common in HIV+ve CD4 <50
  - visual impairment (blurry)
  - fundoscopy: retinal haemorrhages, necrosis ("pizza retina")
  - Mx: IV ganciclovir
- CMV encephalopathy
  - HIV+ve low CD4
- CMV pneumonitis
- CMV colitis

Infectious mononucleosis

- Epstein Barr virus (= HHV4) in 90%
- Adolescents and young adults

S/smx:
- Classic 3: sore throat, cervical lympadenopathy, fever
- Systemic smx
- Palatal petechiae
- Splenomegaly (50%)
- Hepatitis, transient ↑ALT
- Lymphocytosis
- Haemolytic anaemia 2/2 cold agglutinins (IgM)
- Maculopapular, pruritic **rash** in 99% of pts who take **ampicillin or amoxicillin**

Ix: heterophil antibody test (Mono-spot) in 2nd week to confirm Dx

Mx: smx typically resolve in 2-4w
- supportive tx – rest lots
- simple analgesia
- avoid playing contact sports for 4w to ↓risk of splenic rupture

Dengue fever

- RNA virus (Flavivirus)
- *Aedes aegypti* mosquito incubates for 7d

S/smx of dengue fever
- fever, retro-orbital HA, myalgia, bone pain, arthralgia ("break-bone fever"), pleuritic pain
- facial flushing • maculopapular rash

Warning signs
- Abd pain, hepatomegaly
- Persistent vomiting
- Clinical fluid accumulation (ascites, pleural effusion)

Dengue haemorrhagic fever
= DIC: thrombocytopaenia, spontaneous bleeding
- +ve tourniquet test, petechiae, purpura, ecchymosis, epistaxis
- 20-30% develop dengue shock syndrome

Ix: FBC (↓WCC, ↓platelets), LFT (↑ALT)
- Dx: serology, NAAT, NS1 antigen

Mx: supportive (fluid resus, blood transfusion, etc)

Ebola virus

- Part of Filoviridae family
- Human to human – direct contact (broken skin, mucous membranes), blood, secretion, organs. Fomites.
- Healthcare workers

S/smx:
- Incubation 2-21d
- Pt not infectious until smx develop
- First smx: fever, fatigue, myalgia, HA, sore throat
- Next: vomiting, diarrhoea, rash, renal dysfunction, liver dysf, smx of internal and external bleeding

Mx: supportive, isolate!!
± broad spectrum abx if severe

Herpes simplex virus

D: infection with HSV1 or 2 causing oral (herpes labialis), genital and ulcers and skin lesions

R: HIV, immunosuppression, high-risk sexual behaviour

A/P: acquired at mucosal surfaces or breaks in skin
- virus replicates in the epidermis, then infects sensory or autonomic nerve endings
- travels by retrograde axonal transport to sensory ganglia
- enters latent state, causing lifelong infection + reactivation later on

S/smx: lesions (cold sores, fever blisters), lymphadenopathy, tingling sensation

Ix: clinical Dx ± wound swabs

Mx: PO antivirals (eg aciclovir)
- preferred to topical
- short course eg aciclovir 200 mg five times a day for 5d
- for pts with recurrences, long-term tx necessary (eg aciclovir 400 mg bds for 12mo)

- Contact tracing: inform partners
- Daily antivirals + condom use to ↓risk of transmission
- Avoid sexual activity when prodromal smx or genital lesions are present
- Pregnant women should inform Dr
  - elective C-sec if 1° episode occurs during pregnancy >28w
  - in women with recurrent episodes, tx with suppressive therapy – low risk transmission

see also genital herpes [→08.08]

EBV-associated conditions
- Malignancies
  - Burkitt's lymphoma
  - Hodgkin's lymphoma
  - Nasopharyngeal carcinoma
  - HIV-associated central nervous system lymphomas
- Non-malignant: hairy leukoplakia

Measles

D: caused by RNA paramyxovirus
- Spread by aerosol transmission. Very infectious. Incubation 10-14d.
- Pt is infective from **prodrome until 4d after rash starts**

S/smx
- Prodromal phase: irritability, conjunctivitis, fever
- Koplik spots: white spots ('grains of salt') on buccal mucosa; typically develops *before* rash
- Rash – starts from the head then spreads to the whole body
  - discrete maculopapular rash becoming blotchy and confluent
  - desquamation may occur after a week; spares palms and soles
- Diarrhoea in 10%

Ix: IgM abs detected within a few days of rash onset

Mx: mainly supportive
- Consider admission in immuno-suppressed (or pregnant)
- ! notifiable disease

- If unimmunised child comes into contact with measles, offer MMR
  - vaccine-induced abs develop more rapidly than natural infxn
  - give within 72h

Complications
- Otitis media: most common comp
- Pneumonia: most common cause of death
- Encephalitis: typically occurs 1-2w following the onset of the illness
- Subacute sclerosing panencephalitis: very rare, may present 5-10y after illness
  - S/smx: Δ behaviour, myoclonus, choreoathetosis, dystonia, dementia, coma, death
- Febrile convulsions
- Keratoconjunctivitis, corneal ulceration
- Diarrhoea
- ↑incidence of appendicitis
- Myocarditis

Mumps

- RNA paramyxovirus
- Droplets
MOA: Spreads to respiratory tract epithelial cells → parotid glands → other tissues
Incubation: 14-21d
Infective: 7d before, 9d after parotid swelling starts

S/smx: fever, malaise, myalgia, parotitis (earache, pain on eating) – unilateral then bilateral in 70%

Mx: MMR prevents in 80%
- Rest, analgesia • ! Notifiable !

Complications
- Orchitis – 25-35% of post-pubertal males, 4-5d after start of parotitis
- Sensorineural hearing loss – unilateral and transient
- Meningoencephalitis
- Pancreatitis

Novovirus

- Non-encapsulated RNA virus
- Faecal-oral route, virus becomes aerosolised when pt vomits or toilet flushing. Fomites, food prep.

S/smx: develops within 15-50h
- Nausea, vomiting, diarrhoea + HA, low-grade fevers, myalgia

Dx: history, stool viral PCR

Mx: supportive (ORS); self-limiting ~72h
- Isolate infxn, good hand hygiene
  - Alcohol gel not as effective

DDx:
- Rotavirus: similar, but tends to affect children <5yo
- Salmonella: 6-72h incubation
  - exposure to contaminated food products, eg milk
  - bloody diarrhoea + high fever
- E coli: longer incubation (≤10d)
  - bloody diarrhea and severe abdo pain

Parvovirus B19

Aka erythema infectiosum, slapped
cheek syndrome · 💧 droplets
! Pt is infectious 3-5d before rash

S/smx: · Mild fever
· Rose-red rash on cheeks
  - Peaks after a week
  - Heat will trigger rash
  - Once rash appears, child is not
    infectious – no need to exclude from
    school
· Athralgia in adults

In pregnancy
· Before 20w: check maternal IgM and
  IgG
· Can cross placenta → ↓erythropoiesis
  → hydrops fetalis
  - HF 2/2 severe anaemia
  - Accumulation of fluid in fetal serous
    cavities – ascites, pleural, pericardial
    effusion
  - Mx: intrauterine blood transfusion

Other presentations
· Can be asymptomatic
· In immunosuppressed pts:
  pancytopaenia
· In chronic haemolytic anaemia (eg
  sickle cell disease): aplastic crises
  - 2/2 viral suppression of erythropoiesis
    (~1w)

HMFD

· 🦠 intestinal viruses coxsackie
  A16 and enterovirus 71

S/smx: · mild systemic upset:
          sore throat, fever
· oral ulcers
· vesicles on palms and soles

Mx: · symptomatic tx – analgesia and
  hydration
· children do not need to be excluded
  from school unless they feel unwell
· reassure that not linked to disease in
  cattle

Rabies

· 🦠 RNA rhabdovirus
· 🐕 Dog, rat, raccoon, skunk bites
· 🌍 Rural areas of Africa and Asia
  – children especially
· MOA: bite → retrograde movement of
  virus up the CNS
· Negri bodies – cytoplasmic inclusion
  bodies in infected neurons

S/smx:
· Prodrome: HA, fever, agitation
· Hydrophobia: water provokes muscle
  spasms
· Hypersalivation

Mx: wash the wound
· Immunised: 2 doses more
· If not: human rabies immunoglobulin
  given (around the wound) + full course
  of vaccination
· If not tx: fatal :(

Yellow fever

· 🦠 RNA virus (yellow fever virus)
· 🦟 mosquitoes Aedes aegypti

S/smx: incubation for 2-14d
· Mild flu-like illness ~1w
· Classic description:
  - phase 1: sudden onset high fever,
    rigors, nausea, vomiting ± bradycardia
  - phase 2: jaundice, haemetemesis,
    oliguria
  - Councilman bodies (inclusion bodies)
    seen in hepatocytes

Mx: supportive ± ICU
Vax: protection 10d after vax

Rubella   ≈ German measles

· 🦠 togavirus · winter & spring
· 💧 respiratory droplets
· Incubation 14-21d
· Individuals infectious 7d before smx
  appear to 4d after rash starts

S/smx:
· Prodrome: fever
· Rash: maculopapular, face → whole
  body; fades after 3-5d
· Lymphadenopathy: suboccipital and
  postauricular

Complications: · arthritis
· thrombocytopaenia
· encephalitis   · myocarditis

In pregnancy
· Risk highest in first 8-10w
· Damage rare after 16w

Congenital rubella syndrome
· Sensorineural deafness
· Congenital cataracts
· Congenital heart disease (e.g. patent
  ductus arteriosus)
· Growth retardation
· Hepatosplenomegaly
· Purpuric skin lesions
· 'Salt and pepper' chorioretinitis
· Microphthalmia
· Cerebral palsy

Dx: IgM. Check parvovirus B19 also
(difficult to differentiate)

Mx: ! Notifiable disease !
· Offer MMR in post-natal period
  - Do NOT offer before/during pregnancy

Viral exanthema
· First disease: Measles
· Second: Scarlet fever
· Third: Rubella
· Fourth: Dukes' disease
  - ?? non-existent, or used as a generic
    term to describe other viral rashes
· Fifth: Parvovirus B19
· Sixth: Roseola infantum [15.03]

Human immunodeficiency virus   HIV

· 🦠 Retrovirus that replicates in human
  lymphocytes and macrophages
  ÷ HIV1, HIV2
· 🩸 Blood, sexual fluids, breast milk

Seroconversion – smx in 60-80%
· Sore throat
· Lymphadenopathy
· Malaise, myalgia, arthralgia
· Diarrhoea
· Maculopapular rash
· Mouth ulcers
· Rarely, meningoencephalitis

Mx: ART = 3 drugs, typically 2 NRTI +
  1 PI or 1 NNRTI
· Start as soon as Dx confirmed

Entry inhibitors – prevents HIV1
  from infecting immune cells
· Maraviroc [binds to CCR5]
· Enfuvirtide [binds to gp41]

Nucleoside analogue reverse
  transcriptase inhibitors (NRTI)
· Zidovudine, lamivudine, tenofovir
· General SE: peripheral neuropathy

Non-NRTI (NNRTI)
· Nevirapine, efavirenz
· SE: P450 inducing, rashes

Protease inhibitors (PI)
· indinavir, nelfinavir, ritonavir
· SE: DM, hyperlipidaemia, buffalo
  hump, central obesity
· indinavir: renal stones, asmymptomatic
  ↑bilirubin
· ritonavir: potent P450 inhibitor

Integrase inhibitors:
· Raltegravir, elvitegravir
· Blocks integration of viral genome into
  DNA of host cell

See 15.03 for HIV in children

Notes:
· Toxoplasmosis (protozoan) →05.06
  + 16.06 for maternal toxoplasmosis
· Hepatitis viruses →03.03
· VZV/chickenpox, Shingles →09.07

CD4 200-500
· Oral thrush: Candida
· Shingles: Herpes zoster
· Hairy leukoplakia: EBV
· Kaposi sarcoma: HHV-8
  - Purple papules or plaques on the skin
    or mucosa → ulcers
  - Radiotherapy, resection

CD4 100-200
· Cryptosporidiosis
  - most common cause of diarrhoea in
    HIV
  - Ix: stool sample – acid-fast stain of the
    stool may show red cysts
  - Mx: supportive
· Cerebral toxoplasmosis
· Progressive multifocal leuko-
  encephalopathy: JC virus
  - Widespread demyelination
· Pneumocystis jirovecii pneumonia
  (see also 02.03)
  - CD4 count <200 should receive PCP
    prophylaxis
  - S/smx: dyspnea, dry cough, fever, few
    chest signs
  - Pneumothorax common
  - Extrapulmonary: hepatosplenomegaly,
    lymphadenopathy, choroid lesions
  - Ix: CXR, exercise-induced desats,
    bronchoalveolar lavage
  - Mx: cotrimox, IV pentamidine ±
    steroids if hypoxic
· HIV dementia (aka AIDS dementia
  complex), caused by HIV itself

CD4 50-100
· Aspergillosis :· A. fumigatus
· Esophageal candidiasis
  - Sx: dysphagia, odynophagia
  - Mx: fluconazole, itraconazole
· Cryptococcal meningitis
· Primary CNS lymphoma :· EBV

CD4 <50
· Cytomegalovirus retinitis
  - 30-40% of pts in this category
· Mycobacterium avium-intracellular
  - Sx: fever, sweat, abd pain, diarrhoea
  - Mx: rifabutin, ethambutol,
    clarithromycin

Amoebiasis

- 🦠 Protozoa *Entamoeba histolytica*
- 📧 Faecal-oral route
- 📊 Children. 10% world chronic

Amoebic dysentery
- profuse, bloody diarrhoea
  - ± long incubation period
- stool microscopy of hot stool (w/in 15 min) may show trophozoites
- Mx: PO metronidazole + diloxanide furoate ("luminal agent")

Amoebic liver abscess
- usually single mass in right lobe; can be multiple
- contents: "anchovy sauce"
- S/smx: fever, RUQ pain, malaise
  - hepatomegaly
- Ix: US • Serology +ve in >95%
- Mx: PO metronidazole + diloxanide furoate ("luminal agent")

Cryptosporidiosis

- 🦠 *Cryptosporidium hominis*
  Cryptosporidium parvum
- 📧 Faecal-oral route
- 📊 Young children, immunocompromised. Most common cause of protozoal diarrhoea

- Ix: Ziehl-Neelsen stain of the stool – characteristic red cysts

- Mx: supportive
  - if HIV +ve, start antiretroviral
  - for immunocompromised, nitazoxanide or rifaximin

Cutaneous larva migrans

- 🦠 Dog hookworm *Ancylostoma braziliense*

- S/smx: intensely itchy and creeping rash 2/2 subcutaneous migration of larvae

- Mx: albendazole, ivermectin

Giardiasis

- 🦠 *Giardia lamblia*
- 📧 Faecal-oral route
- 📊 Travellers, esp those who swim or drink in contaminated water, MSM

S/smx: often asmx
- Non-bloody diarrhoea + steatorrhea, bloating, abdo pain
- Lethargy, flatulence, wt loss
- Malabsorption and lactose intolerance

Ix: stool microscopy (65% sens)
- stool antigen detection assay: more sensitive and faster

Mx: PO metronidazole

Leishmaniasis

- 🦠 intracellular *Leishmania*
- 📧 sandfly bites

Cutaneous leishmaniasis
- *L tropica* or *L mexicana*
- Crusted lesion at site of bite
- Underlying ulcer
- Dx – punch biopsy

Mucocutaneous leishmaniasis
- *L braziliensis*
- Skin lesion spreads to involve mucosae or nose, pharynx, etc

Visceral leishmaniasis
- *L donovani*
- Mediterranean, Asia, S America, Africa
- S/smx: fever, sweats, rigors
- Massive hepatosplenomegaly
  ↳ pancytopaenia
- Poor appetite, wt loss
- Grey skin – "kala-azar" (black sickness)
- Dx: bone marrow or splenic aspirate aspirate

Mx: w&w, topical or systemic antifungals (eg amphotericin)

Malaria

- 🦠 *Plasmodium* • falciparum: severe :(
  - vivax, ovale, malariae
- 🦟 female *Anopheles* mosquito
Protective factors: sickle cell, G6PD def, HLA-B53

- 🦠 *Plasmodium* falciparum
  → most common, most severe
- S/smx: • blood film: schizonts
  - parasitaemia > 2%
  - hypoglycaemia • T>39°C
  - acidosis • anaemia

Complications
- cerebral malaria: seizures, coma
- AKI: blackwater fever, 2/2 intravascular haemolysis
- ARDS • DIC • hypoglycaemia

Mx:
- Artemisinin-based combination therapies (ACT), eg. artermether + lumefantrine, etc
- If parasite count >2%, IV artesunate
- >10%: exchange transfusion
- Shock indicates bacterial septicaemia: tx accordingly (resus, etc)

- 🦠 Malaria: non-falciparum
  → most common *vivax*
- S/smx: fever, HA, splenomeg
- Vivax/ovale: cyclical fever 48h
- Malariae: fever every 72h
  + nephrotic syndrome
- Mx: ACT except in pregnant women
  + Primaquine to prevent relapse

Trypanosomiasis

- 🦠 *Trypanosoma gambiense*
  Trypanosoma rhodesiense
- 🦟 tsetse fly bites

T. rhodesiense:
- Trypanosoma chancre – painless squamous nodule at site of infxn
- Intermittent fever
- Posterior cervical LN enlargement
- Later: CNS involvement e.g. somnolence, HA, mood changes, meningoencephalitis
- Mx of early disease: IV pentamidine or suramin
- Mx of late disease or CNS involvement: IV melarsoprol

T. cruzi = **Chagas disease**
- American trypanosomiasis
- Early phase: 95% asmx
  ± chagoma (erythematous nodule at site of infxn)
  ± Periorbital edema
- Chronic disease
  - Myocarditis
  - GI: mega-esophagus, megacolon → dysphagia, constipation
- Mx: eg benznidazole, nifurtimox in acute phase
- Chronic phase – Mx of complications

Schistosomiasis

- 🦠 Parasitic flatworm
- 📧 Contaminated water

Acute infection
- Swimmers' itch
- Katayama fever: + urticaria, athralgia myalgia, cough, diarrhoea, eosinophilia

Schistosoma haematobium
- Worms deposit egg clusters in bladder leads to inflammation
- Swimmers' itch, obstructive uropathy, kidney damage → frequency, haematuria, bladder calcification
- Risk factor for squamous cell bladder cancer!!
- Mx: PO praziquantel

S. mansoni and *S. japonicum*
- Worms mature in liver → portal system → distal colon
- Hepatosplenomegaly 2/2 portal vein occlusion
- Liver cirrhosis, variceal disease, cor pulmonale

Chikungunya virus
- 🦠 Alphavirus. Incubates ~15d
- 🦟 Aedes species of mosquito
- S/smx:
  - Sudden onset of high fever (>38.5°C) lasts btwn 2-7d
  - Polyathralgia & polyarthritis – lasts longer than fever (1-3w)
  - Rash and other skin problems
  - Photophobia, retro-ocular pain, conjunctivitis, and other eye problems
  - Lymphadenopathy
  - 1/5 neuropathic-type pain
- Mx: Supportive
  - Arthritis: NSAIDs or DMARDs

West Nile virus
- 🦠 Flavivirus. Incubates 2-6d
- 🦟 Mosquito, contact with infected blood
- S/smx:
  - Sudden onset fever, malaise
  - Arthralgia, myalgia, rash
  - Lymphadenopathy
  - Visual disturbances, conjunctival injection, chorioretinitis, inflammatory vitritis
  - ❗ Neuroinvasive disease: encephalitis, meningitis, poliomyelitis
- Ix: serology
- Mx: supportive

Filariasis
- 🦠 Caused by nematode parasites transmitted via mosquitoes (incl Aedes)
- Chronic disease – adult worms proliferate in the lymphatics → occlusion of lymph nodes disrupt the lymphatic drainage
  - Can also ↑risk of 2ndary infxns (eg strep and fungal infxns)
  - More infxns → more damage to lymphatics → can lead to elephantitis
- S/smx: fever, malaise
  - Abscess and granuloma formation
  - Lymphedema
  - Tropical pulmonary eosinophilia (pulmonary restrictive lung disease – immune rxn to filarial infxn)
- Ix: blood smear, PCR, scrotal US
- Mx: diethylcarbamazine + ivermectin + albendazole (combination therapy)
  - Surgical tx to debulk skin and create lymphovenous anastomosis
  - Long-term pt may require compressive bandage. Encourage skin hygiene

Bacterial vaginosis

- 🦠 anaerobic *Gardnerella vaginalis* 👥 women

MOA: overgrowth of *G. vaginalis* leads to fall in aerobic lactobacilli producing lactic acid → ↑pH → problems :(

Ansel's criteria for Dx of BV (≥3 of 4)
- thin, white homogenous discharge
- clue cells on microscopy: stippled vaginal epithelial cells
- vaginal pH > 4.5
- +ve whiff test (addition of KOH results in fishy odour)

Mx: PO metronidazole for 5-7d
- 70-80% initial cure, relapse >50% within 3mo
- 💊 topical metronidazole or topical clindamycin

Complications – in pregnancy
- Preterm labour, low birth weight, chorioamnionitis, late miscarriage
- Tx still low dose PO metronidazole

Trichomonas vaginalis

S/smx: • Vaginal discharge: offensive, yellow/green, frothy
- Vulvovaginitis – **strawberry cervix**
- pH >4.5
- In males: asmx or urethritis

Ix: microscopy of wet mount shows mobile trophozoins

Mx: PO metronidazole 5-7d or one-off 2g metronidazole

Donovanosis aka granuloma inguinale

- 🦠 *Klebsiella granulomatis*
- Not common in the developed world

S/smx: • Small, painless and enlarging nodules usually on area of contact (eg penis, labia, perineum)
- Nodules then burst open → fleshy, red ulcers with rolled edges → ❗ bleeding

Mx: abx (azithromycin, doxycycline, etc)

Genital warts

- 🦠 HPV 6 & 11 most common HPV 16, 18, 33 cancer

S/smx: small (2-5mm) fleshy protuberances, slightly pigmented; may bleed or itch

Mx: • if multiple, non-keratinised warts: topical podophyllum
- solitary, keratinised: cryotherapy
- 💊 topical imiquimod
- Genital warts can be resistant and recurrent
- Most clear without intervention ~1-2y

Chlamydia

- 🦠 obligate intracellular *Chlamydia trachomatis*
- 👥 Most common STI in UK ~1 in 10 young women

S/smx: asmx in 70%F and 50%M, incubation 7-21d
- F: cervicitis (discharge, bleeding), dysuria
- M: urethral discharge, dysuria

Ix: 💊 NAAT using urine (first void) in M, vulvovaginal swab in F
- Carried out 2w post-exposure

Mx: 💊 doxycycline 7d
- 💊 azithromycin 3d
- 💊 if pregnant: azithromycin, erythromycin or amoxicillin
- Partner notification, treating then testing (based on exposure)
  - M with urethral smx: all contacts 4w 4w before and since
  - F and asmx M: most recent sexual partner

Complications: • epididymitis
- PID → perihepatitis (FHC) • infertility
- endometritis
- ↑risk ectopic pregnancies
- reactive arthritis

For candidiasis (thrush), see 17.07

Genital herpes

🦠 HSV1, HSV2

S/smx: • painful genital ulceration
- a/w dysuria and pruritus
- Primary infection is often more severe than recurrent episodes
  - systemic features (HA, fever, malaise) more common in primary episode
- ± tender inguinal lymphadenopathy, urinary retention

Ix: NAAT, ?HSV serology

Mx: saline bathing, analgesia, topical anaesthetic agents
- PO aciclovir – some pts may benefit from longer term course
- Genital warts can be resistant and recurrent

Pregnancy
- elective C-sec if 1° episode occurs during pregnancy >28w
- in women with recurrent episodes, tx with suppressive therapy – low risk transmission

see also Herpes simplex virus [→08.05]

Lymphogranuloma venereum

- 🦠 *Chlamydia trachomatis* serovariants L1, L2 and L3
- 👥 MSM, HIV, ?tropics

Stage 1: small painless pustule which later becomes an ulcer
Stage 2: Painful inguinal lymphadeno-pathy → fistulating buboes
Stage 3: proctocolitis

Mx: doxycycline

Chancroid

- 🦠 G-ve *Haemophilus ducreyi*

S/smx: painful genital ulcer
- Ulcer – sharply defined, ragged, undermined border
- unilateral, painful inguinal LN enlargement

Mx: • check for HIV
- 💊 azithromycin 1g single dose
- Tx Sexual partners within 10d – based on exposure (no testing req)

Gonorrhoea

- 🦠 Gram-ve diplococcus *Neisseria gonorrhoeae*

S/smx: • GU, rectal, pharynx
- Incubates 2-5d
- M: urethral discharge, dysuria
- F: cervicitis, vaginal discharge
- Rectal and pharyngeal: asmx

Ix: swabs (NAAT and culture)

Mx: 💊 IM ceftriaxone 1g
- 💊 PO cefixime 400mg + azithromycin 2g

Complications:
- Urethral strictures, epididymitis, sapingitis → infertility
- Disseminated gonococcal infxn
  - tenosynovitis
  - migratory polyarthritis
  - dermatitis (maculopapular / vesicular)

Syphilis

- 🦠 *Treponema pallidum*

Primary stage
- Chance – painless
- Local non-tender lymphadenopathy

Secondary stage (~6-10w)
- systemic: fevers, lymphadenopathy
- rash on trunk, palms and soles
- buccal 'snail track' ulcers (30%)
- condylomata lata (painless, warty lesions on the genitalia)

Tertiary stage
- gummas (granulomatous lesions of the skin and bones)
- ascending aortic aneurysms
- general paralysis of the insane
- tabes dorsalis
  - slow degeneration of nerves (↓propioception)
- Argyll-Robertson pupil [→05.05]
  - small, irregular pupils that do not constrict to lights but to accommodation

Congenital syphilis

- Blunted upper incisor teeth (Hutchinson's teeth), 'mulberry' molars
- Rhagades (linear scars at the angle of the mouth)
- Keratitis   • Saber shins
- Saddle nose   • Deafness

Dx based on clinical features, serology and microscopic exam

Non-treponemal tests
- E.g. rapid plasma reagin, VDRL
- Ax quantity of antibodies produced; becomes -ve after tx
- False +ve in - pregnancy
  - SLE, antiphospholipid
  - TB   - leprosy
  - HIV   - malaria

Treponemal-specific tests
- E.g. TP-EIA, TPHA
- Qualitative only, reported as 'reactive' or 'non-reactive'

Negative non-treponemal test + positive treponemal test
= successfully treated syphilis

Mx: 💊 IM benzylpenicillin
- 💊 doxycycline
- Monitor RPR/VDRL after tx
  - 4x ↓ in titres (eg 1:16 → 1:4) indicates adequate response
- Jarisch-Herxheimer reaction
  - fever, rash, tachycardia in response to abx
  - no tx required usually

STI: ulcers

Painful
- Singular: chancroid
- Multiple: genital herpes (HSV)

Painless
- Singular: chance in syphilis
- LGV – small painless pustule which later forms an ulcer
- Multiple: genital herpes (HSV), *Klebsiella granulomatis* (aka donovanosis; see 08.05)

Other causes of genital ulcers
- Behcet's disease
- Carcinoma

Animal & human bites

Animal bites
· *Pasteurella multocida*

Human bites
· Aerobic and anaerobic bacteria:
  Strep, Staph, Eikenella,
  Fusobacterium, Prevotella
· Consider risk of HIV, hep C

Mx: clean wound, do not suture
close unless thorough washout
  ⚕ co-amoxiclav
  ⚕ doxy + metronidazole

Lemierre's syndrome

= infectious thrombophlebitis of
the internal jugular vein

2/2 bacterial sore throat caused by
Fusobacterium necrophorum
→ peritonsillar abscess

· Neck pain, stiffness, tenderness
· Systemic: fever, rigors
· ± septic pulmonary emboli

Post-splenectomy sepsis

· Vaccinations
  - pneumococcal   - HiB
  - meningococcal type C
· Administer 2w before
  splenectomy or 2w after
· Annual influenza vaccination
· Abx prophylaxis immediately
  following splenectomy
  - penicillin V 500 mg BD
  - amoxicillin 250 mg BD

Pyrexia of unknown origin

= fever >3w, resisting Dx after 1w
in hospital

2/2 neoplasm · Lymphoma
· Preleukemia · Atrial myxoma
· Hypernephroma

2/2 infxn · TB   · Abscess

2/2 connective tissue disorders

Cellulitis

D: infection of the dermis and deeper
sq tissues

A: *Strep pyogenes, S. aureus*

Eron classification
Class I: - no signs of systemic toxicity,
no uncontrolled comorbidities
II: - systematically unwell, or
  - comorbidity (eg peripheral
    arterial disease)
III: - severe systemic upset
  - unstable comorbidity that may
    interfere with response to tx
  - life-threatening infection due to
    vascular compromise
IV: - sepsis
  - severe life-threatening infxn, eg
    necrotising fasciitis

Mx of Eron Class I & II
  ⚕ PO flucloxacillin
  ⚕ clarithromycin, erythromycin
    (in pregnancy) or doxy
· Class II: IV may be needed, try to
  treat in community

Eron Class III / IV
· Admit if - rapidly deteriorating
  - <1yo - immunocompromised
  - significant lymphedema
  - facial / periorbital area
  ⚕ PO/IV co-amoxiclav
  ⚕ PO/IV clindamycin, IV cefuroxime,
    or IV ceftriaxone

Necrotising fasciitis

Classifications
Type 1: mixed anaerobes and
  aerobes – often occurs post-op
  in diabetics
Type 2: *Strep pyogenes*

R: recent trauma, DM (esp if tx with
SGLT-2I), IVDU, immuno-
suppression

S/smx:
· most commonly affects the
  perineum (= Fournier's gangrene)
· Acute onset of pain, swelling,
  erythema
  ≈ rapidly worsening cellulitis
  - pain out of keeping with physically
    features
· Skin necrosis and crepitus are late
  signs
· ± Fever and tachycardia (absent or
  late)

Mx: urgent surgical debridement, IV
abx

Prognosis: avg mortality 20%

See also 09.01

Antimicrobial SE

Aminoglycosides	Rifampicin	Trimethoprim
· Haematologic SE incl agranulocytosis	· RNA polymerase inhibitor	· Myelosuppression
· Ototoxicity	· Revs up P450 (inducer)	· Transient ↑creatinine due to competitive inhibition
	· Red pee	
Cotrimoxazole	· Hepatitis	· Teratogenic risk in 1st trim – avoid during pregnancy
· HyperK · HA	· Flu-like smx	
· Rash (incl SJS)	Tetracyclines	
Metronidazole	- eg doxycycline	Vancomycin
· disulfiram-like rxn with alcohol	· Discolouration of teeth; do not use in <12yo, pregnant, bfeeding	· nephrotoxicity
· ↑anticoagulant effect of warfarin	· Photosensitivity	· ototoxicity
	· Angioedema	· thrombophlebitis
	· Black hairy tongue	· red man syndrome

Sepsis

= life-threatening organ dysf caused
by a dysregulated host response to
infxn

Quick screening to identify pts at
↑risk of sepsis – qSOFA
· RR > 22   · SBP <100
· Altered mentation

Sepsis 6
3 in
· O2: aim sats >94%
· Broad spectrum abx
· IVF: 500 mL crystalloid over 15 min
3 out
· Blood cultures
· Measure serum lactate
· Measure urine output hourly

Within ICU, a full SOFA score is
used
  ↳ SOFA >2 – ↑mortality by 10%
    compared to other pts
· PaO2
· Platelets   · Bilirubin
· Cardiovascular MAP, use of
  vasopressors
· GCS
· Creatinine   · UO per day

Spinal epidural abscess

= collection of pus superficial to the
dura mater. ❗ medical emergency

A: usually S. aureus

P: contiguous spread from adjacent
structures (eg discitis), haematogenous spread (eg bactaeremia from
IVDU), or direct infxn (eg surgery)

S/smx: fever, back pain, focal neuro
deficits according to segment of cord
affected

Ix: bloods, blood cultures, infection
screen (incl CXR, urine cultures),
MRI whole spine

Mx: long-term abx (broad spectrum,
then refined based on culture
results)
· Surgical evacuation if large or non-
  responding

Nematodes

Ancylostoma braziliense
· most common cause of cutaneous
  larva migrans
· Central, South America

Strongyloides stercoralis
🔲 percutaneously e.g. walking
  barefoot
· Causes pruritus and larva currens
  - similar apperance to cutaneous
    larva migrans
  - moves through the skin at a far
    greater rate
· abdo pain, diarrhea, pneumonitis
· may cause Gram-ve septicaemia
  due to carrying of bacteria into
  bloodstream
· eosinophilia sometimes seen
Mx: thiabendazole, albendazole,
  ± ivermectin, esp in chronic infxn

Toxocara canis
🔲 ingesting eggs from soil
  contaminated by dog faeces
· commonest cause of visceral larva
  migrans
· eye granulomas, liver/lung
  involvement

Threadworms (aka pinworms)
🪱 Enterobius vermicularis
🔲 Ingesting eggs 👤 Children
· S/smx: - asmx in 90%
  - Perianal itching, esp at night
  - Girls may have vulval smx
· Dx: usually clinical Dx. If confirmation
  needed, apply tape to perianal area
  ("swab") → sending for microscopy to
  find eggs
· Mx: antihelmintic for whole household
  - ⚕ Mebendazole (single dose)
  - With hygiene measures

Diarrhoea

Infectious: non-inflammatory
- Viruses: Norwalk virus, rotavirus, adenoviruses, astrovirus, coronavirus
- Preformed toxin (food poisoning): Staph aureus, Bacillus cereus, Clostridium perfringens
- Toxin production: enterotoxigenic E.coli, Vibrio cholerae, Vibrio parahaemolyticus
- Protozoa: Giardia lambia, Crypto-sporidium, Cyclospora, Isospora

Infectious: inflammatory / invasive
- Shigella, Salmonella, Campylobacter, enteroinvasive E.coli, E.coli O157:h7, Yersinia enterocolitica, C. difficile, Entamoeba histolytica, N. gonorrhoea, Listeria monocytogenes

Noninfectious
- Inflammatory: Ulcerative colitis, Crohn's disease
- Malabsorption
  - Coeliac disease   - Radiation
  - Blind loop syndrome
  - Short bowel syndrome
- Neoplastic: carcinoma, villous adenoma
- Other intestinal
  - Diverticular disease
  - Irritable bowel syndrome
  - Faecal impaction (overflow diarrhoea)
  - ! Ischaemic colitis
  - Ileocolic fistula
- Gastric: post-vagatomy
- Pancreatic
  - Chronic pancreatitis
  - Cystic fibrosis
  - Carcinoma ± pancreatic resection
- Endocrine
  - Diabetes   - Thyrotoxicosis
  - Carcinoid syndrome
  - Zollinger-Ellison syndrome
  - VIPoma   - Medullary thyroid cancer
- Drug-induced
  - Antibiotics   - Laxatives
  - Magnesium-containing antacids
  - Cytotoxic agents
- Others: anxiety, diet

Gastroenteritis   Sorted by incubation time

Organism/source	Incubation	Source of infection	Diarrhoea	Vomiting	Pain	Fever	Others
			Diarrhoea	Vomiting	Pain	Fever	
Heavy metals, eg zinc	5min – 2h	Work exposure, paint, etc		V	P	F	Delayed fever, flu-like features.
Scrombotoxin	10-60 min	Fish (eg tuna, mackerel)	D				Flushing, sweating
Mushrooms	15min – 24h	Mushrooms	D	V	P		Fits, coma, LFT derangements
Red beans	1-3h	Red beans	D	V			
Bacillus cereus	1-5h	Rice	D	V			Vomiting type onset within 6h
							Diarrheal type onset after 6h
Staph aureus	1-6h	Meat	D	V	P		Hypotension
Campylobacter	2-5h	Milk, poultry, water	Bloody D		P	F	Peritonism. Flu-like prodrome. A/w Guillain Barre.
Vibrio cholerae	2h – 5d	Water	Profuse D	V		F	Rapid dehydration
E. coli – enterotoxigenic	6-48h	Water, food, soil	D	V	P	F	= Traveller's diarrhoea
C. perfringens	8-24h	Meat	D		P		
Vib. parahaemolyticus	12-24h	Seafood	Profuse D	V	P		
C. botulinum	12-36h	Processed food		V			Paralysis
Salmonella	12-48h	Meat, eggs, poultry	D	V	P	F	Septicaemia
Noroviruses (eg Norwalk virus)	12-48h	Faecal oral	D	Projectile V	P	F	"Winter vomiting illness". Remains contagious 48h after smx resolve
E. coli O157:H7 – enterohaemorrhagic	12-72h	Water, food, soil	Bloody D		P+/-		Typhoid-like features, haemolytic uraemic syndrome
E. coli – enteropathogenic	12-72h	Water, food, soil	D	V		F	Especially in infants
Y. enterocolitica	24-34h	Milk	D	P		F	
C. difficile	1-7d	Antibiotic-associated Hospital-acquired	Bloody D	P			Gut perforation, toxic megacolon
Rotavirus	1-7d	Food/water	D	V		F	Malaise
Shigella	2-3d	Any food	Bloody D		P	F	Headache, neck stiffness
Listeria monocytogenes	2-9d	Cheese, pates	D	V		F	Meningoencephalitis, flu-like smx, miscarriages.
Cryptosporidium	4-12d	Cow → water → man	D in HIV				
Giardia lamblia	1-4w	Nappies, cats, dog, crows	D				Malabsorption. Prolonged course. Weight loss. Can affect other organ systems
Entamoeba histolytica	1-4w	Food/water	Bloody D		P		

Table adapted from OHCS

Bloody infectious diarrhoea (notifiable)
- Campylobacter
- E.coli enterohaemorrhagic
- C. difficile
- Shigella
- Entamoeba histiolytica

Other infections
- Ascending cholangitis [03.01]
- Breast abscess/mastitis
- Conjunctivitis [05.03]
- Croup [15.04]
- Cutaneous warts [09.06]
- Encephalitis [04.04]
- Epididymo-orchitis [07.06]
- Folliculitis [09.05]
- Head lice [09.05]
- Infective endocarditis [01.07]
- LRTI / pneumonia [02.03]
- Meningitis [04.04]
- Septic arthritis [12a.01]
- Spontaneous bacterial peritonitis [03.02]
- Tinea / dermatophyte infections [09.06]
- Tuberculosis [02.03]
- Varicella zoster (chickenpox) [09.07]
- Vaginal candidiasis / thrush [17.07]

Dermatological emergencies

Acute urticaria and angioedema

D: **Urticaria** (aka hives) is a skin condition characterised by erythematous, blanching, oedematous, non-painful, pruritic lesions that typically resolve within 24 hours and leave no residual markings.
Angio-oedema is a sudden, pronounced swelling of the subdermis or mucous membranes.

A/P: usually allergic, IgE-mediated or mast cell degranulation. Most common allergens are drugs and foods.

R: +ve FHx, exposure to food/ drug trigger, recent viral infxn, recent insect bite/sting

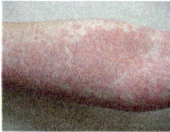

Ix: bloods (FBC, ESR, CRP, C4 level), others as indicated eg skin prick test

Mx:
- (if anaphylaxis) IM adrenaline, IV antihistamine ± corticosteroid
- allergen identification, avoidance
- investigate underlying disorder?
- 2nd gen antihistamine
- ref to dermatologist if necessary, advice to ↓scratching

Erythroderma: ≥95% of skin involved

photo from Wikipedia

Stevens-Johnson syndrome
Toxic epidermal necrolysis

D: SJS is a severe skin detachment with mucocutaneous complications.
- SJS has <10% total body surface area (TBSA) involvement
- SJS/TEN overlap: 10-30% TBSA
- TEN: >30% TBSA involvement

R: pts with active cancer, drugs (anticonvulsants, antibiotics, etc), recent infxn, SLE, HIV, radiotherapy, HLA and genetic predisposition, smallpox vaccination

A/P: detachment of epidermis from the papillary dermis at the epidermal-dermal junction; manifests as a papulomacular rash and bullae as a result of keratinocyte apoptosis

S/smx: · rash - maculopapular (wide-spread) + target lesions
  - may develop into vesicles or bullae
  - Nikolsky's sign - blisters and erosions appear when skin is rubbed gently
- Mucosal involvement
- Systemic smx: fever, arthralgia

Ix: · Skin biopsy key to Dx
- Blood cultures to r/o toxic shock and scalded skin syndromes
- FBC, blood glucose, U&Es (incl Mg, PO4, bicarb), ESR, CSR, LFT
- ABG   · CXR
- Coagulation studies - r/o DIC
- Skin swab - 2ndary skin infxn

Mx: · Admit ± burns/ITU
- Find and remove causative agent
- Supportive care + careful wound care (= 2nd degree burn)
- Fluid Mx, pain Mx

P: worse if >50yo, high TBSA, not in burns centre, sepsis + abx use, pulmonary issues. Higher mortality in children also.

Eczema herpeticum

D: disseminated HSV-1 or HSV-2 infxn characterised by fever and clusters of itchy blisters or punched-out erosions

A/P: HSV-1/2 infection superimposed on pre-existing skin condition, most commonly in infants and children with atopic dermatitis (∴ ↓immunity)

S/smx:
- clusters of itchy and painful blisters
- most commonly on face/neck
- new patches form and spread over 7-10d, rarely widely disseminated
- a/w fever, swollen LN, malaise
- blisters are monomorphic ± filled with clear yellow fluid or thick purulent material ± blood stained
- blisters may weep or bleed, then start to crust and form sores
- may form scars in long term

Ix: · swab - serology, PCR or MC&S
- ? skin biopsy

Mx: · aciclovir PO 400-800 mg 5x/d for 10-14d or until lesions heal
- If pt is severely unwell, IV aciclovir
- 2ndary bacterial infxn - abx
- Topical steroids not recommended
- Ref to ophthalmologist if ocular involvement

Cutaneous vasculitis

D: cutaneous manifestation of vasculitic disorders

S/smx: purpura (±palpable)

Mx: DMARDs, steroids for underlying vasculitis

Staph scalded skin syndrome

D: severe, superficial blistering skin disorder which is characterised by the detachment of epidermis ∴ exotoxin release from *Staph aureus*.

R: <5yo (peak 2-3yo), ↓immunity

A/P: toxigenic S. aureus producing exfoliative toxins A and B bind to desmogleins in the epidermis → desmoglein-1 is broken down → epidermis detaches → blistering

** desmoglein-1 is NOT present in mucosa, therefore mucosa is spared in SSSS

S/smx:
- Usually starts out with non-specific smx in children - fever, unwell, etc
- Red rash with wrinkled tissue or paper-like consistency
- Formation of large fluid-filled blisters (can be cloudy or pus)
- Blisters rupture easily → skin peels off as large sheets → burned appearance
- Nikolsky's +ve

Ix: · clinical Dx
- Skin & wound swabs MC&S
- Blood cultures if sepsis
- Skin biopsy if concerned about other causes

Mx: admit
- IV abx eg flucloxacillin, ceftriaxone
- Supportive: IVF, pain relief, skin care (gentle washing with soap substitute, apply emollients, burn dressings if needed)

C: scarring, hypothermia, hypovolaemia/ electrolyte abn, 2ndary infections (sepsis, cellulitis, pneumonia), renal failure
P: if tx promptly, should resolve within 2w

Necrotising fasciitis

D: life-threatening subcutaneous soft-tissue infection

R: inpatient contact with index case, VZV infxn, cutaneous injury, surgery, trauma, non-traumatic skin lesions, IVDU, ↓immunity (eg DM, PVD, etc)

A/P:
- Type I - polymicrobial infxn caused by anaerobe + facul anaerobe
- Type II - monomicrobial infxn most commonly GAS, MRSA
- Type III - monomicrobial, fresh-water infxn (rare)
- Type IV - monomicrobial fungal; mucormycosis
- Infxn is introduced into and spreads along the fascial plane, but does not spread into muscle layer

S/smx:
- Systemic signs (∴ bacterial toxins): fever, tachycardia, hypotension
- May develop over a few days (acute) or few hours (fulminant)
- **Pain out of proportion to clinical findings, or numbness**

Ix: if suspected, surgical exploration asap to r/o
- 'Finger test' can be performed under LA for Dx - make 2cm incision down to deep fascia
  - minimal resistance to finger dissection (+ve)
  - absence of bleeding
  - presence of necrotic tissue
  - murky or greyish dishwasher fluid
- Blood, tissue cultures, Gram stain
- Bloods: FBC (WCC breakdown), U&Es, CRP, CK, LFTs, clotting screen, ABG

Mx: emergency surgical debridement + empirical abx tx
- ITU Mx post-op

P: poor if end organ damage or shock (50-70%)

Melanoma

D: malignant tumour arising from melanocytes

R: FHx, PMH (melanoma, actinic damage, atypical naevi), white skin, red/blond hair colour, light eye colour, high freckle density, sun exposure, sunbed use, large congenital naevi, immunosuppresion, xeroderma pigmentosum

Clinical classifications
- Superficial spreading melanoma
  - 70-80% - spreads superficially before extending to dermis
- Nodular melanoma 9-15%
  - poorer prognosis
- Lentigo maligna melanoma 5-15%
  - slower growing
- Acral lentiginous melanoma 1-3%
  - in darker skin, on palms, soles and nail apparatus
- + other rarer variants

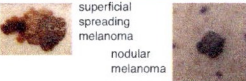

superficial spreading melanoma

nodular melanoma

S/smx:
- ABCDE rule
  - **Asymmetry of lesion**
  - **Border irregularity**
  - **Colour variability**
  - **Diameter >6mm**
  - **Evolution**
- Any lesion that looks atypical in appearance in comparison to surrounding skin should raise suspicion - "ugly duckling sign"
- Melanoma of the nail
  - persistent single-nail melanonychia striata
  - Hutchinson's sign (melanoma extends into the proximal/ lateral nail fold)
- Bleeding of the lesion

Marjolin's ulcer: cutaneous malignancy arising in the setting of previous damage

Ix: dermoscopy, skin biopsy, immunohisto-chemistry + sentinel LN biopsy, bloods, CT/PET scans

Mx: Excision biopsy (may need further excision depending on pathology report). **Breslow thickness** will determine margin of excision
- 0-1mm thick → 1cm margin
- 1-2mm thick → 1-2cm margin
- 2-4mm thick → 2-3cm margin
- >4mm thick → 3cm margin

P: **Breslow thickness** is the single most impt factor in predicting prognosis
- <0.75mm → 95-100% 5y survival
- 0.76 - 1.50mm → 80-96%
- 1.51 - 4mm → 60-75%
- >4mm → 50%

Risk factors for metastasis:
- >55yo • Acral or head/neck tumour
- Breslow's >4mm
- Vascular invasion
- Absence of regression
- TERT promotor & BRAF mutations

Melanoma - DDx

Benign/dysplastic melanocytic naevi
- more uniform in shape and colour
- less likely to itch or bleed

Seborrhoeic keratosis
- waxy, "stuck on" often hyperkeratotic appearance
- dermoscope: + horned cysts, hairpin shaped blood vessels

Pigmented basal cell carcinoma
- pearly appearance, less pigmented
- prominent telangiactic vessels
- dermoscope: leaf-like areas of pigmentation, arborising vessels

Pigmented actinic keratosis
- more hyperkeratosis and erythema
- less pigmented, usually smaller
- ± painful

Intracorneal haematoma
- can be pared away with scalpel blade

Dermatofibroma
- skin dimpling on palpation
- scar-like appearance
- typically localised to extremities

Subungual haematoma
- reddish-black globules of pigment that grows out distally as nail grows
- usually hx of trauma
- -ve Hutchinson's!

Tinea nigra = superficial infection
- on hands, feet; usually not itchy, more homogenous pigmentation
- can be pared away with scalpel blade

Pyogenic granuloma
- lobular haemangioma usually in children
- bright red in colour → becomes fleshly pink after some time

Seborrhoeic keratosis

D: benign skin tumour, usually multiple over torso and forehead

R: >50yo, light skin, FHx, sun/UV

A/P: skin aging

S/smx:
- Appears "stuck on" with wart-like texture
- Subtypes: flat, raised, filiform and pedunculated   *Filiform = threadlike*
- Variable colours and surface may have greasy scale overlying it
- Painless, but can be very itchy
- A/w blepharitis (eyelid inflam)

Ix: dermoscopy (milia-like cysts and comedo-like openings)

Mx: conservative or shave excision

Benign naevi

D: benign collection of melanocytes in the epidermis, dermis, or both

R: genetic predisposition, fair skin, age - older children and young adults

Congenital melanocytic naevi
- >1cm diameter
- ↑risk of malignant transformation
Junctional melanocytic naevi
- Circular macules
- May have heterogenous colour
- Most naevi of the palms, soles, mucous membranes are this kind
Compound naevi
- Domed pigmented nodules ≤1cm in diameter
- Arise from junctional naevi, usually have uniform colour + smooth
Spitz naevi
- Usually develop over a few months in children
- Pink or red in colour, most common on face and legs
- May grow ≤1cm ± rapid growth
Atypical naevus syndrome
- ± autosomal dominant inheritance
- some ↑risk of melanoma, esp if they have a parent/sibling with melanoma

Dermatofibroma

D: solitary dermal fibrous nodules

A/P: ? can develop after minor trauma to skin (eg shaving)

S/smx: • young adults, F>M
- usually <1cm, on extremities
- feels like small rubbery buttons lying just under surface of skin
- pink to brown in colour forming a ring around the knot of tissue

Mx: conservative or excision

Pyoderma gangrenosum

D: non-infectious, inflammatory disorder resulting in painful ulcers

A/P: neutrophilic dermatosis; dense infiltration of neutrophils in the affected tissue
A/w IBD in 10-15%
- rheum disorders (RA, SLE)
- haematological disorders (myeloproliferative, lymphoma, myeloid leukaemias, MGUS)
- Wegener's
- Primary biliary cirrhosis
- 50% idiopathic

S/smx:
- Location: typically on the lower limb
  - often at site of minor injury (pathergy)
- Usually starts quite suddenly as a small pustule, red bump or blood-blister
- Later, the skin then breaks down resulting in an ulcer which is often painful
  - edge of ulcer is purple, violaceous and undermined
  - ulcer may be deep and necrotic
- May be a/w fever and myalgia

Ix: clinical Dx ± histology to r/o other causes of ulcer

Mx: • PO steroids
- in difficult cases, ciclosporin and infliximab may have a role
- surgical options delayed until disease is relatively under control to prevent further damage

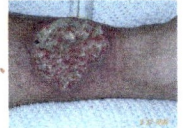

Basal cell carcinoma = rodent ulcer

D: neoplasm of the skin related to exposure to sunlight

R: UV, sunlight, XR exposure, arsenic exposure, xeroderma pigmentosum, childhood cancer survivor, transplant pts

S/smx:
- Nodular: pearly white with telangiectasias
- "Rolled borders"
- Small crusts and non-healing wounds
- May later ulcerate with central crater
- Sun-exposed sites, esp H&N
- Other types eg superficial, pigmented
  ↳ atypical presentations

Ix: Biopsy. Exact histopathology will determine need for further treatment.

Mx: standard excision or cryosurgery or non-surgical topical therapies (imiquimod, fluorouracil), radiotherapy.
- Mohs surgery (with intraoperative frozen slices to ensure margins are clear)
- !! strict sun protection measures + frequent skin checks

P: high risk factors for recurrence:
- tumour >2cm + located central face
- poorly defined margins
- high risk histological sub-type
- histological features of aggression; perineural or perivascular location
- failure of previous tx
- *immunosuppression*

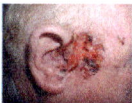
Ulcerated BCC

Squamous cell carcinoma

D: proliferation of atypical, transformed keratinocytes in the skin with malignant behaviour
- precursor lesions are known as **actinic keratosis** (AK)
- in situ tumours are known as **Bowen's disease**
- invasive tumours
- metastatic disease

R: UV, solid organ transplant recipient, immunosupp, light skin, FHx, ↑age, M>F, XR/radiotherapy, carcinogens, actinic keratosis, previous skin cancer, long standing leg ulcers (Marjolin's ulcer)

Features
Actinic keratoses
- small, crusty or scaly, lesions
- pink, red, brown or same colour as skin
- typically on sun-exposed areas
- multiple lesions may be present

Bowen's disease (SCC in situ)
- Red, scaly patches often 10-15mm in size, slow-growing

SCC
- Tumour grows over 3-6mo
- Painless, ulcerating ± bleeding
- Cauliflower-like appearance
- Keratoacanthoma - dome-shaped, central keratin-filled crater; involutes after 2-3mo
- Verrucous carcinoma - locally destructive but rarely metastatic; grows outwards, fungus/wart-like

Ix: biopsy
- AK intraepidermal keratinocytic dysplasia, esp in basal layer
- Bowen's disease - full-thickness atypia, confined to epidermis, intact basement membrane
- Invasive disease - crosses basement membrane

Mx of actinic keratosis
- prevention of further risk: e.g. sun avoidance, sun cream
- fluorouracil cream: typically 2-3w course
  - ! warn pt skin will become red and inflamed but to continue
  - can prescribe steroid cream to help with inflammation
- topical diclofenac: may be used for mild AKs – moderate efficacy, much fewer side effects
- topical imiquimod: trials have shown good efficacy
- cryotherapy
- curettage and cautery

Mx of Bowen's disease
- as with actinic keratosis
- fluorouracil cream: bd for 4w
  - warn pt that skin will become red and inflamed but to continue
  - can prescribe steroid cream to help with inflammation
- cryotherapy
- curettage and cautery

Mx of SCC
- Surgical excision with 4mm margins if lesion <20mm.
- If tumour >20mm then margins should be 6mm.
- Mohs micrographic surgery may be used in high-risk patients and in cosmetically important sites

P: good prognosticators incl well-differentiated, <20 mm diameter, <2mm deep, no immunosuppression

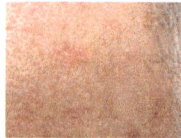
Actinic keratosis

Acne vulgaris

D: skin disease affecting the pilosebaceous unit

R: puberty, FHx/genetics, greasy skin or ↑sebum production, medications (androgens, steroids, anti-epileptics, isoniazid, lithium, hormones)

A/P: follicular epidermal hyperprolifera-tion → formation of keratin plug → plug obstructs the pilosebaceous follicle
- Activity of sebaceous glands may be controlled by androgen
  - levels often normal in pts with acne
  - colonisation by the anaerobic bacterium *Propionibacterium acnes*
- Inflammatory cascade

Features
- **Comedones** are due to a dilated sebaceous follicle
  - whitehead: top is closed
  - blackhead: top is opened
- **Inflammatory lesions** are due to follicle bursting, releasing irritants
  - Papules
  - Pustules
- Excess inflammation can cause nodules or **cysts**
- **Scarring** can result – ice-pick scars or hypertrophic scars
- **Drug-induced acne**: often monomorphic (eg steroids often cause pustules)
- **Acne fulminans**: very severe acne a/w systemic upset, often requires hospital admission + steroid tx

- Mild: open and closed comedones ± sparse inflammatory lesions
- Moderate: widespread non-inflam matory lesions, numerous papules and pustules
- Severe: extensive inflammatory lesions (incl nodules), pitting and scarring

Ix: clinical Dx ± hormonal evaluation, swabs for bacterial culture

Mx: step-wise approach
- **Single topical therapy** (retinoids, benzoyl peroxide)
- **Combi topical therapy** (abx, benzoyl peroxide, retinoid)
- **Oral abx**: tetracyclines (lymecycline, oxytetracycline, doxycycline)
  - avoid in pregnant/bfding women and in children <12yo
  - use erythromycin in pregnancy
  - use for max 3mo
  - co-prescribe with topical retinoid or benzoyl peroxide to ↓risk of resistance developing
  - risk of Gram-ve folliculitis – use high dose PO trimethoprim
- **COCP** are an alternative to oral abx in women
  - use in combi with topical retinoid or benzoyl peroxide
  - Dianette has ↑risk of VTE as compared to other COCPs therefore 2nd line, given only for 3mo, and counsel about risks
- **PO isotretinoin** – only under specialist
  - absolute CI in pregnancy, hyperlipidaemia

Discuss with pt
- Can take 4-8w for initial response, full response can take months
- Adhere to tx even if no early response
- With isotretinoin
  - regular blood tests may be needed
  - safety netting: stop and seek tx if severe HA, ↓night vision, significant liver enzyme or lipid elevations, or adverse psychiatric events
  - do not donate blood during tx or 30d after
  - do not get pregnant – pregnancy tests and monthly while on tx
  - dry skin and chapped skin common, use moisturiser

photos from Wikipedia

Eczema

D: inflammatory skin condition characterised by dry, pruritic skin with a chronic relapsing course

R: filaggrin gene mutation, <5yo, FHx, allergic rhinitis, asthma

A/P: loss of function mutation of filaggrin gene mutation predisposes to breaks in the epidermal barrier → ↑exposure & sensitisation to allergens + environment factors → inflammatory reaction

Phases & features
· Infantile phase (birth to 2yo)
  - dermatitis on cheeks, forehead, scalp and extensor surfaces
  - prominent vesicular component
  - oedema, weeping, crusting
· Childhood phase (2yo to puberty)
  - possibly worse
  - papules and plaques become lichenified ∴ constant scratching
  - antecubital and popliteal fossa, wrists, hands, ankles, and feet
· Adult phase
  - Thickened, dry skin and lichenified plaques

Ix: clinical dx. Allergen testing.

Mx: · Avoid irritants
· Simple emollients
  - large quantities (eg 250g/w), ≈ 10:1 ratio with topical steroids
  - apply emollient, wait 30min, then apply steroid
  - creams soak into skin faster than emollients (oily)
  - emollients can become contaminated with bacteria
· Topical steroids
· Wet wrapping = large amounts of emollient (and sometimes topical steroids) applied under wet bandages
· In severe cases, oral ciclosporin may be used

Steroid creams
· 1 finger tip unit = 0.5g = sufficient to treat skin area about 2x the size of an adult hand
· use weakest potency sufficient to treat pt's smx, do not use for longer than 1-2w at one go

Mild · Hydrocortisone 0.5-2.5%
Mod · Betamethasone 0.025%
       · Clobetasone 0.05%
       · Triamcinolone 0.1-0.2%
Potent · Fluticasone 0.05%
         · Betamethasone 0.1%
V potent · Clobetasone propionate 0.05%

Amount required for applications to different areas
· Face & neck: 15-30g
· Both ears: 15-30g
· Scalp: 15-30g
· Both arms: 30-60g
· Both legs: 100g
· Trunk: 100g
· Groin & genitalia: 15-30g

Adverse effects
· Skin atrophy, striae, rebound smx
  - atrophy esp for face – limit to 1-2w use at a time
· Perioral dermatitis – if applied to face for long periods of time. ↑risk if used with intranasal steroids
· Systemic effects only if applied to large areas
· Potent – limit use to 8w at a go; very potent – limit to 4w
· 4w break before starting another course

Psoriasis

D: chronic inflammatory skin disease characterised by erythematous, circumscribed scaly papules, and plaques

R: FHx/genetic, infection (eg URTI [strep], HIV), local trauma, medications (induce/exacerbate) – βB, lithium, antimalarials, NSAIDs, ACEI, infliximab

A/P: hyperproliferative disorder, involving a complex cascade of inflammatory mediators

Worsened by β-blockers

Classification & features
· Plaque psoriasis (80%)
  - Raised inflamed plaque lesions with a superficial silvery-white scaly eruption
  - Typically on extensor surfaces, scalp, trunk, buttocks, periumbilical areas
  - Clear delineation between good and bad skin
  - Auspitz's sign: if scale is removed, red membrane with pinpoint bleeding points
· Guttate psoriasis
  - Widespread, erythematous, fine, scaly papules - "water drops"
  - Usually a/w Strep URTI in children and adolescents
  - Acute onset over days
  - Most cases resolve spontaneously over 2-3mo; no need for abx
· Pustular psoriasis
· Erythroderma (erythrodermic psoriasis)
  - Generalised erythema + fine scaling
  - often a/w with pain, irritation, and sometimes severe itching
· Psoriatic arthritis [→12.01]
  - a/w athralgia, joint deformities, nail changes
· Reactive arthritis [→12.02]
  - "can't see can't pee can't climb a tree"

Ix: clinical Dx

Mx: step-wise approach
⚬ Potent corticosteroid cream OM + vitamin D analogue ON
  - eg betamethasone with calcipotriol
  - apply separately
  - initially for 4w → Ax response
  - trial for at least 8w
⚬ Vitamin D analogue BD
  - trial for 8-12w
3rd: · potent corticosteroid cream BD up to 4w, or
     · coal tar prep OD/BD, or
     · short-acting dithranol

2ndary Mx
· Phototherapy
  - narrowband UVB 3x/w
  - photochemotherapy: psoralen + UVA
  - AE: skin aging, ↑risk of SCC
· Systemic therapy
  - PO MTX esp w joint disease
  - others: ciclosporin systemic retinoids, biologics (DMARDs or others)

Specific areas
· Scalp: potent steroid OD for 4w
  → if no improvement, use different formulation (eg shampoo, mousse) ± topical agent to remove adherent scales before application of corticosteroid
· Face, flexural and genital: mild or mod steroid OD/BD for max 2w

Vitamin D analogue creams
· eg calcipotriol, calcitriol, tacalcitol
· MOA: ↓cell division and differentiation → ↓epidermal proliferation
  - tend to ↓scale and thickness of plaques, but not erythema
· AE are uncommon; can be used long-term
· Avoid in pregnancy
· 100g/w max in adults

Dithranol
· MOA: inhibits DNA synthesis
· Wash off after 30 mins
· AE include burning, staining

Coal tar
· MOA not fully understood; ? inhibits DNA synthesis

Rosacea

D: chronic disorder of the skin characterised by redness, flushing, and other cutaneous findings

R: light skin, hot baths/showers, temp extremes, sunlight, emotional stress, FHx, F>M

S/smx:
· typically affects nose, cheeks and forehead
· flushing is often first symptom
· telangiectasia are common
· later develops into persistent erythema with papules and pustules ± acne vulgaris
· rhinophyma M>F (nose deformity – nodules on the nose)
· ocular involvement: blepharitis
· sunlight may exacerbate smx

Mx
· For all – high SPF sunscreen ± camouflage creams to conceal redness
· Predominant erythema or flushing (limited telangiectasia)
  - ✎ Topical brimonidine gel prn
    ↳ usually ↓redness within 30min, effect lasts for 3-6h
· Mild to moderate papules / pustules
  - ✎ Topical ivermectin
  - ✎ Topical metronidazole, topical azelaic acid
· Moderate to severe disease
  - ✎ Topical ivermectin and PO doxycycline
· Refer to derm if
  - smx not improving – for consideration of laser therapy, esp if ↑telangiectasia
  - rhinophyma

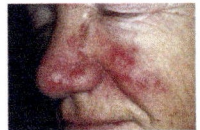
photo from Wikipedia

Impetigo

D: superficial, contagious, blistering infection of the skin caused by the bacteria Staphylococcus aureus and Streptococcus pyogenes

R: ↑humidity, poor hygiene, malnutrition, overcrowding, chronic colonisation with S. aureus (nasal, axillary, pharyngeal, perineal), concomitant skin disease (eg scabies, head lice, atopic eczema)

A/P: GAS → non-bullous type
- formation of thick-walled pustule + erythematous base
S. aureus → bullous
- exfoliative toxin breaks down desmoglein 1 → large blisters in epidermis with neutrophil and bacterial migration into bullous cavity
- bullae = fluid-filled lesions >0.5cm in diameter
Spread is by direct contact with discharges from the scabs of an infected person
↳ mainly by hands, but can spread indirectly by toys, clothing, equipment, environment

S/smx
- "Golden", crusted skin lesions typically found around the mouth
- Vesicles/bullae seen in bullous impetigo – initially clear, then becomes turbid

Ix: clinical Dx

Mx: ▪ H2O2 1% cream
- topical abx creams
  - fusidic acid
  - if resistance or MRSA is suspected, use mupirocin
- In extensive disease, use PO flucloxacillin or erythromycin
- School exclusion: until lesions are crusted and healed, or 48h after commencing abx tx
- Advice bds washing with soap and water – same advice for ppl who have been in contact

Folliculitis

D: inflammatory process involving any part of the hair follicle; it is most commonly 2/2 infection

R: trauma (incl shaving, extraction), topical corticosteroids, DM, immunosuppression

A/P: most commonly infectious in origin – S. aureus, Kleb, Entero-bacter, Proteus, Ps. aeruginosa (hot tub folliculitis). Fungal agents (often in young men), viral (herpes simplex, VZV, Molluscum contagiosum)

S/smx: - red bumps on skin with hx of trauma or other risk factors
- ± pruritus / mild discomfort in early stages
- If the condition worsens, can become very painful with furuncles or carbuncles

Ix: clinical Dx. Consider viral skin swab, skin scraping for microbiology

Mx: uncomplicated folliculitis – usually self-limiting; conservative tx
- Antibacterial soaps, wear loose clothing, cool dry environment, etc
- Careful shaving
Recurrent infectious folliculitis
- PO abx therapy guided by swabs
- ? ▪ flucloxacillin

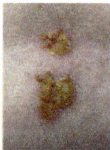
Golden crusted lesions on the chin

Cellulitis & erysipelas

Cellulitis is an infection of the deep dermis and subcutaneous tissue
Erysipelas is more superficial, involving only the upper dermis and superficial lymphatics

R: DM, venous insufficiency, eczema, oedema & lymphoedema, obesity, previous episodes of cellulitis, toe-web abnormalities

A/P: usually S. aureus and GAS – micro-organisms gain entry to dermal and SQ tissues via disruptions in cutaneous barrier

S/smx
- erythema, pain, swelling
- commonly on the shins
- possibly a/w systemic upset

Ix: clinical Dx. ± bloods and blood cultures if sepsis is suspected
Eron classification
Class I: no systemic toxicity, no uncontrolled comorbidities
II: systemically unwell or with co-morbidity that may complicate or delay resolution of cellulitis
III: significant systemic upset (incl acute confusion, ↑HR, ↑RR, hypotension) or unstable co-morbidities that interfere with response to tx, or limb-threatening infection due to vascular compromise
IV: sepsis or life-threatening infxn, eg necrotising fasciitis

Mx: • Class I – PO flucloxacillin (or clarithromycin, erythromycin or doxycycline)
• II: as per class I ± admission
• III & IV: admit + IV abx
  - co-amoxiclav, cefuroxime, clindamycin or ceftriaxone
  - also for rapidly deteriorating pts, <1yo, immunocompromise, significant lymphoedema, facial or periorbital cellulitis

Head lice = pediculosis capitis / nits

D: Infestation of parasitic head louse Pediculus humanus capitis

R: 3-12yo, F>M, close contact with infected ppl, overcrowding or close living conditions

A/P: Head lice grow on hair and feed on human blood
- Eggs are grey or brown, ≈ size of pinhead (diagnostic)
- Eggs are glued to the hair, close to the scalp, and hatch in 7-10d
- Nits are the empty egg shells and are white and shiny - found further along the hair shaft as hair grows

S/smx:
- commonly in children
- cause itching and scratching

Ix: fine-toothed combing of wet or dry hair should reveal eggs, nits or living lice

Mx: tx only indicated if living lice are found – contacts do not need to be treated unless living lice are found
- school exclusion not necessary
  ▪ Dimeticone or cyclomethicone
  - apply, leave for 30min to 8h (depending on product), rinse
  - repeat tx after 8-10d
  ▪ Ivermectin topical lotion
  - apply, leave for 10min, rinse
3rd: Malathion (due to resistance)
  - apply, leave for 8-12h, rinse
- Mechanical removal (esp for <2mo) or wet combing
- Follow instruction of products carefully to prevent recurrence

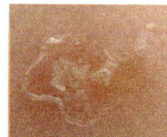
Scabies burrow

Scabies

D: infestation with the ectoparasitic mite Sarcoptes scabiei

R: overcrowding, <15yo or >65yo, sexual contact with new or multiple partners, immunosuppression

A/P: the scabies mite burrows into the epidermis, tunnels through the stratum corneum, and lays 2-4 eggs per day
- Larvae hatch in 2-4d, develop into adult mites ~2w later
- Transmission is via direct and prolonged skin-to-skin contact + fomites (clothes, bedding)
- Host immune response causes pruritus, erythema, papules and nodules – appears 3-4w after initial infestation, but within 1d upon re-infestation
- delayed type IV hypersensitivity

S/smx (clinical Dx):
- widespread pruritus
- linear burrows on side of fingers, interdigital webs, flexor aspects of wrist
- in infants, face and scalp affected
- also, excoriation, 2ndary infxn

Mx: ▪ Permethrin 5% cream applied to all areas incl face & scalp
  - allow to dry and leave on skin for 8-12h
  - re-apply if washed off (eg washing hands)
  - repeat tx 7d later
  - large quantities needed
  - CI in pts allergic to chrysanthemum
  ▪ PO ivermectin or topical malathion 0.5% (24h application)
For all pts,
- avoid close physical contact with others until tx is complete
- all household and close physical contacts should be treated at the same time, even if asmx
- launder, iron or tumble dry clothing, bedding, towels on first day of tx
- advise that itch can last 4-6w post eradication

Tinea / Dermatophyte infections

D: Superficial fungal infection. Dermatophytes are fungal organisms that require keratin for growth.

R: exposure to infected people, animals or soil; exposure to fomites, incl hat, combs, hairbrushes, upholstery; chronic topical or PO steroid use; HIV; DM; occlusive clothing; hot, humid weather; obesity; hyperhydrosis; frequent public bathing + barefoot; deformities of the feet; recent trauma to skin

A/P: fungal organisms (*Microsporum, Trichophyton, Epidermo-phyton spp*) that transmit via direct contact, fomites, soil or animals.
Various sites can be affected
· Hair/hair follicles: **tinea capitis**, tinea barbae, Majocchi's granuloma
· Skin: tinea faciale, **tinea corporis**, tinea curis, tinea manuum, **tinea pedis**
· Nail: tinea unguium
  - onychomycosis is a more inclusive term including nail infxns caused by dermatophytes, yeasts and moulds

Tinea capitis
· often in children, can cause scarring alopecia
· if untreated, a **kerion** may form = a raised, pustular, spongy/boggy mass
· most common cause is *Trychophyton tonsurans*
  - also *Microsporum canis* acquired from cats or dogs
· Dx is clinical ± scalp scrapings – under Wood's lamp, *Microsporum* will glow green
· Mx: PO antifungals
  - terbinafine for *Trychophyton*
  - griseofulvin for *Microsporum* (take after fatty meals OD; req 8-10w course as it is fungistatic)
  - for both: topical ketoconazole for first 2 weeks
    ↳ topical agents not effective as they do not penetrate the hair shaft

Tinea corporis (= ringworm)
· well-defined annular, erythematous lesions with pustules and papules
· Mx: topical agents until no further infxn visible, then apply for 2w thereafter (~2-6w total)
  ± PO azole therapy

Tinea pedis (= athlete's foot)
· Itchy, peeling skin between toes
· Mx: topical terbinafine + disinfect footwear, do not go barefoot in public spaces, etc
· Apply topical agents until no further infxn visible, then apply for 2w thereafter (~2-6w total)

Advise pts:
· Disinfect hairbrushes and combs
· Wear loose-fitting clothing
· Avoid sharing clothes and combs
· Avoid walking barefoot in public areas
· After washing, thoroughly dry any areas that have become infected before dressing
· For tinea pedis: alternating footwear and using foot powders may help ↓risk of relapse

Pityriasis versicolor
aka tinea versicolor
· D: Superficial cutaneous fungal infxn caused by Malassezia furfur
· R: immunosuppression (although can occur in healthy individuals), Cushing's, malnutrition
· S/smx: - Most commonly on trunk
  - Hypopigmented, pink or brown patches ± scale
  - Mild pruritus
· Mx: ✎ Topical antifungal (eg ketoconazole shampoo)
  - ✎ Consider alternative Dx, send scrapings to confirm Dx → if confirmed, PO itraconazole

Candida

D: infection of the skin by *Candida (albicans)*, a yeast-like fungus that is part of the commensal flora of the GIT and vagina

R: skin folds, ↑heat, ↑moisture, trauma, immunocompromise

A/P: colonisation is usually asmx, but can cause infections if barriers are disrupted or immune defenses are lowered

Ix: clinical Dx ± bloods, blood cultures if sepsis suspected

Mx: uncomplicated
· adults: topical imidazole (clotrimazole, ketoconazole, etc) or topical terbinafine
· children: topical imidazole
Inflammation/itch
· topical corticosteroid cream (eg hydrocort 1%) to be used od/bds for max 7-14d
  - reAx to ensure improvement
If *widespread, immunocompromised or refractory to initial tx,*
· PO fluconazole for 2w → reAx
  - consider swabbing, ref to derma
· For children: ref to derma
General hygiene for all pts
· Avoid skin occlusion
· Wash skin regularly with soap substitute, dry adequately
· Lose wt if obesity is contributing factor

For vaginal candidaisis (thrush), see 17.07

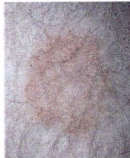
Tinea aka ringworm

Viral warts

D: Warts are elevated, round, hyperkeratotic skin papules with a rough greyish-white or light brown surface

R: water immersion, occupations involving handling of meat or fish, nail biting, <35yo, immuncomp

A/P: HPV1, 2, 3, 27, 57 and 63 infection of keratinocytes causes koilocytosis (viral transformation of the keratinocyte) and proliferation
↳ plantar warts a/w HPV-1

S/smx:
· Round, raised papules that range from pinpoint to 1cm, averaging 5mm in size
· Tiny black dots on the surface of the lesion can be seen after gentle paring with a scalpel
· Often located on fingers or nail folds; filiform warts a/w facial skin
· Warts may fissure, bleed and cause pain, and can also have a rough, scaly appearance

Ix: clinical Dx.

Mx: watchful waiting in immuno-competent pts, esp in children (90% clear in 5y spontaneously)
· ✎ Salicylic acid ± duct tape occlusion, cryotherapy, silver nitrate
· Daily application of salicylic acid-containing compounds ~8w
· AE: tenderness, erosion, superinfection
· Cryotherapy AE: blistering, pain, pigmentation Δ, recurrence
· ✎ Resistant or recurring:
  - Imiquinod: 90% cleared at 4w – daily or every other day application
  - PO zinc sulfate
  - Should be paired with surgical removal or cryotherapy

Molluscum contagiosum

D: long-term infectious condition causing cutaneous lesions

R: close/sexual contact with affected ppl, atopic dermatitis, immunocomp, tropical/humid climate

A/P: molluscum contagiosum virus (MCV), a poxvirus, infects keratinocytes ± mucosa → causes papular lesions
↳ abnormal keratinocytes are termed Henderson-Patterson bodies

S/smx:
· Pinkish/pearly white papules with central umbilication, ≤5mm
· Lesions appear in clusters anywhere on body, *except* palms and soles
· In adults, sexual contact may lead to lesions on genitalia, pubis, thighs and lower abdomen
· Lesions are rarely on the oral mucosa and eyelids

Mx: ✎ conservative ∵ self-limiting
· Spontaneously resolves in ~18mo
· Avoid sharing towels, clothing, baths with uninfected people
· Avoid scratching lesions
  - may need tx for this
· School/social exclusion not needed
· Treatment if desired
· Squeezing (with fingernails) or piercing lesions, then bathe – only a few lesions at once please
· Cryotherapy??
· Eczema/inflammation – emollients, mild steroid (hydrocort), topical abx (fusidic acid)
· Refer if
  - immunocompromised (eg HIV with extensive lesions)
  - eye-lid margin or ocular lesions
  - anogenital (GUM) – r/o other STI

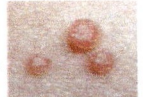
Molluscum contagiosum aka water warts

VZV / chickenpox

D: a childhood exanthem caused by the human α herpes virus (VZV)

R: exposure, 1-9yo, unimmunised status, occupational exposure

A/P: Direct contact or airborne respi droplet spread → virus spreads to regional LN causing 1' viremic phase → spreads to liver, spleen, etc
- 2' viremic phase at ~day 9: mononuclear cells transport the virus to the skin and mucous membranes → classic vesicular rash
- Pts are infectious 2-4d *before* onset of rash, and remain so until lesions are crusted over
- Incubation period is ~14d

S/smx:
- Fever initially ± mild systemic upset
- Rash: itchy, starts on head/trunk
  - macular → papular → vesicular
- Severe disease a/w complications such as pneumonia, neurological sequelae, hepatitis, secondary bacterial infxn

Mx: supportive
- Keep cool, trim nails, calamine lotion
- School exclusion until lesions have crusted over
- Do not give NSAIDs - ? ↑risk of secondary bacterial infxns
  - secondary invasive GAS infections can result in necrotising fasciitis
- at risk pts: PO/IV antiviral therapy
  - give within 72h of onset

Post-exposure prophylaxis (PEP)
→ varicella zoster immunoglobulin (VZIG) for PEP
- Significant exposure to VZV/HZV
- Clinical conditions ↑risk of severe varicella, incl pregnant women, immunocompromised pts, neonates
- No abs to VZV

VZV in pregnancy
- mother: 5x risk of pneumonitis
- fetal varicella syndrome
  - 1% risk if before 20w gest
  - skin scarring, eye defects (micro-phthalmia), limb hypoplasia, microcephaly, learning disabilities
- shingles in infancy: 1-2% risk if maternal exposure in 2nd/3rd trim
- severe neonatal varicella: fatal in 20% cases

VZV prophylaxis/Mx in pregnancy
- if in doubt, check maternal blood for varicella antibodies
- if ≤20w and not immune, give VZIG asap – effective 10d post-exposure
- if >20w and not immune, either VZIG or PO antivirals from day 7 to 14 post-exposure

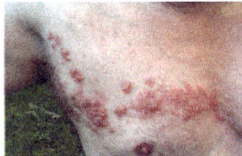
Shingles rash on a single dermatome (?T2)

Herpes zoster / shingles

D: reactivation of VZV, characterised by dermatomal pain and papular rash

R: >50yo, F>M, HIV, chronic steroid use, chemotherapy, malignancies

A/P: reactivation of latent VZV from dorsal root or CN ganglia, present since primary infection
- Latent infection is established by evading the immune system

S/smx:
- Prodromal period: burning pain for 2-3d + 20% pts fever, HA, fatigue
- Vesicular eruption follows in the dermatomal distribution of infected ganglion (usually T1 to L2)
  - pain (localised, stinging), pruritus, rash (erythematous maculopapular rash → clear vesicles → crusted over)
  - does not cross the midline
- Corneal ulceration if CN V

Mx: • advise pts they are potentially contagious; avoid pregnant women and immunosuppressed
  - until vesicles have crusted over, usually 5-7d following onset
  - covering lesions ↓risk
- Analgesia: paracetamol & NSAIDs
  - ↖ neuropathic agents
  - PO corticosteroids in first 2w if immunocompetent
- Antivirals: w/in 72h of onset
  - benefits: ↓incidence of post-herpetic neuralgia, esp in old ppl
  - aciclovir, famciclovir, valaciclovir

Complications
- Post-herpetic neuralgia 5-30% – resolves w/in ~6mo, may be longer
- Ophthalmic involvement
- Ramsay Hunt syndrome (ears): ear lesions and facial paralysis

See also Ophthalmic shingles 05.03

Pityriasis rosea

D: inflammatory skin disease with unclear aetiology

R: 10-35yo, F>M

S/smx:
- In some individuals, there may be a Hx of recent viral infxn
- Herald patch
  - Usually on trunk
  - Usually about 2w before main rash
- Erythematous, oval, scaly patches
  - "Fir-tree" appearance: the longitudinal diameters of the oval lesions run parallel to the lines of Langer

Ix: clinical Dx
- DDx: Guttate psoriasis [→09.04]
  - Guttate psoriasis is usually preceded by Strep throat (2-4w), and presents with 'tear drop' scaly papules on trunks and limbs
  - Either way, both are self-resolving

Mx: Watch & wait – usually resolves spontaneously after 6-12w

See also pityriasis versicolor on 09.06 under Tina / Dermatophyte infxns

Hidradenitis suppurativa

D: chronic inflammatory skin disease that primarily involves intertriginous areas (eg axilla, groin, perineum, etc)

R: obesity, F>M, smoking, FHx

A/P: ? autoimmune disease – repeated inflammation occludes the hair follicles and apocrine glands → nodules, abscesses and scarring

S/smx:
- Recurrent, painful and inflamed nodules, esp on the axillae
- Nodules may rupture, releasing pus
- More severe / complications: rope-like scarring, plaques, sinus tracts, contractures, lymphatic obstruction
- Hurley classification – 3 classes based on severity

Ix: clinical Dx

DDx: acne vulgaris (mainly face, upper chest; →09.03), follicular pyoderma (should respond rapidly to abx), donovanosis (STI, mainly in regions of sexual contact; →08.08)

Mx:
- Good hygiene, loose-fitting clothes
- Smoking cessation, wt loss
- Medical Mx: steroids (injection into lesion or PO), abx (eg flucox)
  - Long-term: topical or PO abx (eg top clindamycin, PO rifampicin)
- Surgical: excision of nodules

P: depends on how well controlled disease is; complete remission may require surgical intervention. May have profound impact on QoL

Pemphigus

D: group of autoimmune blistering diseases that involve the epidermal surfaces of the skin, mucosa, or both
· pemphigus vulgaris
· pemphigus foliaceus
· paraneoplastic pemphigus

R: ↑age, HLA DR4 (PV), DQ1 (PV), DRB1 (PNP), associated malignancy (non-HHV8 Castleman's disease, non-Hodgkin's lymphoma, CLL, thymoma and rare sarcomas)
↑incidence in Ashkenazi Jews

A/P: IgG auto-abs bind to desmoglein 3 or 1 of the desmosome (in skin and mouth), and cause cell detachment and blistering

S/smx:
· Mucosal ulceration 50-70%
· Skin blistering
 - flaccid, easily ruptured vesicles and bullae
 - clear blisters
 - painful but not itchy
 - Nikolsky's +ve (skin peels on gentle rubbing/shearing of the skin)
· On biopsy: acantholysis

Ix: skin biopsy

Mx: ⚕ PO steroid ± azathioprine or mycophenolate
 - steroids to be given with bone protection and PPI
⚕ rituximab ± steroids

P: PV and PF good prognosis if adequately controlled. PNP – mortality can approach 90%

Bullous pemphigoid

D: chronic, acquired autoimmune blistering disease characterised by auto-abs against hemidesmosomal antigens, resulting in the formation of a sub-epidermal blister

R: 60-90yo, HLA DQB1

A/P: Auto-abs against two hemidesmo-somal proteins, BP180 and BP230
· Infiltration of inflammatory cells → release of proteases → inflammatory mediators
· Eosinophilic infiltration

S/smx
· itchy, tense blisters typically around flexures, axillae, groin, abdomen
· pruritus may precede 3-4mo
· blisters heal without scarring
· mouth is spared
 - 10-50% may have mucosal involvement but this is classically a differentiating factor between pemphigus and pemphigoid
· skin biopsy: immunofluorescence shows IgG and C3 at the dermo-epidermal junction

Mx: ref to Derm
· PO corticosteroids or tacrolimus
 - apply sparingly to affected areas bds for up to 2w
· Also topical corticosteroids, immunosuppressants, abx

Insect bites

Local reactions
· Local oedema and pain
· Spider bites may show one or two small fang marks
· Allergic rxns: pain, wheal and flare formation, warmth, pruritus at site
 - usually self-limiting, confined
· Difficult to distinguish between bite and cellulitis acutely
· Delayed allergic rxns are common
 - can cause permanent skin discolouration

Systemic reactions
· Anaphylaxis

Hx taking
· Time course of onset
· Serum sickness: uncommon delayed reaction, usually ~1w after envenom-ation. Fever, myalgias, arthralgias, rash, adenopathy, and HA

Mx:
· Rest, ice, elevate for local pain and swelling
· Clean wound with soap and water
· Fire ant pustules - leave intact. If opened, keep clean and covered
· Ax for tetanus propylaxis
· Stinger removal
 - all should be removed asap
 - scrap the stinger with the edge of a plastic ID card
· Medical tx: corticosteroids, antihistamines, NSAIDs
· Tx secondary infxns accordingly

Others:
· If previous anaphylaxis, ensure Epipen is carried everywhere and pt and family know how to use
· Insect bite or sting can cause redness and itching for ≤10d, try not to scratch to prevent 2ndary infection
Prevention:
· Cover skin, apply DEET, avoid using products with strong scents
· Avoid camping near water
· Keep food/drink covered outdoors
· Inspect skin for ticks/bites at end of day

Flat, non-palpable changes in skin colour

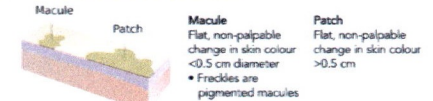

Macule
Flat, non-palpable change in skin colour <0.5 cm diameter
• Freckles are pigmented macules

Patch
Flat, non-palpable change in skin colour >0.5 cm

Elevation due to fluid in a cavity

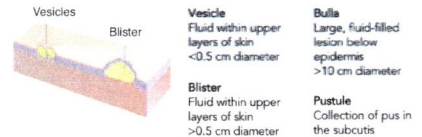

Vesicle
Fluid within upper layers of skin <0.5 cm diameter

Blister
Fluid within upper layers of skin >0.5 cm diameter

Bulla
Large, fluid-filled lesion below epidermis >10 cm diameter

Pustule
Collection of pus in the subcutis

Elevation due to solid masses

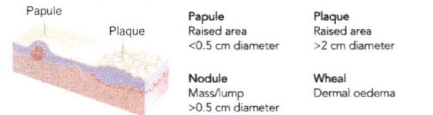

Papule
Raised area <0.5 cm diameter

Nodule
Mass/lump >0.5 cm diameter

Plaque
Raised area >2 cm diameter

Wheal
Dermal oedema

Loss of skin

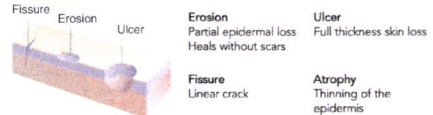

Erosion
Partial epidermal loss Heals without scars

Fissure
Linear crack

Ulcer
Full thickness skin loss

Atrophy
Thinning of the epidermis

Vascular changes

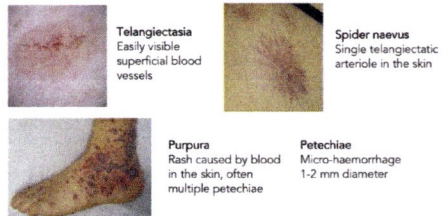

Telangiectasia
Easily visible superficial blood vessels

Spider naevus
Single telangiectatic arteriole in the skin

Purpura
Rash caused by blood in the skin, often multiple petechiae

Petechiae
Micro-haemorrhage 1-2 mm diameter

Diagrams and photos from Wikipedia.
Chart concept derived from Oxford Handbook of Clinical Specialties

Leukemia = **cancer of the WBCs in bone marrow** → marrow failure → ↓RBC / anaemia & ↓ mature WBC and ↓platelets (haemorrhage)

Polycythaemia vera

Lymphoid neoplasms

Acute lymphoblastic leukemia

D: malignant clonal cancer of the **lymphoid progenitor cell**
→ common ALL (75%), CD10+, pre-B phenotype
→ T-ALL (20%) and B-ALL (5%)

R: children <5yo – accounts for 80% of childhood leukemias. a/w Down's.

S/smx *predictable by bone marrow failure*
- anaemia: lethargy and pallor
- neutropaenia: frequent / severe infxns
- thrombocytopenia: easy bruising, petechiae

Other features
- bone pain (2/2 bone marrow infiltration)
- mediastinal mass (T-ALL)
- splenomegaly   • hepatomegaly
- fever – up to 50% of new cases
- testicular swelling (2/2 spread)

Prognosis • Better: t12;21, younger
• Worse: - age < 2yo or > 10yo
   - WBC > 20 at Dx
   - T or B cell surface markers
   - non-Caucasian   - male sex

Chronic lymphoblastic leukemia

D: indolent lymphoproliferative disorder in which **monoclonal B lymphocytes** are predominantly found in peripheral blood

R: >60yo. Most common adult leuk

S/smx: – often asymptomatic
• Systemic signs: anorexia, wt loss
• Bleeding, infxn, lymphadenopathy

Ix: FBC (lymphocytosis – lymph >5; anaemia, thrombocytopaenia), blood film (smudge cells), immunophenotyping (CD5, CD19, CD20 and CD23)

Complications: anaemia, recurrent infxns 2/2 hypogammaglobulin-aemia, warm autoimmune haemolytic anaemia (10-15%)

Richter's transformation
= leukaemia cells enter LNs and change into a high-grade, fast-growing non-Hodgkin's lymphoma (often DLBCL)
→ pt suddenly becomes unwell
S/smx: LN swelling, fever without infxn, wt loss, night sweats, nausea, abdominal pain

Hairy cell leukemia

D: indolent, mature B-cell neoplasm

R: middle age, M>F, whites, ?EBV

Features
- Dry tap on aspiration ∴ marrow fibrosis fibrosis
- Massive splenomegaly
- Pancytopenia
- Histology: fuzzy cells, stains TRAP a/w BRAF mutations

Myeloid neoplasms

Acute myeloid leukemia

D: clonal expansion of **myeloid blasts** in the bone marrow, peripheral blood, or extramedullary tissues

R: >65yo, prev haem disorders, prev chemo, radiation exposure, benzene exposure (paints, petrol, rubber)

S/smx 2/2 bone marrow failure:
- anaemia: pallor, lethargy, weakness
- neutropenia + freq infxns
   - although WBC counts may be very high, functioning neutrophil levels may be low
- thrombocytopenia: bleeding
- splenomegaly   • bone pain

Acute promyelocytic leukaemia
- a/w t(15;17) = fusion of PML and RAR-alpha genes
- a/w younger age, ?Down's
- Histology: Auer rods (seen with myeloperoxidase stain)
- DIC or thrombocytopenia often at presentation
- Good prognosis; responds to all-trans retinoic acid (vit A) and arsenic

Chronic myeloid leukemia

D: malignant clonal disorder of **myeloid stem cells** arising due to the t9;22 mutation (Philadelphia chromosome) resulting in the BCR-ABL fusion gene

R: 65-74yo

S/smx:
- anaemia: lethargy
- wt loss, sweats
- splenomegaly → abd discomfort
- ↑granulocytes at different stages of maturation ± thrombocytosis
- ↓ leukocyte alkaline phosphatase
- may undergo blast transformation (**AML** 80%, **ALL** 20%) "blast crisis"

Mx: tyrosine kinase inhibitors

Polycythaemia vera rubra (PVR)
- primary polycythaemia; clonal proliferation of a marrow stem cell leading to an increase in red cell volume ± ↑neutrophils and platelets
- JAK2 mutation present in ~95%
Relative polycythaemia
→ due to ↓ circulating volume
- Dehydration
- Stress: Gaisbock syndrome (HTN, ↑RBC and plethora without splenomegaly)
Secondary polycythaemia
→ ↑stimulation to produce RBCs
- COPD   • High altitude
- Obstructive sleep apnoea
- Excessive erythropoietin: cerebellar haemangioma, hypernephroma, hepatoma, uterine fibroids
- Iatrogenic / doping

R: (PVR) peak in 60s

S/smx:
- pruritus, typically after a hot bath
- splenomegaly   • hypertension
- hyperviscosity
- arterial and venous thrombosis
- haemorrhage (2/2 abn platelets)

Mx: aspirin, venesection, chemo (hydroxyurea)

Prog: thrombotic events!! 5-15% myelofibrosis, 5-15% acute leukemia (↑risk with chemo)

Myelodysplastic syndromes
- Clonal haematopoietic stem cell disorders characterised by ineffective haematopoiesis, peripheral blood cytopaenias, and risk of progression to AML
- A: 90% primary (typically in >70yo), 10% 2/2 causes such as chemo and radiotherapy (usually 5y after treatment)

• S/smx: can be asmx, otherwise milder version of AML
• Ix: peripheral blood counts, bone marrow exam (dysplastic changes), cytogenic analysis
• Mx: supportive care (eg blood transfusions), DMARDs (eg lenalidomide), immunosupressive therapy, stem cell transplant

Myelofibrosis
- Myeloproliferative disorder characterised by bone marrow fibrosis
- R: radiation exposure, industrial solvent exposure (eg benzene)
- P: thought to be caused by hyperplasia of abnormal mega-karyocytes → ↑platelet derived growth factor → ↑fibroblasts

• S/smx: typically in elderly pts
   - Anaemia (fatigue is the most common presenting smx)
   - Massive splenomegaly
   - Hypermetabolic smx (wt loss, night sweats, etc)
• Ix: bloods (anaemia), blood film (tear drop cells), bone marrow aspirate will be difficult due to 'dry tap'; trephine biopsy will be needed
• Mx: monitoring, may require stem cell transplant if severe

How to interpret blood results
1. Look at lymphocytes
   • ↓ = ALL or AML
2. Look at WBC
   • >100 = likely chronic – ?CML
3. Look at WBC differential
   • Bands = CML
   • Blasts = AML

Non-Hodgkin's lymphomas

- More common than HL
- Generally affects elderly (1/3 cases in >75yo)
- Affects B-cells mainly, T-cell lymphomas less common
- A/w autoimmune disease and viral infxns (worse prognosis)
- S/smx
  - painless lymphadenopathy (non-tender, rubbery, asymmetrical)
  - constitutional B-symptoms: fever, wt loss, night sweats, lethargy
  - extranodal disease: GI, bone marrow, lungs, skin, CNS smx
- Ix
  - ✂ excisional node biopsy
  - CTTAP for staging / PET
  - Serology (HIV, EBV)
  - Other bloods
  - Staging (Ann Arbor system)
    1. One node affected
    2. ≥1 node affected on same side of diaphragm
    3. Nodes affected on both sides of diaphragm
    4. Extranodal involvement (eg spleen, bone marrow, CNS)
    - A = absence of B-symptoms
    - B = presence of B smx
      ↳ eg stage 3B or stage 1A
- Mx: depends on subtype
  - all pts should be offered flu and pneumococcal vaccines
  - pts with neutropaenia may require abx prophylaxis
- Complications
  - bone marrow infiltration (→ pancytopaenic smx)
  - SVC obstruction
  - metastases
  - spinal cord compression

Neoplasms of B cells

Burkitt lymphoma
- Adolescents / young adults
- t8;14   • a/w EBV
- Starry sky appearance, tingible body macrophages
- Jaw lesion endemic in Africa

Diffuse large B-cell lymphoma
- Older adults; 20% children
- BCL2, BCL6
- Most common type of NHL in adults

Follicular lymphoma
- Adults   • t14;18
- Indolent course; waxing, waning lymphadenopathy

Mantle cell lymphoma
- Adults M>F   • t11;14
- Very aggressive; pts present in late stage :(

Marginal zone lymphoma
- Adults   • t11;18
- A/w chronic inflammation, eg Sjogren's, MALT syndrome

Primary CNS lymphoma
- Adults   • a/w EBV, HIV, AIDS
- AIDS-defining. Presents with neuro smx: confusion, seizures, memory loss
- Single, ring-enhancing mass

Neoplasms of T cells

Adult T cell lymphoma
- Adults   • 2/2 HTLV (a/w IVDU)
- Presents w/ cutaneous lesions
- Common in Japan, West Africa, Caribbean

Mycosis fungoides / Sezary syndrome
- Adults
- Presents w/ kin patches, plaques
- CD4+ with cerebriform nuclei and inraepidermal neoplastic cell aggregates
- Sezary = T cell leukemia

LYMPHOMA
= discrete tumour mass arising from lymph nodes

Hodgkin lymphoma

- D: haematological malignancy of **mature B cells** characterised by presence of **Hodgkin's cells** and **Reed-Sternberg cells**
- R: a/w HIV, EBV
- S/smx:
  - Lymphadenopathy (75%)
    ◊ most common in neck (cervical or supraclavicular) > axillary > inguinal
    ◊ usually painless, non-tender, asymmetrical
    ◊ *alcohol-induced LN pain* is charac-teristic of HL but seen in <10% of pts
  - systemic B smx: wt loss, night sweats, fever, pruritus (↓prognosis)
  - other presentations: mediastinal mass
- Ix
  - Bloods: normocytic anaemia, eosinophilia, ↑LDH
  - ✂ LN biopsy
    ◊ Reed-Sternberg cells are diagnostic ("owl eyes"); CD15 and CD30 +ve
- Classification
  - Nodular sclerosis (70%) - good prog
  - Mixed cellularity (20%) - good prog
  - Lymphocyte predominant (5%) - best prognosis
  - Lymphocyte depleted (rare) - worst prognosis
- Staging - Ann Arbor system
- Mx: chemo, radiotherapy
  - if relapsed or refractory, stem cell transplant

8;14: Burkitt lymphoma
11;14: Mantle cell lymphoma
11;18: Marginal zone lymphoma
14;18: Follicular lymphoma
15;17: APML
t9;22: [Philadelphia] CML

Multiple myeloma

D: haematological cancer characterised by clonal proliferation of **plasma cells** in the bone marrow

R: ↑age (median 70yo) MGUS, FHx, ? radiation exposure

P: genetic mutations as B-cells differentiate into mature plasma cells
- ↑production of monoclonal Ig or Ig fragments (paraproteins) in serum and urine
- Normal Ig production impaired, causing relative hypogammaglobulinaemia → predisposes to infxn

S/smx: "CRABBI"
- Calcium: hyperCa (>2.75)
  - 2/2 osteoclastic bone resorption → "bones stones moans groans" + constipation & confusion
- Renal issues
  - light chain deposition within renal tubules → renal damage → dehydration, ↑thirst
  - amyloidosis, nephrocalcinosis, nephrolithiasis
- Anaemia
  - 2/2 bone marrow crowding suppressing erythropoeisis
- Bleeding
  - 2/2 thrombocytopaenia
- Bones: lytic bone lesion
  - pathological fractures
- Infection
  - due to defective and decreased Ig
- Others   - Hyperviscoscity
           - Neuropathy
           - Amyloidosis

Ix: Bloods (FBC, peripheral blood film [rouleaux formation!], U&Es, bone profile (↑Ca)
- Protein electrophoresis, urinalysis (Bence Jones proteins)
- Bone marrow aspiration
- Imaging - whole body MRI
  ↳ 'rain drop skull'

Dx criteria
- 1 major + 1 minor; or 3 minor

Major • Plamacytoma
         • 30% plasma cells in bone marrow sample
         • ↑M protein in blood or urine

Minor • 10-30% plasma cells
         • Minor ↑M protein
         • Osteolytic lesions on imaging
         • ↓ antibodies in blood

Mx:
- W&w if "smouldering MM"
- Stem cell transplant
- Supportive care to ↓complications
  - Hydration
  - Bisphosphonate infusions for bone pain and osteolytic bone lesions
  - Denosumab

P: incurable if no stem cell transplant. Relapse at ~2-5y tx. Median survival 29-62 mo depending on stage at Dx.

Other plasma cell problems
Waldenstrom's macroglobulinaemia
- Disorder 2/2 overproduction of IgM
- S/smx:
  - Peripheral neuropathy
  - Hyperviscosity syndrome: HA, blurry vision, Raynaud's, retinal haemorrhages
- Ix: Bone marrow: >10% small lymphocytes with IgM inclusions
- Complications: thrombosis
Monoclonal gammopathy of undetermined significance
- Overproduction of any Ig type
- S/smx: usually asmx
  - 10-30% have a demyelinating neuropathy
- Ix: bone marrow <10% monoclonal plasma cells
- Complications: 1-2% risk of transforming to multiple myeloma

Neutrophils / Phagocytes

Chronic granulomatous disease
- D: ↓NADPH oxidase → ↓ ability of phagocytes to produce reactive oxygen species
- S/smx:
  - Recurrent pneumonias and abscesses by catalase +ve bacteria (eg Staph aureus) and fungi (eg Aspergillus)

Chediak-Higashi syndrome
- D: Microtubule polymerization defect → ↓phagocytosis
- Autosomal recessive
- S/smx: "PLAIN"
  - progressive neurodegeneration
  - lymphohistiocytosis
  - partial albinism
  - recurrent pyogenic infections
  - peripheral neuropathy
- Ix: neutrophils and platelets have giant granules, pancytopaenia, mild coagulation defects

Leukocyte adhesion deficiency
- D: Defect of LFA-1 integrin (CD18) protein on neutrophils
- Autosomal recessive
- S/smx:
  - recurrent skin and mucosal bacterial infxn with no pus
  - impaired wound healing
  - delayed separation of umbilical cord
- Ix: ↑neutrophils in blood, but absence of neutrophils at infxn sites

B-cell disorders

Common variable immunodeficiency (CVID)
- Defect in B-cell differentiation
- S/smx
  - presents after 2yo
  - ↑risk of autoimmune disease, bronchiectasis, lymphoma, heart and lung infections
- Ix: ↓IgG, IgM, IgA

X-linked (Bruton) agamma-globulinaemia
- Defect in BTK (tyrosine kinase gene) → no B cell maturation
- X-linked recessive
- S/smx:
  - presents ~6mo (↓maternal IgG)
  - recurrent bacterial and enteroviral infxns
- Ix: absent B cells in peripheral blood, ↓Ig of all classes. Absent or few LN and tonsils
- ❗ live vaccines contraindicated

Selective IgA deficiency
- Maturation defect in B cells
- Most common primary antibody deficiency
- A/w coeliac disease (may cause false -ve coeliac ab screen)
- S/smx: - most pts are asmx
  - recurrent sinus and respi infxns
    ↳ ↑susceptibility to giardiasis
  - anaphylactoid reaction in response to blood transfusions
- Ix: ↓IgA (but normal IgG, IgM)

T-cell disorders

DiGeorge syndrome
- Absent thymus and parathyroid glands due to 22q11 microdeletion (results in failure to develop 3rd and 4th pharyngeal pouches)
- S/smx: "CATCH-22"
  - Cardiac defects
  - Abnormal facies
  - Thymic hypoplasia
  - ◊ giving rise to T-cell deficiency and recurrent viral and fungal infxns)
  - Cleft palate
  - Hypocalcaemia 2/2 parathyroid aplasia → tetany
- Velocardiofacial syndrome is similar

Job syndrome
- STAT3 mutation → deficiency of Th17 cells → impaired recruitment of neutrophils to sites of infxn
- S/smx:
  - cold abscesses
  - baby teeth retained
  - coarse facies
  - dermatological problems
  - ↑IgE
  - bone fractures from minor trauma

Chronic mucocutaneous candidiasis
- T cell dysfunction → impaired cell-mediated immunity against Candida
- S/smx:
  - non-invasive Candida albicans infxns of skin and mucous membranes

B & T-cell disorders

Severe combined immunodeficiency (SCID) →15.15 for more
- Several types including X-linked recessive defective IL-2 receptor, autosomal recessive adenosine deaminase deficiency
- S/smx - failure to thrive
  - chronic diarrhoea
  - thrush
  - recurrent viral, bacterial, fungal and protozoal infxns
- Mx
  - live vaccines contraindicated
  - antimicrobial prophylaxis and IVIG
  - bone marrow transplant

Ataxic telangiectasia
- Defect in ATM gene → defect in DNA repair enzymes → accumulation of mutations
- Autosomal recessive
- S/smx:
  - Cerebellar defects → ataxia
  - Spider angiomas (= telangiectasia)
  - IgA deficiency
  - ↑sensitivity to radiation

Wiskott-Aldrich syndrome
- Defect in WASP gene → leukocytes and platelets cannot recognise actin skeleton → defective antigen presentation
- X-linked recessive
- S/smx: "WA-TER"
  - Thrombocytopaenia
  - Eczema
  - Recurrent pyogenic infxns
  - ↑risk of autoimmune disease and malignancy
- Ix: ↓IgM levels

Hyper IgM syndromes
- CD40 gene mutation → IgM cannot switch to other classes
- S/smx:
  - severe pyogenic infxns early in life
  - opportunitistic infxn with Pneumo cystis, Cryptosporidium, CMV
- Ix: normal or ↑IgM, ↓↓IgG, IgA or IgE

Acute intermittent porphyria

D: partial deficiency of porphobilinogen deaminase → accumulation of porphyrin precursors and porphyrins
→ defective haem synthesis
- Autosomal dominant

R: FHx, F>M (5:1)
Exacerbators:
- drugs (eg phenytoin, progestins, metoclopramide, sulfonamide abx)
- ↓caloric intake
- Smoking (more frequent attacks)

S/smx:
- Classically presents in 20-40yo
- Abdominal pain, vomiting
- Neuro: motor neuropathy
- Psychiatric: depression
- HTN and ↑HR

Ix:
- ↑urinary porphobilinogen and total porphyrins (esp during attacks)
  ◊ urine will turn deep red on standing
- ↑serum porphobilinogen (PBG) and delta-aminolaevulinic acid (DALA)
- Assay of red cells for porphobilinogen deaminase

Mx: • Avoid triggers
- During acute attacks,
  - IV haemin / haem arginate
    ↳ specialist treatment
  - IV glucose (if IV haemin not available)
    – ≥300g dextrose (10% glucose)
- Other options: givosiran (↓PBG and ↓DALA), liver transplant

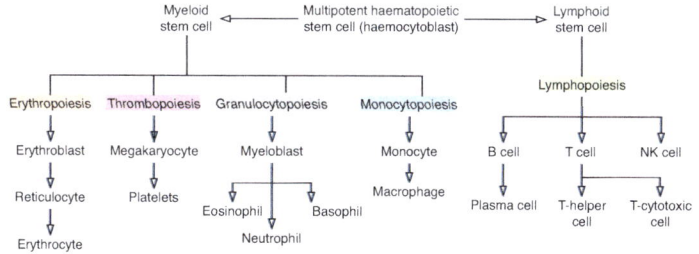

Myeloid stem cell ⟷ Multipotent haematopoietic stem cell (haemocytoblast) ⟷ Lymphoid stem cell

Erythropoiesis · Thrombopoiesis · Granulocytopoiesis · Monocytopoiesis · Lymphopoiesis

Erythroblast → Reticulocyte → Erythrocyte

Megakaryocyte → Platelets

Myeloblast → Eosinophil, Basophil, Neutrophil

Monocyte → Macrophage

B cell → Plasma cell

T cell → T-helper cell, T-cytotoxic cell

NK cell

Highlighted ones come up more in exams

Anaemia — Hb < 120 g/L in non-pregnant females / Hb <130 g/L in males

Branches:
- **Microcytic (MCV <80 fL)**
  - Thalassemias
  - Anaemia of chronic disease
  - Iron deficiency
  - Lead poisoning
  - Sideroblastic anaemia
- **Normocytic (MCV 80-100 fL)**
  - **Nonhaemolytic** — reticulocyte index ≤2%
    - Iron deficiency (early)
    - Anaemia of chronic disease
    - Aplastic anaemia
    - Chronic kidney disease
  - **Haemolytic** — reticulocyte index >2%
    - **Intrinsic**
      - Membrane defects
        - Hereditary spherocytosis
        - Paroxysmal nocturnal haemoglobinruia
      - Enzyme deficiencies
        - G6PD deficiency
        - Pyruvate kinase def
      - Haemoglobinopathies
        - Sickle cell anaemia
        - HbC disease
    - **Extrinsic**
      - Autoimmune (÷warm, cold)
      - Microangiopathic
        - TTP/HUS
        - DIC
        - Malignancy
        - Pre-eclampsia
      - Macroangiopathic
        - Prosthetic heart valves
      - Infections
        - Malaria
- **Macrocytic (MCV >100 fL)**
  - **Megaloblastic**
    - Folate deficiency
    - Vitamin B12 deficiency
    - Fanconi anaemia
  - **Non-megaloblastic**
    - Liver disease
    - Alcohol
    - Hypothyroidism
    - Pregnancy
    - Reticulocytosis
    - Myelodisplasia
    - Drugs, eg cytotoxics

Iron studies

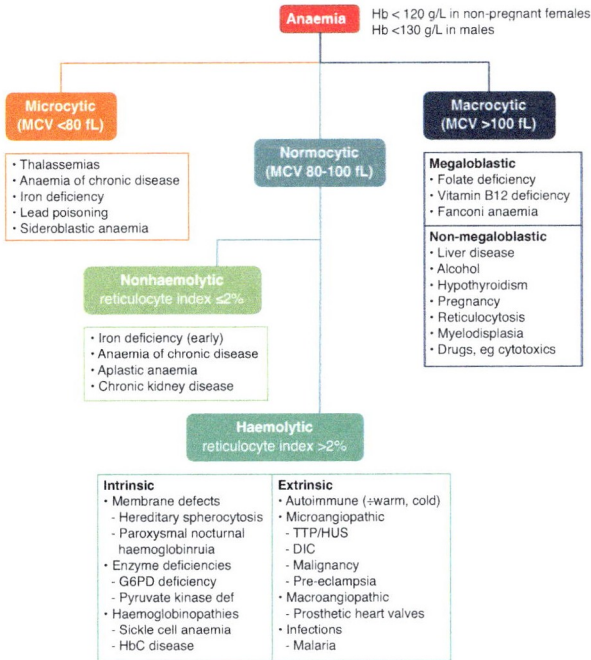

Iron studies	Serum iron	Transferrin/ TIBC	Ferritin	% transferrin saturation
Iron deficiency	↓ <8	↑	↓	↓↓
Chronic disease	↓ <15	↓	↑	-
Haemochromatosis	↑	↓ (screening)	↑	↑↑

- Primary disturbance is highlighted in pink
- Transferrin transports iron in blood
- TIBC = total iron binding capacity; indirect measure of transferrin
- Ferritin functions as iron storage but is also a marker of inflammation

Microcytic (MCV <80 fL)

Anaemia of chronic disease
- D: Anaemia 2/2 inflammation-mediated ↓RBC production ± ↓RBC survival
- A/w autoimmune disorders, malignancy, infxn, critical illness, major trauma, or major surgery with delayed recovery, other chronic disease states (eg CKD, HF, COPD)
- Mx: treat underlying disease
  - blood transfusion, erythropoiesis stimulating agents, supplemental iron

Iron deficiency anaemia
- Causes: inadequate dietary intake (eg vegans), poor intestinal absorption, ↑iron requirements (eg pregnancy), blood loss (eg menorrhagia)
  - in low-income countries, hookworm infxns (Ancylostoma)
- In older adults esp w hx of GI bleed, IDA = malignancy until otherwise proven
- Ix: blood films may show RBC of different sizes/shapes, target cells, and pencil poikilocytes
  - Endoscopy to r/o malignancy
- Mx: treat underlying cause
  - PO ferrous sulfate (can cause abdo pain, GI upset)
  - Iron-rich diet

Lead poisoning
- S/smx: abd pain, peripheral neuropathy (mainly motor), neuro-psychiatric features, fatigue, constipation
  - blue lines on gum margin (20% of adult pts, rare in children)
- Ix: blood lead levels, blood films will show basophilic stippling
- Mx: DMSA, D-penicillamine, EDTA, dimercapol (all of these are chelating agents)

Sideroblastic anaemia
- Disorder where RBC cannot form haem in the mitochondria → deposits of iron in the mitochondria = ring sideroblast
- Causes: congenital, myelodysplasia, alcohol, lead, anti-TB meds

β-thalassemia
- D: Genetic syndrome of ineffective erythropoiesis caused by mutations of the beta-globin gene
- R: FHx
- A/P: ineffective erythropoiesis.
  - ↓β-chains can lead to ↑α-chains and precipitation, causing RBC damage
  - Erythroid hyperplasia → bony changes in skull, extra-medullary haematopoiesis (liver, spleen)
- S/smx:
  - Presents in 1st year of life with failure to thrive, hepatosplenomegaly
  - Expansion of bony skull rarely
  - Microcytic anaemia
  - ↑HbA2 and HbF, absent HbA
- Mx: - Transfusion dependent
  - Iron chelation (desferrioxamine) to prevent iron overload (→ organ failure)

α-thalassemia
- D: Genetic syndrome of ineffective erythropoiesis caused by mutations of the alpha-globin gene
- R: FHx
- A/P: ineffective erythropoiesis (similar to β-thalassemia)
- S/smx:
  - if only 1-2 α-globulin alleles are affected, pts are usually asmx
  - if 3 α-globulin alleles are affected (= Hb H disease), pts have variable smx
    ◊ anaemia, jaundice, gallstones, hepatosplenomegaly
  - if all 4 α-globulin alleles are affected, this is incompatible with life (fetus dies in utero)
- Mx: - If asmx, no tx necessary
  - If severe, blood transfusion, splenectomy, consider stem cell transplant

- Ix: bloods, iron studies (↑ferritin, ↑iron, ↑transferrin saturation), blood film (basophilic stippling of RBCs), bone marrow aspiration
- Mx: supportive, tx underlying cause ± pyridoxine (B6)

Normocytic (MCV 80-100 fL)

Nonhaemolytic
reticulocyte index ≤2%

Iron deficiency anaemia (early)

Anaemia of chronic disease

Aplastic anaemia
- Pancytopaenia with hypocellular marrow and no abnormal cells
- Causes: idiopathic, congenital (eg Fanconi anaemia), drugs (cytotoxics, chloramphenicol, sulphonamides, phenytoin, gold), toxins (benzene), infxns (parvovirus B19, hepatitis), radiation
- ≥2 of the following must be present:
  - Hb <100 g/L
  - platelets <50 x 10⁹/L
  - neutrophils < 1.5 x 10⁹/L
- Mx: if not severe, monitoring ± steroids or IVIG may be sufficient
  - if severe or congenital, pts may need stem cell transplant

Chronic kidney disease
- 2/2 ↓erythropoietin levels due to declining renal function
- Usually becomes apparent when GFR <35 mL/min
- Mx: optimise iron status and give erythropoiesis-stimulating agents

Hereditary spherocytosis

- inherited abnormality of the RBC caused by defects in structural membrane proteins (autosomal dominant in 75%)
- P: sphere-shaped RBC due to cytoskeleton defects → ↓surface area of RBC + RBCs are destroyed by the spleen
- S/smx: - failure to thrive, jaundice, gallstones, splenomegaly
  - aplastic crisis precipitated by parvovirus B19 infxn
- Ix: bloods (↑mean corpuscular Hb concentration), blood films (spherocytes)
- Dx: clinical based on Hx and labs
- Mx: - acute crisis: supportive ± blood transfusion
  - longterm: folate replacement, splenectomy

G6PD deficiency

- enzyme deficiency (X-linked recessive), more common in Mediterranean and African populations
- Precipitating drugs: antimalarials (primaquine), ciprofloxacin, sulph-group drugs (eg sulphonamides, sulphasalazine, sulfonylureas)
- S/smx: neonatal jaundice
  - intravascular haemolysis
  - ± gallstones, splenomegaly
- Ix: blood films (Heinz bodies, bite and blister cells), definitive Dx with G6PD enzyme assay (done 3mo after acute episode of haemolysis)
- Mx: avoid triggers
  - if chronic + severe: splenectomy

Paroxysmal nocturnal haemoglobinuria

- Acquired disorder of the blood characterised by intravascular haemolysis and thrombophilia 2/2 absence of anchor proteins on membrane of RBCs
- Triad of Coombs -ve haemolytic anaemia, pancytopaenia, venous thrombosis (eg Budd-Chiari syndrome)
- Mx: eculizumab, stem cell transplant

Autoimmune haemolytic anaemia

- Decompensated acquired haemolysis caused by the host's immune system attacking its own RBCs
- Ix: bloods, Coombs +ve

Warm AIHA

- Antibody usually IgG
- Haemolysis most at body temp and at extravascular sites (eg spleen)
- Causes: idiopathic, autoimmune disease (eg SLE), neoplasia (eg lymphoma), drugs (eg methyldopa)
- Mx: treat underlying disorder
  - steroids ± rituximab

Cold AIHA

- Antibody usually IgM
- Haemolysis most at 4°C; complement mediated at intravascular sites
- Associated s/smx: Raynaud's and acrocyanosis (painless bluish discolouration of both hands)
- Causes: neoplasia (eg lymphoma), infections (eg mycoplasma, EBV)
- Mx: less responsive to steroids

Macroangiopathic haemolytic anaemia

- Mechanical shearing damage to RBCs
- Causes: prosthetic heart valves, aortic stenosis
- Ix: blood films (schistocytes)

Thrombotic thrombocytopaenic purpura

- Clinical syndrome of microangiopathic haemolytic anaemia and thrombocytopaenic purpura
- A: post-infxn (eg GI), pregnancy, drugs (eg penicillin, COCP), tumours, SLE, HIV
- P: absence of ADAMTS-13 (vWD factor cleaving enzyme) → large vWD multimers → platelet plugs within vessels
- S/smx: - anaemia + thrombocytopaenia
  - microemboli can cause fluctuating neuro signs and renal failure
  - fever
- Mx: plasma exchange + steroids
  - following resolution of acute episode, pts can be given aspirin to ↓risk of platelet aggregation

Haemolytic uraemic syndrome

- Syndrome comprising of microangiopathic anaemia, thrombocytopaenia and AKI
- Causes:
  - classically Shiga toxin-producing E.coli (O157:H7) esp in children
  - Others: pneumococcal infxn, HIV, SLE, drugs, cancer
- P: endothelial injury → microvascular injury and anaemia
- S/smx: no specific s/smx apart from infective diarrhoea preceding HUS
- Ix: FBC (Coombs -ve anaemia), blood films (schistocytes and helmet cells), U&Es (AKI), stool culture / PCR (looking for E.coli, Shiga toxins)
- Mx: supportive (fluids, transfusion)
  - no role for abx

Hb C disease

- Mutation in gene coding for β-globin – glutamic acid to lysine
- Causes extravascular haemolysis
- Pts with HbSC (1 normal allele, 1 mutated allele) have milder disease
- Ix: blood film (crystals inside RBCs, target cells)

Sickle cell disease

- D: autosomal-recessive disorder causing production of sickle cell Hb and subsequent complications
- R: FHx / genetic
- A/P: Hypoxia & acidosis triggers polymerisation of HbS → rigid sickle shaped RBC
  - Occlusion in small vessels or adhesion to vessels
  - Deformed cells → haemolysis → anaemia :(
  - ± Activation of WBC
  - Anaemia leads to high blood flow can cause cardiomegaly ± HF
- Dx: Hb electrophoresis
- Acute Mx of crises
  - **Analgesia** must be offered within 30min of presentation
    ↳ titrate to pt's pain, may range from paracetamol to opioids
  - Resus: fluid rehydration, oxygen as needed
  - Abx as needed
  - Blood transfusion if >20g/L drop from baseline Hb level
  - Exchange transfusion reserved for stroke and acute chest syndrome

Disseminated intravascular coagulation

- Activation of coagulation pathways results in formation of intravascular thrombi and depletion of platelets and coagulation factors
- Causes: sepsis, trauma, obstetric complications (eg HELLP syndrome), malignancy
- Ix: bloods (↓platelets, ↓fibrinogen, ↑PT, ↑APTT, ↑D-dimer), blood film (schistocytes)
- Mx: treat underlying disorder
  - if platelets <20 or <50 + active bleeding, platelet transfusion
  - fresh frozen plasma to replace coagulation factors

Infections, eg malaria

- ↑destruction of RBCs

Sickle cell disease (cont)

- Long-term Mx (preventative)
  - Hydroxyurea (↑HbF to prevent painful episodes)
  - Prophylactic penicillin if frequent pneumococcal infxns (lifelong)
    ↳ erythromycin if pen allergy
  - Folic acid supplementation if deficient and poor diet
  - Pneumococcal polysaccharide vaccine q5y (∴ hyposplenism)
  - Sickle cell disease does not protect against malaria – they still need prophylaxis

Sickle cell crises

Thrombotic crises

- aka painful / vaso-occlusive crises
- triggered by infxn, dehydration, deoxygenation (e.g. high altitude)
- clinical Dx; r/o other possibilities
- infarcts can occur in bones, eg avascular necrosis of hip, hand-foot syndrome in children, lungs, spleen and brain (stroke)

Acute chest syndrome

- vaso-occlusion within the pulmonary microvasculature → infarction in the lung parenchyma
- S/smx: dyspnoea, CP, pulmonary infiltrates on CXR, ↓pO2
- Mx: analgesia, O2 ± abx
- transfusion: improves oxygenation
- ** most common cause of death in sickle cell *after* childhood

Aplastic crises

- 2/2 infection with parvovirus
- sudden fall in Hb
- ◊ bone marrow suppression causes ↓reticulocyte count

Sequestration crises

- sickling within organs such as the spleen or lungs causes pooling of blood with ↓Hb
  ↳ a/w an ↑reticulocyte count

Macrocytic (MCV >100 fL)

Megaloblastic anaemias affect DNA synthesis and inhibit nuclear division → causes large size of RBCs (megaloblasts)

B12 deficiency
- B12 is needed in the development of RBCs and also the maintenance of the CNS
- Causes of B12 deficiency
  - pernicious anaemia (autoimmune)
  - post-gastrectomy or ileocaecal resection
  - dietary deficiency (eg vegan)
  - disorders or surgery of the terminal ileum, eg Crohns
- Features of B12
  - Macrocytic anaemia
  - Sore tongue/mouth (glossitis)
  - Neurological smx (see subacute combined degeneration)
  - Neuropsychiatric disturbances, eg mood disturbances
- Mx
  - if no neurological involvement, IM B12 is sufficient
  - ! replace B12 deficiency before folic acid (prevents precipitating subacute combined degeneration)

Folate (B9) deficiency
- Causes: ↑requirements (eg preg), ↓absorption (eg alcoholics), drugs (eg methotrexate, phenytoin)
- S/smx: no neurologic smx (as opposed to B12 deficiency)

Fanconi anaemia
- Autosomal recessive of bone marrow failure characterised by pancytopaenia
- S/smx:
  - Aplastic anaemia
  - ↑risk of acute myeloid leukaemia
  - Neurological smx
  - Skeletal abnormalities: short stature, abnormalities of the thumb, radius and ulna, lower limb abnormalities
  - Cafe au lait spots
- Mx: supportive (blood transfusions), stem cell treatment

Normoblastic anaemias

Anaemia in liver disease
- 2/2 many causes, including GI haemorrhage, hypersplenism (due to portal hypertension)
- A/w clotting disorders due to severe liver disease

Anaemia in alcohol use
- Dose dependent effects
- Also linked to nutritional deficiency
- ↓RBC production + structurally abnormal RBCs
- a/w ↓WBC, ↓platelets as well

Anaemia in hypothyroidism
- (can cause different types of anaemia)
- 2/2 bone marrow suppression, ↓EPO or comorbid disease

Methaemoglobinaemia

D: Hb which has been oxidised from Fe2+ to Fe3+ causing tissue hypoxia

Causes
- Congenital - HbM, HbH, NADH methaemoglobin reductase deficiency
- Acquired
  - drugs: sulphonamides, nitrates, dapsone, sodium nitroprusside, primaquine
  - chemicals, eg aniline dyes

S/smx:
- Chocolate brown blood
- Cyanosis
- Dyspnoea, anxiety, HA
- Severe: acidosis, arrythmias, seizures, coma
- "Refractory hypoxaemia"
  - pulse oximetry constant at 85%
  - pO2 on ABG will be falsely normal (machine cannot differentiate between normal Hb and metHb)
  - Saturation gap should hint towards haemaglobinopathy

Mx: · Ascorbic acid if congenital
· IV methylene blue if acquired

Thrombophilia

D: abnormality of blood coagulation that ↑risk of thrombosis
- Factor V Leiden – most common
- Prothrombin gene mutations
- Antithrombin III deficiency
- Protein C or S deficiency
- Antiphospholipid syndrome
- Combined oral contraceptive pill

Factor V Leiden
- Prevalence of up to 6% in white people, rare in other ethnicities
- Gain of function in factor V Leiden protein → ↑↑activity of factor V
- Aka activated protein C resistance as protein C inactivates factor V much more slowly
- Heterozygotes 4-5x risk of VTE, homozygotes 10x risk

S/smx:
- Asymptomatic until VTE occurs

Ix: Screening is not recommended even after VTE because previous Hx of VTE is already considered a risk factor for further events – no need to specifically screen for clotting disorders

Mx: · Generally does not require tx in day to day life
· Prophylaxis in hospitalisation, cancer or surgical procedures
  - early mobilisation
  - LMWH, DOAC or aspirin are options if there is no excessive bleeding risk
  - If ↑bleeding risk, mechanical thromboprophylaxis (eg compression stockings, intermittent pneumatic compression)
· If VTE occurs, prophylactic DOAC for 3mo (6mo if not provoked)
  - see DVT and PE Mx [→01.07]

Antiphospholipid syndrome APS

D: association of persistent antiphospholipid abs with thromboses and pregnancy-related morbidity
Antibodies include
- lupus anticoagulant
- anticardiolipin antibody
- anti-beta2-glycoprotein I

R: PMH of SLE (30% of pts with SLE are +ve for APS abs) and other auto-immune disorders

S/smx: "CLOT"
- Clots - venous/arterial thrombosis
- Livedo reticularis (mottled skin)
- Obstetric complications
  - **Recurrent miscarriages**
  - Pulmonary HTN
  - Pre-eclampsia
- Thrombocytopaenia

Ix: antibodies as above, bloods and clotting screen (↓platelets and ↑APTT)

Mx
- Primary thromboprophylaxis: aspirin 75 mg
- Secondary thromboprophylaxis (after an event has occured)
  - lifelong warfarin (target INR 2-3)
  - if arterial thrombosis, warfarin (target INR 2-3)
  - if recurrent events, consider adding aspirin
- Mx in pregnancy
  - Low dose aspirin once pregnancy is confirmed
  - Add on LMWH (eg enoxaparin) once fetal heart is seen on US, usually discontinued at 34w

Thrombocytosis

D: platelets >400 x 10⁹/L

Causes
- Reactive
  - platelets are an acute phase reactant; ↑inflammation → ↑platelets
  - eg iron deficiency anaemia, surgery, severe infxn
- Malignancy
- Hyposplenism
  - ↓ability of the spleen to destroy circulating platelets
- Essential thrombocytosis (aka essential thrombocythaemia)

Essential thrombocytosis
- D: chronic myeloproliferative neoplasm a/w ↑number or ↑size of platelets
- R: JAK2 mutation in 50% of pts
- S/smx:
  - platelets >600 x 10⁹/L
  - arterial or venous thrombosis
  - burning sensation in hands
- Mx
  - Life-threatening thrombosis: platelet-pharesis
  - 75 mg aspirin to ↓thrombotic risk
  - Hydroxyurea (hydroxycarbamide) to ↓platelet count
  - Interferon-α in younger pts

Immune thrombocytopenia ITP

D: aka immune thrombocytopenic purpura; autoimmune disorder with isolated ↓platelets in the absence of an identifiable cause

R: women of childbearing age, <10yo or >65yo

A: autoimmune
P: abs are directed against glycoprotein IIb/IIIa or Ib-V-IX complex → destruction of platelets in spleen → ↓platelet count

S/smx:
- Can be asmx; picked up on bloods
- Petechiae, purpura
- Bleeding, eg epistaxis
- Rarely, catastrophic bleeding (eg ICH)

Ix: FBC (isolated platelets <100 x 10⁹/L + no other abnormality)
- Bone marrow exam only if there are atypical features (eg splenomegaly) or failure to respond to tx

Mx:
- Life/organ-threatening bleed
  ↳ IVIG + **prednisolone** + platelet transfusion
- If platelets <30 or bleeding:
  ↳ prednisolone ± IVIG
- If mild and no other risk factors, consider observation
  - in children, 80% resolve within 6mo with or without treatment
  - in adults, only 5-10% – monitor
- Advice to avoid activities that may result in trauma, eg contact sports

Other platelet disorders
- Bernard-Soulier syndome
  - Large platelets (**b**ig **s**uckers)
  - Defect in adhesion of platelets due to ↓GpIb
- Glanzmann thrombasthenia
  - Defect in aggregation due to ↓GpIIb/IIIa

Thrombocytopaenia

D: platelets <100 x 10⁹/L
- Normal range: 150-400 x 10⁹/L

Severe thrombocytopaenia
- ITP   · DIC   · TTP
- Haematological malignancy

Moderate thrombocytopaenia
- Heparin-induced thrombocytopaenia
  - immune-mediated: antibodies against platelet factor 4 and heparin complex
  - develops 5-10d after tx
  - ↓platelets ~50%, thrombosis, skin allergy
  - Mx: stop heparin ± protamine sulfate (if overdose)
    - if pt still needs anticoagulation, use direct thrombin inhibitor (eg argatroban) or low molecular weight heparinoid (daparanoid)
- Drug-induced (eg quinine, diuretics, sulphonamides, aspirin, thiazides)
- Alcohol and liver disease
  - portal hypertension → sequestration of platelets in the spleen
  - ↓thrombopoietin production in liver
- Hypersplenism
  - sequestration of platelets in the spleen
  - viral infxns (eg EBV, HIV) can lead to hypersplenism
- Pregnancy
- SLE / antiphospholipid syndrome
- Vitamin B12 deficiency

Mx: · Treat underlying disorder
- Platelet transfusions (*see section on blood products – platelets*)

Haemophilia

D: X-linked recessive deficiency of coagulation factor resulting in a bleeding disorder
- Haemophilia A: ↓factor VIII (A-8)
- Haemophilia B: ↓factor IX (aka Christmas disease)
- Note: up to 30% of pts have no FHx of condition

S/smx:
- Hx of recurrent or severe bleeding
  - eg prolonged bleeding after trauma or surgery
- Musculoskeletal bleeding
  - Haemarthroses (into joints)
  - Bleeding into muscles
- Pseudotumours: recurrent bleeds into soft tissues → chronic encapsulated cystic mass
- Intracranial bleeding
  - 3-5% of newborn boys with severe haemophilia

Ix: bloods (↑APTT + normal PT, other normal tests)
- Plasma factor VIII & IX assay will show ↓ or absent factors
- Mixing study
  - pt plasma + normal plasma will show corrected APTT
  - 10-15% of pts with haemophilia A will develop antibodies to factor VIII tx

APTT measures the intrinsic coagulation pathway of which factors VIII and IX are part of; PT measures the extrinsic coagulation pathway which is not affected in haemophilia

Mx:
- Prophylaxis
  - regular infusion of plasma-derived factors
  - emicizumab in haemophilia A (mimics action of factor VIII)
- Life or limb threatening bleed
  - factor concentrate + supportive care as needed
  - if pt has antibodies to factor VIII, they need a bypassing agent

---

von Willebrand disease vWD

D: inherited bleeding disorder due to either a quantitative or qualitative abnormality of von Willebrand factor (vWF)
- 80% have type 1 disease which is autosomal dominantly inherited
- Type 2 and 3 are more severe

Type 1: partial ↓vWF
Type 2: abnormal form of vWF
Type 3: complete absence of vWF
  ↳ autosomal recessive

R: FHx, consanguineous parents (esp for type 3 vWD)

P: · vWF mediates platelet adhesion to exposed subendothelium at sites of vascular injury
- Also functions as a carrier molecule for factor VIII
- Problems with vWF → ↓platelet adhesion → bleeding problems

S/smx:
- Excessive or prolonged bleeding from minor wounds or post-op
- Easy and excessive bruising
- Menorrhagia

Ix: bloods: ↑bleeding time, ↑APTT (or normal) ± factor VIII
  ↳ normal PT, normal FBC usually
- Defective platelet aggregation with ristocetin

Mx:
- In severe active haemorrhage: vWD-*containing concentrate ± platelet* transfusion
- In less acute settings
  - tranexamic acid
  - desmopressin (MOA: induces release of vWF from Weibel-Palade bodies in endothelial cells)

Neutropaenia

D: neutrophils <1.5 x 10⁹/L
- Normal range: 2.0 - 7.5 x 10⁹/L
- Mild neutropenia: 1.0 - 1.5 x 10⁹/L
- Moderate: 0.5 - 1.0 x 10⁹/L
- Severe: <0.5 x 10⁹/L
- Agranulocytosis: <0.1 x 10⁹/L

Causes
- Viral: HIV, EBV, hepatitis
- Drugs: cytotoxics, carbimazole, clozapine
- Benign ethnic neutropaenia
  - common in black or Afro-Carribean ethnicities
  - no treatment required
- Haematological malignancies
  - myelodysplasia
  - aplastic anaemia
- Rheumatological conditions
  - Felty's syndrome (RA + splenomegaly + neutropaenia)
- SLE (2/2 anti-neutrophil abs)
- Severe sepsis
- Haemodialysis

Mx:
- Treat or remove cause
  ↳ stop offending drugs
- Refer to haematology
- Abx prophylaxis
- Granulocyte colony stimulating factor (GCSF) can be used

See also neutropaenic sepsis [→10.10]

Packed red cells

- Each unit is ~300 mL
  - whole blood is collected from donor, and then plasma is removed
- Each bag should raise the pt's Hb by approximately 10 g/L (3% haematocrit)
- Requires G&S and **cross-match** before administration

Indications for giving
- Acute major haemorrhage
- Regular transfusions for chronic anaemia
- In most other settings, transfusion thresholds
  - In pts without acute coronary syndrome (eg STEMI), <70 g/L
  - In pts with ACS, <80 g/L

- Store at 4°C prior to infusion
- In non-urgent scenario, a unit of RBC is usually transfused over 90-120 minutes
- Shelf life of ~42 days

Platelets

- Platelet-rich plasma
- Platelet concentrate – high speed centrifugation
- Highest risk of bacterial contamination compared to other blood products

Indications for giving
- Active bleeding
  - if platelets <30 x10⁹ with clinically significant bleeding, eg melaena
  - if platelets <100 x 10⁹ with severe bleeding or bleeding at critical sites (eg CNS)
- Before invasive procedure
  - aim for >50 x 10⁹ in most pts
  - >50-75 if high risk of bleeding
  - >100 if surgery at critical site
- If no active bleeding or planned invasive procedure, threshold for platelet transfusion is <10 x 10⁹ if there are no alternatives

CMV -ve and irradiated blood

- CMV -ve blood is essentially blood without leucocytes as CMV is transmitted in leucocytes
- Irradiated blood products are depleted of T cells, and are used to avoid transfusion-associated graft versus host disease

Indications for giving CMV-ve blood
- Granulocyte transfusions
- Intra-uterine transfusions
- Neonates ≤28d post expected date of delivery
- Pregnancy: elective transfusions during pregnancy (not during labour or delivery)

Indications for giving irradiated blood
- Granulocyte transfusions
- Intra-uterine transfusions
- Neonates ≤28d post expected date of delivery
- Bone marrow or stem cell transplants
- Immunocompromised (eg chemo or congenital – but not HIV)
- Pts with current or previous Hodgkin lymphoma

Fresh frozen plasma   FFP

- Each unit is around 150-220 mL
  - in warfarin reversal, 30 mL/kg needed
  - give along with ≥1L fluid in 70kg person (caution in fluid overload states; may not be suitable)
- Prepared from single units of blood. Contains clotting factors, albumin and immunoglobulin
- Requires G&S and **cross-match** before administration
- Universal donor is AB blood

Indications for giving
- Pts with clinically significant but no major haemorrhage with a PT:APTT >1.5
- Prophylaxis for surgery if there is significant risk of bleeding

Cryoprecipitate

- Each unit is 15-20 mL
- FFP is centrifuged → liquid that remains on top (= supernatant) is cryoprecipitate)
- Contains Factor VIII and fibrinogen among other clotting factors
  - clinically used to replace fibrinogen
- Requires G&S and **cross-match** before administration

Indications for giving
- Pts with clinically significant but no major haemorrhage with fibrinogen concentration <1.5 g/L
  ↳ eg DIC, liver failure, trauma
- Emergency situations for haemophiliacs and von Willebrand disease
- Prophylaxis for surgery if there is significant risk of bleeding and where fibrinogen <1.0 g/L

Prothrombin complex   PCC

- aka factor IX complex, contains factors II, IX and X ± VII
- Dose: Bereplex 50 U/kg
- Main indication is emergency reversal of anticoagulation in pts with severe bleeding or head injury with suspected ICH
- Rarely for prophylaxis

Cell saver devices

- Device collects pts blood during surgery and re-infuses it
  - some devices wash the RBCs prior to re-infusion (↓risk of contamination) but they are more expensive
- May be acceptable to Jehovah witnesses
- CI in malignant disease due to risk of ↑disease dissemination

Warfarin – Mx of high INR

STOP WARFARIN IN ALL PATIENTS
Major bleeding
- IV Vit K 5mg
  - takes 4-6h for effect
- PCC or FFP
  - give with Vitamin K
INR >8 + minor bleeding
- IV Vit K 1-3 mg
- if INR high after 24h, repeat IV vit K
- INR <5: restart warfarin

INR >8 + no bleeding
- PO vit K 1-5 mg
- if INR high after 24h, repeat PO vit K
- INR <5: restart warfarin
INR 5-8 + minor bleeding
- IV Vit K 1-3 mg
- INR <5: restart warfarin
INR 5-8 + no bleeding
- withhold 1-2 doses
- reduce subsequent maintenance dose

Blood product transfusion complications

Acute haemolytic reaction
- D: acute onset of intravascular haemolysis due to **ABO-incompatible blood** trf resulting in complement activation and inflammatory cascade. RBC destruction 2/2 IgM abs
- S/smx: onset within minutes of trf, fever, abd pain, hypotension.
  - If severe: DIC, ARDS
- Mx: stop transfusion, check blood product (identity, blood type, Coombs test), repeat cross-match, fluid resuscitation

Non-haemolytic febrile reaction
- D: acute onset immune-mediated reaction to blood products
- A/P: **abs against fragments** from cells (?contamination) or WCC, formation of immune complexes
- A/w: RCC transfusion (1-2%), platelet transfusions (10-30%)
- S/smx: fever, chills
- Mx: slow or stop transfusion, paracetamol and monitor

Minor allergic reaction
- D: acute onset of minor allergic reaction, possibly due to foreign plasma proteins
- S/smx: pruritus, urticaria
- Mx: temporarily stop transfusion, antihistamines, monitor

Anaphylactic reaction
- D: acute onset of IgE-mediated major allergic reaction. Anaphylactoid reaction in pts with IgA deficiency who have anti-IgA abs
- S/smx: hypotension (shock), dyspnoea, wheezing, angioedema
- Mx: stop transfusion, IM adrenaline, oxygen, fluid resus

Transfusion-related acute lung injury (TRALI)
- D: Non-cardiogenic pulmonary oedema ?2/2 ↑vascular permeability ∴ host neutrophils activated by substances in donated blood
- S/smx: Hypoxia, pulmonary infiltrates on CXR, fever, ↓BP
- Mx: Stop transfusion, O2, support as needed

Transfusion-associated circulatory overload (TACO)
- D: hypervolaemia 2/2 excessive transfusion, seen esp in pts with pre-disposing conditions such as HF
- S/smx: pulmonary oedema, ↑BP
- Mx: slow or stop transfusion, consider IV furosemide, support as needed

Hereditary angioedema

D: ↓plasma levels of complement C1 inhibitor protein → uncontrolled release of bradykinin → oedema of tissues
· Autosomal dominant

S/smx:
· Painless, non-pruritic swelling of subcutaneous / submucosal tissues (=angioedema)
· May affect upper airways, skin or abdominal organs
· Painful macular rash may preceed
· Rarely urticaria

Ix: ↓C1 inhibitor during attacks, ↓C2 and C4 all the time

Mx: · 🔪 IV C1-inhibitor concentrate
· 🔪 FFP if not available
· No response to IM adrenaline, antihistamines or glucocorticoids

Hyposplenism

D: ↓ spleen's function (due to structural or functional causes)

Causes
· Splenectomy
· Sickle cell disease
  - can cause splenomegaly, but hyposplenism is more common
· Coeliac's disease   · Graves' disease
· SLE   · Amyloid deposits

Ix: on blood films – Howell-Jolly bodies, siderocytes (RBCs containing non-haemoglobin iron, usually removed by spleen)

Splenomegaly

D: ↑size ± function of spleen

Causes of massive splenomegaly
· Myelofibrosis
· Chronic myeloid leukaemia
· Visceral leishmaniasis (kala-azar)
· Malaria
· Gaucher's syndrome (inherited disorder of lipid metabolism)

Other causes
· Portal HTN
· Lymphoproliferative disease e.g. CLL, Hodgkin's
· Haemolytic anaemia
· Infection: hepatitis, glandular fever infective endocarditis
· Thalassaemia
· Felty syndrome (in rheumatoid arthritis)

Thymoma

D: neoplasm of the epithelial cells of the thymus gland located in the anterior mediastinum

R · **Myasthenia gravis** (30-40% of pts with thymoma)
· RBC aplasia   · Dermatomyositis
· SLE   · SIADH

S/smx: · generally asmx, 1/3 cases identified incidentally on imaging
· Large tumours can cause chest discomfort, cough, dyspnoea – can cause death if it compresses the airway or heart (cardiac tamponade)

Ix: chest MRI + tissue biopsy

Mx: surgical resection if possible + post-op radiotherapy. if recurrent, chemotherapy may be indicated

Lymphadenopathy

D: lymph nodes abnormal in size (>1cm), consistency or number

Causes (↑inflammation)
· Infective
  - infectious mononucleosis
  - HIV (including seroconversion)
  - Eczema with 2ndary infxn
  - Rubella   - Toxoplasmosis
  - CMV   - Tuberculosis
  - Roseola infantum
· Neoplastic – leukaemia, lymphoma
· Others
  - Autoimmune conditions (eg SLE)
  - Graft versus host disease
  - Sarcoidosis
  - Drugs (eg phenytoin, allopurinol, isoniazid)

Bilateral hilar lymphadenopathy
· **Sarcoidosis**
· **Tuberculosis**
· Lymphoma or other malignancies
· Pneumoconiosis
· Fungi, eg histoplasmosis

Anticoagulants

Direct oral anticoagulants

Indications
· prevention of stroke in AF
· prevention of VTE following hip and knee surgery
· treatment of DVT and PE

Dabigatran
· MOA: direct thrombin inhibitor
· Mainly renal excretion
· Reversal: Idarucizumab

Rivaroxaban
· MOA: direct factor Xa inhibitor
· Mainly liver excretion
· Reversal: andexanet alfa

Apixaban
· MOA: direct factor Xa inhibitor
· Mainly faecal excretion
· Reversal: andexanet alfa

Edoxaban
· MOA: direct factor Xa inhibitor
· Mainly faecal excretion
· Reversal: ? andexanet alfa

Warfarin

· MOA: prevents vitamin K activation
· Indications - mechanical heart valves
  - 2nd line after DOACs
· Monitoring
  - INR (= international normalised ratio, the ratio of pt's prothrombin time over normal prothrombin time)
· Factors *potentiating* warfarin
  - liver disease
  - P450 enzyme inhibitors, eg amiodarone, ciprofloxacin
  - Drugs that displace warfarin from plasma albumin, eg NSAIDs
  - Drugs that inhibit platelet function, eg NSAIDs, aspirin
  - Cranberry juice
· Side effects
  - Haemorrhage
  - Teratogenic (but can be used in breastfeeding mothers)
  - Skin necrosis (avoid by concurrent heparin administration during initial phase)
  - Purple toes

Unfractionated heparin (UFH)

· MOA: activating antithrombin III → inhibits thrombin, factors X, IX, XI, and XII (intrinsic pathway)
· IV administration, short half life
· Monitor using APTT
· Indications
  - anticoagulation needed but high risk of bleeding – UFH can be rapidly terminated + antidote
  - renal failure
· Antidote: protamine sulfate
· Side effects - thrombocytopaenia (HIT)
  - osteoporosis, ↑risk fractures
  - hyperkalaemia

Low molecular weight heparin

LMWH · Eg enoxaparin
· MOA: activates antithrombin III → inhibits only factor Xa
· Subcut admin, long half-life
· Indications   - ACS
  - VTE treatment and prophylaxis
· No antidote, and not routinely monitored (fewer side effects)

Antiplatelets

Aspirin
· MOA: blocks COX1 and COX2 enzymes → ↓prostaglandin, prosta-cyclin and thromboxane synthesis → ↓platelet aggregation
· Indications
  - first line for ischaemic heart disease (ACS prevention)
· Contraindications: children <16yo due to risk of Reye's syndrome
  - except in Kawasaki disease
· SE: as per NSAIDs
  - also potentiates effects of oral hypoglycaemics, warfarin, steroids

P2Y12 inhibitors
eg clopidogrel, ticagrelor, prasugrel
· MOA: inhibits P2Y12 receptor on platelets → ↓platelet aggregation
· Indications
  - first line in TIA, ischaemic stroke and peripheral arterial disease
  - second line or combined with aspirin in other conditions
· SE: GI upset

Tranexamic acid

· Synthetic derivative of lysine
· MOA: reversibly binds to lysine receptor sites on plasminogen or plasmin → prevents plasmin from degrading fibrin ∴ *anti-fibrinolytic*
  ↳ essentially, prevents clots from breaking down
· Indications
  - Menorrhagia
  - IV bolus in major haemorrhage (proven benefit if administered within first 3h)

Neutropenic sepsis

aka febrile neutropaenia

D: medical emergency; presence of fever in a neutropenic patient

R: 7-14d after chemo, immunosup, prior episode, ECOG>1, etc

A: infxn, most often Gram+ve (S aureus, S epidermidis); and Gram-ve (E.coli, Klebsiella, Ps aeruginosa).
P: Chemo-induced immunosup
· Mucosal breaches, lines, catheters, etc as routes of entry

S/smx: Mainly fever, but any other s/smx of sepsis
· ! ASK "when was your last chemo?" - most likely ~10d post-chemo, but can be any time <6w

Ix: FBC (neutrophils <0.5), blood cultures, lactate, LDH, etc

Mx: · Sepsis 6
 - Abx: piptazo to cover. Only 30% of cultures come back +ve, so go broad spectrum
· If pt still febrile and unwell after 48h, add meropenem ± vancomycin
· If not responding in 4-6d, order Ix for fungal infxn (eg HRCT)
· ± GCSF if appropriate

Superior vena cava obstruction SVCO

D: Oncological emergency caused by the compression of the SVC

A: lung cancer (esp SCLC), non-Hodgkin's lymphoma, other cancers
· Non-malignant causes: aortic aneurysm, mediastinal fibrosis, goitre, SVC thrombosis

P: Compression of SVC → ↓drainage of blood from top of the body (head, neck, arms)

S/smx: · Dyspnoea
· Swelling of face, neck and arms
· HA (worse in mornings)
· Visual disturbances (? 2/2 cerebral oedema)
· Pulseless jugular venous distention

Mx: · Endovascular stenting to provide symptomatic relief
· Radical chemo or chemo-radiotherapy in some cancers
· ± glucocorticoids (weak evidence)

Not much explanation as to why SVC obstruction causes visual disturbances in the literature

Tumour lysis syndrome

D: oncological emergency caused by the rapid breakdown of cancer cells and the subsequent release of large amounts of intracellular content into the bloodstream.

R: haematological cancer, large tumour burden, tx sensitive tumours, recent cancer tx, pre-existing renal impairment, dehydration, volume depletion, nephrotoxic drugs

P: ↑K, ↓Ca, ↑PO, ↑urate, ↑LDH
· LDH is a prognostic factor – indicates rate/level of cell death

S/smx: · Most often occurs in children and young adults
· Most often when chemo starts
 ↳ 12-72h after
· NVD, anorexia, muscle weakness, muscle cramps, tetany, flank pain, lethargy, paraesthesia, and laryngeal spasm

Ix: U&Es, etc

Mx: · Fluid resus
· Manage hyperkalaemia
· IV rasburicase for high risk pts
 ↳ breaks down uric acid
· Allopurinol for lower risk pts

Graft versus host disease GVHD

D: major complication following allogeneic haematopoietic cell transplantation, occurring when donor T cells respond to histioincompatible antigens on host tissues

÷ acute and chronic
· Acute GVHD – classically within 100d of transplantation
· Chronic – follows acute disease or arises de novo after 100d

R: HLA disparity (↑degree of mismatch → ↑risk of GVHD)
· ↑age of donor or recipient
· female donor with male recipient
· advanced malignant condition
· graft source (bone marrow or peripheral blood source a/w ↑risk vs umbilical cord blood)

P: acute GVHD – antigen presenting cells activate donor T cells → target tissue destruction. Chronic GVHD is not as well understood.

S/smx of acute GVHD
· skin (80%): painful maculopapular rash (often neck, palms, soles) ± erythroderma or toxic epidermal necrosis-like syndrome
· liver (50%): jaundice
· GIT (50%): watery or bloody diarrhoea, persistent NV
· culture -ve fever
· there are scoring systems that take into account the degree of involvement (grades I to IV)

S/smx of chronic GVHD
· skin: poikiloderma (pigmented skin disorder), scleroderma, vitiligo, lichen planus, etc
· eyes: keratoconjunctiva sicca, corneal ulcers, scleritis
· GI: dysphagia, odynophagia, oral ulcers, ileus
 - oral lichenous changes are characteristically seen early on
· lungs: obstructive or restrictive lung disease

Dx is based primarily on clinical s/smx
· Tissue biopsy with histiopathological confirmation if aetiology is not clearly determined
· Other Ix guided by systems affected

Billingham criteria for diagnosis of GVHD:
1. Transplanted tissue contains immunologically functioning cells
2. Recipient and donor are immunologically different
3. Recipient is immunocompromised

Mx
· Prophylaxis
 - calcineurin inhibitor (eg ciclosporin or tacrolimus)
 - AND low-dose methotrexate or mycophenolate
· Mx of acute grade I (skin only)
 - topical corticosteroid (eg hydrocort cream) + calcineurin inhibitor
· Mx of acute grade II to IV
 - systemic (IV/PO) corticosteroid + calcineurin inhibitor
· Mx of chronic GVHD
 - systemic (IV/PO) corticosteroid + calcineurin inhibitor
 - AND abx prophylaxis (eg azithromycin)
 - AND pneumocystis prophylaxis (eg tmp-smx)
 - AND vaccinations

P: in acute GVHD, complete response rates ~20-40%. Most impt predictor of long-term survival is primary response to therapy.
In Chronic GVHD, if treated early most cases resolve within 5y. 2y survival was 74% in one study.

Organ transplant

· Allograft transplants = organ transplanted from one individual to another
· Isograft = transplant between identical twins
· Autograft = transplant to one's own self (eg skin graft)
· Xenograft = transplant from another species (eg porcine heart valve)
· Sources of organs
 - Live donor
 - DBD = donor brain dead
 - DCD = donor cardiac dead

Matching organ donor to recipient
· Matching antigens
 - ABO groups
  ◊ incompatibility will result in hyperacute rejection
 - Human leucocyte antigens (HLA A, B, C, DR alleles)
  ◊ ideally all 8 alleles are matched
  ◊ ↑degree of mismatch → ↑risk of rejection
 - Major histocompatibility antigens

Types of organ rejection
· Hyperacute
 - immediately, due to pre-formed antigens (eg ABO incompatibility)
 - greatest risk in renal transplants
· Acute
 - within first 6mo, T-cell mediated
 - tissue infiltrates + vascular lesions
 - all types of organ transplants are susceptible, can occur in up to 50% of cases
· Chronic
 - after first 6mo
 - vascular changes mainly → organ ischaemia, eg in cardiac transplants, rapid coronary artery disease
 - ↑risk with previous acute rejections

Common cancers (UK specific)

Most common cancers in males
1. Prostate (27%)
2. Lung (13%)
3. Bowel (12%)
4. Head and neck
5. Kidney
6. Melanoma
7. NHL
8. Bladder
9. Oesophagus
10. Leukaemia

Most common cancers in females
1. Breast (30%)
2. Lung (13%)
3. Bowel (10%)
4. Uterus
5. Melanoma
6. Ovary
7. CNS
8. NHL
9. Pancreas
10. Kidney

Most common causes of **cancer death**
(in the whole population)
1. Lung
2. Bowel
3. Prostate
4. Breast
5. Pancreas
6. Unknown primary
7. Oesophagus
8. Liver
9. Bladder
10. CNS

Data obtained from Cancer Research UK,
which has collected data from 2016-2019.

Carcinogens
- Aflatoxin (from *Aspergillus*) → liver (hepatocellular carcinoma)
- Aniline dyes → bladder (transitional cell carcinoma)
- Asbestos → mesothelioma and bronchial carcinoma
- Nitrosamines (found in some processed foods) → oesophageal and gastric cancer
- Vinyl chloride (chemical used to make PVC) → hepatic angiosarcoma

Tumour markers
- Ca125: ovarian cancer
- Ca19-9: pancreatic cancer
- Ca15-3: breast cancer
- Prostate specific antigen (PSA): prostatic carcinoma
- Alpha-feto protein (AFP): hepatocellular carcinoma and teratoma
- Carcinoembryonic antigen (CEA): colorectal cancer
- S-100: melanoma, schwanomma
- Bombesin: SCLC, gastric cancer, neuroblastoma

Genetic conditions that predispose to cancer

Li-Fraumeni syndrome
- D: cancer predisposition disorder due to germline mutations to p53 tumour suppressor gene
- Autosomal dominant
- Cancers: Sarcomas, leukaemias
- Tends to be diagnosed when pt develops sarcoma <45yo
- Pt may be diagnosed on screening when another family member develops cancer <45yo, or sarcoma at any age
- Mx: no cure, pts should adhere to preventive screening

BRCA 1 and 2 mutations
- BRCA 1 is on chromosome 17
  BRCA 2 is on chromosome 13
- 55-72% of women with BRCA1 and 45-69% of women with BRCA2 will develop breast cancer by 70-80yo
  ↳ in contrast to 13% in general population (4-6x prevalence)
- Also a/w ↑risk of developing breast cancer in contralateral breast after first breast cancer Dx
- 39-44% of women with BRCA1 and 11-17% of women with BRCA2 will develop ovarian cancer by 70-80yo
  ↳ in contrast to 1.2% in general population
- BRCA2 a/w prostate cancer in men
  Data from this website.

Von Hippel-Lindau disease
- D: disease characterised by growth of cysts and/or tumours (benign or malignant)
- Autosomal dominant
- Tumours: haemangioblastomas, renal cell carcinoma, pancreatic NETs, phaeochromocytomas, etc
  - Depending on where these are found, they cause different smx
  - Eg in CNS tumours can cause ataxia
- Mx: Surgical removal of tumours

Lynch syndrome
- D: aka hereditary non-polyposis colo-rectal cancer syndrome – a predisposition to developing colorectal cancer (and endometrial cancer)
- Autosomal dominant
- Amsterdam criteria to help identify pts at high risk
  - ≥3 family members with confirmed Dx of Lynch syndrome-related cancer (colorectal, endometrial, small bowel, ureter or renal pelvis)
  - ≥1 is a first-degree relative of the other two
  - ≥2 successive affected generations
  - ≥1 colon cancers Dx at <50yo
  - Familial adenomatous polyposis has been excluded
- Risk Mx
  - eg, colonoscopy starting at 20yo, repeat every 1-2y
  - colectomy if surveillance measures are not possible

Familial adenomatous polyposis
- D: cancer predisposition disorder where numerous adenomatous polyps lining the intestinal mucosal surface with a high potential for malignancy
  - one variant is known as Gardner syndrome
- Autosomal dominant
- Mutation of APC gene located on chromosome 5
- **Gardner syndrome:**
  - numerous colonic polyps
  - skull osteoma
  - thyroid cancer
  - epidermoid cysts
  - desmoid tumours in 15% (soft tissue tumour aka aggressive fibromatosis)
- Mx: many pts undergo colectomy ± proctectomy to ↓risk of colorectal cancer

Prescribing for common problems in cancer and palliative care

Pain prescribing
SIGN guidelines 2008 - cancer
- breakthrough dose of morphine is **one-sixth** the daily dose
- laxatives for all pts on opioids
- in renal impairment
  - in mild-mod: oxycodone preferred
  - in severe: alfentanil, buprenor-phine, fentanyl preferred
- for metastatic bone pain
  - options: strong opioids, bisphosphonates, radiotherapy
  - maybe denosumab
  - consider referral to oncologist
- when ↑dose of opioids, increase by 30-50%
  - **1.5x** the dose for both regular and breakthrough
- SE: nausea and drowsiness tend to be transient; constipation usually persistent

Conversion between opioids
Oral preparations
- codeine → morphine = ÷10
- tramadol → morphine = ÷10
- morphine → oxycodone = ÷2

Transdermal patches
- 12 mcg fentanyl patch ≈ 30 mg morphine PO
- 10 mcg buprenorphine patch ≈ 24 mg morphine PO

Subcutaneous delivery
- PO → SQ morphine = ÷2
- PO morphine → SQ diamorphine = ÷3
- PO oxycodone → SQ diamorphine = ÷1.5

Hiccups
- Chlorpromazine
- Haloperidol, gabapentin ± Dexamethasone, esp if hepatic lesions

Agitation and confusion
- Haloperidol
- Chlorperazine, levomepromazine

Secretions
- Educate family that the pt is likely not troubled by secretions
- Hyoscine (= Buscopan)
- Glycopyrronium

Nausea and vomiting
- ↓gastric motility: metoclopramide, domperidone
- chemically mediated: ondansetron, haloperidol, levomepromazine
- visceral/serosal: cyclizine, levopromazine ± buscopan
- ↑ICP: cyclizine, dexamethsaone ± radiotherapy if 2/2 lesion
- vestibular: cyclizine, metoclopramide, prochlorperazine, atypical antipsychotics (olanzapine)
- cortical, eg anticipatory: lorazepam, cyclizine

Breast cancer

D: ductal or lobular carcinoma
– carcinoma in situ vs invasive
Most common types
· Invasive ductal carcinoma:
  most common
  ↳ 'No Special Type (NST)'
· Invasive lobular carcinoma
· Ductal carcinoma-in-situ (DCIS)
· Lobular carcinoma-in-situ (LCIS)

R: ↑age, F>M, FHx, genetics, oestrogen exposure (endo and exogenous), alcohol, radiation

S/smx:
· Lump: hard, irregular, fixed in place
  ± tethered
· Nipple retraction   · Discharge
· Skin dimpling
· **Paget's disease of the breast**
  - eczematoid change of the nipple
  - a/w underlying breast cancer
· Inflammatory breast cancer
  - cancer cells block LN drainage

Ix: *2ww ref* for
· unexplained breast or axilla lump
  in pts ≥30yo
· Unilat nipple Δ in pts ≥50yo
· suspicious skin Δ
> Non urgent ref for unexplained breast
  lumps in pts ≤30yo

Triple Ax
· Clinical Ax (based on history &
  physical exam)
· Imaging (US for ≤30yo, and
  mammogram for all others)
  - hypoechoic mass
  - irregular + internal calcification
  - enlarged axillary LN
· Histology (needle aspiration/core
  biopsy)

Others
· hormone receptor testing
· HER2 testing
· CT or PET if mets suspected

Mx: *Before surgery*
· No palpable axillary LN – pre-op US →
  if +ve, sentinel node biopsy
· Palpable axillary LN – axillary node
  clearance (a/w lymphadenopathy and
  ↑risk infections)

Surgical options
· **Mastectomy** if multifocal tumour,
  central tumour, large lesion in small
  breast, DCIS >4cm
· **Wide local excision** (WLE) if solitary
  tumour, peripheral, small lesion, DCIS
  <4cm
· Offer reconstructive surgery

Radiological options
· For WLE: whole breast RT rec –
  ↓recurrence by 66%
· For mastectomy: T3 and T4 tumours
  and/or ≥4 +ve nodes

Hormonal options
· If pt is +ve for hormone receptors
· Pre- and peri-menopausal: tamoxifen
  - SE: ↑risk of endometrial cancer, VTE,
    menopausal smx
· Post-menopause: aromatase inhibitors,
  eg anastrazole
  - MOA: ↓peripheral synthesis of
    estrogen

Biological options
· For HER2 +ve (20-25% tumours):
  trastuzumab (Herceptin)

Chemotherapy
· Neoadjv to downstage 1' lesion
· Axillary node disease

P: · Men have higher mortality
· Various prognostic tools
· Biomarkers: CEA

Cysts: round, smooth and well-
defined borders, mobile,
possibly fluctuant
– a/w pain due to mastalgia

Fibroadenoma

D: benign tumour of stromal/ epithelial
breast duct tissue that develops from a
whole lobule – 12% of all breast masses

R: young (20-40yo), hormone exposure
(estrogen & progestrogen)

S/smx
· ≤3cm, round, smooth and well-defined
  borders, firm, mobile, and painless
  ("breast mouse")

Mx: conservative – monitoring
· Over 2y period, ≤30% get smaller
· No increased risk in malignancy unless
  FHx or ?complex
Surgical – if ≥3cm in diameter

Fibrocystic breast changes

aka fibroadenosis, benign mammary dysplasia

D: non-specific term; continuum of
physiological to pathological changes

R: 30-50yo, ↑hormone exposure

A/P: the stroma, ducts and lobules
respond to female sex hormones and
become fibrous and cystic – may
fluctuate within menstrual cycle

S/smx – often occur prior to menses
(within 10d) and resolve once menses
begins
· Lumpiness ± fluctuation of breast size
  ± nipple discharge
· Mastalgia – cyclical or non-cyclical

Mx: r/o cancer
· Advice: wear supportive bra, avoid
  caffeine, apply heat to area
· Rx: NSAIDs, hormonal tx under
  specialist guidance

P: mastalgia likely chronic, relapsing
(~12y). Cysts ~1/4 pts experience
recurrence in 1y

Fat necrosis

D: localised degeneration and scarring of
fat tissue in the breast

A/P: often triggered by localised trauma,
radiotherapy, surgery → inflammatory
reaction → fibrosis and fat necrosis

S/smx:
· firm, irregular, fixed in local structures,
  painless
· a/w skin dimpling, nipple inversion
· a/w oil cyst containing liquid fat

Ix: since it presents similarly to breast Ca
– triple Ax required
· Imaging can show similar appearance
  to breast Ca
· Histology may be req to confirm Dx and
  r/o Ca

Mx: conservative – may resolve
spontaneously with time. Surgical
excision if symptomatic

Lipoma

D: slow-growing, benign, mesenchymal
tumours made of adipocytes

S/smx:
· 1 in 1000, usually middle-aged pts
· Smooth, soft, mobile, painless
· Not a/w skin changes.

Mx: conservative – converstion to
liposarcoma is very rare.
Surgical excision, liposuction or lipolysis
indicated for
· Cosmetic reasons
· Symptomatic: painful, bothersome
· ↑size or concern for conversion
  - size >5cm   - pain
  - deep anatomical location
  - (all 4 features a/w 85% risk)

Site, size and shape
Colour, contour, consistency
Tethering, tenderness
Fluctuance ± transillumination

Phyllodes tumour

D: tumour of the breast stroma

S/smx: · usually F 40-60yo
· Rapid onset, rapid enlargement of
  breast
· 50% benign, 25% borderline, 25%
  malignant – can metastasise, can recur

Mx: wide local excision

Galactocele

D: breast milk-filled cysts occurring due
to blocked lactiferous ducts

S/smx: firm, mobile, painless lump,
usually beneath the areola

Mx: conservative – tend to resolve.
· Drainage with needle if needed
· Abx if infected

Mammary duct ectasia

D: dilatation of the large breast ducts

S/smx: commonly occurs around
menopause + in smokers
· Tender lump around areola
· ± Green nipple discharge
· May cause local inflammation if
  ruptures ≈ plasma cell mastitis

Mx: r/o malignancy, smoking cessation
· If severe smx, total duct excision

Duct papilloma

D: epithelial proliferation in the large
mammary ducts – hyperplastic lesions
that are usually benign

S/smx: · Blood stained discharge,
usually originating from only one duct
· Mass if large enough

Mx: microdochectomy if symptomatic
· No increased risk of malignancy

Septic arthritis

D: infxn of ≥1 joints caused by pathogenic inoculation of microbes

R: underlying joint disease, prosthetic joint, ↑age (esp >80yo), immunosuppression (eg HIV, DM), IVDU, contiguous spread (eg via skin infxn or ulcers), exposure to ticks

A/P: 90% staph or strep - direct or haematogenous inoculation. ❗ Neisseria gonorrhea in young sexually active

S/Smx: hot, swollen, acutely painful joint with restriction of movement = septic arthritis until proven otherwise. Usually single joint, but do not r/o in ≥2 joint. More insidious onset if TB. ± fever.

Ix: synovial fluid sampling (prior to abx if possible; under US guidance), blood cultures, joint imaging. Bloods (WCC, ESR, CRP, etc)

Mx: IV abx covering Gram+ cocci – fluclox or clindamycin IV (2w) then PO. Needle aspiration to decompress joint – "aspirate to dryness". Joint washout may be needed. ❗ Ref to ortho: prosthetics, hip

P: delayed or inadequate tx can cause irreversible joint destruction, fatality

Septic arthritis of a replaced joint
** REF TO ORTHOPAEDICS
- usually Staph epidermidis, other coagulase -ve Staph, or Staph aureus
- Requires aspiration/biopsy in **sterile** environment – 5 samples
- Debridement abx and implant retention
- Two stage revision
  - Op to remove infected replacement and all suspected tissue, joint washout, abx spacer and IV abx
  - Op to remove abx spacer, joint wash out, new total joint replacement inserted
  - Success rates ~88-96%
- Single stage revision - infected replacement removed, washout, and replacement inserted in one op

See also Kocher criteria on 11.10 for paediatric septic arthritis

Compartment syndrome

D: **elevated interstitial pressure in a closed osteofascial compartment** causing **microvascular compromise**

R: **trauma**, bleeding disorder, compression support (e.g. tight casts, dressings), thermal injury (burns), intense muscular activity (chronic)

S/Smx: **6Ps** - pressure (earliest), pain (esp on movement, even passive), parasthesia ± pallor, ↓pulse, paralysis

Ix/Dx: · measure intracompartmental pressure (>20 mmHg is abnormal, >40 mmHg is diagnostic)
· Imaging (eg XR) not useful as pathology unlikely to show up

Mx: · relieve pressure!!
  - Release dressing
  - **Fasciotomy** (within 6h of smx onset)
· Rhabdomyolysis
  - Check CK + U&Es (for kidney function)
  - Aggressive hydration and NaHCO3 ± haemodialysis
· If necrotic tissue found, consider debridement ± amputation

Tendon sheath infection (hand)

Kanavel's cardinal signs
1. Exquisite tenderness over sheath, limited to sheath
2. Finger sits in resting flexed position
3. Exquisite pain on extending finger passively, more marked proximally
4. Fusiform (sausage) swelling of whole finger
If all 4 present, >90% sensitive for flexor tenosynovitis

Mx: REF TO HAND SURGEONS. Elevation, IV abx. Open drainage and washout required

P: delayed tx can lead to fibrosis, joint contracture or extension of infxn to deep palmar spaces and other structures

Spinal cord compression

A: trauma, vertebral fracture, interver-tebral disc herniation, tumours, infection

S/Smx
· **sensory**: Δ sensation below affected level
  - ❗ pain & hemi-sensory loss
· **motor**: weakness or paralysis
· **autonomic** symptoms
  - constipation
  - urinary retention
  - dizziness (hypotension)
  - cold, shivering, drowsiness
  - erectile dysfunction
  - abd pain and distention (ileus)
  - syncope (bradycardia)

BACK PAIN red flags → urgent MRI
► <20yo or >50yo
► Progressive pain
► Night/supine pain that prevents or disturbs sleep, or rest pain
► Pain aggravated by straining
► Thoracic back pain
► Mechanical pain (↑ when standing, sitting, moving)
► Localised spinal tenderness
► Claudication
► No symptomatic improvement with therapy
► Unexplained wt loss
► Past Hx of cancer
► IVDU / steroid use
► S/smx hinting of cauda equina syndrome (see right)

See also NICE's page on red flags for sciatica

Physical exam: Reflexes
↳ **Absent reflexes ↑↑suspicion**
· Anal wink – contraction of anal sphincter on stimulation of perianal area
· Bulbocavernous reflex – tapping the dorsum of penis causes contraction of pelvic floor muscles
· Cremasteric reflex – stimulus to upper thigh causes scrotal elevation
· Babinski's sign +ve is abnormal

Cauda equina syndrome
= refers to any smx below AND radiolo-gical confirmation of compression
· Most commonly caused by central disc prolaps at L4/L5 or L5/S1
· S/Smx:
  - low back pain (common)
  - bilateral sciatica (50% cases)
  - impotence
  - saddle anaesthesia
  - sensorimotor loss in lower extremities
  - neurogenic bladder dysfunction – usually overflow incontinence (later sign that is a/w poorer prognosis)
  - ± bowel dysfunction

Notes on anatomy: conus medullaris ends at L1-L2, and the cauda equina extends from L2 to Co1

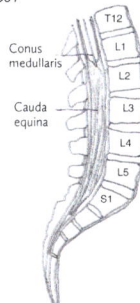

T12
L1
L2
L3
L4
L5
S1
Conus medullaris
Cauda equina

Spinal tumours
· Most often 2/2 metastatic cancer
  ↳ more common in lung, breast, prostate cancers
· S/smx as with other spinal cord lesions
  - back pain is the earliest and most common symptom
· Ix: whole spine MRI
· Mx: high dose PO dexamethasone
  - urgent onco assessment to consider radiotherapy or surgery
  - palliation if not feasible

Open fractures

D: fracture with skin breach

Gustilo-Anderson classification
Type I
· wounds ≤1cm, minimal contamination or muscle damage
Type II
· wounds 1-10cm, moderate soft tissue injury
Type IIIA
· >10cm, high-energy, extensive soft tissue damage + contaminated
· adequate tissue for flap coverage
· farm injuries are automatically at least IIIA
Type IIIB
· same as type 3a but with extensive periosteal stripping
· inadequate tissue for flap coverage
Type IIIC
· with vascular injury requiring vascular repair (regardless of degree of soft tissue injury)

Mx
· ABCDE - full exposure to look for associated injuries
· Abx required + tetanus booster (if no booster in last 5y)
· Definitive Mx is surgical
  - ideally in theatre within 6h of injury
  - remove foreign material
  - remove devitalised tissue
  - extensive irrigation of wound
  - stabilise & set fracture

Mx of closed fractures
· Immobilise fracture including proximal and distal joints
· Monitor and document neurovascular status esp after reduction and immobilisation
· No abx needed if closed

Shoulder

Adhesive capsulitis
aka frozen shoulder
- D: chronic fibrosing condition causing slowly progressing restriction of the shoulder's range of movement
- R: 40-70yo, DM, prior Hx of adhesive capsulitis, previous shoulder surgery, conditions that predispose to shoulder immobility
- S/smx:
  - external rotation affected more than internal rotation or abduction
  - both active and passive movement affected
  - 3 phases: freezing, adhesive, recovery
  - bilateral in 20%
  - episode typically between 6-24mo
- Dx: clinical ± imaging (eg MRI)
- Mx: NSAIDs, physio, oral corticosteroids and intraarticular steroids

Rotator cuff injury
- D: spectrum of injuries including tendinopathy, partial and full tears
  - subacromial impingement
  - calcific tendonitis
  - rotator cuff tears
  - rotator cuff arthropathy
- R: >60yo
- A: acute trauma, or repetitive ± vigorous overhead activity, or age-related degeneration
- P: trauma + poor blood supply (and ∴ lack of healing) → chronic injury
- S/smx: shoulder pain worse on abduction
  - painful arc of abduction (typically 60° to 120°
  - pain over anterior acromion
- Ix: XR, US/MRI
- Mx: - surgical if significant impact on ADLs and fit for surgery
  - others: conservative (NSAIDs, physio), arthroscopic debridement

Acromioclavicular joint injury
- A: trauma, usually due to fall on shoulder or fall on outstretched hand
- ÷ Grades I to VI
- Mx: - Grade I-III: conservative, sling
  - Grade IV-VI: surgery

Shoulder dislocation
- D: dislocation of the humeral head from the glenoid cavity of the scapula (accounts for 50% of all major joint dislocations)
- Anterior >95% cases
  - arm is usually abducted and externally rotated + prominent acromion
- Posterior (2-4%)
  - arm is in adduction and internal rotation + pt cannot rotate externally
- S/smx: as above
  - check for neurovascular compromise (eg axillary nerve injury)
  - r/o associated fractures
- Mx: - Reduction ± sedation
  - Can generally be done in the ED with some CI (eg humeral fracture, arterial injury, etc)

Humeral factures
- Proximal humeral fractures
  - usually seen in older pts with osteoporosis after fall on outstretched hand
  - a/w axillary nerve injury
- Mid-shaft fractures
  - a/w radial nerve injury (both due to injury and 2/2 surgical manipulation) – 85-90% imprrove over 3mo of observation
    ↳ radial nerve injury will present as wrist drop

Biceps (tendon) rupture
- D: the separation of the long or short tendon of the biceps from its attachment site or the full-width tear of one of these tendons
- R: M>F (3:1), ↑age
- A: heavy overhead activities, shoulder overuse, smoking, corticosteroids
- S/smx: - sudden pop or tear at the shoulder → pain, bruising, swelling
  - Weakness in shoulder
  - 'Popeye' deformity: bulge of muscle in middle of upper arm
- Ix: exam + MRI
- Mx: RICE + NSAIDs
  - Conservative, esp if elderly
  - Surgery

Elbow+

Cubital tunnel syndrome
- D: compression of the ulnar nerve (C8 & T1) as it passes through the cubital tunnel
- S/smx: numbness, tingling ± pain of the 4th and 5th finger
  - intermittent then constant
  - ± weakness and muscle wasting
  - pain worse when leaning on elbow
  - ± Hx of OA or trauma to area
- Ix: clinical Dx ± nerve conduction
- Mx: - avoid aggravating motions
  - physio, steroid injections, surgery

Radial tunnel syndrome
- D: compressive neuropathy of the posterior interosseous nerve (PIN) at the level of proximal forearm
- S/smx: pain 4-5cm distal to lateral epicondyle, ± worse on extending elbow and pronating forearm

Medial epicondylitis (golfer's elbow)
- D: chronic tendinosis of the wrist flexors and pronators that attach to the medial epicondyle
- S/smx: pain at the medial epicondyle worse on wrist flexion and pronation (door knock movement)
  - ± numbness, tingling in 4th and 5th finger due to ulnar nerve

Lateral epicondylitis (tennis elbow)
- D: tendinosis of the common extensor tendons
- S/smx: pain when extending wrist and elbow against resistance
  - acute pain 6-12w, chronic phase between 6mo and 2y
- Mx: rest, ice, physio, NSAIDs

Olecranon bursitis
- D: swelling over posterior aspect of elbow
- Typically in middle-aged males
- S/smx: a/w pain, warmth, redness

Pulled elbow
- D: subluxation of the radial head
- Most common children <6yo
- S/smx: elbow pain, limited supination and extension of elbow
- Mx: analgesia + passive supination of the elbow joint while elbow is flexed to 90°

Colles' fracture

- Classically follows a fall onto an outstretched hand (aka FOOSH)
- Distal radius fracture with dorsal displacement of fragments

Classical Colles' fractures:
- Transverse fracture of the radius
- 1" proximal to the radio-carpal joint
- Dorsal displacement and angulation

Early complications
- *median nerve injury*: acute carpal tunnel syndrome presenting with weakness or loss of thumb or index finger flexion
- compartment syndrome
- vascular compromise
- malunion
- rupture of the extensor pollicus longus tendon

Late complications
- osteoarthritis
- complex regional pain syndrome

Monteggia's fracture

- Ulna fracture and dislocation of proximal radio-ulnar joint
- Mechanism: FOOSH + forced pronation

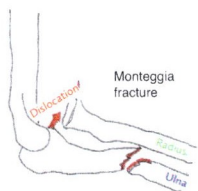

Monteggia fracture

Smith's fracture

- Mechanism: falling on the dorsal (back) side of the hand when the wrists are flexed
  ↳ hand is "inward"
- Volar (palmar) angulation of distal radius – "garden spade" deformity

Colles' fracture

Smith's fracture

Barton's fracture

- Distal radial fracture (Colles' or Smith's) a/w radiocarpal dislocation
- Mechanism: fall onto extended and pronated wrist

Galeazzi fracture

- Radial shaft fracture and dislocation of distal radio-ulnar joint
- Mechanism: fall on hand with rotational force

Galeazzi fracture

Carpal tunnel syndrome
- D: compression of median nerve in the carpal tunnel
- R: 40-60yo, ↑BMI, F>M, fractured wrist, DM, pregnancy, RA
- S/smx:
  - pain, pins and needles in thumb, index and middle finger
  - classically worse at night, pt might shake their hand to obtain relief
  - weakness of thumb abduction
  - wasting of thenar eminence
  - Tinel's sign: tapping carpal tunnel causes paraesthesia
  - Phalen's sign: flexion of wrist causes smx
- Ix: electrophysiology will show prolongation of action potential
- Mx: 6w trial of conservative tx (corticosteroid injection, wrist splint at night)
  - If severe or refractory, surgical decompression (flexor retinaculum division)

De Quervain's tenosynovitis
- D: inflammation of the sheath containing the extensor pollicis brevis and abductor longus tendons
- S/smx: - pain on radial side of wrist
  - tenderness over radial styloid
  - abduction of thumb against resistance is painful
- Finkelstein's test: "teapot test" +ve
- Mx: - analgesia ± steroid injection
  - immobilisation with thumb splint
  - if refractory, surgery

Trigger finger
- D: stenosing tenosynovitis of the fingers ± thumbs
- R: F>M, RA, DM
- S/smx:
  - more common in thumb, middle or ring finger
  - initially stiffness, snapping when extending a flexed digit ("trigger")
  - ± nodule at base of finger
- Mx: steroid injection ± finger splint
  - if refractory, surgery

Scaphoid fracture
- Classically follows a fall onto an outstretched hand (=FOOSH) or contact sports
- S/smx: pain along radial aspect of wrist, loss of grip/pinch strength
  - maximal tenderness over anatomical snuffbox – 90-95% sensitive, but poorly specific
  - ± wrist joint effusion
  - pain elicited by telescoping the thumb (pain on longitudinal compression)
  - tenderness on scaphoid tubercle
  - pain on ulnar deviation of wrist
- Ix: XR (↑sensitivity after 1w) ± MRI
- Mx: immobilisation with Futuro splint or standard below-elbow backslab
  - Ref to ortho for imaging 7-10d
  - Undisplaced fractures: cast for 6-8w + imaging later on
  - Displaced fractures: surgical fix
  - Proximal scaphoid pole fractures: surgical fixation
- Complications: non-union, avascular necrosis
  - 80% of blood supply of the scaphoid is derived from the dorsal carpal branch (branch of radial artery) in retrograde manner; disruption risks avascular necrosis of the scaphoid

Dupuytren's contracture
- D: myofibroblastic disease affecting the palmar and digital fascia of the hand (most commonly fourth and fifth fingers)
- A: genetic disorder (autosomal dominant), manual labour, phenytoin, alcoholic liver disease, DM, trauma to hand
- Mx: Surgical tx when pt cannot flatten hand on table (Hueston table top test)

Boxer fracture
- D: Minimally displaced fracture of the fifth metatarsal, usually after punching a hard surface
- S/smx: sunken knuckle
- Mx: Conservative – usually involving immobilisation; refer to hand surgeons

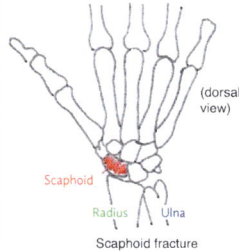

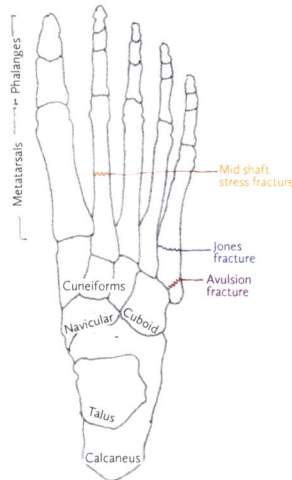

Ganglion
- D: synovial cyst filled with gelatinous mucoid material
- S/smx:
  - Firm, well-circumscribed mass that transilluminates
  - Most commonly on dorsal aspect of wrist, ± pain
- Mx: conservative – most of them resolve spontaneously
  - Surgical excision if severe smx or neurovascular smx

(dorsal view)

Scaphoid

Radius   Ulna

Scaphoid fracture

Phalanges

Metatarsals

Mid shaft stress fracture

Jones fracture

Avulsion fracture

Cuneiforms

Navicular Cuboid

Talus

Calcaneus

Club foot

aka talipes equinovarus
- D: fixed inversion and plantarflexion of the foot
- 1:1000 births, 50% bilateral

R: M>F (2x), spina bifida, cerebral palsy, Edward's syndrome, oligohydramnios, arthrogryposis (=congenital joint contracture)

Dx: clinical – no imaging needed

Mx:
- Ponseti method: manipulation and progressive casting soon after birth
  - Usually results in correction after 6-10w → maintain correction with night-time braces until child is 4yo
  - Also requires Achilles tenotomy in 85%, can be done under local anaesthesia
- Surgery, esp if child presents late

Metatarsal fracture

D: fracture of one or more of the metatarsal bones
  ↳ proximal 5th metatarsal most commonly fractured
- Stress fracture: 2/2 repeated mechanical stress

5th metatarsal fracture
- Proximal avulsion fracture
  - proximal tuberosity
  - usually a/w lateral ankle sprain, after inversion injuries of the ankle
- Jones fractures: transverse fracture at metaphyseal-diaphyseal junction

Metatarsal stress fractures
- Usually in otherwise healthy athletes
- Most commonly at the 2nd metatarsal shaft

S/smx: - pain and bony tenderness
  - swelling   - antalgic gait (limp)

Ix: XR (AP & lateral view)
- Repeat XR may be needed for stress fractures as they may appear normal at first, but 2-3w later, periosteal reaction may show
- Isotope scan or MRI may show stress fracture

Plantar fasciitis

- D: inflammation of the plantar fascia
- S/smx: pain around medial calcaneal tuberosity
  - usually on onset of activity
- Mx: - rest where possible
  - wear shoes with good arch support and cushioned heels
  - feet stretching before exercise

Hip / NOF fractures

R: osteoporosis, osteopenia, ↑age, falls, ↓BMI, F>M, high energy trauma

S/smx: pain ± rhabdomyolysis / AKI
- **shortened, externally rotated leg**
- if fracture is not too severe, pt may still be able to wt bear

Classification by location
- **intracapsular** (subcapital): from the edge of the femoral head to the insertion of the capsule of the hip joint
- **extracapsular**
  - trochanteric or subtrochanteric
  - lesser trochanter as the dividing line

Garden system classification
- Type I: Stable #, with impaction in valgus
- II: Complete fracture but undisplaced
- III: Displaced fracture, usually rotated and angulated, but still has bony contact
- IV: Complete boney disruption
→ blood supply disruption in III and IV

Mx of suspected NOF#
- 1' survey + determine nature of injury
- Request AP pelvis and lateral view XR
- Pain score + appropriate analgesia
- IV access + bloods (including G&S)
- If NOF# confirmed or still suspected, MRI (gold standard) or CT (if MRI CI or not available within 24h)

Mx of undisplaced intracapsular fractures
- internal fixation, or hemiarthroplasty if unfit

Mx of displaced intracapsular fractures
- arthroplasty (THR or hemiarthroplasty)
- THR favoured if
  - pts able to walk independently out of doors with only stick
  - no cognitive impairment
  - medically fit for anaesthesia and op

Mx of extracapsular fractures
- stable intertrochanteric fractures: dynamic hip screw
- reverse oblique, transverse or subtrochanteric #: intramedullary device

Also: pain Mx, rehab, ↓falls risks, med review

Hip dislocation

Posterior dislocation (90%): shortened, adducted, internally rotated

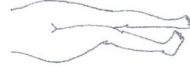

Mx · ABCDE + analgesia
- **reduction under GA within 4h to ↓risk of avascular necrosis**
- long-term physio

Complications
- Sciatic or femoral nerve injury
- Avascular necrosis
- OA esp in older pts
- Recurrent dislocation due to ligament damage

P: 2-3mo for healing, best prognosis when reduced <12h post-injury, ↓damage to joint

Anterior dislocation: abducted and externally rotated. No leg shortening

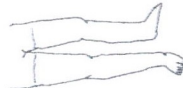

NOF#: shortened & externally rotated

C: VTE, avascular necrosis, non-union
P: 30% mortality at 1yr; up to 75% may not regain pre-morbidity level of function

Avascular necrosis of the hip

- D: loss of blood supply resulting in death of bone tissue
- A: long-term **steroid** use, **chemo**, alcohol excess, trauma
- S/smx: - initially asmx
  - pain in affected part
- Ix: XR may be normal at first
  - Later on – osteopenia, microfractures
  - Crescent sign when there is collapse of articular surface
  - MRI imaging of choice
- Mx: joint replacement

Acetabular labral tear

aka hip labral tear
- A: trauma, degeneration, etc
- S/smx:
  - hip/groin pain
  - snapping sensation around hip
  - ± sensation of locking
- Ix: XR ± MRI
- Mx: conservative (rest, NSAIDs, physio ± steroid injection)

Meralgia paraesthesica

- D: entrapment neuropathy of the lateral femoral cutaneous nerve
- R: 30-40yo, M>F, DM, obesity, tense ascites, trauma
- Can also be caused iatrogenically (eg lap hernia repair)
- S/smx: burning sensation over antero-lateral aspect of thigh
  - others: numbness, deep muscle ache, coldness, shooting pain
  - smx worse on standing, relieved by sitting
  - smx reproducible by deep palpation over the ASIS (pelvic compression test is highly sensitive) and extension of the hip
- Ix: clinical ± nerve conduction
- Mx: injection of nerve with local anaesthetic will abolish pain (also confirms Dx) – US guided injection

Pubic symphisis dysfunction

aka pelvic girdle pain
- D: syndrome arising from pubic symphisis ligament laxity, most commonly in pregnancy due to hormonal changes
- S/smx:
  - pain over pubic symphisis with radiation to groins and medial aspect of thighs
  - ± waddling gait
- Mx: usually resolves on giving birth
  - analgesia, physio (eg pelvic floor physical therapy)

Idiopathic transient osteoporosis of the hip

- D: temporary loss of bone in femoral head and neck
- R: M>F (3:1), 40-55yo men, women in 3rd trim of pregnancy
- S/smx:
  - absence of trauma in hx
  - progressive hip and groin pain over several weeks
  - may not be able to bear weight
  - local tenderness + usually normal hip range of movement
- Ix: XR, MRI
- Mx: avoid weight bearing to avoid stress fractures; resolves spontaneously in 6-8mo

Greater trochanteric pain syndrome

aka trochanteric bursitis
- A: repetitive activity, mechanical overload
- P: repeated movement of fibroelastic iliotibial band
- S/smx: pain on lateral side of hip or thigh + tenderness on palpation of greater trochanter
- Ix: XR to r/o pathology
- Mx: activity modification, physio, wt loss, steroid injection, NSAIDs

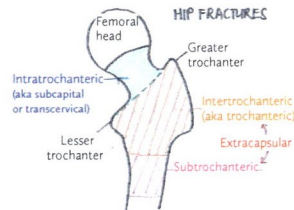

HIP FRACTURES

Femoral head

Greater trochanter

Intratrochanteric (aka subcapital or transcervical)

Intertrochanteric (aka trochanteric)

Lesser trochanter

Extracapsular

Subtrochanteric

Knee

Ligament and meniscal injuries

Unhappy triad
- Usually 2/2 lateral blow to knee
- ACL + MCL + meniscus (medial or lateral)

ACL injury · 2/2 twisting injuries
- +ve anterior drawer & Lachman's

PCL · Dashboard injuries

MCL
- Damage commonly from skiing and valgus stress
- Usually causes passive knee abduction

LCL · Isolated injury uncommon

Menisci · 2/2 twisting injuries
- Locking and giving way common
- Thessaly's test: wt bearing at 20° of knee flexion, +ve if pain on twisting knee

Ix: MRI needed to visualise ligaments and menisci
Mx: refer to orthopaedics
- arthroscopic or open surgical Mx

Bursitis & cysts

Infrapatellar bursitis: a/w kneeling (aka Clergyman's knee)

Prepatellar bursitis: a/w kneeling (aka Housemaid's knee)

Baker cyst
- D: distension of the gastrocnemius-semimembranosus bursa
  - 1°: no underlying pathology
  - 2°: underlying problem eg OA
- S/smx: bulge behind the knee
  - if rupture, may cause smx similar to DVT (but can also be asmx)
- Mx: in children, no tx required
  - in adults, tx underlying cause

Patella fracture
- A: direct injury (eg fall, dashboard injury); indirect injury caused by forceful contraction of the quadriceps, eg when trying to prevent a fall)
- S/smx:
  - swelling and bruising
  - look for associated fractures
  - pain and tenderness aroudn the knee, well localised to patella
  - test whether pt can still extend their leg
- Ix: XR (AP & lateral)
- Mx:
  - undisplaced + intact extensor mechanism: do not require surgery; hinged knee brace for 6w + ask pt to fully weight bear
  - otherwise, surgical mx likely required

Iliotibial band syndrome
- D: inflammation of the iliotibial band
- R: runners (1 in 10 people who run regularly)
- S/smx:
  - burning pain at or just under the lateral femoral epicondyle
  - tenderness 2-3cm above the lateral knee joint line
- Mx: activity modification and iliotibial band stretches ± physio

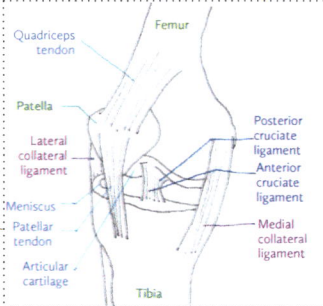

Quadriceps tendon
Femur
Patella
Lateral collateral ligament
Meniscus
Patellar tendon
Articular cartilage
Tibia
Posterior cruciate ligament
Anterior cruciate ligament
Medial collateral ligament

Ankle fractures

Ottawa Rules for XR of ankles
- pain in the malleolar zone
- bony tenderness at the lateral malleolar zone (from the tip of the lateral malleolus to include the lower 6 cm of posterior border of the fibular)
- bony tenderness at the medial malleolar zone (from the tip of the medial malleolus to the lower 6 cm of the posterior border of the tibia)
- inability to walk four weight bearing steps immediately after the injury and in A&E

Weber classification
- A: below the syndesmosis
- B: fractures start at the level of the tibial plafond and may extend proximally to involve the syndesmosis
- C: above the syndesmosis which may itself be damaged
- Subtype known as a Maisonneuve fracture may occur with spiral fibular fracture that leads to disruption of the syndesmosis with widening of the ankle joint, surgery is required.

Mx depends upon stability of ankle joint and patient co-morbidities.
- All ankle fractures should be **promptly reduced** to remove pressure on the overlying skin and subsequent necrosis
- Young patients with unstable, high velocity or proximal injuries will usually require surgical repair
- Elderly patients – conservative Mx better

Ankle sprains

A sprain is a stretching, partial or complete tear of a ligament.
In the ankle, ÷
- high ankle sprains involving the syndesmosis
- low ankle sprains involving the lateral collateral ligaments

Low ankle sprains (90%)
- injury to the ATFL most common
- inversion injury most common mechanism
- pain, swelling, tenderness over affected ligaments ± bruising
- patients usually able to weight bear unless severe

| Grade I (mild): microtear of ligament |
| II (mod): partial tear |
| III (severe): complete tear |

Ix: XR by Ottawa rules ± MRI

Mx: RICE ± orthosis (cast, crutches).
Severe – ?surgery

High ankle sprains (10%)
- usually 2/2 eversion mechanism
- wt bearing difficult
- Hopkin's squeeze test: pain when tibia and fibula squeezed together mid-calf

Ix: XR by Ottawa rules ± MRI

Mx: · if no separation: non-wt bearing orthosis or cast until pain subsides
- if separation: ORIF

Achilles tendon

R: quinolones (e.g. **ciprofloxacin**) a/w tendon disorders. hypercholesterolaemia a/w tendon xanthomata

Tendinitis
- gradual onset of posterior heel pain; worse following activity
- morning pain and stiffness
Mx: supportive
- analgesia
- ↓precipitating activities
- physio: calf eccentric exercises

Tendon rupture
- pop + sudden pain + inability to walk / continue playing
- Simmon's triad:
  - ask pt to lie down, feet hanging off bed
  1. rupture may lead to ↑dorsiflexion
  2. feel for gap in tendon
  3. squeeze calf muscle, rupture will cause muscle to stay in neutral position
- Dx by US!
- Urgent ref to orthopaedics

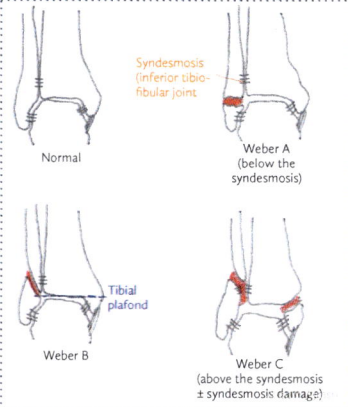

Normal
Syndesmosis (inferior tibio-fibular joint)
Weber A (below the syndesmosis)
Tibial plafond
Weber B
Weber C (above the syndesmosis ± syndesmosis damage)

Cervical spondylosis

aka degenerative cervical spine disease, degenerative disc disease
- Specific term for OA of the spine
- Can lead to radiculopathy and cervical myelopathy

R: >40yo, smoking

S/smx: • neck pain ± spasm
- referred pain can cause HA around occipital area
- ± radiating arm pain (rare)

Ix: cervical XR ± MRI (if pain >4-6w and not amenable to tx)

Mx: ↓ physio, NSAIDs
- Consider muscle relaxants eg baclofen, diazepam

Degenerative cervical myelopathy

D: spinal cord compression 2/2 degenerative changes to the cervical spine (further manifestation of cervical spondylosis)

S/smx: as above, plus
- Loss of motor function (eg ↓digital dexterity – pt cannot button shirt)
- Loss of sensory function causing numbness (eg carpal tunnel syndrome)
- Loss of autonomic function (eg urinary or faecal incontinence)
  - r/o cauda equina syndrome
- Hoffman's sign +ve
  - Hold pt's middle finger by the DIP, and watch the thumb and index finger
  - Flick the middle finger down
  - If the thumb and index finger twitch (come closer together), then this is Hoffman +ve
  - ? UL equivalent of Babinski sign

Mx: • refer to neurosurgery or orthopaedic spinal surgery
  → decompressive surgery

Spinal stenosis

aka lumbar spondylosis
D: degenerative condition of the lumbar spine causing narrowing of the spinal canal

R: >40yo, previous back surgery, previous injury, achondroplasia, acromegaly
Weaker risk factors: manual labour, FHx, smoking, DM, peripheral vascular occlusive disease

A: degenerative changes
P: narrowing of spinal canal → compression of nerve roots of cauda equina → s/smx

S/smx: • Lower back pain
- Claudication-like s/smx (eg calf pain, pain on walking, leg numbness, pain radiating down leg)
  - pain with spinal stenosis tends to improve on sitting, and pts find it easier to walk uphill than downhill

Ix: XR + MRI (will show canal narrowing)

Mx:
- r/o cauda equina syndrome
  ↳ surgical emergency
- if not severe: analgesics
- definitive tx: surgery (laminectomy)

- **Spondylosis** = degenerative changes to the spine (eg OA)
- **Spondylolysis** = (stress) fracture of the vertebra; usually referring to fracture through the pars interarticularis of the lumbar vertebrae
- **Spondylolisthesis** = displacement of one vertebra over an adjacent vertebra

Scheuermann's kyphosis

D: Condition of hyperkyphosis where there is anterior wedging of the vertebral bodies >5° in ≥3 adjacent vertebral bodies
- most commonly affecting the thoracic spine
- M>F 2:1, 12-17yo (aka juvenile kyphosis)

S/smx: • postural deformity
- subacute thoracic pain (in the absence of trauma, worse with activity)
- Rigid hyperkyphotic curve that does not resolve with lying down

Ix: XR (should show anterior wedging ± epiphyseal plate disturbance)

Mx: minor - physio, analgesia
- severe - may require bracing or surgical stabilisation

Scoliosis

D: structural spinal deformity, with evidence of ≥10° lateral curvature with vertebral rotation on a standing upright radiograph of the spine

R: FHx, peak adolescent growth spurt

S/smx:
- postural deformity: usually identified on screening
- scoliometer measurement >5° at any paraspinal prominence

Ix: clinical Dx ± XR (to calculate Cobb angle which quantifies spinal curvature ≈ degree of severity)

Mx:
- minor scoliosis: watch and wait
- Cobb angle 21-45°: bracing
- >45°: consider surgical spinal arthrodesis (spinal fusion)

Discitis

D: infection of the intervertebral disc space

R: children, immunocompromise, IVDU, alcoholics, malignancy

A: usually due to haematogenous seeding – bacterial (*Staph aureus* most common), viral, TB, aseptic

S/smx: • back pain
- general: fever, rigors, septic shock
- neuro: change in lower limb neurology if epidural abscess develops

Ix: MRI, CT-guided biopsy + MCS to guide abx choice

Mx: • Abx (6-8w IV abx)
- Choice dependent on culture
- Ax for endocarditis with trans-thoracic echo

Complications: • Sepsis
- **Epidural abscess**
  - collection of pus superficial to the dura of the spinal cord
  - Long-term abx (as above)
  - May require surgical drainage of the abscess

Autonomic dysreflexia

- 2/2 spinal cord injury at/above **T6**
- S/smx: extreme hypertension, flushing, sweating above level of cord lesion, agitation → haemorrhagic stroke
- Mx: removal/control of stimulus, tx of life-threatening hypertension ± bradycardia
  - stimulus may be faecal impaction or urinary retention

Rib fractures

R: blunt chest trauma (eg RTA), CPR, physical abuse in children, osteoporosis, contact sports
Weaker risk factors: cancer / metastasis

S/smx:
- severe, sharp chest wall pain
  - esp with deep breaths, coughing
- significant chest wall tenderness over site of fracture ± bruising
- Auscultation: crackles ↓breath sounds if there is underlying lung injury
- ↓ventilation if pt is in pain or underlying lung injury
- Pneumothorax ▶ : ↓chest expansion, ↓breath sounds, hyper-resonant percussion
- Flail chest ▶
  - occurs when there is ≥2 rib fractures along ≥3 consecutive ribs (resulting in a "detached" segment of rib bones)
  - this flail segment moves paradoxically during respiration and impairs ventilation ± contusional injury to lung

Ix: CT for major trauma / metastases
- CXR as 1st line but can miss up to 50% of rib fractures
- In physical abuse for children, non-acute rib fractures may show up as periosteal reactions
  - rib fractures in children are assumed as non-accidental injury until otherwise proven
  - refer to safeguarding
  - skeletal survey + CT head (if <1yo, external evidence of head trauma, or neurological s/smx)

Mx:
- Conservative: analgesia (to prevent breathing problems)
  - inadequate ventilation can ↑risk of chest infxns
  - consider nerve blocks
- If severe or refractory to conservative Mx, may require surgical fixation
- Flail chest: immediate referral to cardiothoracics

Dermatomes

C2 Posterior half of the skull (cap)
C3 High turtleneck shirt
C4 Low-collar shirt
C5 Ventral axial line of upper limb
C6 Thumb + index finger
    Make a 6 with your left hand by touching
    the tip of the thumb + index finger
    together - C6
C7 Middle finger + palm of hand
C8 Ring + little finger

T4 Nipples
T5 Inframammary fold
T6 Xiphoid process
T10 Umbilicus

L1 Inguinal ligament
L2, L3 Anterior & medial thigh
L4 Knee caps
    Down on all fours · L4
L5 Big toe, dorsum of foot
    (except lateral aspect)
    L5 = Largest of the 5 toes

S1 Lateral foot, small toe
    S1 = the smallest one
S2, S3 Genitalia

Fat embolism

D: presence of fat particles that can result in a systemic manifestation

A: most commonly due to trauma (eg fracture of long bones, post-op complication, soft tissue damage, crush injury), non-traumatic causes (eg fatty liver)

S/smx: · Depends on organ that is affected by the fat emboli
· Respi (similar to PE): ↑HR, ↑RR, dyspnea, hypoxia (usually ~72h following injury), fever
· Skin: red/brown impalpable petechial rash, subconjunctival and oral petechiae
· CNS: confusion, agitation
  - retinal haemorrhages and intra-arterial fat globules on fundoscopy

Ix: imaging may be normal; high degree of suspicion required

Mx
· Prompt fixation of long bone fractures
· DVT prophylaxis
· Supportive care

Osteomalacia

D: Metabolic bone disease characterised by incomplete mineralisation of the underlying mature organic bone matrix
· Rickets – in children [→11.10]
· Osteomalacia – in adults

R/A: ↓Ca and Vit D in diet, **CKD**, ↓sunlight, inherited disorders of Vit D and bone metabolism, anticonvulsant therapy, coeliac disease, liver disease

S/smx: · Bone pain ± muscle tenderness
· Fractures, esp femoral neck
· Proximal myopathy → "waddling gait"

Ix: bloods (↓Vit D, ↓Ca, ↓PO4, ↑ALP), XR (translucent bands, pseudofractures)

Mx: · Vit D supplementation
  - Loading dose usually needed
· Ca supplementation if needed

Osteomyelitis

D: infection of the bone

A: · Staph. aureus most common
· Salmonella spp most common in pts with sickle cell disease
P: · Haematogenous spread
  - 2/2 bacteraemia
  - most common form in children
  - R: sickle cell anaemia, IVDU, immunosuppression, infective endocarditis
· Non-haematogenous spread
  - Contiguous spread (from adjacent soft tissues), or from direct innoculation (eg via trauma)
  - more often polymicrobial
  - R: pressure sores, DM, peripheral arterial disease

S/smx: · Hot, erythematous swelling over affected bone + bone pain

Ix: MRI

Mx: Abx according to local guidelines
· NICE recommends flucloxacillin for 6w (clindamycin if penicillin allergy)
  - Consider adding fusidic acid or rifampicin for initial 2w
· If MRSA cultured, switch to vancomycin

Charcot joint

· D: joint damage 2/2 loss of sensation (aka neuropathic joint)
· R: DM, neurosyphillis
· S/smx
  - swollen, red and warm joint
  - less pain than expected (due to sensory loss)
· Ix: XR ± others
· Mx: immobilisation (casting)
  - orthotics to prevent recurrence
  - surgical intervention if severe deformity

Osteochondritis dissecans

D: acquired idiopathic lesion of subchondral bone resulting in delamination and sequestration ± articular cartilage involvement and instability
· Tends to affect adolescents

R: repetitive throwing / valgus stress, gymnastics or wt bearing on upper extremities, ankle sprain / instability, competitive athletics

S/smx:
· Most commonly affects knee
  - pain, swelling worse on activity
  - joint catching, locking ± giving way
  - painful clunk when flexing or extending joint
  - joint effusion
  - tenderness on palpation of articular cartilage
   ↳ pain on anteromedial aspect of knee when flexed to 90°

Ix: XR (may show subchondral crescent sign [= osteochondral lesion] or loose bodies)
· MRI (evaluate cartilage, visualise loose bodies, stage and Ax stability of joint)

Mx: · Refer to orthopaedics
· If no joint malalignment, conservative Mx (NSAIDs, watch and wait) may be enough
· If joint malalignment or unstable, arthroscopy + surgery may be needed

	Sensory loss	Motor weakness	Reflexes	Test
L3	Anterior thigh	Hip flex, hip abd, knee ext	↓ knee reflex	+ve femoral stretch test
L4	Ant knee, medial malleolus	Knee ext, hip add		
L5	Dorsum of foot	Foot and big toe dorsiflex	Reflexes intact!!	+ve sciatic stretch test
S1	Posterolat leg, lat foot	Plantarflex of foot	↓ ankle reflex	

	Sensory loss	Motor weakness
Femoral	Ant, medial thigh and leg	Knee ext, thigh flex
Obturator	Medial thigh	Thigh adduction
Lat cutaneous	Lat, posterior thigh → meralgia paraesthetica	
Tibial	Sole of foot	Plantarflex & inv of foot
Common peroneal	Dorsum of foot + lateral leg	Foot dorsiflex, eversion + foot drop
Superior gluteal	None	Hip abduction +ve Trendelenburg
Inferior gluteal	None	Hip ext, lateral rotation

a/w sciatic nerve injury
difficulty rising from seated position

Joint replacements = arthroplasty

Hip replacements
· cemented hip replacement
  - metal femoral component is cemented into the femoral shaft and
  - cemented acetabular polyethylene cup
For younger, more active pts,
· uncemented hip replacements more common but more expensive
· hip resurfacing
  - metal cap is attached over the femoral head
  - preserves femoral neck for conventional arthroplasty if req later on

Post-op recovery
· physio, home exercises
· walking sticks or crutches for 6w post-op in hip and knee replacements

Advice to ↓risk of dislocation
· avoid flexing the hip > 90 degrees
· avoid low chairs
· do not cross your legs
· sleep on your back for the first 6w

Complications
· wound and joint infections
· VTE: LMWH for 4w post hip replacement
· dislocation

Pagets disease of the bone

D: chronic localised bone remodelling disorder characterised by ↑bone resorption, bone formation, and remodelling

R: FHx, >50yo, M>F

A: unknown, ?genetics
P: localised areas of metabolic hyperactivity of the bone
· 3 phases
  - bone resorption (↑osteoclastic activity)
  - mixed osteoclastic and osteoblastic activity → deposition of structurally abnormal bone
  - sclerotic phase (bone formation > bone resorption)

S/smx: · 95% asymptomatic
· most commonly affects skull, spine/pelvis, long bones of lower extremities
· classic pt: older male with bone pain and isolated ↑ALP
· bone pain
· if untreated, can cause bowing of tibia and bossing of skull (protuberance of the frontal bones)

Ix: · bloods: ↑ALP, normal Ca, PO4
· XR: osteolysis in early disease, mixed lytic/sclerotic lesions in later disease
· Bone scan: ↑isotope uptake at active bone lesions

Mx: · treat only if bone pain, skull or long bone deformity, fracture, or periarticular location
· ⚡ Bisphosphonate
  - PO risedronate or IV zoledronate
· Calcitonin less commonly used

Complications
· Deafness (2/2 CN entrapment)
· Bone sarcoma   · Fractures
· High-output cardiac failure (2/2 ↑blood flow within bone and surrounding limb tissue)

Osteoporosis

D: ↓bone density and bone micro-deformities causing ↑bone fragility and susceptibility to fracture

R: F>M, ↑age, ↓BMI, RA, post-menopause, smoking, ↑alcohol use, FHx of hip fracture, **glucocorticoid** use, white ancestry, CKD, testosterone deficiency, etc

S/smx:
· asymptomatic until fracture occurs

Ix: · XR for fractures
· Risk Ax with FRAX score - 10y risk of fracture (alternative: QFfracture)
  - intermediate risk, offer DEXA scan
  - high risk, offer bone protection
· DEXA scan
  - may not be required in F≥75yo according to clinician judgment
  - T-score: based on bone mass of young reference population
    ↳ <-2.5 = osteoporosis
  - Z-score: adjusted for age, gender and ethnic factors

Mx:
· In women confirmed to have osteoporosis, start tx
· ⚡ Alendronate
  - 25% cannot tolerate this; offer risedronate or etidronate
  - if bisphosphonates cannot be tolerated, offer strontium ranelate or raloxifene
· Calcium & Vit D supplementation
· Other options
  - HRT: ↓incidence of vertebral and non-vertebral fractures, but there are concerns about ↑risk of heart disease and breast cancer
  - hip protectors: helps esp in nursing home pts, but may be uncomfortable ∴ low compliance
  - Falls risk Ax
! For pts on glucocorticoids
  - if it is anticipated that pt will be on ≥3mo of steroids (equivalent of prednisolone 7.5 mg), start bone protection asap
    - eg in polymyalgia rheumatica
    - bisphosphonate

Bisphosphonates
· MOA: inhibits osteoclasts
· AE: - oesophageal reactions
  - osteonecrosis of the jaw
  - atypical stress fractures (alendronate)
  - acute phase response: fever, myalgia
  - hypoCa (usually clinically unimportant)
· Counselling: swallow whole with plenty of water on empty stomach ≥30min before breakfast
  - sit/stand upright for ≥30min after taking medicine
· Correct vitamin D deficiency before giving bisphosphonate
· Stop bisphosphonates at 5y if
  - Pt <75yo
  - Femoral neck T-score > -2.5
  - Low risk according to FRAX/NOGG

Pathological fractures

· **Osteogenesis imperfecta**
  - Defective osteoid formation 2/2 congenital inability to produce adequate intercellular substances like osteoid, collagen and dentine
  - Failure of maturation of collagen in all the connective tissues.
  - XR: translucent bones, multiple fractures, particularly of the long bones, wormian bones (irregular patches of ossification) and a trefoil pelvis
> types of osteogenesis imperfecta
  I: normal quality, ↓quantity
  II: ↓quality, ↓quantity
  III & IV: ↓quality, normal quantity
· **Osteopetrosis**: Autosomal recessive; bones are harder and denser. XR: marble bone

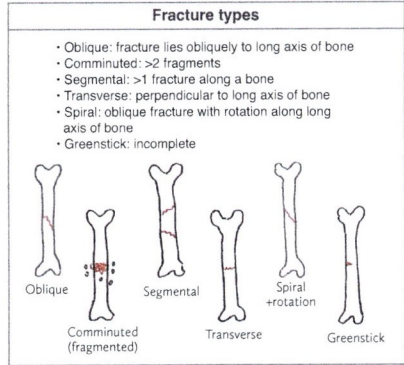

Fracture types

· Oblique: fracture lies obliquely to long axis of bone
· Comminuted: >2 fragments
· Segmental: >1 fracture along a bone
· Transverse: perpendicular to long axis of bone
· Spiral: oblique fracture with rotation along long axis of bone
· Greenstick: incomplete

Oblique   Segmental   Spiral +rotation

Comminuted (fragmented)   Transverse   Greenstick

S/Smx: non-mechanical pain, swelling ± pathological fracture ► ► ►

```
DDx – 1' or 2'        Dx leads
bone tumour          (1) age distribution
                     (2) PMHx
                     (3) location of pain
                     (4) imaging
```

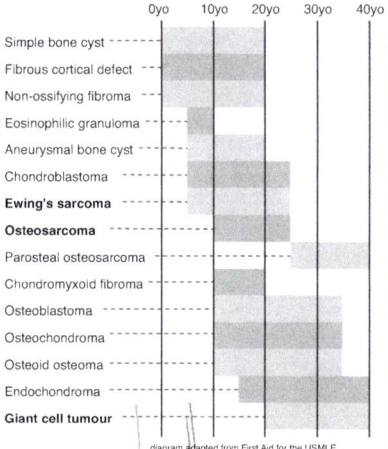

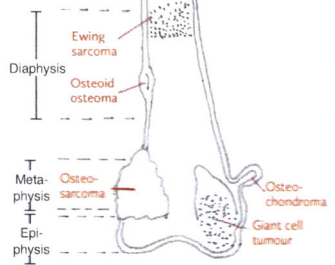

	0yo	10yo	20yo	30yo	40yo
Simple bone cyst					
Fibrous cortical defect					
Non-ossifying fibroma					
Eosinophilic granuloma					
Aneurysmal bone cyst					
Chondroblastoma					
Ewing's sarcoma					
Osteosarcoma					
Parosteal osteosarcoma					
Chondromyxoid fibroma					
Osteoblastoma					
Osteochondroma					
Osteoid osteoma					
Endochondroma					
Giant cell tumour					

diagram adapted from First Aid for the USMLE

Diaphysis — Ewing sarcoma, Osteoid osteoma

Meta-physis — Osteosarcoma, Osteochondroma

Epi-physis — Giant cell tumour

Osteosarcoma

D: primary osseous malignant neoplasm composed of mesenchymal cells producing osteoid and immature bone

R: 10-25yo, ?M>F, Paget's disease, radiotherapy, Rothmund-Thomson, familial retinoblastoma, Li-Fraumeni

A/P: ↑ osteoid production by osteoblasts

S/Smx: **bone pain** (gradual worsening), esp in 10-25yo + swelling (usually firm to touch), limping, ↓ROM ± skin ulceration

Ix: XR of affected limb
- radiolucent lesion
- periosteal rxn (Codman's triangle, spiculations)
± soft tissue swelling.
• MRI, CT thorax, radionuclide bone scan
• Bloods – ↑ALP and ↑LDH
• Bone biopsy to confirm histology

Mx: chemo + surgical resection

Chondrosarcoma

D: malignant cancer of the cartilage
• 30-60yo
• affects the flat bones (ilium, ribs)

Mx: wide local resection ± chemo/radio

Bone mets (PBKTL): **Prostate, breast, kidneys, thyroid and lungs**

· Most common sites of metastases: spine, pelvis, ribs, skull, long bones
· S/smx:
- bone pain
- pathological fractures
- hypercalcaemia (moans, stones, bones, groans)
- ↑ALP

Ewing's sarcoma

D: small round blue cell tumour
• <15yo, M>F
• a/w t(11;22) translocation

S/smx: • affects bones around knee
• Pt may present with fever and hot swelling – often mistaken for osteomyelitis

Ix: XR may show onion skin periosteal reaction + lung mets

Mx: 12w neoadjv chemo + re-evaluate, re-stage + wide local resection / amputation

P: poor – 50% 5-y survival

Giant cell tumour

D: tumour of multinucleated giant cells within a fibrous stroma
• most of them are locally aggressive but benign. ~10% transform to malignant tumours (aka osteoclastoma)
• 20-40yo, F>M

S/smx: bony prominence around the knee; other locations include wrist, hip, shoulder or lower back)

Ix: XR will show "soap bubble appearance"

Mx: local excision, replace defect with cement or bone graft

P: recurrence is common

Trauma

Thoracic trauma
· Haemothorax
  - 2/2 laceration of blood vessel
  - Mx: ✄ wide bore chest drain
    ✄ Thoracotomy if >1.5L blood loss initially, or >200 mL/h loss for >2h
· Mediastinal traversing wounds
  - Entrance in one side of the thorax, exit in the other side
  - Haematoma indicates ↑likelihood of great vessel injury
  - Ix: CTPA, oesophageal contrast swallow
  - Mx: ?thoracotomy
· Traumatic aortic disruption
  - Most common cause of death after RTA
  - 98% will show up on XR
· Cardiac contusions
  - Result in cardiac arrhythmias + sternal fracture
  - Ix: echo
  - Mx pericardial effusions or tamponade accordingly
· Pulmonary contusion
  - Common. Insidious onset, but lethal
  - Mx: early intubation & vent
· Diaphragmatic injury
  - Usually on left side
  - Mx: gastric tube passing into thoracic cavity, then surgical repair
· Simple pneumothorax →02.04
· Tension pneumothorax →02.04
· Flail chest → 11.06
· Cardiac tamponade →01.09

Splenic trauma
· Small injuries (eg small haematoma, little blood loss) can be Mxed conservatively
· Laparotomy with conservation if
  - ↑Intraabdominal blood
  - Moderate haemodynamic compromise
  - Tears or lacerations affecting <50% of spleen
· Resection (removal of spleen) if
  - Hilar injuries
  - Major haemorrhage + shock
  - Major associated injuries

Lower genitourinary tract trauma
· Urethral injury
  - Bulbar rupture often 2/2 straddle type injuries → urinary retention, perineal haematoma, blood at the meatus
  - Membranous rupture usually 2/2 pelvic fracture → penile or perineal oedema/haematoma
  - Ix: Ascending urethrogram
  - Mx: Suprapubic catheter
· External genitalia injuries
  - Often 2/2 penetration, blunt trauma, devices, mutilation
  - Uro/plastics input required
· Bladder injury
  - -Intra- or extra-peritoneal
  - S/smx: haematuria, suprapubic pain
  - Ix: IV urethrogram or cystogram
  - Mx: laparotomy if intraperitoneal injury, conservative Mx if extraperitoneal

Liver trauma
· Laceration of blood vessels can cause haematoma (subcapsular or intrapernchymal), or bleeding into the abdomen
· Injury to bile duct more likely to occur in severe injuries, central injuries or penetrating trauma
· S/smx: RUQ pain, right shoulder tip pain, ↓BP, shock
· Ix: ↑ALT/AST, CT
· Mx: Maintain haemodynamic stability; 80% can be treated non-surgically

Head injuries
See →04.12

Ocular trauma
· Presents as hyphema (blood in anterior chamber of eye), eye pain/swelling, proptosis, 'rock hard' eyelids, and RAPD
· ↑risk of vision loss due to ↑IOP
· Mx: - Immediate ref to ophthal
  - Admit + strict bed rest
  - Urgent lateral canthotomy to decompress the orbit

Juvenile idiopathic arthritis

D: chronic paediatric inflammatory arthritides characterised by onset before 16yo and the presence of objective arthritis (in ≥1joints) for ≥6w

R: F>M, HLA polymorphisms, FHx of autoimmunity

A: Autoimmune disorder
P: Chronic inflammation of synovium

S/smx:
• Systemic onset:
 - Fever   - Salmon-pink rash
 - Arthritis   - Lymphadenopathy
 - **Uveitis** - Anorexia, wt loss
• Pauciarticular (60% cases) – ≤4 joints affected, usually medium sized joints eg knees and ankles

Ix: ANA, rheumatoid factor -ve

Mx:
• Pauciarticular / oligoarticular (≤4 joints):
 ⚕ Intra-articular corticosteroids
 - Consider use of NSAIDs and DMARDs if severe
• Polyarticular (≥5 joints)
 - DMARDs, ⚕ Methotrexate
 - Consider use of NSAIDs, biological agents if appropriate

Paeds fractures

• Complete fracture: both sides of cortex are breached
• Toddlers fracture: oblique tibial fracture in infants
• Plastic deformity: stress on bone resulting in deformity without cortical disruption
• Greenstick: unilateral cortical breach only
• Buckle / torus: incomplete cortical disruption resulting in periosteal haematoma (bulging of cortex)

Transient synovitis of the hip

• D: self-limiting inflammatory disorder of the hip – more common in young children
• R: 2-12yo, M>F 2:1 ± hx of recent URTI
• A/P: non-specific inflammation, possibly 2ndary reaction post-viral infection
• S/smx: - limited movement + pain
 - limp (but weight bearing)
 - +ve log roll (involuntary muscle guarding in affected limb)
 - pt may keep hip in abduction and external rotation
• Ix: XR (typically normal)
• Mx: activity restrictions, bed rest, analgesia (NOT aspirin in young children)
 - Safety netting advice for parents

Septic arthritis vs transient synovitis
Kocher criteria for dx of septic arthritis
- fever >38.5°C   - non-wt bearing
- ↑ESR >40   - ↑WCC >12
If 3-4 criteria are present, PPV is >90% for septic arthritis.

Growth plate fractures

I: Fracture through physis only
II: through physis + metaphysis
III: physis + epiphysis + joint
IV: physis + metaphysis + epiphysis
V: crush injury involving physis

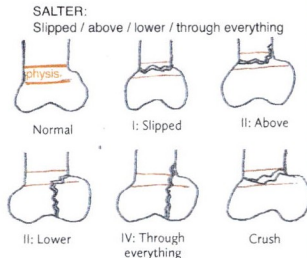

SALTER:
Slipped / above / lower / through everything

Normal   I: Slipped   II: Above

II: Lower   IV: Through   Crush
             everything

Developmental dysplasia of the hip

D: spectrum of conditions affecting the proximal femur and acetabulum
• Affects 1-3% newborns, L>R hip more often affected, but 20% cases bilateral

• Hip dysplasia = radiographic finding showing femoral head is not fully interacting with the acetabulum
• Hip subluxation = partial articulation of joint surfaces – usually shows up as hip that has ↑laxity with provocative testing
• Hip dislocation = femoral head sits outside acetabulum
• Fixed antenatal dislocation = hip cannot be reduced

R: F>M (6x ↑risk), **breech** presentation, FHx, firstborn child, oligohydramnios, birth wt >5kg, congenital calcaneovalgus foot deformity

A: not fully understood
P: incorrect anatomical relationship between femoral head and acetabulum leads to abnormal development

Screening and testing
• Screening by US if
 - 1st degree FHx of hip problems in childhood
 - Breech presentation at or after 36w gestation
 - Multiple pregnancy
• All other children are screened at newborn check and 6w check by clinical exams
 - **Barlow test**: attempts to dislocate an articulated femoral head
 - **Ortolani test**: attempts to relocate a dislocated femoral head
 - Symmetry of leg length
 - Level of knees when hips and knees are all flexed
 - Restricted abduction of the hip in flexion
• If any clinical suspicion
 ⚕ US if ≤4.5 months
 ⚕ XR if >4.5 months old
• Mx: - Monitor until 6w old
 - If no improvement, Pavlik harness if child <4-5mo, or surgery if older

Perthes' disease

D: Self-limiting degenerative condition affecting hip joints of children (4-8yo)
• M>F (5x more common)
• 10% bilateral

A/P: **Avascular necrosis** of the femoral epiphysis → collapse, repair, remodelling → self-limiting disorder

S/smx: • Hip pain (progressive)
• Limp
• Stiffness, ↓range of hip movement

Ix: Hip XR (↑joint space, ↓femoral head size), bone scan or MRI if normal XR but worsening smx

Mx: • Cast or braces to stabilise joint
• If <6yo: watch and wait
• If >6yo or severe: consider surgical Mx

Slipped capital femoral epiphysis

D: Anterosuperior displacement of the femoral *metaphysis* due to weakness in the growth plate.

R: Obesity, puberty, M>F

A/P: stress around the hip joint + shear forces cause slip of the growth plate

S/smx: • Most commonly in 10-15yo
• Hip, groin, medial thigh or knee pain
• Loss of internal rotation of leg in flexion
• Occurs bilaterally in 20%

Ix: XR (AP & lateral, typically frog-leg views) will show slipped epiphysis

Mx: Internal fixation of the hip

Complications: OA, avascular necrosis of the femoral head, chondrolysis, leg length discrepancy

Rickets

D: Condition arising from deficient mineralisation at the growth plate of long bones, presenting in childhood

R: ↓Ca and Vit D intake (eg developing countries or lower socioeconomic status), prolonged breastfeeding, unsupplemented cow's milk formula, ↓sunlight exposure

A/P: ↓Ca, ↓Vit D, and/or ↓PO4 – disrupts normal process of bone mineral deposition, esp at the growth plate
• If condition goes on for a long time, bone deformity occurs

S/smx:
• Bone pain, arthralgia
• Lower limb abnormalities
 - Genu varum (bow legs) in toddlers
 - Genu valgum (knock nees) in older children
• Kyphoscoliosis
• Craniotabes (soft skull bones)
• Harrison's groove: horizontal groove along lower border of thorax

Ix: bloods (↓Vit D, ↓Ca, ↑ALP)
• XR may show 'rickety rosary' – swelling at the costochondral junction

Mx: Vit D supplementation

Club foot →11.03

Rheumatoid arthritis

D: chronic, erosive arthritis. Affects ~1% of population.

R: F>M, FHx (main), ?smoking

A/P: **Inflamed synovium** → infiltration of inflammatory cells + cytokines → erosions

Earlier s/smx:
- **Symmetrical** arthritis >6w (insidious development; small → large joints)
- Swollen, painful joints in hands/feet
- Stiffness worse in the morning
- ± systemic disturbances

Later s/smx:
- Deformities: swan neck, boutonniere, Z-thumb, ulnar deviation
- +ve squeeze test

Others: relapsing/remitting monoarthritis of different large joints (palindromic rheumatism)

Dx: clinical + lab confirmation
- Rheum screen: RF (70%), anti-CCP (90-95%)
- X-rays of hands & feet (NICE rec)
  - early: loss of joint space, juxta-articular osteoporosis, soft-tissue swelling
  - periarticular erosions, subluxation

Am College of Rheumatology criteria
- joint involvement
  - more points for more joints
  - ≥1 small joint must be involved
- serology (+ve ↑↑RF, anti-CCP)
- acute phase reactants (↑CRP, ESR)
- duration of smx (>6w)

Mx:
- **Start DMARD asap!!**
  - **monotherapy** ± short-course of bridging prednisolone
- Monitoring: CRP + DAS28 score

Flares: • Corticosteroids PO/IM

(Mx cont) DMARDs
- **MTX** - monitor FBC, LFTs
  - AE: myelosuppression, liver failure, pneumonitis
- Sulfasalazine
  - AE: rashes, oligospermia, heinz body anaemia, ILD (lung)
- Leflunomide
  - AE: liver failure, interstitial lung disease, HTN
- Hydroxychloroquine
  - AE: Retinopathy, corneal deposits
- Gold – AE: Proteinuria
- Penicillamine – AE: proteinuria, ↑MG

TNFα inhibitors
> indicated if inadequate response to ≥2 DMARDs including MTX
- Etanercept = recombinant protein, acts as decoy receptor for TNF-α
  - SQ admin
  - AE: demyelination, reactivation of TB
- Infliximab = (mab) binds to TNF-α and prevents it from binding TNF receptors
  - IV admin
  - reactivation of TB
- Adalimumab: (mab) SQ admin

Rituximab
- anti-CD20 mab, ↓B cell
- two 1g IV infusion, 2 weeks apart
- AE: infusion reactions

Abatacept (not recommended by NICE)
- Fusion protein that modulates key signal required for activation of T-cells; ↓T cell prolif, ↓cytokines
- IV infusion

P: following a/w ↓prognosis
- RF   • anti-CCP   • HLA-DR4
- poor functional status at presentation
- X-ray: early erosions (<2y)
- Extra-articular features
- Insidious onset   • ?F sex

Complications / extra-articular manifestations
- Ocular manifestations in 25%: keratoconjunctivitis sicca, episcleritis, sleeritis, corneal ulceration, keratitis
- Respi: pulmonary fibrosis, pleural effusion, pulmonary nodules, bronchiolitis obliterans, pleurisy
- Osteoporosis (2/2 steroids?)
- Ischaemic heart disease
- ↑risk of infections (2/2 DMARDs?)
- Depression   • Amyloidosis
- Felty's syndrome: RA + splenomegaly + neutropenia

Osteoarthritis

D: degenerative joint disorder, the result of mechanical and biological events that destabilise the normal process of degradation and synthesis of articular cartilage chondrocytes, extracellular matrix, and subchondral bone

R: >50yo, F>M, obesity, genetic factors, knee alignment, ↑activity, post-trauma

S/smx: pain, functional difficulties, ↓ROM, malalignment. Knee > hip > hand

OA of the hip
- chronic hx of groin ache; ↑by exercise, ↓by rest - "C sign"
- Oxford Hip Score to Ax severity

OA of the hand
- ?+ve FHx, F>M, >55yo, ↑risk for hip, knee OA
- R: hypermobility, ↑working with hands
- Usually bilateral, basal thumb joint (CMC), DIPs
- Episodic joint pain (intermittent), stiffness (short)
- painless nodes - Heberden's (DIP), Bouchard's (PIP) - 2/2 osteophytes
- Squaring of the thumbs (causes fixed adduction of thumb)

► rest pain, night pain, morning stiffness >2h → ?alt cause

Ix: XR of affected joint - **LOSS**
- Loss of joint space
- Osteophyte formation
- Subchondral cysts & sclerosis
r/o RA if needed (FBC, RF, anti-CCP)

Mx: surgical - joint replacement
- For pts with significant pain
- Hips: cemented hip replacement, uncemented HR (in younger, more active pts; more expensive), hip resurfacing (preserves femoral neck)
- Post-op: physio, home-exercises, walking sticks / crutches for ≤6w
- How to avoid dislocation: avoid flexing hip >90', avoid low chairs, do not cross legs, sleep on back for first 6w

Mx: conservative + medical
- wt loss, muscle strengthening
- non-Rx: supports, braces, TENS, shock-absorbing insoles/shoes
  - ◄ paracetamol, NSAIDs
  - ◄ Opioids, capsaicin cream, intra-articular corticosteroids
    - PPI must be prescribed with NSAIDs

Complications:
- VTE, fracture, nerve injury, surgical site infxn: leg-length discrepancy
- Posterior dislocation - presents acutely with clunk, pain, inability to wt bear. O/E internal rotation, shortening of affected leg
- Aseptic loosening (most common reason for revision) + prosthetic joint infxn

---

Psoriatic arthritis

D: chronic inflammatory joint disease associated with psoriasis. Oligo or mono-articular initial pattern + DIP

R: psoriasis, FHx of psoriasis or PA

Exacerbating factors: trauma, alcohol, drugs (βBs, lithium, antimalarials, NSAIDs, ACEI, infliximab), withdrawal of steroids. Strep infxn for guttate psoriasis

A/P: likely genetic, a/w HLA B27. Sero-negative. CD8 T-cells eat away at the joints.

S/smx:
- Symmetric polyarthritis (similar to RA)
- or asymmetrical oligoarthritis (hands and feet – less common than above)
- Sacroiliitis
- **DIP joint disease** (10%)
- Athritis mutilans (severe deformity of hands, 'telescoping fingers')
- **Nail changes** (80-90%): pitting, onycholysis, subungual hyperkeratosis, loss of nail
± Psoriatic skin lesions
± Periarticular disease
  - Enthesitis
  - Tenosynovitis (esp hand flexors)
  - **Dactylitis** - uniquely psoriatic arthritis

Ix: XR - erosive Δs, new bone formation, periostitis, 'pencil in cup' appearance
Bloods - ESR, CRP, RF, anti-CCP

Mx: Tx as for RA
- with mild arthritis, NSAID monotherapy may be sufficient
- Ustekinumab and secukinumab

P: better than RA

Ankylosing spondylitis

D: chronic progressive inflammatory arthropathy of primarily the axial skeleton

R: FHx (97% hereditability), HLA-B27, ERAP1 and IL23R genes, young M>F

New York criteria for Dx
1. low back pain ≥3mo, improved by exercise, not relieved by rest
   · may come on at night; improves on getting up
2. limited lumbar spinal motion
   · Schober's test – ↓forward flexion
3. ↓chest expansion for age/sex
4. XR evidence of sacroiliitis
   · bilateral grade 2 to 4
   · or unilateral grade 3 to 4
Passmed's – other features 'A's
· Apical fibrosis   · Anterior uveitis
· Aortic regurg   · Achilles tendonitis
· AV node block   · Amyloidosis
· Cauda equina   · Peripheral arthritis

Ix: XR – Δ apparent only in later disease
· Sacroiliitis: subchondral erosions, erosions
· Squaring of lumbar vertebrae
· 'Bamboo spine' – late, uncommon
· Syndesmophytes 2/2 ossification of annular fibrosus
· CXR - apical fibrosis

If XR -ve, MRI may capture earlier changes
Spirometry – restrictive defect

Mx: · regular exercise, physio
·   NSAIDs
·   anti-TNFα drugs if refractory
· DMARDs only useful if peripheral joint involvement

Gout

D: mono/oligo-articular inflammatory microcrystal synovitis

A/P: chronic hyperuricaemia
(>450umol/L) ↑risk of crystal formation

R: ↑age (>40), M>F, menopause, consumption of meat, seafood, alcohol, Rx (diuretics, ciclosporin, tacrolimus, pyrazinamide, aspirin), FHx, ↑cell turnover rate

FHx – Lesch-Nyhan syndrome (enzyme deficiency, X-linked recessive [M>>F], with gout, renal failure, neuro deficits, learning difficulties, self-mutilation)

S/S/mx: 70% in first MTP, rapid onset severe pain, joint stiffness, swelling and joint effusion, tenderness ± tophi

Ix: synovial fluid analysis [needle shaped negatively birefringent MSU crystals under polarised light], serum uric acid levels [check after 2w after acute episode], XR

ACUTE Mx
  · NSAIDs, colchicine
· colchicine has slower onset, also causes diarrhea
  · PO steroids (e.g. prednisolone 15 mg/d) or intra-articular steroids
** if pt is already on allopurinol, continue

Indications for urate-lowering therapy
** after first attack of gout
esp if ≥2 attacks in 12mo, tophi, renal disease, uric acid renal stones, prophylaxis if on cytotoxics or diuretics

PROPHYLACTIC Mx
  · Allopurinol 100 mg OD, titrate to uric acid <300 umol/L
? start after acute episode is over
+ colchicine / NSAID cover (≤ 6mo)
  · febuxostat
3rd: (refractory) uricase, IV pegloticase

Pseudogout

more accurately acute calcium pyrophosphate crystal deposition disease

D: microcrystal synovitis caused by the deposition of calcium pyrophosphate dihydrate crystals in the synovium

R: ↑age. RF for pseudogout at <60yo: haemochromatosis, hyperPTH, ↓Mg, ↓PO4, acromegaly, Wilson's disease

S/Smx: painful and tender joints. knee, wrist and shoulders most commonly affected. Chronic form mimics OA/RA, a/w variable degrees of inflammation.

Ix: arthrocentesis with synovial fluid analysis [weakly-positively birefringent rhomboid-shaped crystals], XR [chondrocalcinosis]

Mx: arthrocentesis (exclude septic arthritis), NSAIDs ± intra-articular, intra-muscular or PO steroids as for gout

Reactive arthritis

D: inflammatory arthritis that occurs after exposure to certain GI and GU infections

one of the HLA-B27 associated seronegative spondyloarthropathies

A/P: a/w Shigella, Salmonella, Yersinia, Campylobacter, Chlamydia. ?triggered by bacterial DNA in synovial tissue

R: M>F, HLA-B27, preceding chlamydial or GI infection

S/smx: "cannot see, cannot pee, cannot climb a tree" (urethritis, conjunctivitis, arthritis)

Ix: Hx taking, bloods (ESR, CRP, ANA, RF, ?HLA-B27).

Mx: symptomatic - analgesia, NSAIDs, intra-articular steroids
persistent disease - sulfasalazine, MTX

P: smx rarely last >12mo

Polymyalgia rheumatica

D: an inflammatory rheumatologic syndrome. A/w GCA in some pts

R: ≥50yo, GCA, ?F>M

A/P: unknown / unclear

S/smx
· Rapid onset (<1mo)
· Aching, morning stiffness in proximal limbs (✗ weakness)
· Others: mild polyarthralgia, lethargy, depression, low-grade fever, anorexia, night sweats

Ix: ↑ESR (>40). Normal CK and EMG.

Mx: prednisolone (e.g. 15 mg OD) - pt usually responds dramatically and w/in 24h. If no response, consider other dx.
· continue until ESR/CRP resolves
· Taper slowly. Tx usually ~1y

Fibromyalgia

D: chronic pain syndrome diagnosed by the presence of widespread body pain

R: FHx, rheumatological conditions, 20-60yo, F>M

A/P: CNS – pain or sensory amplification; "nociplastic pain". Centralisation of pain.

S/smx: · hyperalgesia, allodynia
· Multiple sites; "pain all over"
· Lethargy, cognitive impairment, 'fibro fog', sleep disturbances, HA, dizziness

Dx is clinical; normal bloods.

Mx: bio-psycho-social model
· Pt education on condition   · CBT
· Aerobic exercise (most evidence)
· Pregabalin, duloxetine, TCAs

Chronic fatigue syndrome

aka myalgic encephalomyelitis
D: Condition characterised by disabling fatigue affecting mental and physical function more than 50% of the time for at least 3 mo
· Smx not better attributed to other disorder

R: F>M, lower socioeconomic status, ↑BMI, ↑physiological toll (eg pregnancy, inadequate rest), chronic health conditions (eg DM, cancer), psychological stress (eg depression)

Cause & pathology not well understood

S/smx: · Tiredness/fatigue
· Sleep problems – ↑ or ↓ sleep
· Myalgia, arthralgia
· HA   · Painful LN
· Sore throat   · "Flu-like" smx
· Cognitive dysfunction (eg inability to concentrate)
· Dizziness, nausea
· Palpitations

Ix – to r/o other conditions, esp cancer
· "Tired all the time" (TATT) bloods: FBC, U&Es, LFTs, TFTs, ESR/CRP, HbA1c, IgA TTE, CK, bone profile + consider Vit D, Vit B12 & folate, iron studies, monospot test, HIV test, hepatitis serology, early morning cortisol
  ↳ CK will be normal
· Other tests: urine dip, CXR, sputum samples for TB

Mx: · Refer to specialist CFS service
· Energy Mx: help with managing energy levels to continue functioning
· Physical activity & exercise
  - Under advice of ME/CSF specialist team
  - Graded exercise therapy not recommended by NICE
· Cognitive behavioural therapy

Systemic lupus erythematosus

D: chronic multisystem disorder characterised by presence of ANA

R: F>M, >30yo, African descent in Europe/US & Asians, drugs (sulfasalazine, isoniazid, phenytoin, carbamazepine)

A/P: type III HS rxn, a/w HLA B8, DR2, DR3. 😊 immune system dysregulation → immune complex formation → affects any organ

S/smx: RASH or PAIN
· Rash: malar, discoid
  - discoid: scaly, red, well-demarcated rash in sun-exposed areas
· Arthritis, athralgia
· Serositis: pleuritis, pericarditis
· Haematologic: cytopenias, ITP, etc
· Oral, nasopharyngeal ulcers
· Renal disorders, Raynaud's
· Photosensitivity
· ANA+ve
· Immunoglobulins – anti-dsDNA, anti-Smith, antiphospholipids
· Neurologic: seizures, psychosis

Ix: autoimmune screen (99% ANA, 70% anti-dsDNA, 30% anti-Smith, etc). ESR monitored; ↑CRP may indicate infection. ↓complement levels during active disease. ? anti-dsDNA titres to monitor disease development if +ve

Mx: NSAIDs, sunblock, 😊 HCQ! If internal organ involvement, 😊 prednisolone, cyclophosphamide

Lupus nephritis
WHO classification
· class I: normal kidney
· II: mesangial glomerulonephritis
· III: focal, segmental proliferative GN
· IV: diffuse proliferative GN
  - most common, severe
  - 'wire-loop' appearance, thickened capillary wall, immune complex deposits, granular appearance
· V: diffuse membranous GN
· VI: sclerosing GN

Mx: · Treat HTN
· Initial therapy for class III and IV: glucocorticoids + mycophenolate or cyclophosphamide
· Subsequent therapy: mycophenolate, azathioprine
P: can result in ESKD requiring transplant. Urine dipstick to monitor, r/o proteinuria

Systemic sclerosis ≈ scleroderma

D: multi-system, autoimmune disease, characterised by functional and structural abnormalities of small blood vessels, fibrosis of skin and internal organs, and production of auto-abs

R: FHx, immune dysregulation (e.g. +ve ANA), F>M (4:1)

LeRoy classification and features:
· Diffuse cutaneous systemic sclerosis: skin thickening on the proximal extremities or the trunk + face and distal extremities
  - a/w Scl-70 antibodies
  - respi involvement – 80% interstitial lung disease, pulmonary artery HTN (most common cause of death)
  - also renal disease, HTN
  - poor prognosis :(
· Limited cutaneous systemic sclerosis: skin thickening confined to sites distal to the elbows and knees ± face
  - a/w anti-centromere abs
  - CREST: calcinosis, Raynaud's, esophageal dysmotility, sclerodactyly, telangiectasia
· Sine scleroderma: no skin involvement
· 'Pure' scleroderma: no internal organ involvement
  - Tightening and fibrosis of skin
  - Plaques (morphea) or linear

Ix: serum auto-abs, full bloods, ESR, CRP, pulmonary function tests, ECG, echo, CXR, barium swallow, etc

Mx: according to smx (e.g. ACEI for renal disease, CCB for Raynaud's). 😊 DMARDs for advanced/severe disease

P: mean survival ~12y after Dx

Dermatomyositis

D: idiopathic autoimmune inflammatory myopathy characterised by distinctive skin manifestations

R: FHx, children or >40yo, F>M, black ethnicity, UV radiation
May be a/w underlying malignancy (typically ovarian, breast, lung) – screen for underlying cancer

A/P: autoimmune; autoantibodies present, evidence of T-cell mediated muscle injury, complement-mediated vascular damage

S/smx – myositis
· Proximal muscle weakness ± tenderness
· Raynaud's
· Respiratory muscle weakness
· Interstitial lung disease
· Dysphagia, dysphonia
S/smx – skin lesions
· Photosensitive
· Macular rash over back, shoulder
· Periorbital heliotrope rash
· Gottron's papules
· Mechanic's hands – extremely dry and scaly hands with linear cracks
· Nail fold capillary dilatation

Ix: ↑↑CK, serum aldolase, muscle and skin biopsy (vasculitis), EMG abn, 70% ANA+ve. Remainder have abs to anti-Jo-1, anti-SRP, anti-Mi2

Mx of acute flares:
· IV corticosteroids ± IVIG
· DMARD, rituximab
Mx of ongoing disease: PO steroids
· sun protection
· topical steroids for skin lesions ± tx malignancy

Polymyositis

D: idiopathic autoimmune inflammatory myopathy characterised by only muscle inflammation

Similar to dermatomyositis apart from not having skin lesions

Sjogren syndrome

D: chronic inflammatory and auto-immune disorder characterised by diminished lacrimal and salivary gland secretion

R: F>M, SLE, RA, scleroderma, HLA II markers, 20-30yo or after menopause

A/P: immunological, genetic, hormonal, and viral components ± estrogen involvement

S/smx
· dry eyes: keratoconjunctivitis sicca
· dry mouth
· vaginal dryness   · arthralgia
· Raynaud's, myalgia
· sensory polyneuropathy
· recurrent episodes of parotitis
· RTA (usually subclinical)

Ix: RF 50%, ANA 70%, anti-Ro (SSA) 70%, anti-La (SSB) 30%, Schirmer's test – filter paper near conjunctival sac to measure tear formation. Histology: focal lymphocytic infiltration. ± hypergamma-globulinaemia, low C4

Mx: artificial tears and saliva ± pilocarpine to stimulate saliva

P: ↑↑ lymphoid malignancy (40-60x)

Antiphospholipid syndrome

→ See 10.06

Wegener's — Granulomatosis with polyangiitis

· D: autoimmune condition a/w a necrotizing granulomatous vasculitis, affecting both the upper and lower respiratory tract and kidneys
· S/smx
  - URT: epistaxis, sinusitis, nasal crusting
  - LRT: dyspnoea, haemoptysis
  - Rapidly progressive glomerulonephritis nephritis ('pauci-immune', 80% of cases)
  - Saddle-shape nose deformity
  - Also vasculitic rash, eye involvement (e.g. proptosis), CN lesions
· Ix
  - cANCA >90%, pANCA in 25%
  - CXR: wide variety
  - Renal biopsy: epithelial crescents in Bowman's capsule
· Mx: - steroids
        - cyclophosphamide
        - Plasma exchange
· P: median survival 8-9y

Churg-Strauss — Eosinophilic granulomatosis with polyangiitis

D: autoimmune condition associated with a necrotizing granulomatous vasculitis, affecting the respiratory tract (?only)

S/smx
· asthma
· blood eosinophilia (e.g. > 10%)
· paranasal sinusitis
· mononeuritis multiplex
· pANCA positive in 60%

Wegener's (left circle): renal failure, epistaxis, haemoptysis, cANCA

(overlap): vasculitis, sinusitis, dyspnea

Churg-Strauss (right circle): asthma, eosinophilia, pANCA

See next pg for microscopic polyangiitis

Vasculitis

D: inflammation of the blood vessels. Usually refers to autoimmune systemic vasculitides. ÷vessel sizes

R: age>50, white ancestry, sex (depending on disorder)

A/P: autoimmune. Fibrinoid necrosis of the vessel wall with fragmentation of chromatin into unstructured granules and RBC extravasation.

S/Smx: constitutional smx
General: abdo pain, foot drop, wrist drop, ulcers, haematuria, purpura, nasal smx, sinus pain, wheeze
· See specific conditions for s/smx

Ix: ESR, CRP, ANCA, U&E, urinalysis, biopsy of affected tissue

Mx: corticosteroids + bone protective agents, cyclophosphamide

P: likely lifelong Mx required

Large-vessel vasculitis
· Takayasu's arteritis
· Giant cell arteritis
Medium-vessel vasculitis
· Polyarteritis nodosa
· Kawasaki's disease
Small-vessel vasculitis
· Wegener's
· Microscopic polyangiitis
· Churg-Strauss syndrome
· Cryoglobulinaemic vasculitis
· Henoch-Schönlein purpura
· Leukocytoclastic angiitis
Variable vessel vasculitis
· Cogan syndrome
· Behçet's disease.
Single organ vasculitis
· Cutaneous leukocytoclastic angiitis
· Cutaneous arteritis
· Primary central nervous system vasculitis
· Isolated aortitis

Giant cell arteritis

D: granulomatous vasculitis of large and medium-sized arteries

R: >50yo, F>M, ?FHx

S/smx:
· Site: branches of external carotid artery, esp temporal artery, skip lesions
· Onset: <1mo
· Character: tender, palpable temporal artery + HA (85%), jaw claudication (65%), ocular complications (majority anterior ischemic optic neuropathy)
 · Fundoscopy: swollen pale disc and blurred margins
 · ! amaurosis fugax → permanent blindness [→05.01]
· A/w: PMR (50% – aching, morning stiffness in prox limbs)
· Also: also lethargy, depression, low-grade fever, anorexia, night sweats

Ix: ↑ESR >50, possibly ↑CRP
· Temporal artery biopsy
 - Histology: multinucleated giant cells
? Duplex US of temporal artery: hypoechoic halo sign
 ! CK and EMG should be normal

Mx: ! urgent 60mg prednisolone PO
· if no visual loss, high dose pred
· if visual loss, IV methylprednisolone before PO prednisolone
 - there should be a dramatic response for pts with visual smx
· same-day ophthalmology review
· if tx with steroids, + bisphosphonate
· ?low-dose aspirin

P: Tx usually required for 1-2y.
Early neuro complications: vision loss, CVA. Late complications: relapses, CVA, aortitis leading to aortic aneurysm and aortic dissection.

Takayasu's arteritis

D: chronic granulomatous vasculitis affecting large arteries: primarily the aorta and its main branches

R: FHx, F>M, <40yo, Asian (Jap)

S/smx
· systemic features of a vasculitis, eg malaise, headache
· unequal BP in the upper limbs
· carotid bruit and tenderness
· absent or weak peripheral pulses
· UL or LL claudication on exertion
· aortic regurgitation (~20%)
· a/w renal artery stenosis

Ix: ↑ESR (>50), ↑CRP, CTA or MRA (shows segmental narrowing or occlusion of affected vessels)

Mx: prednisolone (high to low dose), aspirin, alendronate

P: relapsing disease. Cardiac failure is a common cause of death.

Microscopic polyangiitis

D: small-vessel ANCA vasculitis

S/smx:
· renal: ↑Cr, haematuria, proteinuria
· fever, lethargy, myalgia, weight loss
· rash: palpable purpura
· cough, dyspnoea, haemoptysis
· mononeuritis multiplex

Ix: pANCA 50-75%, cANCA 40%

Polyarteritis nodosa

D: necrotising inflammation of medium-sized or small arteries without glomerulo-nephritis or vasculitis in arterioles, capillaries or venules

R: HBV, 40-60yo, M:F 2:1

A/P: triggers – immune complexes, endothelial dysfunction, etc → intimal proliferation → thrombosis → ischaemia or infarction of organ/tissue ± aneurysm

S/smx: · fever, malaise, athralgia, wt loss, HTN
· mononeuritis multiplex, sensorimotor polyneuropathy [→04.09]
· testicular pain
· livedo reticularis
· haematuria, renal failure
· ANCA (20%) in 'classic' PAN
· Hep B serology +ve (30%)

Ix: CRP, ESR, FBC, rheum screen, etc

Mx: PO prednisolone, DMARD – cyclophosphamide ± IVMP

Henoch-Schonlein purpura

D: IgA mediated small vessel vasculitis. A/w IgA nephropathy.

S/smx:
· palpable purpuric rash (+ localized oedema) over buttocks and extensor surfaces of arms and legs
· abdominal pain
· ± IgA nephropathy: haematuria, AKI

Mx: analgesia, supportive tx of nephropathy. inconsistent support for steroids and DMARDs

P: generally good, self-limiting in children. Monitor BP and urinalysis. 1/3 pts have relapse

See 15.14 for more details

Behcet's syndrome

D: complex multisystem disorder a/w presumed autoimmune-mediated inflammation of the arteries and veins

R: eastern Mediterranean, M>F, young adults (20-40yo), HLA-B51, FHx

S/smx:
· classic triad: oral ulcers, genital ulcers, anterior uveitis
· thrombophlebitis and DVT
· arthritis   · erythema nodosum
· neurological involvement (e.g. aseptic meningitis)
· GI: abd pain, diarrhoea, colitis

Ix: Clinical Dx.
· Pathergy test – needle prick → puncture site becomes inflamed with small pustule – suggestive

Mx: · prednisolone + azathioprine (or other DMARDs).
· Ulcers – topical triamcinolone paste
· VTE prevention, etc

Causes of otalgia (painful ear)

Otitis externa + malignant OE

Otitis media – acute or chronic

Furunculosis = painful Staph abscess arising in hair follicle within the canal
- Lance with sucker fine end
- Tx with oral abx
- Check with DM

Barotrauma
- Severe pain ± 2ndary effusion as a transudate or haemotympanum
- Prevent: don't fly with URTI, decongestants, repeatedly yawn, swallow, move jaw

TMJ dysfunction
- Earache, facial pain, joint clicking related to teeth-grinding + stress!
- Conservative tx ± analgesia

Causes of discharging ear

Otitis externa + malignant OE

Otitis media – acute or chronic

Eustachian tube dysfunction
- Closed (blocked) vs constantly open (patulous; "sniffing")
- Blocked Mx: Grommet insertion, balloon dilation
- Patulous Mx: topical intranasal irritants → oedema of Eustachian tube orifice. Also surgery

Cholesteatoma
- peak incidence 5-15yo
- S/smx: discharge ± deafness, HA, pain, facial paralysis, vertigo → impending CNS compromise
- Mx: mastoid surgery

Mastoiditis
- S/smx: fever, tenderness, swelling, redness behind pinna, protruding auricle
- CT to Dx
- Mx: abx, myringotomy ± mastoidectomy

Otitis externa

D: diffuse inflammation of the external ear canal

R: external canal obstruction, high environmental humidity/ temp, swimming, local trauma, allergy, skin disease, DM, immunocompromise

A/P: most commonly P. aeru or S. aureus. Can be 2/2 seborrhoeic dermatitis, contact dermatitis

S/smx + Ix
- **ear pain, itch, discharge**
  - tragal tenderness is quite specific
- otoscopy: red, swollen, eczematous canal
- Swab if repetitive + ref to ENT

Mx ⚡ topical abx ± steroid
- mild: hydrocortisone cream to pinna, EarCalm spray (2% acetic acid to ↓pH)
- mod: Otosporin, etc
- If TM is perforated, avoid amino-glycosides (risk of ototoxicity)
- clear out canal debris
- if canal very swollen, consider ear wick
- ⚡ oral abx if infxn spreading
- ?? empirical use of antifungal
3rd: if no response to topical abx, refer to ENT for further Ix

Administration of topical abx
- Lie down + affected ear up
- Put as many drops required to fill the ear canal, massage the ear canal and pinna to help drops go in
- Remain in this position for ≥5m
- Don't expose ear to water

Complications
- Malignant OE (see sticky note on right)
- CN VII palsy (poor prog)
Prog: 65-90% have resolution within 7-10d

Otitis media

D: inflammation/infection involving the middle ear space

R: day care attendance, older sibs, young age, FHx, supine feeding, craniofacial anomaly, immunocomp

A/P: usually preceded by URTI. Most infxns are bacterial – S pneumoniae, H. influenzae and M. catarrhalis.

S/smx • Otalgia due to bulging TM
- Ear discharge if TM ruptures – less or no otalgia
- Fever in 50%   • Hearing loss
- Recent URTI (usually viral)

Ix: Otoscopy
- Bulging TM → loss of light reflex
- Opacification / erythema of TM
  ↳ indicates middle ear effusion
- Perforation + purulent otorrhea

Mx • Analgesia alone; 60% cases resolve in 24h without abx
  - consider delayed prescription
- Abx if - smx ≥4d, no improvement
  - systemically unwell
  - immunocompromised
  - <2yo with bilateral OM
  - OM with perforation + discharge
  - Abx: ⚡ amoxicillin 5-7d,
    ⚡ erythromycin or clarithromycin

Complications
- Perforation of TM → can cause COM (if >6w)
- Hearing loss • Labyrinthitis
Can lead to cholesteatoma, which can lead to these complications
- Mastoiditis   • Meningitis
- Brain abscess   • CN VII palsy

Glue ear

= otitis media with effusion
or serous otitis media

R: M>F, sibs with glue ear, spring/winter, bottle feeding, day care attendance, parental smoking

S/smx: • Peaks at 2yo
- Hearing loss in 80% – most often noticed by parents/teachers
  - poor listening, poor speech, language delay, inattention, etc
- Can be painless

Otoscopy:
- Variable appearance of TM
  - dull, grey, yellow
- Bubbles or fluid level
- Otoscopic Dx is very inaccurate

Ix: ref for formal Ax of hearing
- Audiograms: conductive defects
- Tympanometry: look for flat type B

Mx: Active observation for 3mo
  - 50% of children with bilateral hearing loss of 20dB likely to resolve in 3mo
  - reAx hearing at 3mo
  - ❗ if Down's or cleft palate, ref to ENT urgently (∴ ↑risk of infxns)
- Autoinflation of Eustachian tube
- Surgery
  - for persistent bilat OME + hearing level in better ear of 25-30 dBHL or worse over 3mo
  - **grommets**: allows air to pass through to middle ear
    ◊ risk of infxn, tympanosclerosis
    ◊ aural cleaning, topical abx
    ◊ may require removal
    ◊ swimming ok, no diving, use ear plugs, swim hats
    ◊ extrude after 3-12mo, recheck hearing; 25% need re-insertion
  - tympanostomy for adults
- Hearing aids for persistent bilateral OME and hearing loss if surgery not acceptable
- Topical or systemic abx NOT rec; also not rec: Δ diet, antihistamines, decongestants, steroids, acupuncture

Chronic otitis media
- D: TM perforation in the setting of recurrent / chronic infections (>6w)
- Types: benign COM (dry), chronic serous OM, chronic suppurative OM
- S/smx: hearing loss, otorrhoea, fullness, otalgia
- Mx: topical or PO abx, aural cleaning, water precaution, follow up appts
- ± surgery (grommets, etc)
- Complications: cholesteatoma

Malignant otitis externa
- D: Osteomyelitis of the skull base
- **R: DM, immunocompromise**
- A: Ps. aeruginosa most commonly
- P: Infxn spreads from soft tissues of external auditory meatus → bony ear canal → temporal bone / skull base
- S/smx:
  - Severe, unrelenting, deep otalgia
  - Temporal HA
  - Purulent discharge
  - ± Dysphagia, hoarseness, CN VII dysfunction
- Ix: CT head
- Mx: urgent referral to ENT
  - IV abx (covering Pseudomonas)

Hearing loss

Conductive hearing loss

Normal otoscopy
- Otosclerosis
- Congenital
- Eustachian tube malfunction

Abnormal otoscopy

External ear	Middle ear
· Earwax (cerumen) · Foreign body · Otitis externa · Congenital (atresia) · Benign mass (polyp, osteoma, exostosis) · Tumour (SCC) · Dermatologic (eg moles)	· Otitis media · Tympanic membrane perforation · Cholesteatoma · Barotrauma · Tumours (glomus, adenoma) · Eustachian tube dysfunction

Sensorineural hearing loss

Assymetric
- Neoplasm (vestibular schwannoma)
- Iatrogenic (radiation, surgery)
- Idiopathic

Symmetrical

Congenital	Central (CNS)	Cochlear
· Hereditary hearing disorders · TORCH infxns - Toxoplasmosis - Others (syphillis, Hep B) - Rubella - Cytomegalovirus - Herpes simplex · Teratogenic drugs · Alcohol	· Infection (eg meningitis) · Stroke / TIA · Multiple sclerosis	· Presbycusis · Loud noise · Cochleitis · Ototoxic drugs (eg aminoglycosides) · Meniere's diseaes · Autoimmune disorders

Tinnitus

Ix: audiometry, tympanogram.
· If unilateral, MRI to r/o vestibular schwannoma
Mx: treat underlying cause. Hearing aids, psych support, CBT

Subjective (only pt hears it)

Unilateral
- Vestibular schwannoma
- CN VIII lesion
- Brain stem lesion
- Multiple sclerosis
- Infarction
- Meniere's

Bilateral

No hearing loss	Somatosensory
· Metabolic - thyroid dysf - Vit A, B zinc def · Psychogenic, anxiety, depression · Drugs - **salicylates** · Idiopathic	i.e., pt can modify tinnitus by moving head, jaw, or eyes, or pressure on face · TMJ · Bruxism · Whiplash · Skull fracture · Closed head injury

With hearing loss

Conductive HL	SNHL
· Ear wax impaction · Otitis media · Otosclerosis · External or middle ear lesion	· Loud noise · Ototoxic drugs - propanolol - levodopa - loop diuretics · Presbycusis · Congenital

Objective (pulsatile/rhythmic)

Muscular
- Stapedius, tensor tympani, palatal muscle spasm
- Degenerative disease of H&N
- Eustachian tube dysfunction

Vascular

Arterial	Venous
· Normal blood flow in artery near ear · Congenital - persistent stapedial artery · Atherosclerosis · Idiopathic intracranial HTN · Systemic HTN acute exacerbation · Glomus tympanicum (benign tumour)	· AV shunt · High jugular bulb · Glomus jugulare (tumour) · Hyperthyroidism

Vertigo

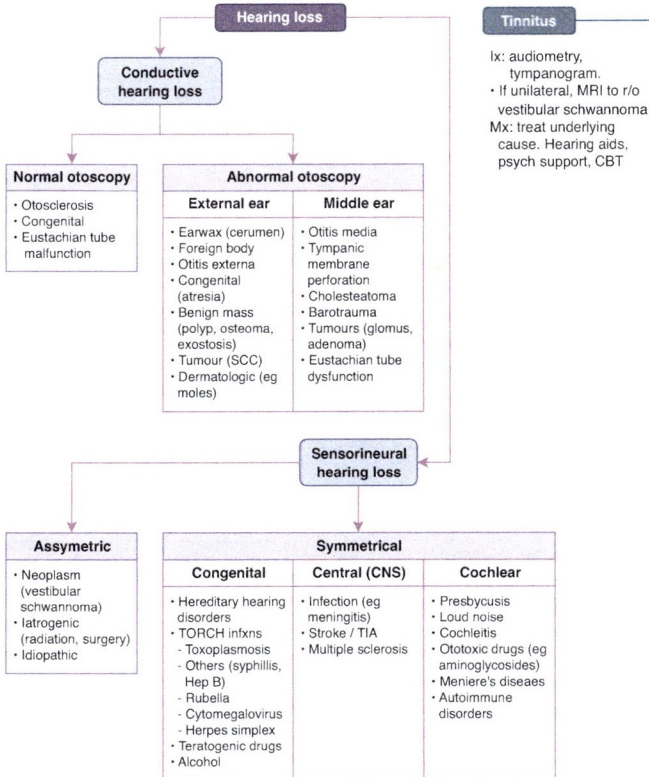

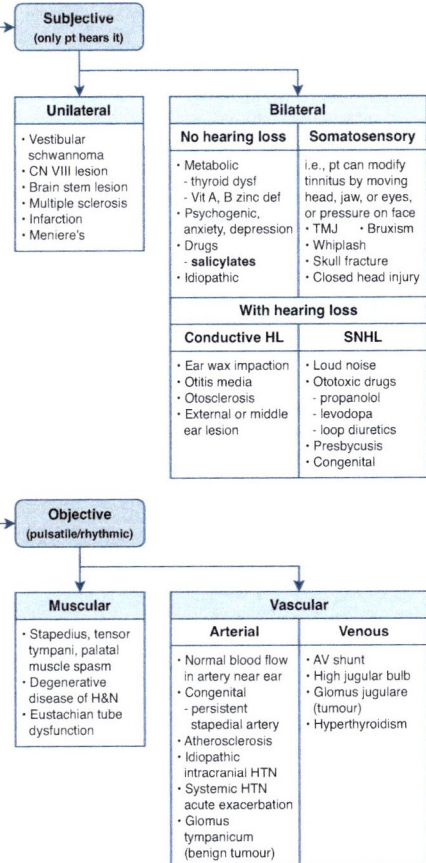

D: True vertigo is the illusion of rotary movement of either the body or the environment

Central vestibular dysfunction

- Vertigo 2/2 CNS causes
- S/smx: imbalance, **bidirectional** nystagmus, ± neurological s/smx

Causes
- Vascular: stroke/TIA at the brainstem, vertebrobasillar insufficiency, basilar artery migraine
  - vertebrobasilar ischaemia is usually seen in elderly pts who become dizzy when they bend their neck backwards
- Infxn: meningitis, cerebellar or brainstem abscess
- Inflammation: multiple sclerosis
- Intoxication: barbiturates, EtOH
- Trauma: cerebellar contusion
- Lesions: infratentorial tumours, cerebellopontine angle tumours, glomus tumours

Peripheral vestibular dysfunction

- Vertigo 2/2 peripheral nervous system causes (i.e. causes that affect CN VIII alone)
- S/smx: **unidirectional** nystagmus, imbalance, etc

Causes
- BPPV
- Labyrinthitis (± HL ± tinnitus)
  - Hx of recent viral infxn
- Vestibular neuronitis
  - Hx of recent viral infxn
  - **no** hearing loss
- Meniere's
- Vestibular schwannoma
- Ototoxicity (eg 2/2 drugs)
- Otitis media
- Temporal bone fractures

Childhood deafness

1 in 500 newborns has bilateral permanent SNHL ≥40dB
÷ 50% genetic, 25% non-genetic, 25% idiopathic(?)

Genetic hearing loss (50%)
÷ conductive HL or SNHL

Non-genetic hearing loss (25%)
· Intrauterine TORCH infxn, eg CMV, rubella, toxoplasmosis, HSV, syphilis
· Perinatal: prematurity, hypoxia, intraventricular haemorrhage, kernicterus
· Infxns: meningitis, encephalitis, measles, mumps
· Others: ototoxic drugs, acoustic or cranial trauma

Universal newborn hearing screening
within weeks of birth
· Otoacoustic emissions
· Auditory brainstem responses
Subjective hearing tests in older children
· Distraction testing (6-18mo)
· Visual reinforced audiometry (6-30mo)
· Speech discrimination (24-60mo)

Mx: support, advice, info
· Hearing aids or cochlear implants
= multichannel electrode inserted surgically into cochlear that directly stimulates auditory nerve to produce electrical signals

Deafness in adults

<u>Sudden SNHL</u> is defined as
· Loss of ≥ 30dB
· in 3 contiguous pure tone freqs
· over 3d

Ix/Mx: · immediate specialist ref
· work up includes MRI (to r/o acoustic neuroma), otherwise Dx as idiopathic sudden SNHL
· **High-dose steroids** (pred 60mg OD for 7d, then 7d tapering)

Prognosis: -ve factors include <15yo or >65yo, ↑ESR, vertigo, HL in opposite ear, severe HL

<u>Conductive HL</u>: cause is 'always' found - infxn, occlusion, trauma, fracture, etc

Otosclerosis

D: abnormal bone remodeling in the middle ear where bone tissue is replaced by vascular spongy bone

A: unknown; ?AD; 50% FHx, 85% bilat, F>M 2:1
P: spongy bone forms around stapes footplate. Calcification leads to fixation → progressive CHL

Smx: · starts early adult life, may be accelerated by pregnancy
· ~75% tinnitus ± vertigo
· 10% Schwartze's sign: flamingo pink blush in posterior segment
· Audiometry: Carhart's notch

Mx: w&w, hearing aid, or surgery to replace fixed stapes, cochlear
· Careful selection for surgery ∴ can be complicated by complete SNHL
- surgery only on worse hearing ear; contralateral SNHL is CI !

Vestibular schwannoma

= acoustic neuroma
D: benign cerebellopontine angle tumour that grows from the superior vestibular component of the vestibulocochlear nerve

R: Neurofibromatosis type 2

S/smx according to affected CN
· CN VIII: vertigo or balance problems (20%), unilateral SNHL (70%), unilateral tinnitus (50%)
· CN V: absent corneal reflex
· CN VII: facial palsy
· Bilateral in NF type 2
· Larger tumours: mass effect (eg ↑ICP)

Ix: urgent ref to ENT
· MRI of cerebellopontine angle
· Audiometry

DDx: meningioma 10%, epidermoid tumours 5%

Mx: w&w with interval MRI scans in small, slow growing tumours
· Surgical removal for large or rapidly growing tumours
- stereotactic radiosurgery

BPPV — Benign paroxysmal positional vertigo

D: peripheral vestibular disorder that manifests as sudden, short-lived episodes of vertigo elicited by specific head movements

R: ↑age, F>M, head trauma, vestibular neuronitis or labyrinthitis, migraines, inner ear surgery, Meniere's

S/smx: · vertigo triggered by change in head position ± nausea
· 10-20 second episodes
· Dx: Dix-Hallpike manouvre - vertigo and rotatory nystagmus

Mx: w&w - self-resolving in weeks to months usually
· Epley manouvre
· Brandt-Daroff exercise
· Meds (eg betahistine) limited value

Meniere's disease

D: disorder of inner ear of unknown cause, characterised by excessive pressure and progressive dilation of the endolymphatic system

P: ? over-production or impaired absorption of endolymph

S/smx:
· classic triad: ≥2 episodes of vertigo, tinnitus, and SNHL
- Vertigo: 20min to 12h ± NV
- Tinnitus: "roaring"
· Aural fullness: sensation of pressure and fullness in ear
· "Drop attacks" - sudden loss of balance (but no LOC)
· Bilateral in 30-50%

Mx: · ENT referral
· Inform DVLA - current advice is to cease driving until satisfactory control of smx
· Acute attacks: buccal or IM prochlorperazine ± admission
· Prevention: betahistine, vestibular rehab exercises

Vestibular neuronitis

D: peripheral disorder of vertigo caused by inflammation of the vestibular nerve

R: recent viral illness (esp URTI)

S/smx: · Vertigo, nausea, vomiting, unsteadiness
· NO hearing loss or tinnitus
· Nystagmus (fine horizontal)
· ± Positive head impulse test

Ix: clinical Dx

Mx: · Advice on safe driving + working
· If severe smx
🔸 Cyclizine, prochlorperazine, cinnarizine or promethazine
- PO usually sufficient
- can offer IM or buccal if pt wants
❗ Short course only otherwise pt may get rebound smx
· Advice usually self limiting (4-6w)
· Chronic illness: 🔸 vestibular rehabilitation exercises

(Viral) labyrinthitis

D: peripheral disorder of vertigo and hearing loss caused by inflammation of the otic capsule (the labyrinth)

R: URTI (viral), chronic suppurative otitis media, acute OM, cholesteatoma

S/smx: · Vertigo, dizziness, NV
· Nystagmus (fine horizontal)
· **Hearing loss** (may be uni or bilateral)
· **Tinnitus**
· ± Positive head impulse test

Ix: clinical Dx

Mx: same as vestibular neuronitis

Rhinosinusitis

D: inflammation in the nose and paranasal sinuses with ≥2 smx:
· nasal blockage / obstruction / congestion
· Nasal discharge
· Facial pain / pressure
· Reduction or loss of smell
· Endoscopic or CT signs of sinus or middle meatus obstruction

Acute or chronic (>12w)

Severe if ≥3 smx:
· Discoloured discharge
· Severe local pain
· Fever   · ↑ESR/CRP
· Double sickening (deterioration after initial milder phase)

DDx: migraine, TMJ dysf, dental pain, neuropathic pain, temporal arteritis, herpes zoster

Acute rhinosinusitis
Mx of mild rhinosinusitis (≈ common cold): self-limiting
· Analgesia, nasal saline irrigation, decongestants
· If smx >10d, trial intranasal corticosteroids (eg mometasone)
· If smx >14d further, ref to ENT

Mx of mod rhinosinusitis
· Intranasal steroid spray
· If smx >14d, ref to ENT

Mx of severe rhinosinusitis
· Topical steroids & abx
· ReAx at 48h - if improvement, continue Tx for 14d
· If no improvement, ref to ENT

Complications of sinusitis
· Orbital cellulitis/abscess
· Intracranial involvement
 - Meningitis, encephalitis, cerebral abscess, cavernous sinus thrombosis
· Mucoceles
· Osteomyelitis
· Pott's puffy tumour (subperiosteal abscess arising from frontal osteomyelitis)

Chronic rhinosinusitis

D: >12w of rhinosinusitis

Predisposing factors:
· atopy: hay fever, asthma
· nasal obstruction e.g. septal deviation or nasal polyps
· recent local infection e.g. rhinitis or dental extraction
· swimming/diving   · smoking

S/smx:
· facial pain: typically frontal pressure pain which is worse on bending forward
· nasal discharge: usually clear if allergic or vasomotor. Thicker, purulent discharge suggests 2ndary infxn
· nasal obstruction: e.g. 'mouth breathing'
· post-nasal drip: may produce chronic cough (DDx GORD)

Ix: endoscopy to look for nasal polyps, culture, imaging.

Mx:
· avoid allergens
· Intranasal corticosteroids
· Nasal irrigation with saline solution
· If indicated by culture, long-term abx may be needed, eg 12w course of macrolide abx

Mx of rhinosinusitis with polyps
· Children: r/o neoplasms, CF, meningocele/ encephalocele
· Mild disease in adults
 - intranasal steroids + review at 3mo
· Moderate: trial steroid spray ± doxycycline for 20d. Review 1mo.
· Severe: topical steroids ± short course of PO steroids, review at 1mo
 - if no improvement, CT scan ± surgery

▶ RED FLAGS ▶
· Unilateral smx
· Persistent smx despite 3mo of tx
· Epistaxis   · Numbness

Nasal fractures

Dx: · New nasal deformity
· a/w facial swelling, black eyes
· ❗ r/o head or C-spine injury
· Look for **septal haematoma** – boggy swelling of the septum causing near-total nasal obstruction
 - if present, requires urgent I&D

Mx: · Treat epistaxis
· Analgesia, ice
· Close skin injury
· ReAx 5-7d post injury once swelling has resolved
· If manipulation under anaesthesia required, do this 10-14d after injury (before nasal bones are set)

CSF rhinorrhea

A: ethmoid fractures disrupting dura and arachnoid, ▶ tumour

Dx/Ix: CSF sampling (+ve for glucose, β2 transferrin)

Mx: · if traumatic, conservative Mx: usually spontaneously resolves
 - 7-10d bedrest with head elevated 15-30° ± lumbar drain
 - Avoid coughing, sneezing, nose-blowing
 - Cover with abx and pneumococcal vaccine

Epistaxis

D: bleeding from the nostril, nasal cavity, and/or nasopharynx and may be classified as anterior or posterior

R: dry weather, nasal trauma, 1' coagulopathy (and other conditions predisposing to bleeding, incl cancer)

A: 95% bleeding originates in Little's area, located in the anterior inferior septum (Kiesselbach plexus)

Management
· ABCDE, resus if needed
· Hx: which side, trauma, quantify loss, on warfarin or aspirin? PMH.
· Ask pt to apply pressure by **pinching the lower part of nose for 10min**. Repeat if still bleeding.
· Breathe through mouth, sit forward, spit blood into bowl.
· Place ice pack on dorsum of nose or suck on ice
· If still bleeding, cauterise with silver nitrate
 - use headlight and speculum
 - remove clots with suction
 - apply cotton ball soaked in 1:200,000 adrenaline for 2min or use local anaesthetic spray
 - find bleeding points ("small volcanoes"), apply cautery for 2s at a time
 - cauterise base of vessel before hitting the active bleeding point
· If bleeding point cannot be identified, ref to ENT: may try exploration under anaesthesia, arterial ligation, or embolisation

Management (cont)
· If bleeding continues,
 - anterior nasal pack - advance into nose horizontally and parallel to hard palate
 - remove after 24h
· If bleeding still continues, pack the other nostril ± pressure
· If still, use postnasal pack or Foley urinary catheter (??)

Post-bleeding Mx
· Don't pick or blow nose!!!
· If you sneeze, send it through your mouth
· Avoid bending, lifting, or straining
· No hot food or drink
· If bleeding restarts, apply ice to bridge of nose and hold soft lower part continuously for 20min

Cancer of the paranasal sinuses
· Suspect when chronic sinusitis presents for the first time in later life
· Blood-stained nasal discharge
· Nasal obstruction
Ix: MRI/CT ± endoscopy & biopsy
Types: SCC (50%), lymphoma (10%), AC, etc.
Mx: radiotherapy ± radical surgery

Nasopharyngeal cancer
· E: rare except in individuals from southern China
· S/smx: neck lump (90%), nasal smx (bleeding, obstruction, discharge), hearing loss (usually unilat), unilat serous otitis media, CN palsies due to base of skull extension
· Dx/Ix: endoscopy + biopsy
 - Staging by MRI
· Mx: RT + chemo + surgery
· P: >80% 5y survival for stage I; <30% for advanced tumours

Sore throat

= pharyngitis, tonsillitis, laryngitis

A: viral (25%), bacterial

Dx: **CENTOR CRITERIA**
↳ to determine which pts likely have bacterial infxns and ∴ will benefit from antibiotics
- Presence of tonsillar exudate
- Tender anterior cervical lymphadenopathy or lymphadenitis
- Hx of fever
- Absence of cough
- 0-2: 3-17% · 3-4: 32-56% likely
- If all 4 absent, negative predictive value is 80%

Dx: **FeverPAIN criteria**
↳ similar to Centor criteria; to identify pts likely to have Strep pharyngitis
- Fever > 38°
- Purulence (pharyngeal / tonsillar)
- Attend rapidly (≤3d)
- Inflamed tonsils (severe)
- No cough or coryza
- 2-3: 34-40% · 4-5: 62-65% likely

Mx: · Symptomatic relief: ibuprofen ± paracetamol for fever & pain
· Consider mouthwash or spray
· Abx only indicated if
  - Centor / FeverPain +ve
  - Features of marked systemic upset 2/2 to acute sore throat
  - Unilateral peritonsillitis
  - Hx of rheumatic fever
  - ↑risk of acute infxn
· If abx indicated, use phenoxymethyl-penicillin (penV) or clarithromycin 7-10d course
· ! avoid amoxicillin – causes rash if pharyngitis is caused by EBV
· ! if pt on DMARDs or carbimazole, check FBC urgently

DDx of unilateral tonsillar enlargement
· Peritonsillar abscess
· Malignancy (perform excision biopsy to r/o)

Complications of tonsillitis
· Otitis media · Sinusitis
· Peritonsillar abscess (quinsy)
  - Sore throat, dysphagia, peritonsillar bulge, uvular deviation, trismus (lockjaw), muffled voice
  - Mx: abx, aspiration
· Parapharyngeal abscess
  - Diffuse swelling in neck, dysphagia, head turned towards side of abscess
  - Mx: CT/US, IV abx, I&D under GA
· Lemierre syndrome
  - Acute septicaemia and jugular vein thrombosis 2/2 infxn with Fusobacterium + septic embolism

P: if uncomplicated, smx resolve in 40% within 3d, and within 1w in 85%

TONSILLECTOMY
· Only done if recurrent sore throats are due to tonsillitis, and these episodes are disabling
  - ≥7 well-documented, clinically significant, adequately tx sore throats in preceding year
  - ≥5 episodes in each of last 2y
  - ≥3 episodes in each of last 3y
· Other indications: children with obstructive sleep apnoea, suspicion of malignancy
· Complications
  - 1' haemorrhage (<24h) - return to theatre asap
  - 2' haemorrhage (>24h)
    ◊ 2/2 infxn of tonsillar fossae
    ◊ ENT emergency
    ◊ ABCDE, resus ± theatre
    ◊ if bleeding stops, admit for H2O2 gargles and IV abx

Scarlet fever: see full entry →08.03

Obstructive sleep apnoea

D: Episodic partial or complete airway obstruction during sleep

R: obesity, M>F, post-menopause, chronic snoring, macroglossia (eg hypothyroidism), large tonsils, etc

S/smx: · Daytime somnolence
· Partner may notice episodes of apnoea, gasping, restless sleeping
· Compensated respiratory acidosis

Ix/Dx:
· Epworth Sleepiness Scale (questionnaire for pt ± partner)
· Multiple Sleep Latency Test – measures time to fall asleep in a dark room
· Polysomnography

Mx: · Wt loss
· CPAP (for mod to severe OSA)
· Intra-oral devices (eg mandibular advancement) if CPAP not tolerated, or if mild smx
· Inform DVLA if excessive daytime sleepiness + advice pt not to drive

---

Stridor

Stridor = inspiratory high-pitched noise inspiration 2/2 partial obstruction at larynx or large airway
Stertor = inspiratory snoring noise 2/2 obstruction of pharynx

Causes
· Congenital: laryngomalacia, web/ stenosis, vascular rings
· Inflammation: laryngitis, epiglottitis, croup, anaphylaxis
· Tumours: haemangiomas, laryngeal papilloma (HPV-related)
· Trauma: thermal, chemical, intubation-related

Croup

= laryngo-tracheo-bronchitis

E: 6mo to 6yo, autumn, ?M>F

A: usually parainfluenza viruses

S/smx	Mild	Mod	Severe
Barking cough	Occasional	Frequent	Frequent
Stridor at rest	None	Easily audible	Prominent
Chest wall recession	None or mild	Present at rest	Marked
General behaviour	Happy, E+D, playing	Can be placated, interested in surroundings	Significant distress, lethargic or restless

---

Acute epiglottitis

D: infxn of the supraglottis with the potential to cause airway compromise

A: *Haemophilus influenzae* type B most common, but also *Strep pneumoniae*, *S aureus*, MRSA. Less commonly, viral, fungal, traumatic

P: inflammatory pathways lead to localised oedema of the airway → ↑airway resistance

S/smx: · rapid onset
· high temp, generally unwell
· stridor · drooling saliva
· 'tripod' position: pt finds it easier to breathe if leaning forward

Dx: only by airway trained staff – direct visualisation. XR lateral view may show thumb sign, PA view may show steeple sign

Mx: · O2 + keep pt upright
· immediate senior involvement (ENT, anaesthetics) – endotrach intubation may be needed
· If suspected, DO NOT examine throat or distress pt
· IV abx to resolve

Mx:
· Admit any child with mod to severe croup, or if <6mo, known airway abn, uncertainty about Dx
· Regardless of severity, single dose of PO dexamethasone (0.15mg/kg)
  ↳ alt: prednisolone

Emergency tx
· High flow O2
· Nebulised adrenaline

Laryngomalacia

D: congenital abnormalities that predisposes to dynamic supraglottis collapse during inspiration

A/w: GORD (50%), neurological abn (up to 20%), M>F (2x), genetic syndromic disorders (eg Down's)

S/smx: onset within 2-4w of birth, resolution by 2y. Normal cry (differentiates from vocal cord palsy or laryngeal webs)

Ix: flexi laryngoscopy

Mx: w&w if mild.
· If mod (stridor, ↑work of breathing, etc), w&w or surgery
· Severe (10-15%): endoscopic supraglottoplasty

P: 85% spontaneously improve by 12-24mo.

Dysphonia (hoarseness)

Hoarseness = difficulty producing sound, with change in voice pitch or quality

Laryngeal cancer
- Ix all hoarseness >6w - hoarseness is the chief (and often only) presentation of laryngeal carcinoma. Esp in smokers

Vocal cord palsy
- Weak, breathy voice
- Often due to cancer

Laryngitis
- Usually viral, maybe bacterial
- Can be 2/2 GORD or autoimmune disease (eg RA)
- Mx: supportive ± abx if indicated

Reinke's oedema
- Chronic cord irritation from smoking ± voice abuse → gelatinous fusiform enlargement of cords
- Conservative Mx (stop smoking), laser therapy

Vocal cord nodules
- 2/2 vocal cord abuse usually
- Fibrous nodules (often bilat) form at junction of anterior 1/3 and posterior 2/3 of cords
- Speech therapy or surgical excision

Disorders of speech articulation
- Spasmodic dysphonia ≈ "blepharospasm" of the vocal cords
- Muscle tension dysphonia - functional disorder
- Children with functional speech disorders (difficulty pronouncing certain sounds)

Dysphagia

= difficulty swallowing
Odynophagia = painful swallowing

Q&A
- Can fluids be drunk as per normal?
  - YES: stricture?
  - NO: motility disorder?
- Is it difficult to make the swallowing movement?
  - YES: bulbar palsy (esp if pt coughs on swallowing)
- ► Is the dysphagia constant and painful?
  - YES: malignant stricture?
- Does the neck bulge or gurgle on drinking? - YES: pharyngeal pouch?

Malignant causes
- Oesophageal cancer
- Pharyngeal cancer
- Gastric cancer
- Extrinsic pressure, eg from lung cancer or node enlargement

Neurological causes
- Bulbar palsy
- Lateral medullary syndrome
- Myasthenia gravis • Syringomyelia

Others
- Benign stricture • Pharyngeal pouch
- Achalasia • Systemic sclerosis
- Oesophagitis • IDAnaemia

Ix: Bloods (FBC, ESR), CXR, barium swallow, endoscopy + biopsy, esophageal motility studies

Pharyngeal pouch

= Zenker's diverticulum; a posteromedial diverticulum through Killian's dehiscence
- R: ↑age, M>F 5:1
- S/smx: dysphagia, regurgitation, aspiration, neck swelling (gurgles on palpation), halitosis
- Ix: barium swallow combined with dynamic video fluoroscopy
- Mx: surgery

Benign esophagial stricture

- A: reflux, swallowing corrosives, foreign body, trauma
- Mx: dilatation

Oesophageal carcinoma

D: neoplastic mucosal lesions ÷ SCC or AC (rarely other kinds)

R:	ACs (lower 1/3)	SCCs (upper 2/3)
	• GORD	• Smoking
	• Barrett's	• Alcohol
	• Smoking	• Achalasia
	• Obesity	• Plummer-Vinson
		• ↑nitrosamines

► S/smx: dysphagia, anorexia, wt loss, vomiting, odynophagia, melaena, cough

Ix/Dx: upper GI endoscopy for Dx. Endoscopic US for locoregional staging. CT or PET-CT for initial staging (mets). Laparoscopy to detect occult peritoneal disease

Mx: • Operable disease: surgical resection
  ↳ risk of anastomotic leak
• Adjuvant chemo • Palliation :/

P: very poor. Even localised disease has <50% 5y survival.

Barrett's esophagus

- D: metaplasia of the lower oesophageal mucosa (columnar epithelium replacing squamous epithelium)
- R: GORD, M>F (7:1), smoking, central obesity
- S/smx: GORD smx; Barrett's itself is asmx
- Ix: endoscopy and biopsy required for histology Dx
  - Metaplasia = cell transformation (ie squamous to columnar)
  - Dysplasia = replacement of mature cells with less mature ones
  - See also 03.08 GORD for when pts get endoscopies for GORD
- Mx: high dose PPI (? evidence)
  - if metaplasia confirmed: endoscopic surveillance with biopsies every 3-5y
  - if dysplasia, offer endoscopic interventions including radiofrequency ablation and endoscopic mucosal resection

Globus pharyngeus

aka Globus hystericus
= sensation of lump in the throat most noticed when swallowing saliva
- A: unknown; ? excess muscle tension in the pharynx or ↑acid exposure at laryngopharyngeal junction
- Mx: Reassure. Endoscopy may be needed to exclude malignancy (esp with red flag smx)

HNSCC Head and neck squamous cell carcinoma

Umbrella term including oral cavity cancers, cancers of pharynx, and cancers of the larynx. 90% are SCC.

R: >80% in >50yo. A/w smoking (10x risk), HPV 70% of oropharyngeal Ca, ↑alcohol, Vit A & C def, nitrosamines in salted fish, GORD, deprivation

S/smx ► • Neck pain/lump
- Hoarse voice >6w
- Sore throat >6w
- Mouth bleeding • Numbness
- Sore tongue • Painless ulcers
- Patches in the mouth
- Earache/effusion
- Lumps (lip, mouth, gum)
- Speech change • Dysphagia

Ix/Dx: Ref urgently to ENT. Endoscopy, FNA/biopsy, CT/MRI, etc

Mx: Surgery, chemo/radio

HPV-related cancer (HPV 16)
- Linked to cancer of tongue, tonsil and pharynx
- Most commonly transmitted during oral sex
- Occur in younger people, better prognosis (compared to smoking)
- Vaccination may ↓risk

Bell's palsy

D: acute, sudden-onset, unilateral facial palsy of probable viral aetiology

R: intranasal influenza vaccination, pregnancy (3x), DM (5x)

A: probable reactivation of HSV-1 within geniculate ganglion, correlation with Covid-19
P: Infxn/inflammation leads to demyelination and neural inflam

S/smx: • Paralysis of 1/2 face
- UMN palsy spares the forehead
- LMN palsy affects whole face
- Others: post-auricular pain, change in taste, dry eyes, hyperacusis

Mx: • PO prednisolone within 72h of onset of Bell's palsy
  - 25mg/12h for 10d, or
  - 60mg/24h for 5d, then taper by 10mg every day
- Antivirals alone not recommended; may be added if severe
- ! Eye care - artificial tears and eye lubricants ± tape eyelids shut at night
- ► If no improvement in 3w, refer urgently to ENT ± plastics ± ophthalmology (if eye problems)
- ► Also ref to ENT or neuro if
  - recurrent Bell's (7%)
  - bilateral facial palsy: Lyme disease, GBS, leukaemia, sarcoidosis, EBV, trauma, myasthenia gravis

P: 80% full recovery within 3-4mo. If untx, 15% have permanent mod to severe weakness

Lumps in the neck

Q&A
- "How long has the lump been present?"
  - if <3w, reactive lymphadenopathy from self-limiting infxn is likely
- "Which tissue layer is the lump in?"
  - Intradermal: sebaceous cyst, lipoma, etc

Ix · US ± **FNAC** · CT
· Virology and Mantoux test · CXR

DDx: Midline lumps
- <20yo: dermoid cyst
- If moves up on protruding tongue: thyroglossal cyst
  = fluid-filled sac resulting from incomplete closure of thyroid's migration path
- >20yo: thyroid mass
- Bony hard: chondroma?

DDx: Submandibular triangle
- <20yo: reactive lymphadenopathy
- >20yo
  - r/o malignant lymphadenopathy (eg firm, non-tender; any B-smx)
- r/o TB!!
- If it's not a node, consider submandibular salivary stone, tumour or sialadenitis

DDx: Anterior triangle
- Lymphadenopathy
- Branchial cyst [Mx: excision]
- >40yo: parotid tumour?
- Laryngoceles
  - painless, M>F, made worse by blowing
- If lump is pulsatile
  - Carotid artery aneurysm
  - Tortuous carotid artery
  - Carotid body tumour [rare]

DDx: Posterior triangle
- Cervical rib
- Pharyngeal pouches (usually on L)
- Cystic hygromas: macrocystic lymphatic malformations; bright transillumination
- Small lumps: think of lymphadenopathy 2/2 TB, viruses, metastases

Xerostomia

Typical causes
- Drugs: Hypnotics & TCAs, psychotics, β-blockers, diuretics
- Mouth breathing · Dehydration
- ENT radiotherapy
- Sjogren syndrome, SLE and scleroderma, sarcoidosis
- HIV/AIDs · Parotid stones

S/smx:
- Dry, atrophic, fissured oral mucosa
- Discomfort → difficulty eating, speaking and wearing dentures
- No saliva pooling in floor of mouth

Comp: dental caries, candida infxn

Mx: ↑PO fluids, frequent sips
- Good dental hygiene – no acidic drinks or foods
- Try saliva substitutes or dry mouth products

Salivary gland problems

Sialadenitis
= acute infxn of submandibular or parotid glands
- R: elderly or debilitated pts who are dehydrated ± poor oral hygiene
- S/smx: painful diffuse swelling of gland and fever. Pus may leak out of duct
- Mx: abx + good oral hygiene
  - Sialogogues are helpful
  - Surgical drainage may be required
- Comp: chronic or recurrent attacks may lead to strictures or salivary gland stones :(

Sialolithiasis
- Salivary stones; usually affect the submandibular gland (↑Ca, thicker)
- S/smx: pain, tense swelling of gland during/after meals ± palpable stone on floor of mouth
- ± Ix: plain XR or sialogram
- Mx: small stones may pass spontaneously; may need surgery for larger stones

Salivary gland tumours
- 80% rule: 80% in parotid gland, 80% benign pleomorphic adenomas, 80% in superficial lobe
- RF for malignancy: neck radiation, smoking
- ► S/smx: hard, fixed mass ± pain, a/w facial nerve palsy
- Ix: US/MRI, FNAC, biopsy
- Mx: surgery, radiotherapy

Specific tumours:
- Pleomorphic adenoma = slow-growing benign tumour; middle-age, may turn malignant if present for a long time
- Warthin's tumour: elderly men, may be bilateral. Mx: partial parotidectomy
- Mucoepidermoid carcinoma: aggressive high-grade - excision + RT
- Adenoid cystic tumours: painful slow-growing tumours that tend to spread along nerves ("perineural infiltration") + distant mets and late recurence. Mx: surgical excision, post-op RT

Dentistry for doctors

Teeth problems: is the pain...
- worse with sugar and heat?
- worse/better with cold?   Tooth is alive (pulpitis)
- intermittent?
- worse with percussion?
- constant/uninterrupted?   Tooth is dead (osteitis/abscess)
- exacerbated by movement btwn finger and thumb?   Abscess

Trismus = when opening the mouth is difficult because of spasm or pain
- Sign of severe infxn :(→ always req maxfax ref

Facial swellings due to dental infxn
- If related to lower jaw, Ax for airway obstruction
- If spreading to eye, Ax CN II
- Usually subsides with PO Abx

Systemic disease complicating dental infxn
- Ref any pt that is immunocompromised, at risk of endocarditis, or at risk of bleeding (eg coagulopathy)

Peridontal disease
- Vincent's angina (necrotising ulcerative gingivitis) a/w smoking, HIV
  - Foul-smelling, caused by anaerobes (Fusobacteria) ± spirochetes (eg Borellia)
  - Mx: amoxicillin 500mg/8h PO + metronidazole 400 mg/8h PO + dental ref

Cannabis

- Aka marijuana, pot, weed, etc
- THC is considered the primary psychoactive compound, but there are 500+ chemicals in cannabis

---

CNS & psych – dependent on individual:
- In some individuals: euphoria, relaxation, sedation, ↑appetite, ↓short-term memory, ↓concentration, ↓coordination
- In others: anxiety, panic attacks, paranoia, psychosis (incl delusions, hallucinations) – esp at higher doses

Cardiovascular: ↑HR, ↑BP, chest pain, palpitations, ECG changes

Renal: AKI

Muscular: hypertonia, myoclonus, muscle jerking and myalgia

Others: cold extremities, dry mouth, dyspnoea, mydriasis, vomiting and hypokalaemia, conjunctival injection

Mx: • Supportive treatment for smx
- Psychosocial support for reducing and controlling use
- No approved medications

MDMA/Ecstasy

- MOA: stimulates the release of dopamine, norepinephrine, serotonin

CNS: ataxia

Psych: agitation, anxiety, confusion

Cardiovascular: ↑HR, ↑BP

Renal: hyponatraemia (2/2 SIADH or ↑water intake)

Others: hyperthermia, rhabdomyolysis

Mx: supportive treatment
- Dantrolene if severe hyperthermia

Methamphetamine works similarly

Cocaine

- Alkaloid derived from coca plant
- MOA: blocks uptake of dopamine, noradrenaline and serotonin

CNS: seizures, mydriasis (enlarged pupil), hypertonia, hyperreflexia

Psych: agitation, psychosis, hallucinations

Cardiovascular: ! coronary artery spasm (which can cause MI), ↑HR or ↓HR, ↑BP, ECG changes (QT prolongation, widening), aortic dissection

Others: ischaemic colitis, hyperthermia, metabolic acidosis, rhabdomyolysis

Mx: ⚕ benzodiazepines
- Chest pain: benzos + GTN
  - If MI, do PCI [→01.01]
- HTN: benzos + sodium nitroprusside
  - ▶ DO NOT give β-blockers

Nitrous oxide

- Aka whippets, balloons, laughing gas
- MOA: dissociative anaaesthetic, blocks the NDMA receptors (↓pain), induces euphoria and relaxation + ↑release of endogenous opioids and dopamine

CNS: HA, dizziness, incoordination, numbness, tremors

Psych: euphoria, altered perceptions, hallucinations, anxiety, paranoia

Others: hypoxia, hypothermia, ↑HR, ↑BP

Long-term effects
- ! Vitamin B12 deficiency → subacute combined degeneration of the spinal cord & anaemia
- Psychological issues
- Direct harm from inhaling gas – lung damage, barotrauma, frostbite, etc

Lysergic acid diethylamide (LSD)

- Synthetic hallucinogen that has psychedelic effects – distorts sensory stimuli and enhances feelings & introspection

CNS: tremors, paresthesias, mydriasis, hyperreflexia, HA, drowsiness

Psych: acute reactions ("bad trips"), impaired judgment (→injury), euphoria or dysphoria, agitation, psychosis

Cardiovascular: ↑HR, ↑BP, palpitations

Others: NV, dry mouth, pyrexia

Mx: • According to smx
- Agitation: if reassurance fails, ⚕ benzo
- Psychosis: may require antipsychotics
- Massive ingestions may require ITU care (eg intubation & ventilation)

Opioid misuse

- Includes wide range of drugs (morphine, heroin, codeine, buprenorphine, methadone, fentanyl, etc)
- MOA: stimulates mu, kappa and delta-opioid receptors to mediate analgesia pre- and post-synaptically

S/smx of opioid misuse
- Pinpoint pupils (miosis), drowsiness, ↓RR, rhinorrhea, ± needle track marks
Complications
- Viral infxn 2/2 sharing needles, eg HIV
- Bacterial infxn 2/2 sharing needles, eg infective endocarditis, septic arthritis
- VTE • Respi depression, coma, death

Acute Mx
- IV or IM naloxone: 400 mcg, then 800 mcg (up to 2 doses at 1min intervals), then 2 mg (1 dose), then 4 mg

Long-term Mx
- ⚕ Methadone or buprenorphine
  - Methadone: full agonist of μ-opioid receptor; helps to relieve withdrawal smx and cravings
  - Buprenorphine: partial agonist at μ-opioid receptor, antagonist at κ-receptor; similar effect to methadone and helps ↓ depressive and dysphoric states
- Compliance monitored by urinalysis
- Detox for 4w in inpatient facility, then 12w in community

Overdose / Poisoning Mx

Benzodiazepines
- Antidote: flumazenil
- Otherwise, supportive Mx

β-blockers
- If HR<40 or unstable, ⚕ atropine ± glucagon

Carbon monoxide
- 100% oxygen
- Hyperbaric oxygen

Cyanide
- Hydroxocobalamin (Vitamin B12)
- Combination of amyl nitrite, sodium nitrite, and sodium thiosulfate

Digoxin
- S/smx: generally unwell, anorexia, confusion, yellow-green vision, arrythmias, gynaecomastia
- Toxicity may be precipitated by hypokalaemia (and ↓Mg, ↑Ca, ↑Na, acidosis), renal failure, MI, hypoalbuminaemia, hypothyroidism
- Drug-drug interactions: quinidine, verapamil, diltiazem, spironolactone, ciclosporin, thiazides, loop diuretics
- Mx: Digibind, correct potassium levels and manage arrythmias

Ethylene glycol & Methanol
- ⚕ Fomepizole – inhibits alcohol dehydrogenase
- ⚕ Ethanol (if fomepizole not available)
- Haemodialysis if refractory to Mx

Heparin
- Protamine sulphate

Iron
- Desferrioxamine – iron chelating agent

Lead poisoning
- Dimecaprol, calcium edetate

Lithium
- Volume resuscitation (IV fluids)
- Haemodialysis if severe
- ± IV sodium bicarbonate

Organophosphates (insecticides)
- ⚕ Atropine ± ?pralidoxime

Paracetamol
- → 03.04 (NAC, activated charcoal)

Salicylates (eg aspirin)
- S/smx: respiratory alkalosis (2/2 hyperventilation) then metabolic acidosis, tinnitus, GI upset/bleeding, seizures, coma
- ⚕ IV bicarbonate (urinary alkalinisation)
  - Charcoal if presenting early
- Haemodyalisis

Tricyclic antidepressants
- ⚕ IV bicarbonate – ↓risk of seizures and arrythmias
- If arrythmias develop, DO NOT use class 1a and 1c antiarrhythmics, avoid class 3 drugs

Warfarin
- → 10.08 (Vitamin K, PTC, FFP, etc)

Depression

D: Major depressive disorder is a clinical syndrome characterised by persistent low mood + loss of interest and enjoyment, among other symptoms

R: postnatal, PMH or FHx of depression or suicide, dementia, drugs (eg corticosteroids, propran-olol, COCP), comorbidities, F>M

A: poorly understood
P: many theories, including neuro-transmitter dysfunction

Dx - Screening
- Patient Health Questionnaires
  - Scale of 0 to 3
    ◊ 0 = not at all
    ◊ 3 = all the time
- PHQ-2, "Over the last 2 weeks, how often have you been bothered by these problems?"
  - Little interest/pleasure in things?
  - Feeling down/depressed/hopeless?
- If PHQ-2 score ≥3, follow-up with PHQ-9

Dx - DSM-5 criteria [PHQ9]
↳ ≥5 smx present within same 2w period, represents Δ from baseline, ≥1smx *must* be (1) or (2)
(1) depressed mood
(2) ↓↓ interest/pleasure in activities
(3) wt loss / wt gain (or appetite)
(4) insomnia / hypersomnia
(5) psychomotor agitation or retardation
(6) fatigue / ↓ energy
(7) ↓ability to think/concentrate, or indecisiveness
(8) feelings of worthlessness or inappropriate guilt
(9) recurrent thoughts of death, suicidal ideation (± plan), attempt

Ix (in all pts with new Dx of MDD): TFTs, U&Es, FBC ± B12/folate - to r/o potentially reversible causes

---

Mx of less severe depression (PHQ9 <16)
- NICE discourages antidepressants as first-line
- Offer guided self-help, CBT, counselling, etc
- If pt prefers medications, SSRIs can be offered

Mx of more severe depression (PHQ9 ≥16)
- Combi CBT + antidepressant
  - SSRI, SNRI or other antidepressants if indicated based on prev Hx
- Other modes of therapy available based on what suits the pt best

Mx - switching antidepressants
- If pts stop antidepressants abruptly, they are likely to experience smx
  - GI upset, "brain zaps", etc
  - gradual ↓ over 4w (except fluoxetine)
- Switching between SSRIs: stop one SSRI before starting the other (except fluoxetine)
- Switching from **fluoxetine** to SSRI or TCA: stop fluoxetine → wait 4-7d before starting next SSRI/TCA
  - fluoxetine has a long half-life
- Switching SSRI to TCA
  - Slowly ↓SSRI while ↑TCA (=cross tapering)

SSRIs [→06.06 for more]
= selective serotonin-reuptake inhibitors
AE · ❗ all SSRIs can theoretically ↑risk of suicide – pts must be reviewed at 1w after starting
- ❗ GI upset – NVD
- ↑risk of GI bleeding
  - If pts is also on NSAID, + PPI
- Hyponatraemia
- Drug-drug interactions:
  - NSAIDs or aspirin (see above)
  - warfarin/heparin - consider mirtazapine instead
  - Triptans – avoid SSRIs
- Counsel pt to watch for ↑anxiety and agitation after starting SSRI
- Citalopram & escitalopram can ↑QTc - avoid in pts with heart problems + watch out for older pts or pts with liver impairment

---

Suicide

D: the act of taking one's own life

Risk factors "SADPERSONS"
- S: male sex (males more likely to complete suicide, but females more likely to attempt)
- Age: >45yo / advancing age
- Depression or other mental health disorder
- Previous attempt + Hx of deliberate self-harm
- Excessive alcohol/substance use
- Rational thinking loss
- Social supports lacking
  - Unemployment
  - Social isolation or living alone
- Organised plan
- No spouse (unmarried, divorced, or widowed) – includes individuals whose partners have committed suicide
- S: Chronic sickness

Risk factors a/w completion of suicide at a future date
- Planned attempt
- Efforts to avoid discovery
- Leaving a written note
- Final acts such as sorting out finances
- Violent method

Protective factors
- Family support
- Having children at home
- Religious belief

Mx: · Good hx required – compassionately done but detailed
- In acute setting, medical / surgical stabilisation, then ref to psych liaison team
- Ref to safeguarding
- Mx of underlying problems if possible, eg comorbidities
  ↳ seldom possible, but worth trying

Seasonal affective disorder
- Depression predominantly in the winter months
- Treat as per depression
  - do not give sleeping pills
  - little evidence for light therapy

Note regarding SADPERSONS
- Developed in 1983, and is useful as a mnemonic but is not particularly sensitive
- This version of Sadpersons has been merged with data on other risk factors

---

Bipolar disorder

Bipolar I = mania and depression
↳ more common
Bipolar II = *hypo*mania and depression

Manic episode
- Distinct period of abnormally and persistently elevated, expansive or irritable mood
- + persistently ↑ goal-directed activity or energy
- Lasting ≥1w and present most of the day, nearly every day
- During this period, ≥3 smx:
  - ↑self-esteem or grandiosity
  - ↓need for sleep
  - more talkative than usual or pressure to keep talking (= "pressured speech")
  - flight of ideas (or subjective experience that thoughts are racing)
  - distractibility
  - ↑goal-directed activity or psychomotor agitation
  - excessive involvement in activities that have high potential for painful consequences (eg unrestrained shopping sprees)
- Mood disturbance is sufficient to cause severe marked impairment in social or job functioning
  - or necessitates admission

Hypomanic episode
- ≥4 consecutive days
- ≥3 smx as above
- Change in mood/functioning that is uncharacteristic of the individual BUT *not severe enough* to cause social or job functioning and does not require admission

R: typically develops in late teen years, lifetime prevalence of 2%

Mx of acute manic episode
- ✎ **antipsychotic** (eg quetiapine, olanzapine, etc)
- ✎ valproic acid or lithium
- unless this has been used before and there is evidence of benefit
- lithium may take up to 3w for effectiveness, therefore not ideal for acute setting
- If pt presents to GP
  - Hypomania: routine ref to community mental health team (CMHT)
  - Mania: urgent ref to CMHT

Mx of depressive episode
- Ensure pt is on prophylaxis (and is compliant) + check serum levels
- Consider adding SSRI (along with mood-stabilising prophylaxis)
  - SSRIs should not be used alone in bipolar disorder due to risk of triggering manic episode
- Quetiapine is also licensed to treat depression in bipolar disorder

Prophylactic Mx
- ✎ lithium ± valproate
- ✎ valproate, olanzapine, or quetiapine
  - valproate not for females of childbearing potential
- Aim for single agent, but most pts will require mood stabiliser + low-dose antipsychotic, or mood stabiliser + antidepressant

Generalised anxiety disorder

D: ≥6mo excessive worry about everyday issues disproportionate to any inherent risk, causing distress or impairment. Pt finds it difficult to control the worry.

+ ≥3 of these smx most of the time:
· Restlessness or nervousness
· Easy fatigueability
· Poor concentration
· Irritability · Muscle tension
· Sleep disturbance
(in children ≥1 smx)

R: FHx of anxiety; physical or emotional stress (eg bullying); Hx of physical, sexual or emotional trauma (eg sexual abuse, loss of loved one); other anxiety disorder (eg panic disorder, social phobia); chronic physical health condition; F>M (2:1)

S/smx: as above
· Others include muscle aches, sweating, dizziness, dyspnoea, chest pain, NVD (or other GI complaints)

Ix: to r/o physical health conditions that may be causing GAD
· TFT to r/o hyperthyroidism
· ECG to r/o arrhythmias (eg if pt complains of palpitations)
· Ask pt about medications / habits that may contribute to anxiety, eg salbutamol, caffeine / theophylline, corticosteroids, antidepressants

Mx (NICE's step-wise approach):
· Education about GAD + active monitoring
  - encourage pt to ↓caffeine, to ↓triggers that may contribute to anxiety
· Low-intensity psych interventions, eg self-help, support groups
· High-intensity psych interventions, eg CBT or applied relaxation or drug tx
  - ⚖ sertraline
  - ⚖ alternative SSRI (eg fluoxetine) or SNRI (eg duloxetine or venlafaxine)
  - 3rd: consider pregabalin

Mx (continued)
❗ warn pt of risk of ↑suicidal thinking and self-harm with medications – follow up in 1mo or sooner depending on risk
· Highly specialist input (eg multi-agency teams)
  - if pt is at high risk of self-harm or suicide, may require admission

Panic disorders

D: recurring unexpected panic attacks over a 1mo period
· ≥1 attack followed by 1mo period in which individual worries about having additional attacks or their implications
  - eg pt is worried they might be having heart attack
· and/or individual has changed their behaviour in a maladaptive way
  - eg pt stops going out

Panic attacks are characterised by ↑↑fear or physical discomfort, reaching a peak within a few minutes
· ≥4 of following smx
  - Palpitations, pounding heart, ↑HR
  - Sweating   - Trembling/shaking
  - Sensations of shortness of breath or smothering
  - Feelings of choking
  - Chest pain or discomfort
  - Nausea or abdominal distress
  - Feeling dizzy, unsteady, light-headed or faint
  - Chills or heat sensations
  - Paresthesias
  - Derealisation (feelings of unreality) or depersonalisation (being detached from oneself)
  - Fears of losing control or 'going crazy'
  - Fear of dying

Ix: as per GAD

Mx: · similar to that of GAD
· ⚖ CBT or drug treatment
  - SSRI offered first
  - if CI or no response after 12w, offer imipramine or clomipramine

Obsessive-compulsive disorder

D: Obsessions – recurrent and persistent thoughts, urges, or images that are experienced as intrusive and unwanted
Compulsions – repetitive behaviours or mental acts that an individual feels driven to perform in response to an obsession, or according to rules that must be applied rigidly

Dx – obsessions and compulsions
· These are time-consuming, or cause clinically significant distress, or impair social and job functioning

R: FHx, paediatric autoimmune neuropsychiatric disorders a/w streptococcal infxn (PANDAS)

S/smx: · peak onset 10-20yo, or during perinatal period
· Pt may have hx of abuse, bullying or neglect
· Obsessions and compulsions as above – they may not necessarily be "visible" (eg repeating a certain phrase in one's mind)
· Scored with Y-BOCS scale

Mx:
· If mild functional impairment
  ⚖ CBT, exposure and response prevention (ERP)
  ⚖ Offer SSRI
· If moderate impairment
  ⚖ SSRI (fluoxetine specifically for body dysmorphic disorder)
  ⚖ Consider clomipramine if pt has had good prior response
· If severe impairment
  - refer to 2ndary mental healthcare team for Ax
  - while awaiting Ax, offer SSRI and CBT or consider clomipramine
· ERP involves exposing pt to anxiety-provoking situation and stopping their compulsions
· SSRI – usually requires higher dose and longer period for initial response (≥12w)

Post-traumatic stress disorder

Diagnostic criteria
A. Exposure to actual or threatened death, serious injury, or sexual violence
  - involves direct experience, witnessing event, learning about the event, or repeated exposure
B. Presence of ≥1 intrusive smx a/w traumatic event
  - recurrent, involuntary, and intrusive distressing memories of traumatic event
  - recurrent distressing dreams in which content or affect of dream are related to traumatic event
  - dissociative reactions (eg flashbacks) in which individual feels/acts as if the traumatic event were recurring
  - intense or prolonged psychological distress or marked physiological reactions at exposure to internal or external cues that symbolise or resemble the traumatic event
C. Persistent avoidance of stimuli a/w traumatic event
D. Negative alterations in cognition and moods (≥2 of following)
  - inability to remember important aspect of event
  - persistent and exaggerated negative beliefs about oneself, others or the world
  - persistent distorted cognitions about cause or consequences of the traumatic event (blaming oneself)
  - persistent negative emotional state (eg fear, horror, anger, guilt)
  - markedly ↓interest or participation in significant activities
  - feelings of detachment or estrangement from others
  - persistent inability to experience positive emotions
E. Marked alterations in arousal and reactivity (≥2 of following)
  - irritable behaviour or angry outbursts
  - reckless or self-destructive behaviour
  - hypervigilance
  - exaggerated startle response
  - problems with concentration
  - sleep disturbance

· A + ≥1mo of BCDE + clinically significant distress or impairment in social and job functioning

Mx:
· Following traumatic event, single session individual debriefing is NOT recommended (no evidence of benefit)
· If mild smx <4w, watchful waiting
· Trauma-focused CBT or eye movement desensitisation and reprocessing (EMDR) therapy may be used in more severe cases
· Drug tx not first-line, but if given, use venlafaxine or SSRI
  - if severe, trial of risperidone

Acute stress disorder

D: psychological stress reaction that occurs <4w after a person has been exposed to a traumatic event
· diagnostic criteria are similar to PTSD apart from the timeframe

Mx:
· ⚖ Trauma-focused CBT
· Benzodiazepines may be used for acute smx but have to be used with caution

Eponymous syndromes
· **Charles Bonnet**: audio/visual hallucinations occurring in clear consciousness
  - pt is usually aware these hallucinations are not real, and there are no other significant neuro-psychiatric disturbances
  - "Lilliputian" hallucinations – seeing small people/things
  - a/w ophthalmologic disorders (eg ARMD, glaucoma, cataracts)
· **Cotard**: pt believes part or all of their body is either dead or non-existent (a/w severe depression and psychotic disorders)
· **De Clerambault**: erotomanic delusion (eg believing a famous person is in love with you)
· **Othello**: pathological jealousy without real proof of infidelity

summary of DSM-V

Features that define psychotic disorders

as per DSM-V

Delusions
- Fixed beliefs not amenable to change in light of conflicting evidence
- Types: persecutory, referential, grandiose, erotomanic, nihilistic, somatic
- Termed *bizarre* if they are clearly implausible and not understandable to same-culture peers
- Also encompasses
  - thought withdrawal
  - thought insertion
  - delusions of control

Hallucinations
- Perception-like experiences without an external stimulus
- May occur with any sensory modality, but auditory hallucinations are most commonly a/w SCZ

Disorganised thinking (speech)
= formal thought disorder
- Derailment or loose association (eg Knight's move thinking)
- Tangentiality (obliquely related or completely unrelated answers)
  - Circumstantiality – giving an answer in excessive, unnecessary detail
- Incoherence ("word salad")

Grossly disorganised or abnormal motor behaviour
- Includes under this catatonia, defined as a marked decrease in reactivity to the environment
  - resistance to instructions (negativism)
  - mutism and stupor, etc

Negative symptoms
- blunting of affect
- anhedonia (inability to derive pleasure)
- alogia (poverty of speech)
- avolition (poor motivation)
- social withdrawal

Schizophrenia SCZ

D: mental health disorder in which a person's perception, thoughts, mood, and behaviour are significantly altered

R: strong – FHx
- Parent with SCZ – RR 7.5
- Identical twin with SCZ – RR 50
- Fraternal twin with SCZ – RR 5-15
Less strongly a/w obstetric complications, cannabis use (RR ~2), Black Carribean ethnicity (RR 5.8)

RR = relative risk; ratio of risks for an event for the exposure group versus risks for non-exposure group
eg individuals who have a parent with SCZ are 7.5x more likely to develop SCZ compared to individuals whose parents do not have SCZ

Diagnostic criteria (DSM-V)
A. ≥2 of following for most of 1mo
  - Delusions
  - Hallucinations   ⎤≥1 of these
  - Disorganised speech ⎦
  - Grossly disorganised or catatonic behaviour
  - Negative smx (↓emotional expression or avolition)
B. Significant impact on self-care, social or job functioning
C. Continuous signs of disturbance persist for ≥6mo
  ↳ including ≥1mo of A, + prodromal or residual smx

Schneider's first rank smx
  ↳ useful as triage tool, but not particularly sensitive or specific
- Auditory hallucinations
- Thought disorders (echo, insertion, withdrawal, broadcasting)
- Somatic hallucination
  - false perception of physical experience with the body
- Delusional perception
  - true perception, to which a person attributes a false meaning
  - fixed belief that does not change in light of conflicting evidence
- Feelings or actions experienced as made or influenced by external agents (eg "the CIA is controlling my arm")

Other s/smx of SCZ
- Impaired insight
- Negative smx
- Neologisms (made up words)
- Knight's move thinking
- Catatonia
- Clang associations: ideas only related based on similar sounds or rhymes
- Echolalia: repetition of someone else's speech

Mx:
- • second generation antipsychotics
- offer CBT
- cardiovascular risk-factor modification

P: factors a/w poor prognosis – strong FHx, gradual onset, low IQ, prodromal phase of social withdrawal, lack of obvious precipitant

Psychosis

D: a mental health disorder involving some loss of contact with reality
- Brief psychotic disorder – psychotic s/smx with duration is <1mo
  - not better attributed to other cause
  - with eventual full return to premorbid level of functioning

Can occur in other conditions
- Depression: psychotic depression
- Bipolar disorder
- Puerperal psychosis
- Neurological conditions, eg Parkinson's, Huntington's
- Prescribed drugs, eg steroids
- Illicit drugs, eg cannabis, phencyclidine

S/smx:
- See features that define psychotic disorders
- Others: agitation/aggression, neurocognitive impairment, depression, thoughts of self-harm

Risk factor data from this article, this article, and this article.

Antipsychotics

÷ typical and atypical

Typical antipsychotics
- Dopamine D2 receptor antagonists blocking dopaminergic transmission in mesolimbic pathways
- Cause extrapyramidal side effects and hyperprolactinaemia
- Eg haloperidol, chlorpromazine

Atypical antipsychotics (aka second generation antipsychotics, SGA)
- Act on D2, D3, D4, 5HT (serotonin) receptors
- Fewer extrapyramidal side effects and less hyperprolectinaemia, but can have marked metabolic effects
- Eg olanzapine, risperidone

Side effects

Extrapyramidal side effects (EPSE) "ADAPT"
- **A**cute **d**ystonia [days to weels]
  - sustained muscle contractions
    ◊ torticollis ("wry neck")
    ◊ oculogyric crisis – spasmodic movement of eyeballs into fixed position (usually upwards)
- **A**kasthisia (severe restlessness)
- **P**arkinsonism [weeks to months]
- **T**ardive dyskinesia
  - onset months to years, ~40% of pts
  - choreoathetoid movements, eg chewing, pouting of jaw

Others
- ↑risks in elderly: stroke, VTE
- Antimuscarinic: dry mouth, blurred vision, urinary retention, constipation
- Sedation, wt gain
- ↑prolactin ± galactorrhea
  - 2/2 dopaminergic effects
  - less seen with aripiprazole
- Impaired glucose tolerance
- Neuroleptic malignant syndrome: ↑↑fever, muscle stiffness
- Reduced seizure threshold (esp with second gen antipsychotics)
- Prolonged QT interval (esp with haloperidol)

Side effects (continued)

Clozapine
- Significant risk of agranulocytosis (1%) and neutropaenia (3%)
- Reduced seizure threshold (may induce seizures in up to 3% pts)
- Constipation
- Myocarditis
- Hypersalivation
- Dose adjustment may be necessary if pt starts or stops smoking during tx
- If pt is off clozapine for ≥48h, will require re-titration of dose to prevent toxicity

Monitoring for all antipsychotics

- At start of therapy (baseline)
  - FBC, U&Es, LFTs
  - Lipids, weight/BMI
  - Fasting blood glucose
  - Prolactin
  - Blood pressure   - ECG
- At 3mo
  - Lipids, weight/BMI
- At 6mo
  - Fasting blood glucose
  - Prolactin
- Annually
  - FBC, U&Es, LFTs
  - Lipids, weight/BMI
  - Fasting blood glucose
  - Prolactin
  - Cardiovascular risk Ax
- During dose titration
  - Blood pressure
  ! Clozapine will require initially weekly monitoring of FBC until stabilised on dose

Switching due to side effects
- Tending to cause weight gain: risperidone, olanzapine
  - less likely with aripiprazole and amisulpride, lurasidone
- QTc prolongation
  - less likely with lurasidone

Cluster A
"Odd or eccentric"

Paranoid | *A pattern of distrust and suspiciousness such that others' motives are interpreted as malevolent*

DSM-V criteria – fulfils ≥4 of following
- Suspects that others are exploiting, harming, or deceiving them
- Preoccupation with unjustified doubts about loyalty or trustworthiness of friends
- Is reluctant to confide in others because of unwarranted fear that info will be used against them
- Reads hidden demeaning or threatening messages into benign remarks / events
- Persistently bears grudges
- Perceives attacks on their character or reputation that are not apparent to others, and is quick to react angrily
- Has recurrent suspicions regarding fidelity of spouse or sexual partner without basis

Schizoid | *A pattern of detachment from social relationships and a restricted range of emotional expression*
- Think "android" (robot-like)

DSM-V criteria – fulfils ≥4 of following
- Does not desire or enjoy close relationships (including being part of a family)
- Almost always chooses solitary activities
- Has little interest in sexual experiences with others
- Takes pleasure in few activities
- Lacks close friends or confidants other than first-degree relatives
- Appears indifferent to praise or criticism
- Shows emotional coldness, detachment or flattened affectivity

Schizotypal | *A pattern of acute discomfort in close relationships, cognitive and perceptual distortions, and eccentricities of behaviour*

DSM-V criteria – fulfils ≥5 of following
- Ideas of reference
- Odd beliefs or magical thinking that influences behaviour and is inconsistent with subcultural norms
- Unusual perceptual experiences
- Odd thinking and speech
- Suspiciousness or paranoid ideation
- Inappropriate or constricted affect
- Behaviour or appearance that is odd, eccentric, or perculiar
- Lack of close friends or confidants other than first-degree relatives
- Excessive social anxiety that does not diminish with familiarity and tends to be a/w paranoid fears rather than negative judgments about self

---

Personality disorders
- Refer to enduring patterns of thinking and feeling about oneself and others that significantly and adversely affect how an individual functions in the various aspects of life
- This pattern is stable and of long duration, and its onset can be traced back to at least adolescence or early adulthood
- Thought to affect 1 in 20 people

Mx
- Danger to self or others has to be addressed immediately, eg admission
- Psychological therapies: **dialectical behaviour therapy**
  ↳ a type of talking therapy
- Treat any coexisting psychiatric conditions, eg referrals for substance abuse disorders

---

Cluster B
"Dramatic, emotional, or erratic"

Antisocial | *A pattern of disregard for, and violation of, the rights of others*

DSM-V criteria – fulfils ≥3 of following since 15yo
- Failure to conform to social norms with respect to lawful behaviours (resulting in repeated arrests)
- Deceitfulness (eg repeated lying, conning others for personal profit or pleasure)
- Impulsivity or failure to plan ahead
- Irritability and aggressiveness (eg repeated physical fights or assaults
- Reckless disregard for safety of self or others
- Consistent irresponsibility (eg repeated failure to sustain consistent work behaviour)
- Lack of remorse
! Can only be diagnosed when pt is ≥18yo, but there is often evidence of conduct disorder ≤15yo

Borderline (aka emotionally unstable | *A pattern of instability in interpersonal relationships, self-image, and affects, and marked impulsivity*

DSM-V criteria – fulfils ≥5 of following
- Frantic efforts to avoid real or imagined abandonment
- Pattern of unstable and intense interpersonal relationships characterised by alternating between extremes of idealisation and devaluation
- Identity disturbances – unstable self-image
- Impulsivity in ≥2 areas that are potentially self-damage (eg sex, spending, substance abuse)
- Recurrent suicidal behaviour, gestures, or threats, or self-mutilating behaviour
- Affective instability due to marked reactivity of mood, or anxiety usually lasting a few hours
- Chronic feelings of emptiness
- Inappropriate, intense anger or difficulty controlling anger
- Transient, stress-related paranoid ideation or severe dissociative symptoms

Histrionic | *A pattern of excessive emotionality and attention seeking*

DSM-V criteria – fulfils ≥5 of following
- Uncomfortable with situations in which they are not the centre of attention
- Interaction with others is often characterised by inappropriate sexually seductive or provocative behaviour
- Displays rapidly shifting and shallow expression of emotions
- Consistently uses physical appearance to draw attention to self
- Has a style of speech that is excessively impressionistic and lacking in detail
- Shows self-dramatisation, theatricality, and exaggerated expression of emotion
- Is suggestible
- Considers relationships to be more intimate than they actually are

Narcissistic | *A pattern of grandiosity, need for admiration, and lack of empathy*
- Think Donald Trump

DSM-V criteria – fulfils ≥5 of following
- Grandiose sense of self-importance
- Preoccupation with fantasies of unlimited success, power, brilliance, beauty or ideal love
- Believes that they is "special" and unique and can only be understood by, or should associate with, other special or high-status people
- Requires excessive admiration
- Has a sense of entitlement (ie unreasonable expectations of especially favourable treatment)
- Is interpersonally exploitative (takes advantage of others to achieve their own ends)
- Lacks empathy
- Often envious of others or believes that others are envious of them
- Shows arrogant, haughty behaviours or attitudes

Cluster C
"Anxious and fearful"

Avoidant | *A pattern of social inhibition, feelings of inadequacy, and hypersensitivity to negative evaluation*

DSM-V criteria – fulfils ≥4 of following
- Avoids occupational activities that involve significant interpersonal contact because of fears of criticism, disapproval, or rejection
- Is unwilling to get involved with people unless certain of being liked
- Shows restraint within intimate relationships because of the fear of being shamed or ridiculed
- Is preoccupied with being criticised or rejected in social situations
- Is inhibited in new interpersonal situations because of feelings of inadequacy
- Views self as socially inept, personally unappealing, or inferior to others
- Is unusually reluctant to take personal risks or to engage in any new activities because they may prove embarrassing

Dependent | *A pattern of submissive and clinging behaviour related to an excessive need to be taken care of*

DSM-V criteria – fulfils ≥5 of following
- Has difficulty making everyday decisions without an excessive amount of advice and reassurance
- Needs others to assume responsibility for most major areas of life
- Has difficulty expressing disagreement with others because of fear of loss of support or approval
- Has difficulty initiating projects or doing things alone
- Goes to excessive lengths to obtain nurturance and support from others
- Feels uncomfortable or helpless when alone because of exaggerated fears of being unable to care for themselves
- Urgently seeks another relationship as a source of care and support when a close relationship ends
- Is unrealistically preoccupied with fears of being left to take care of themselves

Obsessive-compulsive | *A pattern of preoccupation with orderliness, perfectionism, and control*

DSM-V criteria – fulfils ≥4 of following
- Preoccupied with details, rules, lists, order, organisation, or schedules to the extent that the major point of the activity is lost
- Perfectionism that interferes with task completion
- Excessive devotion to work and productivity to the exclusion of leisure activities and friendship
- Overconscientious, scrupulous, and inflexible about matters of morality, ethics, or values
- Unable to discard worn-out or worthless objects even when they have no sentimental value
- Reluctant to delegate tasks or to work with others unless they submit to exactly their way of doing things
- Adopts a miserly spending style
- Shows rigidity and stubbornness

Anorexia nervosa

D: Eating disorder characterised by restriction of caloric intake leading to low body weight, an intense fear of gaining weight, and a body image disturbance

R: F>>M, adolescence, obsessive and perfectionist traits, genetic influence (based on twin studies)

Diagnostic criteria
- Restriction of energy intake relative to requirements → significantly low body weight
- Intense fear of gaining weight or becoming fat, even though pt is underweight
- Disturbance in the way in which one's body weight or shape is unexperienced, undue influence of body weight or shape on self-evaluation, or denial of the seriousness of the current low body weight

Other s/smx
- ↓BMI   • Bradycardia
- Hypotension
- Enlarged salivary glands

Ix: bloods
- ↓K   • ↓T3
- ↓FSH, LH, estrogen, testosterone
- ↑cortisol and ↑GH
- impaired glucose tolerance
- ↑cholesterol, ↑carotin

Mx
- If pt is medically unstable, they may require admission ± PO, enteral or parenteral nutrition
  - ❗ If severe, nutrition should be done slowly to prevent refeeding syndrome
  - May also require fluid and electrolyte corrections
- Long term, psychotherapy and structured eating plan with oral nutrition should be discussed

Bulimia nervosa

D: eating disorder characterised by recurrent episodes of binge eating, followed by behaviours aimed at compensating for the binge

R: F>>M; personality disorder; Hx of sexual abuse; impulsivity; FHx of alcoholism, depression, eating disorder

Diagnostic criteria
- recurrent episodes of binge eating (eating an amount of food that is definitely larger than most people would eat during a similar period of time and circumstances)
- a sense of lack of control over eating during the episode
- recurrent inappropriate compensatory behaviour in order to prevent wt gain
  - eg self-induced vomiting, misuse of laxatives, diuretics, or other medications, fasting, or excessive exercise
- the binge eating and compensatory behaviours both occur, on average, at least once a week for ≥3mo
- self-evaluation is unduly influenced by body shape and weight.
- the disturbance does not occur exclusively during episodes of anorexia nervosa

Other s/smx
- Recurrent vomiting may lead to erosion of teeth and calluses on the knuckles (Russell's sign)

Ix: as per anorexia (unlikely to see derangements as nutrition is not as poor as in anorexia)

Mx:
- Referral to specialist care
- Adults: NICE recommends self-help guide first, but if this is not effective, offer CBT
- Children: offer **family therapy**
- High-dose fluoxetine is licensed for bulimia nervosa, but long-term data is lacking

Insomnia

D: difficulty initiating or maintaining sleep, or early-morning awakening that leads to dissatisfaction with sleep quantity or quality

R: F>M, ↑age, chronic medical conditions or pain, psychiatric illness, alcohol/substance misuse, stimulant usage, medicines such as cortico-steroids, poor sleep hygiene, TBI

Ix:
- clinical Dx + risk factor identification
  ↳ pt may need to keep sleep diary
- Actigraphy – sensor device (like a smart watch) worn to measure gross motor activity
- Polysomnography is not routinely indicated
  - consider for pts with suspected obstructive sleep apnoea or periodic limb movement disorder
  - consider if refractory to conventional tx

Mx:
- Identify potential causes, eg poor sleep hygiene, mental health issues
- Pt education: good sleep hygiene
  - no screens before bed
  - limit caffeine intake
  - regular bedtimes
  - avoid daytime naps, etc
- Advise pt not to drive when sleepy
- Only consider use of hypnotics if daytime impairment is severe
  - benzodiazepines
  - z-drugs (zopiclone, zolpidem, etc)
    – but linked to nightmares
  - lowest effective dose for the shortest period of time possible
  - do not give repeat prescription; review after 2w
- Consider referral to CBT

Unexplained symptoms

Somatic symptom disorder
- aka somatisation disorder
- ≥1 somatic smx that are distressing
- preoccupation with health concerns
  - eg excessive time and energy devoted to smx or health concerns
  - pt refuses to accept reassurance or negative test results
- ≥6mo symptomatic

Illness anxiety disorder
- aka hypochondriasis
- preoccupation with having or acquiring a serious illness
- somatic smx are *not present* or only mild
- ≥6mo illness preoccupation

Conversion disorder
- aka functional neurological disorder
- ≥1 smx of altered voluntary motor or sensory function
- clinical findings provide evidence of incompatibility between smx and recognised neurological and medical conditions
- smx is not consciously feigned by pt, and pt is not doing it to seek material gain
- pt may be indifferent to their apparent disorder ("la belle indifference")

Dissociative disorders
- Dissociation is a process of separating oneself off from certain memories, emotions or identities
- This presents with psychiatric smx, including amnesia, depersonalisation, derealisation, etc
- Umbrella term including
  - Dissociative identity disorder (aka multiple personality disorders)
  - Dissociative amnesia
  - Depersonalisation or rerealisation isorder

Factitious disorder
- aka Munchausen's syndrome
- Falsification of physical or psychological s/smx, or induction of injury or disease
- Individual prevents themselves to others as ill or injured
- Deceptive behaviour is evident even in the absence of obvious external rewards
- Imposed on another (= Munchausen's by proxy)
  - eg parent injures their child on purpose to present them as ill

Malingering
- Fraudulent simulation or exaggeration of smx with the intention of financial (or other) gain

Electroconvulsive therapy

D: psychiatric treatment where a generalised seizure is induced in a patient to manage refractory mental disorders

Indications
- Refractory severe depression
  ↳ ~50% response rate
- Life-threatening catatonia
- Prolonged or severe manic episode
- Prior good response

Other points
- Has to be administered under anaesthesia with muscle relaxant
- Cognitive impairment after
  - including retrograde and anterograde amnesia
- Generally regarded as safe for pregnancy

Alternatives
- Transcranial magnetic stimulation
- Vagus nerve stimulation
- Deep brain stimulation

Drugs

Benzodiazepines
- MOA: enhance the effect of GABA, an inhibitory neurotransmitter
- Adverse effects
  - Sedation (including respiratory depression at very high doses or when mixed with other drugs like opioids)
  - Tolerance and dependence can develop → ! should only be prescribed for a short period of time (eg 2-4w) and with regular reviews
- Benzodiazepine withdrawal
  - Taper off slowly (eg drop dose by 1/8th every fortnight)
  - Switch to longer acting benzo (eg diazepam) so that effects are less pronounced
- S/smx of benzo withdrawal syndrome (if withdrawn too fast)
  - insomnia   - irritability
  - anxiety   - tremor
  - loss of appetite
  - perceptual disturbances
  - lowered seizure threshold

Lithium
- MOA: not fully understood
- Narrow therapeutic range: 0.4-1.0 mmol/L; mainly excreted via kidneys
- Adverse effects
  - GI effects: NVD
  - fine tremor
  - nephrotoxicity (diabetes insipidus)
  - hypothyroidism
  - ECG changes
  - weight gain
  - idiopathic intracranial hypertension
  - leukocytosis (↑WCC)
  - hyperparathyroidism
  - hypercalcaemia
- Monitoring
  - Li levels - sample 12h post-dose
  - weekly, and after each dose change until conc are stable
  - dose change: 1 week later, and weekly until conc are stable
  - then 3mo thereafter
  - TFT and renal function q6mo

Mirtazapine
- MOA: α-2 adrenergic blocker → ↑serotonergic and noradrenergic transmission
- Adverse effects (but can be used for good effect!)
  - ↑appetite & weight gain
  - sedation – ?good for insomnia

Selective serotonin reuptake inhibitors (SSRIs)
- Adverse effects
  - GI side effects: NVD
  - ↑risk of GI bleeding
  - ↑risk of anxiety and agitation after starting an SSRI
  - ! For pts <25yo, review after 1w to assess risk of suicide or self-harm
  - Hyponatraemia
- Drug interactions
  - NSAIDs: use PPI
  - Warfarin/heparin: use mirtazapine instead
  - Aspirin: caution (risk-benefit)
  - Triptans and MAOIs: ↑risk of serotonin syndrome
- Citalopram & escitalopram
  - specific concerns re dose-dependent QT prolongation
  - caution in elderly pts, hepatic impairment avoid in pts with known QT prolongation or on medications that prolong QT
- Post-MI: use sertraline
- Children & adolescents: fluoxetine preferred
- Pregnancy:
  - use in 1st trim ↑risk of congenital malformations (esp with paroxetine – DO NOT give)
  - use in 3rd ↑risk of pulmonary hypertension of the newborn
- Discontinuation smx "FINISH"
  - Flu-like smx (eg lethargy)
  - Insomnia (± nightmares)
  - Nausea ± vomiting
  - Imbalance (dizziness, vertigo)
  - Sensory disturbances (paraesthesias, shock-like sensations)
  - Hyperarousal (anxiety, irritability, agitation, aggression, etc)

Serotonin-noradrenaline reuptake inhibitors (SNRIs)
- eg venlafaxine, duloxetine
- Side effect profile similar to SSRIs
- Relatively newer than SSRIs, therefore less evidence base

Tricyclic antidepressants (TCAs)
- MOA: inhibits reuptake of serotonin and noradrenalien
- Adverse effects
  - Anticholinergic effects (eg dry mouth, blurred vision, constipation, urinary retention)
  - Antihistamine effects (eg drowsiness)
    ◊ esp with amitriptyline, clomipramine, dosulepin)
  - Anti-adrenergic effects (eg postural hypotension)
- Amitriptyline is used for neuropathic pain and prophylaxis of migraines

Monoamine oxidase inhibitors (MAOIs)
- MOA: ↑serotonin and noradrenaline in presynaptic receptors
- Not used commonly nowadays due to side effect profile and drug-drug interactions
- Non-selective, eg phenylzine
  - used in treatment of atypical depression
- Selective, eg moclobemide, selegiline, rasagiline
- Adverse effects
  - Hypertensive reactions with tyramine containing foods (eg cheese, pickled herring)
  - Anticholinergic effects (eg dry mouth, constipation, urinary retention, etc)

Zopiclone, zolpidem, zaleplon
- MOA: GABA-receptor agonists
  ↳ similar effect to benzos
- Adverse effects
  - similar to benzos
  - can cause intense dreams and hallucinations in some pts
  - ↑risk of falls in elderly

Mental Health Act: Sectioning

Sectioning refers to (involuntary) detention of a patient under the MHA

Section 2
- Admission for assessment for ≤28d, not renewable
- Requires AMHP + 2 doctors
  - ≥1 doctor must be approved under Section 12(2) ≈ consultant psychiatrist
  - Rarely, the nearest relative (NR) can replace the AMHP in this process, but this is seldom used
- Tx can be administered against pt's wishes

Section 3
- Admission for treatment for ≤6mo, renewable after review
- Requires AMHP + 2 doctors
- Both doctors must review the pt in the last 24h before making their recommendations
- Tx can be administered against pt's wishes
- Can be renewed at 6mo, then 12-monthly thereafter

Section 4
- Admission for assessment for 72h
- Requires GP + AMHP or nearest relative
- Pt is usually admitted to hospital, whereupon section 2 may be started

Section 5(2)
- Detention by doctor for 72h
- Any doctor with full GMC registration (i.e. not FY1 doctors)
- Pt must be hospitalised (not in A&E)

Section 5(4)
- Detention by nurse for 6h

Police powers
- Section 135: break into property to remove a person to a place of safety (usually a hospital or police station)
- Section 136: move someone from a public place to a place of safety
- Valid for 24-36h, during which a MHA assessment (MHAA) should be arranged (thereafter, another section may apply)

Section 17
- Under a "section 17 leave" pts are allowed to leave the hospital and undergo care in the community (Community Treatment Order)
- This is subject to conditions from the responsible clinician
- If the conditions are broken (eg pt is not compliant with regular reviews or taking medication), then the clinician can revoke the leave

MHA Assessment (MHAA)
- Before pts can be sectioned under Section 2 or 3 (ie longer-term sections), they need to undergo an MHAA
- This involves separate interviews with the AMHP and then by the doctors
- Thereafter, the team will submit their paperwork to make the section official
- AMHPs are usually social workers that have undergone specific training and are appointed under the MHA to act as AMHPs

Paediatric BLS

Unresponsive?
→ Shout for help + open airway
Not breathing normally?
→ **5 rescue breaths**
No signs of life?
→ 15 chest compressions
→ then 2 breaths + 15 compressions

Rescue breaths
· Position: neutral for infant, 'sniffing' for child
· Mouth over mouth and nose for infant, mouth over mouth for child
· Watch for chest to rise and fall

Choking algorithim
· If coughing, encourage cough
· If ineffective cough and conscious: 5 back blows, 5 thrusts (chest for infant, abdo for child)

Intraosseous infusion

CI: osteoporosis, osteogenesis imperfecta, infxn at insertion site, vascular injury proximal to insertion site, fracture in target bone, previous IO insertion at site within 48h

Equipment
· manual needle vs semi-automatic
· semi-auto: bone injection gun for children and adults, EZ-IO (reusable drill with 15 mm needle for <39kg, 25 mm needle for >40kg, 45 mm needle)

Prep   · Decontaminate field
· Lidocaine 1% 5 mL if conscious
· Syringe for blood sampling
· Flush · Tape for securing
· Primed infusion set ± 3 way tap

Site of insertion
· Best: prox tibia, anteromedial surface (1-2cm medial to and 1-2cm distal to tibial tuberosity)
· Others: distal femur, distal tibia, proximal humerus)

Paediatric ALS

Unresponsive?
Not breathing / only occasional gasps

CPR: 5 initial breaths then 15:2
Attach defib/monitor

Call resus team
(1 min CPR first if alone)

Ax rhythm

Shockable
(VF or pulseless VT)

Non-shockable
(PEA or asystole)

ROSC

1 shock (4J/kg)

Resume CPR for 2min

Resume CPR for 2min

· after 3rd shock, give adrenaline 10 mcg/kg IV/IO
· repeat alternate cycle
· after 3rd shock, give amiodarone bolus 5 mg/kg IV/IO. Repeat one more time after 5th shock (or later on if relapse)

· Use ABCDE approach
· Control oxygenation and ventilation
· Ix + tx ppt cause
· Temperature control

· Give adrenaline asap
· Repeat on alternate cycles until ROSC

Reversible causes
· Hypoxia
· Hypovolaemia
· Hypo/hyper-K
· Hypothermia
· Tension pneumothorax
· Toxins
· Tamponade, cardiac
· Thromboembolism

Procedure
· Clean with antiseptic, lidocaine
· Insert IO needle at 90° to skin. Advance with screwing motion to marrow cavity
· Correct location = ↓ resistance on entering marrow cavity
· Needle flange should not touch skin to prevent necrosis
· Verify position by aspirating bone marrow or by flushing NaCl without infiltration of surrounding tissue
· Needle should stand upright without support, but secure with tape
· Connect to IV inf via extension ± 3 way tap

Complications: extravasation, dislodgment, local infxn, necrosis, fracture, pain, compartmen syndrome, emboli. More common with prolonged use; d/c once IV access achieved (aim <24h)

Anaphylaxis

Dx: sudden onset, life-threatening problem involving airway, breathing or circulation, and in ~80% skin Δ

Once suspected, chief priority is **adrenaline IM** – strength is 1:1000
↳ best site is anterolateral aspect of middle third of thigh
≤6yo: 0.15 mL (150 mcg)
6-12yo: 0.3 mL (300 mcg)
>12yo: 0.5 mL (500 mcg)
· Repeat in 5min if no improvement

Refractory anaphylaxis
· = ABC problems persisting despite 2 doses of IM adrenaline
· Mx: - IV fluids for shock
  - consider IV adrenaline infusion (only under expert guidance)

Mx after pt's ABC are stabilised
· PO antihistamines in pts with persistent skin smx (urticaria)
· **Ix: serum tryptase levels** – ↑ for ≤12h post-anaphylaxis
· Refer to specialist allergy clinic
· Give 2x epipen + training
· Discharge planning
  - Risk-stratified approach ∴ risk of late reaction in 20% of pts ("**biphasic reactions**")
  - Fast track discharge if pt responds well to first dose of adrenaline, complete resolution of smx, knows how to use epipen, has adequate supervision after discharge
  - Observe for ≥6h if 2 doses of IM adrenaline needed or PMH of biphasic reaction
  - Observe for ≥12h otherwise

Newborn life support

Standby for high risk deliveries
· Emergency C-sec   · Breeches
· Twins/triplets   · Prematurity
· Instrumental delivery · Eclampsia
· Thick meconium-stained liquor

Preparation
· Check and warm the resuscitaire
· Check other equipment – masks, bag valve mask, suction, laryngoscope, ET tubes, O2, ≥2 towels
· Ascertain PMH: gestation, antenatal Hx, antenatal concerns

At birth
· Ax colour, tone, breathing
  - if baby pink and crying: return to mum for 1h of skin-to-skin
  - if not: rub vigorously while drying
· Ax breathing and HR with steth
· if no spontaneous breathing
  - open airway
  - 5 **inflation** breaths via BVM
  - apply pressure of 20-30cmH2O for 2-3s to inflate newborn's lungs
  ↳ goal is to open the lungs

At birth (continued)
· if chest not expanding, readjust head position and try again ± direct inspection of oropharynx & suction
· Key indicator of response is ↑HR – check HR and breathing q30s or establish continuous monitoring
· After 5 inflation breaths and adequate chest expansion, if baby is still not making respiratory effort, continue ventilation breaths 30-40 breaths/min using 4-5 cm H2O of PEEP if available
  ↳ if not pinking up, add O2 stepwise
· If HR not improving and <60 bpm, start compression and ventilation breaths at rate of 3:1

Temperature
· Use resuscitaire while baby is being checked
· Naked, wet newborns cannot maintain body temperature
· A/w ↑mortality in all babies
· Hypothermia = <36.5 for newborns

Thick meconium
· If babies are delivered floppy, apnoeic, and covered in thick viscous meconium – rapidly visualise oropharynx ± suction before stimulation and inflation breaths
· Do not routinely intubate or suction as no evidence

Prematurity
· Preterm infants = <32w gestation
· Require stabilisation and help with temp regulation, feeding, and respiration

APGAR score - 1, 5 ± 10 min of age
· Appearance, pulse, stimulation, muscle tone, respiration – 0, 1, 2
· 7-10 = good; 4-6 = moderate, 0-3 = very low

The ill and feverish child

Ax: ABC, then traffic light Ax

Green light 🟢
- takes most feeds ok
- normal colour (lips, tongues, skin)
- responds to social cues
- content / smiles
- alerts or wakens quickly
- strong/normal cry
- breathing calmly
- normal skin and eyes
- moist mucous membranes

Orange light 🟠
- taking ≤50% feeds · pale
- not responding to social cues
- hard to wake · ↓activity
- no smile · nasal flaring
- ↑RR · sats <95% · crepitations
- CRT >3s · ↓UO
- dry mucous membranes
- rigors · fever >5d · temp ≥39°C
- limb or joint swelling, non-wt bearing, not using extremity

Red light 🔴
- pale / mottled / ashen / blue
- not responding to social cues
- unarousable or doesn't stay awake when aroused
- weak, high-pitched or continuous cry, or grunting
- RR >50, ↑chest indrawing
- ↓skin turgor · non-blanching rash
- bulging fontanelle · neck stiffness
- status epilepticus · focal seizures
- focal neurological signs
- temp ≥38°C if <3mo

Other notes
- If herpes simplex encephalitis suspected, give IV aciclovir
- If >3mo with confirmed bacterial meningitis, give IV corticosteroids
- Children with fever >5d, Ax by paediatrician for Kawasaki disease

Mx of children <3mo
- Ix: urine, FBC, CRP, blood culture ± CXR if respi signs, stool culture if diarrhoea, nasopharyngeal aspirate and throat swab
- LP: perform on all <1mo, 1-3mo + unwell-looking, or 1-3mo + WCC <5 or >15

Mx of children with green features 🟢
- Possibly Mx at home. Always test urine in young children
- Do not prescribe PO Abx if no clear source
- Advice to parents
  - Offer regular drinks or bfding
  - Look for signs of dehydration: dry mouth, no tears, sunken eyes or fontanelle
  - Look for non-blanching rash
  - Check on child at night
  - Do not tepid-sponge or undress child to control fever. Only use antipyretics if child is distressed
  - Keep off school while febrile
  - Seek further help if child becomes more unwell, dehydrated, has a fit, or fever >5d. Go to A&E if non-blanching rash

Mx of children with amber features 🟠
- Ix: urine, FBC, blood culture ± LP if <1yo ± CXR (esp if fever >39°C or WCC >20)

Mx of children with red features 🔴
- Ix: urine, FBC & U&E, blood culture ± LP if <1yo ± CXR ± ABG ± nasopharyngeal & throat swabs
- Fluid bolus: 20 mL/kg IV 0.9NaCl
- Abx: max dose 3rd gen ceph (eg ceftriaxone) if signs of shock, unrousable, signs of meningitis
  - if <3mo, cover for Listeria (eg ampicillin)

Age	RR	HR	SBP 5-50th centile
<1yo	30-40	110-160	65-90
1-2yo	25-35	100-150	70-95
2-5yo	25-30	95-140	70-100
5-12yo	20-25	80-120	80-110
>12yo	15-20	60-100	90-120

Adapted from OHCS

Meningitis

S/smx: poor feeding, lethargy, irritability, NV, HA, myalgia, arthralgia

Meningeal signs come on relatively late – not sensitive or specific
- Neck stiffness · Photophobia
- Kernig's sign: resistance to extending knee when hip flexed
- Brudzinski's sign: hips flex on neck flexion
- Opisthotonus: back arching

Ix: FBC, CRP, U&Es, clotting screen, culture, meningococcal PCR, glucose, ABG. LP if not CI. ± urine, nose/throat swab, stool virology, CXR

CI for LP [any signs of ↑ICP]
- Focal neuro signs · Papilloedema
- Significant bulging of fontanelle
- DIC · Signs of cerebral herniation
- Meningococcal septicaemia
  ↳ do blood cultures & PCR instead

Mx: 1. Abx:
  <3mo: IV amoxicillin + cefotaxime
  >3mo: IV cefotaxime/ceftriaxone
2. Steroids – not for <3mo
  · Consider dexamethasone if LP shows frankly purulent CSF, CSF WBC >1000 ± protein >1g/L, bacteria on Gram stain
3. Fluids: tx of shock
4. Cerebral monitoring: mechanical ventilation if respi impairment
5. Public health notification and abx prophylaxis of contacts – ciprofloxacin
If ↑ICP; tx with hypertonic saline or mannitol
  ↳ discuss with paediatric ITU

Complications:
- acute: seizures, ↑ICP, abscesses, infected subdural effusion
- chronic: hydrocephalus, ataxia, paralysis, deafness (steroids ↓risk), ↓IQ, epilepsy

For bacterial and viral meningitis →04.04

Meningitis: the organisms

Neonatal to 3mo
- GBS: usually vertical transmission. More common in low birth wt babies and following prolonged rupture of the membranes
- E. coli and other Gram-ve
- Listeria monocytogenes

1mo to 6yo
- Neisseria meningitidis (meningococcus)
- Streptococcus pneumoniae (pneumococcus)
- Haemophilus influenzae

>6yo
- Neisseria meningitidis
- Streptococcus pneumoniae

Giving IM benzylpenicillin before hospital admission
- <1yo: 300mg IM
- 1-9yo: 600mg
- ≥10yo: 1200 mg
- When in doubt, give.
- If penicillin-allergic, cefotaxime may be used (50 mg/kg IM stat, if >12yo, 1000mg)

TB meningitis
- Consider in any child with ↓glucose, ↑protein, and ↑WBC in CSF
- Prodromal and meningitic phases
- Staging based on level of consciousness and neuro signs
  1. conscious with no neuro signs
  2. disturbed consciousness ± focal neurology
  3. comatose ± significant neuro deficit
- Complications: communicating hydrocephalus, stroke, ↑ICP
- CSF: first few samples might be normal, or show visible fibrin webs and widely varying cell counts

Encephalitis

S/smx: altered behaviour, cognition or con-sciousness (see also red light signs). High degree of suspicion required – ? odd behaviour

Causes: infective vs non-infective (acute disseminated encephalo-myelitis, ADEM – an acute demyelinating process following a non-CNS infxn)

DDx encephalopathies:
- metabolic (↓glycemia, DKA, ↑NH4), toxic, hypertensive, autoimmune, sepsis
- other CNS infection (meningitis, abscess)
- psychosis, lead or other poisoning
- SAH, malignancy, lupus

Ix: LP CSF opening pressure, protein, lactate, glucose, MC&S, PCR (HSV, VZV, entero-viruses ± EBV, etc)
- Bloods incl NH4, serology & HIV
- Stool culture
- Nose/throat swab (respi PCR)
- Urine (mumps) · MRI or CT
- EEG may be helpful to DDx psychiatric or organic cause

Mx: Start triple therapy with ceftriaxone, clarythromycin and aciclovir while cause is being determined
- HSV: IV aciclovir 14-21d, then repeat LP to confirm CSF is HSV-ve. Do not routinely use corticosteroids. Neuro sequelae common.

For encephalitis in adults →04.04

Measles

D: caused by RNA paramyxovirus
· Spread by aerosol transmission. Very infectious. Incubation 10-14d
· Pt is infective from prodrome until 4d after rash starts

S/smx
· Prodromal phase: irritable, fever, conjunctivitis
· Koplik spots: white spots ('grains of salt') on buccal mucosa; typically develop before rash
· Rash – starts from the head then spreads to the whole body
  - discrete maculopapular rash becoming blotchy and confluent
  - desquamation may occur after a week; spares palms and soles
· Diarrhoea in 10%

Ix: IgM abs detected within a few days of rash onset

Mx: mainly supportive
· Consider admission in immuno-suppressed (or pregnant)
· ❗ notifiable disease

· If unimmunised child comes into contact with measles, offer MMR
  - vaccine-induced abs develop more rapidly than natural infxn
  - give within 72h

Complications
· otitis media: most common comp
· pneumonia: most common cause of death
· encephalitis: typically occurs 1-2w following the onset of the illness)
· subacute sclerosing panencephalitis [for more, see 08.05]
· febrile convulsions
· keratoconjunctivitis, corneal ulceration
· diarrhoea
· ↑incidence of appendicitis
· myocarditis

DDx: See also **Kawasaki disease** on pg 15.06

Mumps

🦠 RNA paramyxovirus
💬 Spread by droplets
MOA: Spreads to respiratory tract epithelial cells to parotid glands to other tissues
Incubation: 14-21d
Infective: 7d before, 9d after parotid swelling starts

S/smx: fever, malaise, myalgia, parotitis (earache, pain on eating) – unilateral then bilat in 70%

Mx: · MMR prevents in 80%
· Rest, analgesia   · ❗ Notifiable ❗

Complications [see 08.05]

Rubella   ≈ German measles

🦠 togavirus   winter and spring
Incubation 14-21d
· individuals infectious 7d before smx appear to 4d after rash starts

S/smx: · Prodrome: fever
· Rash: maculopapular, face to whole body; fades after 3-5d
· Lymphadenopathy: suboccipital and postauricular

Mx: supportive. Notify public health.
Immunisation: live virus

Complications: · arthritis
· thrombocytopaenia
· encephalitis   · myocarditis

See 08.06 for **Congenital rubella syndrome** and more on rubella in adults

Hand foot mouth disease

🦠 intestinal viruses coxsackie A16 and enterovirus 71

S/smx: · oral ulcers
· sore throat, fever
· vesicles on palms and soles

Mx: · symptomatic tx – analgesia and hydration
· no need to exclude children from school unless they feel unwell
· reassure not linked to cattle disease

Erythema infectiosum

caused by Parvovirus B19
= Slapped cheek syndrome
Spread by droplets. Pt is infectious 3-5d before rash appears

S/smx: · Mild fever
· Rose-red rash on cheeks
  - peaks after a week
  - heat will trigger rash
  - once rash appears, child is not infectious – no need to exclude from school
· Can suppress erythropoeisis (aplastic crisis) – serious if RBC lifespan is already short, eg sickle-cell disease.

Dx: IgM (PCR if immunocomp)

Mx: supportive. If aplastic crisis, transfusion and IVIG

More on 08.06

Roseola infantum

= Exanthum subitum, ? 4th disease
🦠 human herpes virus 6
Incubates 5-15d, usually affects children 6mo to 2yo

S/smx:
· **high fever** lasting ~3-5d
· **maculopapular rash follows** fever
· Nagayama spots/ulcers: papular enanthem on the uvula and soft palate
· **febrile convulsions** in ~10-15%
· diarrhoea and cough are also commonly seen
· Rare cause of encephalitis or focal gliosis on MRI. 'Febrile fits' tend to occur after the fever

Mx: supportive. No need to exclude from school

Complications: aseptic meningitis, hepatitis

Chickenpox

D: a childhood exanthem caused by the human α herpes virus (VZV)

R: exposure, 1-9yo, unimmunised status, occupational exposure

A/P: Direct contact or airborne respi droplet spread → virus spreads to regional LN causing 1' viremic phase → spreads to liver, spleen, etc
· 2' viremic phase at ~day 9: mono-nuclear cells transport the virus to the skin and mucous membranes → classic vesicular rash
· Pts are infectious 2-4d before onset of rash, and remain so until lesions are crusted over
· Incubation period is ~14d

Features
· Fever initially ± mild systemic upset
· Rash: itchy, starts on head/trunk
  ↳ macular → papular → vesicular
· Severe disease a/w complications eg pneumonia, neurological sequelae, hepatitis, secondary bacterial infxn

Mx: supportive
· Keep cool, trim nails, calamine lotion
· School exclusion until lesions have crusted over
· Do not give NSAIDs - ? ↑risk of secondary bacterial infxns
  ↳ secondary invasive GAS infxns can result in necrotising fasciitis
· at risk pts: PO/IV antiviral therapy
  ↳ give within 72h of onset

Post-exposure prophylaxis
→ VZIG for PEP
· Significant exposure to VZV/HZV
· Clinical conditions ↑risk of severe varicella, incl pregnant women, immunocompromised pts, neonates
· No abs to VZV

See 09.07 for infection in pregnancy + shingles

HIV in children

· In sub-Saharan countries, ~40% of all under-5 mortality is due to AIDS
· Breastfeeding ↑transmission 50%
· 2/3 infxns occur at delivery

Neonatal Mx
· PEP for 4w starting <4h from birth
  - zidovudine only if maternal viral load <50 copies
  - 3-drug ART otherwise
· Exclusive **formula feeding** from birth
· Initiate PCP prophylaxis with co-trimoxazole from 4w if tests +ve or equivocal
· Delay BCG until confirmed HIV-ve unless high risk of TB exposure
· Other vaccinations per schedule

Neonatal testing
· HIV DNA PCR ± RNA PCR at birth, 6w, 12w. HIV abs at 18mo of age
· Monthly testing if infant is bfding
· Sensitivity of PCR testing ↑ to near 100% at 3mo of age. But interpret with caution
· All clear if tests -ve at 18mo

Consider HIV in children with
· pyrexia of unknown origin
· lymphadenopathy
· hepatosplenomegaly
· persistent diarrhoea
· parotid enlargement
· shingles   · ↓platelets   · clubbing
· extensive molluscum
· recurrent slow to clear infxns
· faltering growth
· TB, pneumocystosis, toxoplasmosis, cryptococcosis, histoplasmosis, CMV, lymphocytic interstitial pneumonia (LIP)
· ❗ rmb seroconversion illness also

Prognosis: by 3yo, ~50% mortality with early-onset opportunistic infxns compared to 3% with no HIV
· Ensure full course of vaccine + pneumococcus + annual influenza

See 08.06 for HIV in adults + more info re medications

URTI in children

Croup = acute laryngotracheobronchitis
· Caused by **parainfluenza virus**, RSV, measles, etc
· Usually in <6yo; peak at 6mo to 3yo. More common in autumn
· S/smx: stridor, barking cough (worse at night), fever, coryzal smx
· Westley Croup Score to stratify into mild, moderate and severe
  ↳ mod-severe: audible stridor at rest; ↑coughing frequency
· Admit if mod-severe, <6mo, known airway abn (eg laryngomalacia), uncertainty about Dx
· Ix: clinical. CXR may show 'steeple sign' in PA view
· Mx: single dose of PO dexamethasone (0.15mg/kg) to all children regardless of severity
  - Emergencies: high flow O2 and nebulised adrenaline

Epiglottitis
· Caused by HiB. ↓incidence due to vaccination, but impt emergency
· S/smx: rapid onset, ↑↑↑T°, unwell, stridor, pooling of saliva, 'tripod' position
· Dx made by Snr clinician. If suspected, **do not approach child**, and **do not examine throat** as this may ppt obstruction. Do not cannulate pt or upset them.
  ↳ CXR may show thumb sign
· May require inhalation of anaesthesia and then endotracheal intubation to protect airway
· Mx: Abx (cefotaxime, ceftriaxone)

Bacterial tracheitis
· Defined by presence of thick muco-purulent exudate and tracheal mucosal sloughing not cleared by coughing
· Risks occluding the airway
· 6mo to 14yo. Viral prodrome for 2-5d then rapid deterioration
· S/smx: stridor, able to swallow oral secretions, very hoarse, mod-high fever, appears toxic, barking cough
· Mx: if severe, early intubation + suctioning of secretions. Abx (cefotaxime + flucloxacillin)

Diphtheria
🦠 Gram+ve *Corynebacterium diphtheriae*
· Spread by contaminated water
· Visitors to Eastern Europe, Russia, Asia
· Risks: homeless/refugee, unimmunised, aged 3-6yo, in 'asocial' families

S/smx:
· Sore throat with 'diphtheric membrane' (grey, pseudo-membrane on posterior pharyngeal wall)
· Bulky cervical lymphadenopathy
  - "bull neck"
· Polyneuritis; often starts with CN
· Heart block. Can cause shock
  - if there is ↑HR out of proportion to fever, suspect myocarditis

Ix: culture of throat swab (Loeffler's media)

Mx: diphtheria antitoxin (10-30k U IM) or 7d erythromycin oral suspension before swabs are known

Stridor
· Croup: barking cough
· Acute epiglottitis
· Inhaled foreign body: sudden onset of coughing, choking, vomiting, stridor
· Laryngomalacia: congenital abn of larynx. Infants typically present at 4w with stridor

Whooping cough ≈ cough of 100 days
· Gram-ve *Bordetella pertussis*
· Immunisation at 2, 3, 4, & 40 mo, but protection is not lifelong
· S/smx - catarrhal phase (≈ URTI smx)
  - paroxysmal phase: 2-8w :(
    ↳ see Dx criteria
  - covalescent phase: cough subsides over weeks to months
· Dx criteria: suspect in a person with cough >14d + ≥1 features:
  - paroxysmal cough   - inspiratory whoop
  - post-tussive vomiting
  - unDx apnoeic attacks in young infants

· Dx confirmed by nasal swab culture, PCR and serology
· Mx: notifiable disease + admit if <6mo
  - oral macrolide indicated if onset of cough was within 21d
    ↳ does not alter the course of illness
  - school exclusion for 48h after commencing abx or 21d from onset of cough if no abx
  - offer household contacts abx prophylaxis
· Complications: subconjunctival haemorrhage, pneumonia, bronchiectasis, seizures
· Vaccination for pregnant women 16-32w

LRTI in children

Bronchiolitis
· Commonest lung infxn in infants
· Most common caused by RSV; also rhinovirus, parainfluenxa, etc
· Age <2yo: peak 3-6mo
· S/smx: coryza (rhinorrhea, stuffy nose, sneezing, sore throat, etc)
  - then cough, ↑HR, wheeze, inspiratory crackles, poor feeding, intercostal recession
  - ± apnea, cyanosis, fever (low grade)
· Illness peaks in 3-5d then resolves; cough may last >3w
· RF for severe disease: congenital heart disease, chronic lung disease, immunodeficiency, etc
· Ix: immunofluorescence of nasopharyngeal secretions
· Mx: supportive
  - humidified O2 via headbox, esp if O2 sats persistently <92%
  - consider NGT, suction

Pneumonia
· *S. pneumoniae* most common
· S/smx: malaise, poor feeding, respi distress. Older children may have typical lobar signs
· Ix: clinical if not severe. Consider CXR, FBC, ABG, blood/sputum cultures
· Mx of mild pneumonia: likely viral, discharge with supportive tx and safety-netting
· Medical Mx: 💊 amoxicillin
  💊 + macrolides if no response, or if mycoplasma or chlamydia suspected
  💊 if a/w influenza, use co-amoxiclav

Asthma in children

D: reversible airway obstruction ± expiratory polyphonic wheeze, dyspnea, or cough. prev 10%

R: birthwt ↓, FHx, bottle fed, atopy, M>F, pollution, past lung disease

Dx: no gold standard.
· spirometry: (FEV1/FVC <70%)
· bronchodilator reversibility test (↑FEV1 ≥12%)
· FeNO

Mx in <5yo
1. newly Dx asthma: SABA
2. newly Dx asthma ≥3w smx or night-time waking
   · SABA + 8w trial of mod dose ICS
   · after 8w, stop ICS and monitor response
     - if smx don't resolve, reconsider Dx
     - if smx restart within 4w of stopping ICS tx, restart ICS at low-dose maintenance
     - if smx restart after 4w, repeat 8w trial of mod dose ICS
3. SABA + low dose ICS + leukotriene receptor antagonist
4. stop LTRA, refer to asthma specialist

Mx in 5-16yo [similar to adults]
1. newly Dx asthma: SABA
2. newly Dx asthma ≥3w smx or night-time waking:
   SABA + paeds low dose ICS
3. SABA + low dose ICS + LTRA
4. SABA + low dose ICS + LABA
5. SABA + switch ICS or LABA for MART that includes low dose ICS
   ↳ MART = ICS + LABA
6. SABA + MART [mod dose ICS]
7. SABA + 1 of following
   - MART [high dose ICS]
   - trial of additional drug (eg theophylline)
   - ref to asthma specialist

See 02.04 for **Cystic fibrosis**

Acute attacks in 2-5yo

Moderate · SpO2 >92%
· no features of severe asthma

Severe · SpO2 <92%
· Too breathless to talk/feed
· HR >140 · RR > 40
· Use of accessory neck muscles

Life-threatening · SpO2 <92%
· Silent chest · Poor respi effort
· Agitation · Cyanosis
· Altered consciousness

Acute attacks in 5-16yo
Attempt to measure PEF

Moderate · SpO2 >92%
· PEF >50% best or predicted
· no features of severe asthma

Severe · SpO2 <92%
· PEF 33-50% best or predicted
· Too breathless to talk/feed or cannot complete sentences
· HR >125 · RR >30
· Use of accessory neck muscles

Life-threatening · SpO2 <92%
· PEF <33% best or predicted
· Silent chest   · Poor respi effort
· Agitation · Cyanosis
· Altered consciousness

Mx of mild to moderate attacks
· Bronchodilator therapy
  · SABA via spacer
    - 1 puff q30-60s, max 10 puffs
    - if smx not controlled, go to A&E
· Steroid therapy for 3-5d
  - dose: 1-2mg/kg OD

Mx of severe to life-threatening attacks
· As above+ sit up, high flow O2
· Get senior input asap ± ITU
· Consider one IV dose of magnesium sulphate 40mg/kg over 20min (≤2g) if poor response to nebs
· Consider IV salbutamol over 10min ± infusion (1-2 mcg/kg/min) or aminophylline (5mg/kg IV over 20min)
· Salbutamol nebs continuously until improving, then ↑intervals.
· Consider starting CPAP in ED

Congenital heart disease

· Occurs in 0.8% live births

L→R shunts / Acyanotic

· VSD (30%)
· ASD
· PDA
· Coarctation of the aorta
· Aortic valve stenosis

R→L shunts / Cyanotic

· Tetralogy of Fallot
· Transposition of the great arteries
· Tricuspid atresia
· Truncus arteriosus
· Total anomalous pulmonary venous drainage (TAPVD)
· Hypoplastic left heart (HLH)

Ventricular septal defect

D: defects in the inter-ventricular septum that allow shunting of blood between the left and right ventricles

R: FHx, Down's (35% of Down's pts will have VSDs)

P: · small defects may spontaneously close
· mod to larger defects can lead to ↑flow into L ventricle and thus into pulmonary circulation

S/smx: Most present in infancy
· Pulmonary hypertension
· Eisenmenger's syndrome
· Murmur: holosystolic at left parasternal border ± palpable thrill

Dx/Ix: echo, CXR, ECG, cardiac MRI

Mx:
· watch and wait for small defects
· Mod to severe: surgical closure
· HF smx must be treated before Sx
· If pt presents with severe pulmonary HTN & Eisenmenger's, closure of VSD is CI
  - pul vasodilators eg bosentan, sildenafil for supportive Tx
  - consider heart-lung transplant :(

Atrial septal defect

Interatrial communications: incomplete separation between the left and right atrium
· 5 types: secundum, ostium primum, sinus venosus, coronary sinus, and vestibular
· Only secundum and vestibular defects are true ASDs

R: F>M (2:1), maternal alcoholism

S/smx:
· Most common congenital heart defect to present in adulthood
· ESM, fixed splitting of S2
· Embolism may pass from venous system to left side of heart causing a stroke

Ostium secundum (70% of ASDs)
· a/w Holt-Oram syndrome (tri-phalangeal thumbs)
· ECG: RBBB with RAD

Ostium primum
· present earlier than ostium 2'
· a/w abn AV valves
· ECG: RBBB with LAD, prolonged PR interval

Mx:
· Young pts with small ASDs - watch and wait; spontaneous closure possible
· If larger or evidence of right atrial enlargement, surgical closure indicated

Patent ductus arteriosus

D: persistence of the ductus arteriosus after birth

R: prematurity (10x), maternal rubella (? 50%), F>M (2:1)

A: · In the fetus, the patency of the ductus arteriosus is maintained by low O2 and circulating PGE2 PG12
· After birth, ↑O2 and ↓prostaglandins (due to removal of placenta and ↑pulmonary blood flow) leads to closure of ductus arteriosus
· Possibly ↓O2 exposure and continued sensitivity to prostaglandins in preterms lead to PDA

P: · Shunting of blood from aorta to pulmonary artery through PDA
· L→R shunting through PDA (oxygena-ted blood goes into pulmonary circulation)
· Can eventually result in late cyanosis in the lower extremities (i.e., differential cyanosis)

S/smx: usually present 2-3mo
· L subclavicular thrill
· Continuous 'machinery' murmur
  - crescendo-decrescendo
· Large volume, bounding, collapsing pulse
· Wide pulse pressure
· Heaving apex beat

Mx if presentation in preterms
· indomethacin or ibuprofen
  - MOA: ↓prostaglandin synthesis, closes connection in majority
· If a/w another heart defect, then prostaglandin E1 (aka alprostadil) is useful to keep duct open until after surgical repair
Mx if older
· Observe until 1yo with echo
· Transcatheter or surgical closure

Coarctation of the aorta

D: narrowing in the aorta, most commonly at the site of insertion of the ductus arteriosus, just distal to the left subclavian artery

R: M>F, Turner's (50%), DiGeorge's, HLHS, Shone's complex, PHACE

· Hypoplastic left heart syndrome (HLHS): underdeveloped LV, mitral and aortic valves ± ASD
· Shone's complex: supravalvular mitral membrane, parachute mitral valve, subvalvular aortic stenosis and coarctation of aorta
· PHACE syndrome: posterior fossa malformations, hemangioma, arterial anomalies, coarctation of the aorta/ cardiac defects, and eye abnormalities

See 15.20 and 15.21 for Turner's and DiGeorge's syndromes

P: effects depend on severity of narrowing and resultant ↑after-load on LV

S/smx:
· infancy: heart failure
· adult: hypertension
  - also a/w bicuspid aortic valve, berry aneurysms and neurofibromatosis
· radio-femoral delay
· mid systolic murmur, maximal over the back
· apical click from the aortic valve
· notching of the inferior border of the ribs (due to collateral vessels)
  - not seen in young children

Mx:
· If not severe, watch and wait
· If critical + risk of HF, prostagladin E is used to keep the ductus arteriosus open while waiting for surgery
· Definitive tx: surgery to correct coarc-tation and ligate the ductus arteriosus

Congenital aortic valve stenosis

D: narrow aortic valve that restricts blood flow from the left ventricle into the aorta

S/smx:
· Mild stenosis may be asmx
· Severe: fatigue, SOB, dizziness, fainting. Usually presents w/in months of birth
· ESM loudest at aortic area
  - crescendo-decrescendo
  - radiates to carotids
· Ejection click, palpable thrill, slow rising pulse and narrow pulse pressure

Dx/Ix: echo, ECG, exercise testing

Mx: percutaneous balloon aortic valvoplasty, surgical aortic valvotomy, valve replacement

Eisenmenger's syndrome

D: shunt reversal (blood flowing from the RV to LV) leading to the distribution of de-oxygenated blood to the systemic arterial circulation

A: ASD, VSD, PDA
P: over time, pulmonary HTN devleops. ↑pul pressure > systemic pressure → reversal of shunt (R>L). This causes deoxygenated blood to bypass lungs and enters into the body → cyanosis :(

S/smx of pulmonary HTN: RV heave, loud P2, ↑JVP, peripheral oedema
· Also: cyanosis, clubbing, SOB, plethoric complexion (a/w polycythaemia)

Mx: only definitive Mx is heart-lung transplant

Tetralogy of Fallot

D: congenital cardiac malformation with these four classic findings:
1. **P**ulmonary stenosis
2. **RV** hypertrophy (concentric)
3. **O**ver-riding aorta
4. **VSD**

R: rubella, ↑maternal age (>40yo), maternal alcoholism, GDM

Pathophysiology due to
- Degree of RV outflow tract obstruction: significant pulmonary obstruction will result in cyanosis
  - Blood will be shunted from RV to the aorta through VSD
- Tet spells are episodes of severe cyanosis a/w hyperpnoea
  - due to pulmonary obstruction → ↓pul blood flow, ↑R-L shunting across VSD

S/smx: · Can be picked up in antenatal scans or newborn check
- Tet spells (as above) – baby turns blue and may faint; triggered by crying, pooping, etc
- Harsh ESM at LLSE
- R-sided aortic arch in 25%
- CXR shows boot-shaped heart, ECG shows RV hypertrophy

Dx/Ix: echo, Doppler, CXR (not often done irl)

Mx of Tet spells
- Squatting / knees to chest
  - ↑ systemic vascular resistance which encourages blood to enter pulmonary vessels
- Supplemental O2
- β blockers – relax RV
- IVF – ↑preload
- Morphine – ↓respi drive, more effective breathing
- Bicarbonate – buffer metabolic acidosis
- Phenylephrine infusion – ↑systemic vascular resistance

Definitive Mx
- Prostaglandin infusion to maintain ductus arteriosus
- Total surgical repair by open heart surgery. 2-stage procedure at 6mo
  ↳ 5% mortality

Transposition of the great arteries

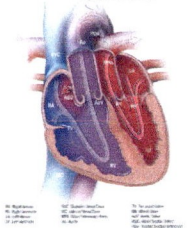

D: attachments of the aorta and the pulmonary trunk to the heart are transposed
- 4.7 per 10,000 live births

R: M>F, diabetic mothers

A/P: embryological discordance between the aorta and pulmonary trunk. Aorta arises from RV, pulmonary trunk arises from LV → two parallel circuits incompatible with life

S/smx:
- Degree of smx depends on other defects, eg PDA, ASD or VSD that allows a shunt for oxygenation
- May be picked up on antenatal US
- Cyanosis, tachypnea
- Loud single S2
- Prominent RV impulse
- Egg-on-side appearance on CXR

Mx:
- Prostaglandin E infusion to maintain ductus arteriosus
- Balloon septostomy - inserting a catheter into foramen ovale via umbilicus, inflate balloon to create large ASD – allows for shunting
- Definitive: open heart surgery

Ebstein's anomaly

D: low insertion of the tricuspid valve resulting in a large atrium and small ventricle. Sometimes referred to as 'atrialisation' of the RV

R: maternal use of lithium.
A/w patent foramen ovale or ASD (80%) resulting in shunt, WPW

S/smx:
- Often present after a few days of birth, after ductus arteriosus closes
- Evidence of HF (e.g. oedema)
- Gallop rhythm heard on auscultation: S3 and S4
- Cyanosis
- SOB and tachypnoea
- Poor feeding
- Collapse or cardiac arrest

Dx/Ix: echo

Mx:
- Medical Mx of arrhythmias and HF
- ? Prophylactic abx to prevent IE
- Definitive Mx by surgical correction

Murmurs and heart sounds in children

- Innocent murmurs in ~80% of children at some time (eg fever, anxiety, etc)
- A flow murmur is the most common
- A venus hum is heard above or below the clavicles, continuous, low pitched
  - abolished pressing the ipsilateral jugular or by lying down
- Still's murmur – heard at LLSE to apex, early systolic, vibratory, loudest on lying flat; child is well

► RED FLAGS ►
- signs of HF · faltering growth
- chest pain · syncope
- unexplained fever · cyanosis
- clubbing · diastolic murmur
- thrills (grade ≥IV) · heave
► Increased suspicion ►
- FHx of CHD

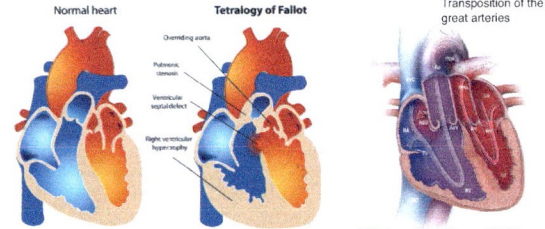

Normal heart / Tetralogy of Fallot / Transposition of the great arteries

Diagrams from Wikipedia

Kawasaki disease

D: Systemic vasculitis that occurs almost exclusively in childhood

R: Asian ancestry (esp Japanese), age 3mo to 4yo

A: ? infection in susceptible host
P: arterial vasculitis and remodelling

Diagnostic criteria
- Classic KD must have 5d of fever refractory to abx therapy (if given) AND ≥4 of the following
- Bilateral conjunctivitis
- Polymorphous rash
- ≥1 mucous membrane change
  - red and cracked lips
  - sore throat / injected pharynx
  - strawberry tongue
- ≥1 extremity change
  - erythema and desquamation of palms/ soles (redness then peeling of skin)
  - periungual desquamation of fingers and toes
- Cervical lymphadenopathy
- Atypical KD may present with fewer of these symptoms

Ix: clinical Dx
Following Dx, pts will need echos to look for coronary artery aneurysms

Mx:
- **High-dose aspirin**
  - 80-100 mg/kg/d PO given in 4 divided doses for 24-72h after fever stops (up to 14d)
  - then 3-5 mg/kg PO OD for 6-8w
- IVIG
- Echo – if coronary artery aneurysms spotted, pt must be referred to paediatric cardiology

Complications
- Coronary artery aneurysms
  - Highest risk in those who do not receive IVIG within 10d of fever onset, and pts who have persistent fever and inflammation despite tx

Abdominal pain - DDx

Acute
- Appendicitis · Gastroenteritis
- Viral illness (eg URTI) a/w mesenteric adenitis
- Constipation · UTI
- Intussusception !
- Torted testis in boys !
- In older girls: consider menses, ovarian cyst, ovarian torsion, PID, ectopic pregnancy

Recurrent
↳ ≥10% of children >5yo suffer recurrent abd pain, with no organic cause in 90%
↳ 4x ↑risk psychological problems in adult life
- Functional abd pain: episodic or continuous pain ≥1x/w for ≥2mo + no evidence of organic disorder
- GI disorders: Coeliac, GORD, IBS, lactose intolerance
- In children with pica, do FBC, iron, ferritin and lead levels
- Psychogenic: stress, depression, family problems, NAI

Rare but serious
- Volvulus · Meckel's diverticulum
- Pancreatitis · Diabetes
- PUD/H pylori infxn · IBD
- Abdominal TB
- Renal stones / gall stones
- Cholecystitis
- Henoch Schonlein purpura

RED FLAGS
- ► wt loss, faltering growth
- ► fever ► GI bleeding
- ► bilious vomiting, lots of vomiting
- ► chronic severe diarrhoea
- ► gross abdo distention
- ► palpable mass or organomegaly
- ► specific tender area
- ► oral ulcers, perianal fistulas, FHx of IBD
- ► back pain

Abdominal pain - DDx

GI obstruction

Air:	· faecal impaction
	· air swallowing
	· malabsorption
Ascites:	· nephrotic syndrome
	· hypoproteinaemia
	· cirrhosis
	· heart failure
Masses:	· Wilm's tumour
	· Neuroblastoma
	· Adrenal tumour
Cysts:	· Polycystic kidney
	· Hepatic cysts
	· Dermoid cysts

Hepatomagaly
- Infxns: mono, CMV, malaria
- Malignancy: leukaemia, lymphoma, neuroblastoma
- Metabolic: Gaucher and Hurler diseases, cystinosis, galactosaemia
- Others: sickle cell disease, haemolytic anaemias, porphyria

Splenomegaly
- as for hepatomagaly, except neuroblastoma

Ix for abd pain / abd distention
- DIP THE URINE
- Ix red flags ± stool for occult blood, US, FBC + CRP/ESR, TTG+IgA, amylase/ lipase, TFTs (if constip), barium studies and consider ref to specialist

Mx if not sinister
- Trial of laxative or antacid if appropriate
- Simple analgesia and antispasmodics
- Avoid dietary interventions unless +ve Hx

See 03.10 for more extensive DDx of abdominal pain

Neuroblastoma

D: malignant tumour arising from the embryological neural crest element of the peripheral sympathetic nervous system – most often at the adrenal medulla
- causes 7-8% of childhood cancer; median age of onset 20mo

S/smx: abdominal swelling
- pallor, wt loss, bone pain, limp, hepatomegaly, paraplegia, proptosis
  - tend to result due to metastasis to LN, scalp, bone

Ix: ↑catecholamines in urine
- Abd XR: calcification
- Biopsy for confirmation

Mx: ref to specialist centre. Excision if possible + chemo

P: depends on genotype. Those <1yo do best. ??Surveillance.

Coeliac disease in children

D: Enteropathy induced by gluten (in wheat, barley, rye)
↳ gluten is a protein found in some grains that acts as a binder

S/smx in children
- Classically presents btwn 6-24mo, after introduction of gluten to diet
- Diarrhoea, anorexia, abd pain and distention, faltering growth ± anaemia
- Signs less obvious in older children – higher level of suspicion req
- A/w other autoimmune disorders, incl T1DM, thyroid disease, JIA; also Down and Turner

Ix: as per adults Ix
Mx: dietary exclusion of gluten
Consider other DDx of malabsorption

See 03.05 for Coeliac disease in adults

Diarrhoea & vomiting

Gastroenteritis
- Rotavirus most common, can cause significant mortality
- Also, norovirus, astrovirus, adenovirus
- Diarrhoea ~5-7d, stops w/in 2w Vomiting ~1-2d, stops w/in 3d

Initial Mx
- Weigh to monitor progress and quantify dehydration
- Start oral rehydration salts (ORS): aim 1mL/kg q5min, continue bfding. Encourage fluid intake if older, ? discourage fruit juices and carbonated drinks

Dx: stool culture if
- septicaemia suspected
- blood/mucus in stool
- immunocompromised child
- ? if child recently abroad
- ? diarrhoea has not improved by d7
- ? uncertain about Dx

Mx of severe dehydration or shock
- Admit for fluids and antiemetics

Chronic diarrhoea
- Most common cause is cows' milk intolerance
- Coeliac disease
- Post-gastroenteritis lactose intolerance (generally resolves after ~7w)

See 08.10 for more extensive DDx of gastroenteritis and diarrhoea

---

Malnutrition

Marasmus: manifestation of severe protein-energy malnutrition which occurs as a result of *total calorie deficiency*
Kwashiorkor: manifestation of severe protein-energy malnutrition a/w *poor-quality diet high in carbs* but low in protein content (child may have sufficient total calorie intake)

Physiologic response to starvation
1. GI absorption of substrate (1-6h)
2. Glycogenolysis (1-2d)
3. Gluconeogenesis (1w)
4. Ketosis (3-4d+)
5. ↑cerebral ketone use (2w+)

S/smx
- wt-for-ht value ≤3x average
- middle-upper arm circumference (MUAC) of <115mm
- specific to Kwashiokor: edema, dermatosis, depigmentation of hair, cheilosis (swelling and fissuring of lips)

Mx
1. Resuscitation & stabilisation
   - rehydrate + prevent infxns, avoid re-feeding syndrome
   - lasts ~1w, pts can be very frail
   - rehydrate with warmed IVF (isotonic)
   - 60-80% of caloric requirement for age, continuous NG feeding at night or small meals at night time, phosphate + vitamin B1
   - monitor closely for refeeding syndrome: arrhythmias, weakness, confusion, etc
2. Nutritional rehabilitation
   - slow increase in caloric intake
   - vaccinations, ↑motor activity
   - lasts 2-6w
3. Follow up, prevent recurrence
   - education, encourage breast-feeding and supplemental feeds
   - educate esp on high protein sources of food

DDx: HIV wasting syndrome (involuntary loss of >10% wt with no other explainable cause), chronic pancreatitis (2/2 Coxsackie B virus, mumps, trauma, CF, etc)

Appendicitis

D: acute inflammation of the vermiform appendix

A: obstruction of lumen of appendix by faecolith, normal stool, or lymphoid hyperplasia
P: obstruction → distension + bacteria multiply

S/smx
· abd pain - starting centrally, then localising to RIF in 1-12h
 - constant with intermittent cramps
 - worse on movement, coughing
 - location of appendix affects location of pain
· use Appendicitis Inflammatory Response (AIR) to quantify risk
 - smx: vomiting, pain in RIF, **migration** of pain to RIF
 - exam: rebound tenderness, guarding, fever
 - bloods: ↑neutrophils, ↑WBC, ↑CRP
· Anorexia is very common; pts unlikely to be hungry
· DRE: boggy sensation, ? right-sided tenderness
· Rovsing's sign (palpation in LIF causing pain in RIF), psoas sign (pain on extending hip if retrocaecal appendix)
· Note: uncommon in <4yo

Dx/Ix:
· Establish IV access
· If ↓BP/septic, catheterise + fluid balance
· Request FBC (Hb, WCC), U&Es, CRP
· Dx can be clinical
 - in children, US first
 - US in females where pelvic organ pathology is suspected
 - CT scan only if inconclusive

Mx: appendectomy (usually lap)
· prophylactic IV abx
· pts with perforated appendicitis require copious abdo lavage
· ? conservative Mx with only abx (depends on surgeon)

Intussusception

D: prolapse of one part of intestine into the lumen of the adjoining distal part, causing intestinal obstruction.

R: M>F, 6-12mo

A: unclear, but likely related to hyperplasia of Peyer's patches and lymphoid tissue in the intestinal wall after antecedent viral infxn
In older children/adults, pathological lead point (anatomical abn eg luminal polyps)
P: telescoping of intestine. Mesen-tery is dragged in, obstructing venous return → oedema, mucosal bleeding, ↑pressure

Features:
· intermittent, severe, crampy, progressive abdominal pain
· inconsolable crying
· during paroxysm the infant will characteristically draw their knees up and turn pale
 - typically infant is relatively settled between bouts of pain
· vomiting
· bloodstained stool - 'red-currant jelly' – is a late sign
· sausage-shaped mass in the RUQ

Dx/Ix: US (donut or target sign), plain XR (soft tissue mass, SBO, free air).

Mx:
· IVF + ensure fluid balance
· Analgesia + sedation (morphine 0.2mg/kg)
· Abx + NGT.   · Xmatch + G&S 2U
· Radiological reduction: air enema works in 75%. If irreducible or perfora-tion, halt and convert to surgical Mx
 ↳ recurrence 5-7%
· Surgical reduction: laparatomy without enema if evidence of peritonitis or perforation. Manual reduction by retrograde squeezing and gentle proximal traction
 - resection and anastomosis if bowel viability is in doubt
 - post-reduction septic shock may occur 2/2 bacterial product
· Resume oral feeding in 24-48h and discharge home in 4-5d

Pyloric stenosis

D: hypertrophy of the pyloric sphincter results in narrowing of the pyloric canal
· incidence 4 in 1000 live births
· M>F 4x. · 10-15% +ve FHx
· first borns more affected

A: no single aetiology. Hypertrophy of pyloric smooth muscle in early infancy (3-6w)
P: prolonged vomiting → ↓Cl-, ↓K+ met alkalosis, etc

S/smx:
· 'projectile' vomiting, typically 30 min after a feed
· ± constipation and dehydration
· ± palpable mass in the upper abdo
· hypochloraemic, hypokalaemic alkalosis 2/2 persistent vomiting
· Test feeding will reveal a pyloric 'tumour' (middle of epigastric)
· Vomit will not have bile, no diarrhoea (constipation will be likely), baby is rarely obtunded

Dx/Ix: clinical. If in doubt, US – thickened (>4mm), elongated (>16mm) pyloric muscle, ↑muscle to lumen ratio with ↓fluid movement.
· Bloods: U&Es, ABG

Mx: · Resus with IVF
· Correct hypovol: 10mL/kg 0.9%NS
· Correct electrolyte imbalance: 0.45% NS / 5% dextrose with KCl at a rate of 120-150 mL/kg/24h
· NGT drainage to prevent aspiration
· Ramstedt pyloromyotomy
 - division of pyloric muscle fibres without opening bowel lumen
· Start feeding within 4-6h post-op, ↑ to full volume by 24h

Hirschsprung disease

D: congenital condition characterised by partial or complete colonic **functional obstruction** associated with the absence of ganglion cells
· 1 in 5000 births
· M>F 3x. A/w Down's syndrome

A: genetic (a/w 24 genes)
P: absence of ganglion cells, presence of hypertrophic nerves, ↑AChE. Failure in the development of tissue derived from the neural crest.

S/smx: · Neonatal period, eg failure or delay to pass meconium
· Older children: constipation, abdo distension

Dx/Ix: · Clinical smx
· Enema XR looking for transition zone
· **Rectal biopsy** + histology

Mx: · Resus + analgesia
· Decompression of colon with regular saline rectal washouts
· Defunctioning stoma if decompression not achieved or if whole colon involved
· Definitive surgery

Gross types
A. Gap between two esophageal blind pouches with no fistula
B. Esophageal atresia with *proximal* tracheoesophageal fistula
C. Esophageal atresia with *distal* tracheoesophageal fistula
D. Esophageal atresia with *proximal and distal* tracheosophageal fistula
E. Tracheoesophageal fistula only

Oesophageal atresia / Tracheo-oesophageal atresia

D: congenital malformations that result from the defective separation of the common embryologic precursors to both the oesophagus and trachea
· 1 in 2500-4500 live births
· can present with other anomalies

Prenatal signs · Polyhydramnios
· small/absent stomach bubble
Postnatal signs
· Respi distress, ↑secretions, aspirating feeds
· Smx depends on anatomy; H-type TOF may present much later

Dx/Ix: antenatal US/MRI, XR chest/abdo will show NGT coiled in upper pouch

Mx: depends on anatomy
· Generally, pts kept NBM with continuous oesophageal pouch suction (Replogle tube).
· Primary surgical repair.
· Consider Mx of other anomalies

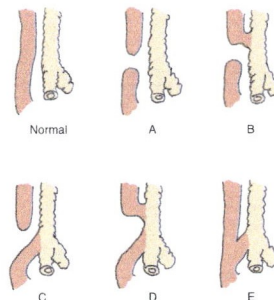

Normal   A   B

C   D   E

Diagram adapted from UCSF Pediatric Surgery website

Congenital diaphragmatic hernia

D: protrusion of abdominal contents into the thoracic cavity due to defect in diaphragm. 1:2400 - only 50% survival

S/smx: usually Dx prenatally by US
- On birth, respi distress, cyanosis, ↓breath sounds + bowel sounds in hemithorax, displaced heart sounds, scaphoid abdomen
- Small hernias may present later on with minor problems
- 61% have other abnormalities

Dx/Ix: · Prenatal US, postnatal CXR

Prenatal Mx:
- fetal tracheal obstruction by balloon, which encourages lung growth and pushes out viscera
Postnatal Mx:
- Intubate, ventilate, paralyse with minimal pressures
- DO NOT use facemask ventilation, as air may enter gut
- Surgery in tertiary centre

Inguinal hernia

D: protrusion of abdominal or pelvic contents through a dilated internal inguinal ring or attenuated inguinal floor into the inguinal canal

S/smx: bulge lateral to pubic tubercle when ↑abdo pressure, eg crying
- R>L   · M>F 5:1
Impt DDx: hydrocele
- Similar etiology, but only allows fluid from peritoneal cavity to pass through. Generally closes during 1st year of life.
- If it persists after 2y, may need surgical closure

Mx: 6-2 rule
- baby <6w: repair within 2d
  ↳ greatest risk of strangulation
- <6mo: repair within 2mw
- <6yo: repair within 2mo

See 03.06 for more hernias

Imperforate anus

D: congenital anorectal malformation where a normal anal opening is absent at birth
- 1 in 5000 births in US. M>F slightly
- a/w some specific syndromes, trisomies. a/w other abnormalities.

S/smx: · Failure to pass meconium within 24h
- Meconium in urine
  - girls may have fourchette fistula
  - boys may have posterior urethral fistula

Dx/Ix: · GU imaging to find other anomalies

Mx: posterior sagittal anorectoplasty

Mid-gut malrotation

D: spectrum of rotational and fixation disturbances that can occur during embryonic development

A: arrested rotation → abn intestinal fixations + malrotation
P: malrotation ↑ susceptibility to volvulus, ischaemia, necrosis.

S/smx of volvulus: 3-7d after birth
- Bilious neonatal vomiting → immediate surgical ref (+NGT)
- Also: epigastric distention, pain, a/w abnormalities of adjacent organs
- ± feeding difficulties
- Blood PR (? mid-gut necrosis) → emergency surgical decompression

Dx/Ix: UGI contrast study - DJ flexure is more medially placed. US may show abn orientation of SMA and SMV

Mx: **Ladd's procedure**

Gastroschisis and omphalocele

D: congenital defects of the abdominal wall resulting in intestinal herniation from the abdominal cavity
- **Gastroschisis** (1 in 3000): para-umbilical defect with evisceration of abdo contents.
- **Omphalocele**: defect of umbilical ring with herniation of abd viscera. Covered by peritoneum and amniotic membrane
  - major >4cm & minor <4cm
  - 72% a/w other malformations
  - a/w Beckwith-Wiedemann, Down's

R: maternal age <20yo (G) or >35 (O), M>F, smoking

Dx/Ix: antenatal US

Mx of gastroschisis:
- Vaginal delivery may be attempted
- Surgical emergency!
- At delivery, cover exposed bowel in cling film, avoid heat and fluid loss
- Theatre asap (within 4h)
- TPN may be required for a while

Mx of omphalocele:
- C-sec to ↓risk of sac rupture
- Staged repair if needed
  - allows sac to granulate and epitheliases over coming weeks
  - as infant grows, the sac contents will be able to fit within the abdo cavity. The shell will then be removed, and abdomen closed

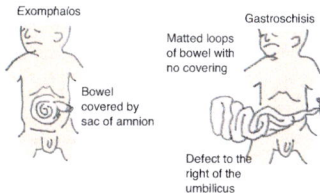

Exomphalos

Bowel covered by sac of amnion

Matted loops of bowel with no covering

Gastroschisis

Defect to the right of the umbilicus

Diagram adapted from OHCS

Meckel's diverticulum

D: Congenital diverticulum of the small intestine – contains mucosa
- Rule of 2s:
  - occurs in 2% of the population
  - 2% are symptomatic
  - 2 times more common in males
  - is 2 feet from the ileocaecal valve
  - 2 inches long

S/smx: generally symptomatic when pt is younger
- Painless rectal bleeding ("currant jelly" coloured stool) in children or melaena in adults
- Abdominal pain – can present similarly to appendicitis

Ix: "Meckel's scan" (usually in kids) – technetium scan, or mesenteric arteriography in more severe cases

Mx:
- if active bleeding + large blood loss, pt may need to have blood transfusion
- Definitively, resection of diverticulum

Infantile colic
- D: Excessive crying and fussing in children. Occurs in 20% of infants
- S/smx: Usually <3mo old
  - Bouts of excessive crying
  - Pulling up legs
  - Usually worse in evening
- Mx: watch & wait. NICE does not recommend use of simeticone or lactase

Infant feeding problems

Cow's milk protein intolerance
- D: Immediate or delayed reaction to proteins present in cow's milk
  - occurs in 3-6% of all children
- S/smx:
  - Presents in first 3mo of exposure to formula milk (containing cow's milk)
  - Regurgitation, vomiting, diarrhoea
  - Urticaria, atopic eczema
  - "Colic" smx: irritability, crying
  - Wheezing, chronic cough
  - Rarely, angiooedema and anaphylaxis
- Ix: usually clinical Dx ± skin prick/patch testing, total IgE and specific IgE for cow's milk protein
- Mx:
  - ⚬ Extensively hydrolysed formula
  - ⚬ Amino acid-based formula
  - If breastfed, continue bfding, eliminate cow's milk from maternal diet + consider use of calcium supplements
    ◊ Use extensively hydrolysed formula when stopping bfding, until 12mo of age and for ≥6mo
- P: usually self-resolving by 3-5yo

GORD in kids
- R: preterm babies, neuro disorders
- S/smx:
  - Presents in first 8w of life
  - Regurgitation, vomiting after feeds or when laid flat
- Ix: usually clinical Dx
- Mx:
  - 30° heads up position while feeding
  - Babies should still sleep on their backs (↓risk of cot death)
  - Ensure baby not overfed, consider trial of smaller and more frequent feeds
  - Trial of thickened formula
  - Trial of alginate therapy (not at the same time as thickened formula)
  - PPI trial *only if*
    ◊ unexplained feeding difficulties
    ◊ distressed behaviour
    ◊ faltering growth

Urinary tract infection

Bacteriuria = bacteria in urine uncontaminated by urethral flora

Vesicoureteric reflux = urine flowing backwards from bladder to kidneys via ureters
· Grade I: incomplete filling of upper urinary tract without dilatation
· II: Complete filling ± slight dilation
· III: Ballooned calyces
· IV: Megaureter
· V: + hydronephrosis

Reflux nephropathy: renal scarring 2/2 reflux (can lead to HTN, ESRD)

· More common in boys until 3mo
· 8% girls, 2% boys UTI in childhood
· Up to 40% have GU abn

Presentation
· Infant: poor feeding, vomitting, irritability
· Younger children: abd pain, fever, dysuria
· Older: dysuria, frequency, haematuria
· UTI: temp >38°C, loin pain/tenderness

Dx/Ix:
· If asmx, DO NOT test urine
· Test urine if
  - s/smx suggestive of UTI
  - unexplained fever ≥38°C
  - with alternative site of infxn but remain unwell
· Urine sample
  - Clean catch preferred, if not use urine collection pads
  - Invasive methods (eg suprapubic aspiration) as last resort

Mx: · Infants <3mo - immediate ref to paediatrician
· If upper UTI: consider admission. PO abx (cephalosporin or coamoxiclav) for 7-10d
· Lower UTI: trimethoprim, nitrofurantoin, cephalosporin, amoxicillin for 3d
  ↳ come back if still unwell 24-48h
· Consider prophylaxis if recurrent

Nephrotic syndrome

Defined as the presence of
1. proteinuria (>3.5g per 24h)
2. hypoalbuminaemia (<30g/L)
3. peripheral oedema
Not a single disease, but a syndrome caused by several renal diseases.

Aetiology
· **Minimal change disease**
  - ? idiopathic
  - 2/2 Hodgkin's L, leukemia, etc
  - peak onset <6yo, M:F 2:1
· Intrinsic kidney disease: FSGS
· 2/2 systemic illness: HSP, diabetes, infection, amyloidosis
Pathophysiology
· Podocytes are affected → glomerular proteinuria
· Urinary loss of albumin 2/2 glomerula damage
  - liver tries to compensate for protein loss, and in the process, there is ↑cholesterol production
· Oedema 2/2 ↓oncotic pressure from hypoalbuminaemia + primary renal Na retention
· Hypercoagulability and thrombosis 2/2 loss of anticoagulant proteins

S/smx: · well child with insidious onset of pitting oedema, initially periorbital, then generalised
· Often Hx of recent URTI
· May progress to anorexia, GI Δ, irritability, ascites, oliguria, SOB
· Risk of infection and thrombosis

Dx/Ix: · Urine: frothy, protein 3+, PCR >200, Na <10
· Blood: albumin <25, U&Es, lipids, C3/C4 (normal), Hb
· MCD: urinalysis will show small molecular wt proteins and hyaline casts
· Note: visible haematuria, HTN, ↑↑Cr not typical features

Mx: · By experienced paediatrician
· High dose steroids (ie pred)
  - pred 60 mg/m2/d (max 80mg) for 4w, then 40 mg/m2 alt days for 4w then taper
  - 80% steroid sensitive, 80% will relapse at some point and require more steroids
  - pts who struggle to wean are referred to as steroid dependant
  - for steroid resistant, use ACEI and immunosuppressants (eg tacrolimus, cyclosporine)
· Low sat diet (high protein diet NOT recommended)
· Diuretics for oedema
· Albumin if prn
· Abx prophylaxis if severe
· Note: live vaccines CI in children receiving high dose prednisolone

Complications
· Hypovolaemia - fluid leaks from intravascular space into interstitial space → oedema and low BP
· Thrombosis - kidneys leak clotting factors
· Infxn - kidney leaks immunoglobulins + use of steroids
· Acute or chronic renal failure
· Relapse: defined as ≥3+ proteinuria for 3 consecutive days

Minimal change disease
· D: the most common form of nephrotic syndrome in children, characterised by minimal histological changes in the kidney
· R: 1-8yo, Hodgkin's lymphoma, leukaemia, recent viral illness
· A: 90% idiopathic
· P: see nephrotic syndrome
· S/smx: · nephrotic syndrome
  · Normotensive
  · Highly selective proteinuria (eg albumin, transferrin)
· Ix: renal biopsy (normal glomeruli, fusion of podocytes, effacement of foot processes)
· Mx: as per nephrotic syndrome
· P: 1/3 have frequent relapses, 1/3 have infrequent relapses

Acute glomerulonephritis

D: glomerular injury usually involving inflammatory changes in the glomerular capillaries and the GBM

A: leukocyte infiltration, antibody deposition, complement activation
· Infections
· Systemic inflammatory conditions eg SLE, RA, anti-GBM disease
· Drugs (eg lithium, PTU, NSAIDs)
· Metabolic disorders (eg DM)
· Malignancy
· Hereditary disorders (eg Fabry's disease, Alport's)
· Deposition diseases (eg amyloidosis)
P: most nephritic syndromes are triggered by immune-mediated injury

Features
· **Haematuria** with red cell casts
  ↳ macro or microscopic
· Proteinuria   · Oliguria
· Hypertension (~50%)
  ↳ more common in nephritic syndrome

Complicated presentations
· Hypertensive encephalopathy: restless, drowsy, severe HA, fits, ↓vision, vomiting, coma
· AKI: acidosis, hyperK, seizure, stupor
· Fluid overload: pulmonary oedema, cardiac failure
· Mixed nephritic-nephrotic syndrome

A patient can have a "nephritic syndrome" (i.e., inflammation of the kidneys) resulting in "nephrotic syndrome" (i.e., the triad of proteinuria, hypoalbuminuria, and peripheral oedema)
↳ this is esp the case if glomerular inflammation results in damage to the podocytes (which then causes severe proteinuria)

Dx/Ix: urinalysis, bloods, throat swabs, CXR (if fluid overload suspected). Renal biopsy if severe.

Mx: supportive
· Tx underlying infxn/cause
· Monitor fluid balance.
  - Fluid restriction if oliguric
  - Diuretics if overloaded
· Check BP often + Mx HTN + low salt
· If encephalopathy, give sodium nitroprusside
· HD if severe renal failure

Post-strep glomerulonephritis
· Most common cause of acute GN in children
· Presents 7-21d after strep infxn (pharyngitis, impetigo)
· S/smx: HTN, haematuria ± oedema, malaise, anorexia, fever, abdo pain
· Dx/Ix: clinical + confirm recent strep infxn with ASO titre, anti-DNAseB, throat swab
· Mx: supportive
  - PO penicillin for 10d to ↓ spread of nephritogenic bacterial strains
  - Oedema usually resolves in 5-10d
  - HTN, haematuria, proteinuria may last for several weeks or months
· Prognosis is very good: 95% recovery

Phimosis

D: non-retractable foreskin with associated scarring that will not resolve spontaneously

A: physiological in boys ≤~4yo. By 11yo, prevalence is <8%.
· Recurrent balanoposthitis, balanitis xerotica obliterans (BXO) – foreskin looks pale, thickened, scarred, repeated forced retraction
P: Circumferential scarring

S/smx: · Non-retractable foreskin
  - May present with ballooning during micturation
· Retention of urine
· Paraphimosis (engorgement)
· Obstruction

Dx/Ix: clinical

Mx: · Analgesia
· Paraphimosis is a medical emergency
  - Manipulation with ice packs, compression, osmotic agent
  - Puncture technique
  - Surgical reduction + circumcision
· Phimosis
  - Wait and see approach
  - Topical corticosteroids (esp before 8yo)
  - Stretching exercises bds x 15d, then od x 15d
· General: personal hygiene!!

Cryptorchidism

D: undescended testis; one or both testes are not present within the dependent portion of the scrotal sac by 3mo.
· D: ≤5% boys at birth; 1-2% at 3mo
· May be a/w other defects

R: FHx, prematurity (15-30%), low birth wt and/or SFGA

A: unknown
P: incomplete migration of testis during embryogenesis from original retroperitoneal position near kidneys to final position in scrotum

Dx/Ix: physical exam in supine position
S/smx:
· malpositioned or absent testis
· palpable cryptorchid testis (unable to be pulled into scrotum, or returns to higher position after pulling)
· non-palpable testis
· ± testicular asymmetry, scrotal hypoplasia
DDx: retractile testis (where testis can be manipulated into scrotum)

Mx:
· Orchidopexy at 6-18mo
  - Inguinal exploration, mobilisation of testis and implantation into a dartos pouch
· If presenting late (eg in teenage years), orchidectomy may be better due to ↑risk of malignancy

Reasons for operating
· ↓risk of infertility
· Allows testes to be examined for testicular cancer
  - undescended testis - 40x as likely to develop seminoma
  - the higher the testis is in the abdomen, the higher the risk is
· Avoid testicular torsion
· Cosmesis

Hypospadias

D: urethra is abnormally located on the ventral surface of the penis
· 1 in 350 male births
· a/w cryptorcidism 10%, inguinal hernia

R: FHx (further male children risk 5-15%)

Features
· Ventral (anterior) urethral meatus
· Hooded prepuce
· Chordee (ventral curvature of the penis) in more severe forms
· Urethral meatus may open more proximally in severe variants (25%)

Mx: · Corrective surgery ~12mo
· DO NOT circumcise before surgery as foreskin may be needed
· In boys with very distal disease, no tx may be needed

Horseshoe kidney

D: fusion defect of the kidneys 2/2 abn position, rotation and vascular supply of the kidneys
· 1 in 500. 90% U shape (lower pole)
· M>F 2:1.
· ?a/w chromosomal disorders

Features:
· Usually asmx, identified incidentally
· May present with abdo pain, UTI infxn

Dx/Ix: US or CT/MRI. CT urogram may help identify stones, blockages and uretopelvic junction blocks.
DDx: crossed fusion renal ectopia or fused pelvic kidney

Mx: symptomatic - regular corrective surgery not rec.
· ↑risk of cancers incl transitional cell tumours (3-4x), Wilms tumour (2x), carcinoid cancer (62-82x)

Wilms' tumour (nephroblastoma)

D: most common childhood renal malignancy; undifferentiated mesodermal tumour of the intermediate cell mass
· presents in children <5yo

A/w: Beckwith-Wiedemann syndrome, WAGR syndrome, hemihypertrophy. 1/3 a/w loss of function mutation in the WT1 gene on chromosome 11.

Features:
· abdominal mass (most common)
  - ballotable, does not move on inspiration
· painless haematuria
· flank pain
· others: anorexia, fever
· unilateral in 95% of cases
· Metastases are found in 20% of pts (most commonly lung)

Staging:
1. Tumour confined to kidney
2. Extrarenal spread, but resectable
3. Extensive abdominal disease
4. Distant metastases
5. Bilateral disease

Dx/Ix: US abdo, CT/MRI (staging, planning op)

Mx: · Urgent (48h) paeds review for children with unexplained enlarged abdo mass
· Nephrectomy
· Chemotherapy
· Radiotherapy if advanced disease

Prognosis is good with 80-90% cure rate. If a/w other genetic conditions, much poorer prognosis

Haemolytic uraemic syndrome

D: microangiopathic haemolytic anaemia, thrombocytopenia, and acute kidney injury
· 90% in children ∴ Shiga toxin-producing E.coli

A: toxin induces damage to endothelium of glomerular capillary bed causing thrombotic microangiopathy
In familial HUS, dysregulation in complement cascade triggers atypical HUS
P: endothelial injury leads to microvascular thrombosis → MAHA, thrombocytopenia, and AKI

Dx/Ix: FBC (anaemia - Hb <8, -ve Coombs test), thrombocytopenia (↓platelets), fragmented blood film (schistocytes and helmet cells), U&Es (AKI), stool culture (looking for STEC infxn, PCR looking for Shiga toxins)

Mx: supportive (fluids, blood trf, dialysis)
· Abx NOT recommended
· ?Plasma exchange - only in severe cases not a/w diarrhea
· Eculizumab ??

Epilepsy

D: tendency to recurrent unprovoked seizures (abn electrical brain activity)
· 1% of children will have a seizure not a/w fever by 14yo
· ÷ generalised, focal, unknown
  ↳ focal further ÷ awareness
· ÷ signs: motor, non-motor

Infantile spasms (West's syndrome)
· Brief spasms ~3-9mo
· Flexion of head, trunk, limbs, then extension of arms - last 1-2s, repeat up to 50x
· EEG: hypsarrhythmia
· Usually 2/2 serious neuro abn (eg tuberous sclerosis, encephalitis, birth asphyxia). May be idiopathic
· Possible tx: vigabatrin, steroids
· Poor prognosis

Lennox-Gestaut syndrome
· ? extension of infantile spasms
· Onset 1-5yo
· Atypical absences, falls, jerks; 90% mod-severe mental handicap
· EEG: slow spike
· Tx: ?ketogenic diet

Absence seizures
· Generalised seizures (i.e., LOC) – pt is unaware of LOC
· Onset 4-8yo.
· Each episode lasts <30s, no warning, quick recovery
· EEG: 3Hz generalised, symmetrical
· Tx: sodium valproate, ethosuximide
· Good prognosis; 90-95% seizure-free in adolescence

Juvenile myoclonic epilepsy (Janz syndrome)
· Typical onset teenage years, F>M
· Infrequent generalised seizures, often in morning or following sleep depri-vation. Daytime absences. Sudden, shock-like myoclonic seizures
· Mx: sodium valproate. Sleep.

See **04.06** for more on seizures, epilepsy and anticonvulsants

Panayiotopoulos syndrome
· 6% of all epilepsies
· Benign focal epilepsy presenting in early childhood 4-7yo
· Autonomic smx dominate: vomiting, sweating, eye deviation, impaired consciousness ± bilat clonic activity. Usually occurs at night.
· May last for >30min
· No brain damage
· EEG: shifting ± multiple foci, occipital predominance
· Mx: remission usually occurs within 2y, medication not needed

Febrile seizures/convulsions
· = single tonic-clonic, symmetrical generalised seizure lasting <15min, occuring as temperature ↑ rapidly in a febrile illness in a normally developing child, occuring only once in 24h
· 3% of children have ≥1 FS, +ve FHx is common

Dx/Ix: find source of infxn, look for signs of meningitis
· MSU, CXR, ENT swabs
· Avoid LP in postictal period

Mx: · O2 + recovery position
· check glucose
· if fit lasts >5min, tx as SE
· Parental education
  - allay fear (child is not dying)
  - FS is a/w ≤3% risk of epilepsy
    ◊ risk ↑ if FHx+ve, complex features (focal onset, >15min, >1 seizure in 24h), developmental abn
  - Recurrence of FS is common
  - If seizure >5min call ambulance

AED options by seizure types
· GTC - M: sodium valproate
  - F: lamotrigine, carbamazepine
  - Adjunctive tx: clobazam, levetiracetam, topiramate
· Absence - 1st: ethosuximide
  - 2nd: sodium valproate
  - Others: lamotrigine, combination
  - Avoid: (all others)
· Myoclonic: sodium valproate, levetiracitam, topiramate
· Tonic or atonic: 1st sodium valproate, 2nd lamotrigine

Status epilepticus Mx

0min:	ABC
· Secure airway   · High flow O2
· Basic obs + glucose
  - if hypoglycemic: 2-5mL/kg IV glucose 10%, repeat glucose
· Secure IV/IO access
· Estimate wt   · Set clock in motion

5min:	· Lorazepam 0.1 mg/kg IV/IO slow bolus, or
· Buccal midazolam 0.5mg/kg (massage btwn lower gum and cheek), or
· Rectal diazepam 0.5mg/kg

15min: · Repeat lorazepam
· Call for senior help
· Reconfirm epileptic seizure
· Prep phenytoin

25min:
· Phenytoin 20 mg/kg IVI over 20 min (monitor ECG), or
· Phenobarbital 20 mg/kg over 20min
· Call PICU and anaesthetist
  - prep for intubation

45min: · RSI with thiopental sodium 4mg/kg IV/IO
· Transfer to PICU

Tests
· Obs + glucose
· Consider - bloods (electrolytes)
  - ABG   - FBC + CRP
  - Septic screen
  - Anticonvulsant levels
  - Toxicology screen, incl CO, lead
  - Blood ammonia
· Consider CT if focal seizures or focal neurologic signs

· Focal: 1st carbamazepine or lamotrigine, 2nd sodium valproate, oxcarbazepine or levetiracetam

Other options
· Ketogenic diet (? can ↓fits by 2/3)
  - SE: constipation, vomiting, etc
· Surgery: if there is an epileptogenic focus
· Vagal nerve stimulation: mainly for focal seizures not for surgery

Stopping anticonvulsants
· Do not stop abruptly
· Taper over ≥6w

Brain tumours

D: malignancy of the brain
· **Medulloblastoma** - midline cerebellar embryonal tumour (inferior vermis)
  - S/smx: causing ↑ICP, speech difficulty, truncal ataxia ± falls
  - Seeding along CSF pathways
  - M>F 4:1; peak age 4yo
· **Brainstem astrocytoma**
  - a/w NF1, prior radiation
  - S/smx: CN palsies, pyramidal tract signs (eg hemiparesis), cerebellar ataxia
  - Most common brain tumour in children
· **Midbrain and 3rd ventricle tumours**
  - may be astrocytomas, pinealomas, or colloid cysts
  - S/smx: posture-dependent drowsiness, behaviour change, pyramidal tract and cerebellar signs, upward gaze defect
· **Suprasellar glioma**
  - S/smx: visual field defects, optic atrophy, pituitary disorders (growth arrest, hypothyroidism, delayed puberty), DI
· **Cerebral hemispheres**
  - usually gliomas, rarely meningiomas
  - S/smx: fits common; other signs depend on the lobe involved
  - Mx seizures, ↑ICP (dexamethasone, CSF shunt), and endocrine abn. Excision if possible, radiotherapy, chemo

▶ RED FLAGS ▶
· HA: >2w that wake child from sleep or occur on waking; persistent HA in any child <4yo; HA a/w confusion or disorientation; persistent HA
· Vomiting: >2w vomiting on waking, persistent vomiting
· Visual system: papilloedema; optic atrophy; new onset nystagmus; proptosis; new-onset paralytic squint or diplopia; reduced visual acuity or visual fields not due to ocular cause
· Motor system: motor skill regression; focal motor weakness; abn gait/ataxia; swallowing difficulties; persistent head tilt without cause; Bell's palsy with no improvement in 4w

When to ref for imaging?
· ≥2 s/smx suggestive of tumour and
· Endocrine s/smx
  - precocious, arrested or delayed puberty
  - galactorrhea   - ammenorrhea
  - growth failure   - DI (polyuria, dipsia)
· Other s/smx
  - ↑head size, macrocepahy
    ↳ most common presenting smx in <4yo - measure head circumference!!
  - Persisting lethargy
  - Behavioural change (new mood disturbance, withdrawal, disinhibition)
  - Dysphagia, dysphasia
  - New focal seizures

Referral
· Discuss with specialist same day if tumour suspected
· Child should be seen within 2w
· Imaging reported <4w
· MRI, contrast CT if MRI unavailable
  ↳ EEG not useful

DDx (space occupying lesions)
· Aneurysms   · Haematomas
· Granulomas   · Tuberculomas
· Cysts (neurocysticercosis)
· Abscess - suspect if ↑ICP, ↑temp, ↑WCC

Spinal tumours
· Consider in children presenting with back or neck pain, gait abn, focal weakness, or scoliosis
· Rare

See **04.07** for more on brain tumours and localisation smx

Neural tube defects

D: spectrum of disorders that can affect the brain or the spinal cord

R: inadequate maternal folate/B12 intake, antenatal exposure to valproate, carbamazepine, isotretinoin or methotrexate, prev affected pregnancy (10x risk), maternal hx of spina bifida or other neural tube defect, maternal obesity or diabetes

A: genetic + environmental factors
P: failure of normal fusion of the neural plate to form the neural tube during the first 28 days following conception

Anencephaly
- Failure to develop most of cranium and brain
- Most infants born stillborn or die shortly after birth
- Can be detected on antenatal US – offer termination of pregnancy

Encephalocele
- Extrusion of brain and meninges through midline skull defect
- Usually a/w cerebral malformations

Spina bifida occulta
- Failure of fusion of vertebral arch
- Aka closed spinal dysraphism
- S/smx:
  - may be asmx (identified incidentally on XR)
  - overlying skin lesion (eg tuft of hair, lipoma, etc) in lumbar region usually
  - **Tethered cord syndrome**
    ◊ ↓ lower limb function: children begin to stumble after they have learnt to walk normally
    ◊ ↓ bladder function: children classically start to dribble after being successfully toilet trained
    ◊ other findings: footdrop, painless sores, scoliosis, back pain exacerbated by exercise in older children

Meningocele
- Herniation of the meninges without involvement of spinal elements
- Apart from visible deformity, there are no neurological smx

Myelomeningocele
- Herniation of both meninges and spinal cord
  - 80% involves lumbar and sacral region
  - A/w Chiari II malformation and hydrocephalus – downward displacement of cerebellar tonsils and medulla (= Chiari II), obstruction of CSF flow through posterior fossa → hydrocephalus
- S/smx
  - Chiari II + hydrocephalus – can cause cognitive deficits, attention deficits, stridor, apnea, etc
  - Neurologic deficits depends on level of lesion; typically affects trunk, legs, bladder and bowel
  - urinary and faecal incontinence affects 97% population
- Ix: Dx on antenatal US or on direct visualisation at birth
- Mx
  - Surgery soon after birth to close up the back lesion
    ◊ in some centres, fetal surgery can be performed during pregnancy
  - Physiotherapy for paralysis and muscle imbalances
  - Skin care required to avoid sores (↓sensation conveys ↑risk)
  - Catheterisation for neuropathic bladder, and regular toileting for bowel incontinence

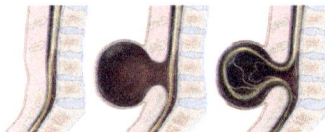

Spina bifida occulta   Meningocele   Myelomeningocele

Autism spectrum disorder

D: lifelong neurodevelopmental condition characterised by persistent impairments in social communica-tion, and restricted, repetitive, and stereotyped patterns of behaviours, interests, or activities

R: M>F (4:1), FHx +ve, valproate exposure in pregnancy

A: genetic element
P: modified brain development → reorganisation of neural networks underlying cognition and behaviour

DSM5 criteria
- Persistent deficits in social communication and interaction across multiple contexts
  - ↓social-emotional reciprocity
  - ↓non-verbal communicative behaviours used for social interaction
  - ↓developing/understanding relationships
- Restricted, repetitive patterns of behaviour, interests or activities
  - Stereotyped or repetitive motor movements, use of objects, or speech
  - Insistence of sameness, inflexible adherence to routines, or ritualised patterns of verbal or non-verbal behaviour
  - Highly restricted, fixated interests that are abnormal in intensity or focus
  - Hyper- or hyporeactivity to sensory input or unusual interest in sensory aspects of the environment

DSM5 criteria (cont)
- Smx must be present in the early developmental period
- Smx cause clinically significant impairment in social, occupational, or other impt areas of current functioning

÷ 3 levels of severity
- Level 1: some support
- Level 2: substantial support
- Level 3: very substantial support

Note: Asperger syndrome has been removed as a diagnostic entity in current classification systems.

Ix: If a child is suspected to have ASD (usually presents around 2-4yo), ref to MDT is needed for assessment

Mx:
- Early educational and behavioural interventions
- Pharmacological
  - SSRI – may help ↓anxiety, depression and repetitive stereotyped behaviour
  - Antipsychotic drugs: ↓aggression, self-harm
  - Methylphenidate: ADHD
- Family support and counselling

Complications / assoc conditions
- Intellectual disability in 40-80%
- Epilepsy: tends to develop in young children or in adolescence
  - higher rates in those with intellectual disability
- Psych: anxiety and depression

Cleft lip and palate
- D: Congenital malformation of the lip and hard palate due to disruption of the embryological growth process
  - 1:1000 births
- Subtypes: isolated cleft lip (15%), isolated cleft palate (40%), combined cleft lip and palate (45%)
- **R: Maternal antiepileptic use**, FHx, genetic or metabolic disorder (eg diGeorge syndrome)
- S/smx:
  - Visible deformity
  - Feeding problems
  - Speech problems
  - ↑incidence of otitis media
- Mx: Surgery – cleft lip repaired before 3mo old usually, cleft palate repaired btwn 6-12mo old

Anaemia

► RED FLAGS ►
- SOB
- Syncope
- Lymphadenopathy
- Hepatosplenomegaly
- Unexplained bone pain
- Haematuria
- Faltering growth
- Fever
- Bruising
- Jaundice
- ↓WCC
- Melaena
- ↓platelets

Ix: FBC, reticulocytes, film, ferritin, CRP/ESR

DDx

Microcytic
- IDA - ↓Fe, ↓ferritin
- Thalassemia
- G6PD deficiency
- Sideroblastic anaemia

Normocytic
- Haemolysis
- Marrow failure
- Thyroid dysfunction
- Anaemia of chronic disease

Macrocytic
- ↓folate (malabs, phenytoin)
- ↓B12 (breast milk from veggie, ↓IF, malabsorption)
- Diamond-Blackfan
- Fanconi's

Eosinophilia + tropics → ?helminth infxn (hookworm, roundworm, etc)

Severe tropical anaemia
- Malaria
- Worms
- ↓B12, G6PD deficiency, malnutrition, sickle cell
- Bacteraemia
- HIV, TB

Haemolysis
- Is malaria or SCD possible?
- Intravascular vs extravascular
  ↳ I: haemoglobinuria
  ↳ E: splenomegaly
- Inborn error or acquired defect?
  ↳ Acquired: Coombs test

See 10.04 for more on Anaemia

Iron def anaemia in children   IDA

- 26% infants worldwide, peak 18mo

S/smx: - less happy baby, ↓ psycho-motor development, poor cognition
- Pallor, lethargy, stomatitis, koilonychia, pica

Dx/Ix: In persistent IDA, suspect bleeding (menorrhagia, IBD, cow's milk protein allergy, Meckel's diverticulum)

Mx: · Trial of iron supp: fumarate syrup
- Aim for Hb rise of >10g/L/mo – response confirms Dx
- Warn of dangers of overdose
- Deworm pts

Prevention:
- No cow's milk if <1yo
- If formula-fed, use iron-fortified, wean at 4-6mo
- Adequate vit C intake, iron supplement if premature

Hereditary spherocytosis

D: inherited abnormality of the RBC, caused by defects in structural membrane proteins → sphere-shaped RBC

R: FHx of splenectomy, anaemia, jaundice, or HS; Northern European ancestry (1 in 5000)

A: autosomal dominant in 75%

P: spherical RBC + less flexibility → ↑fragility → selectively removed and destroyed in the spleen → splenomegaly and ↑bilirubin

S/smx: · failure to thrive
- neonatal jaundice, gallstones
- splenomegaly
- aplastic crisis precipitated by parvovirus infection
- degree of haemolysis variable
- MCHC elevated

Dx/Ix:
- FHx + typical clinical features + labs (blood film – spherocytes, ↑MCHC, ↑reticulocytes)
  ↳ no more tests required
- If Dx equivocal, EMA binding test and cryohaemolysis test
- If atypical presentation, electrophoresis analysis of erythrocyte membranes
- Osmotic fragility test not rec
DDx: hereditary elliptocytosis – RBC are ellipse-shaped. Also autosomal dominant. S/smx and Mx similar

Mx of acute haemolytic crisis
- Supportive ± transfusion prn
Mx long term
- Folate replacement
- Splenectomy ± cholecystectomy if gallstones are an issue

Sickle cell disease

D: autosomal recessive condition that causes sickle-shaped RBCs

R: FHx - if both parents are recessive, child has 1 in 4 chance. African descent. 10% UK Afro-Caribbeans are carriers

A: valine replaces glutamic acid in β globin chain → Hb polymerises within the RBC, forming long stiff fibres of Hb tetramers
P: this is triggered by hypoxia and acidosis → vaso-occlusion in small vessels and hypercoagulability
- Sickle RBCs are more prone to haemolysis → anaemia
- S/smx only show after ~6mo as HbF is present till then and can compensate

Dx/Ix: Hb electrophoresis

See 10.05 for more details

Screening:
- Antenatal screening if parents are known carriers, eg chorionic villus sampling at 8-10w
- Screening in newborns

S/smx after 4-6mo:
- Swelling of joints, esp dactylitis
- Leukocytosis in absence of infxn
- Protuberant abdomen (2/2 enlarged spleen) ± umbilical hernia
- Cardiac systolic flow murmur 2/2 anaemia
- Maxillary hypertrophy with overbite due to extramedullar haematopoiesis (not all)

Mx of crisis
- **Analgesia**, eg opiates
  - must be offered within 30min of presentation. Intranasal fentanyl may be used for children
- Resus as needed: IV fluids for rehydration, oxygen, etc
- Abx if evidence of infxn
- Blood transfusion
  - exchange transfusion only if stroke or acute chest syndrome (requires operating theatre)
Mx long-term
- Hydroxycarbamide: ↑HbF
  - same MOA as hydroxyurea, but approved for children
- Penicillin prophylaxis from 3mo to 5yo (see also NICE guidelines)
  - Erythromycin if pen-allergic
  - Lifelong if ↑risk of infxn
- Folic acid supplementation if nutritionally insufficient
- Pneumococcal polysaccharide vaccine every 5y
- Definitive: haematopoietic stem cell transplantation
  - esp rec if neurological injury, severe/freq pain, recurrent acute chest syndrome

Henoch-Schonlein purpura

aka IgA vasculitis.

R: genetics (Hx of allergy, atopy), M>F 2:1, 2-10yo, **prior infxn (URTI)**
  ↳ ↑age at onset → poorer prognosis

A: IgA immune complexes prompts an autoimmune response
P: tissue deposition of IgA in affected organs (eg skin, kidney)

S/smx:
- **Palpable purpuric rash** (localised oedema) over buttocks and extensor surfaces of arms and legs
- Polyarthritis (75%)
- Abd pain (50%)
- Features of IgA nephropathy, eg haematuria, renal failure (50%)

Dx/Ix: Bloods (FBC, blood film, renal profile, Sr albumin, CRP), blood culturs, urinalysis, urine PCR + obs.
DDx: meningococcal septicaemia, leukaemia, ITP, HUS - r/o!!

Mx: supportive - analgesia, hydration
- Use of steroids is debatable
- Monitor with BP & urine dipstick

P: abd pain usually settles in a few days. Pts without kidney involvement can recover in 4-6w.
- 1/3 pts recur within 9mo
  - more common in older pts, generally milder
- Very rarely, ESRD (5%)

Complications: intussusception, massive GI bleeds, AKI (rare)

Immune thrombocytopenia

Also aka immune thrombocytopenic purpura. An autoimmune haematolo-gical disorder characterised by isolated thrombocytopenia in the absence of an identifiable cause

R: women of childbearing age, <10yo, or >65yo

A: unknown; autoimmune
P: antibodies directed against Gp IIb/IIIa or Ib-V-IX complex. Type II hypersensitivity reaction

S/smx: more acute in children
· Bruising
· Petechial or purpuric rash
· Bleeding is less common; typically presents as epistaxis or gingival bleeding

Dx/Ix: FBC (isolated thrombocyto-paenia; <100), blood film. Bone marrow exam only if atypical features (eg LN enlargement, failure to respond to tx)

Mx: supportive
· ITP resolves in ~80% children within 6mo with or without tx
· Advise to avoid possible trauma
· Advise about concerning signs of bleeding, including persistent HA, melaena, menorrhagia, etc
· If platelet count is very low or significant bleeding,
  - PO/IV corticosteroids
  - IVIG   - Immune inhibitors
  - Platelet transfusions only if emergency, but temporary solution as they will be destroyed by circulating abs
  - Splenectomy, but delay for ≥12mo

Acute lymphoblastic leukaemia

D: malignant clonal cancer of the **lymphoid progenitor cell**
→ common ALL (75%), CD10+, pre-B phenotype
→ T-ALL (20%) and B-ALL (5%)

R: children <5yo – accounts for 80% of childhood leukemias. a/w Down's.

Features *predictable by bone marrow failure*
· **anaemia**: lethargy and pallor
· **neutropaenia**: frequent / severe infections
· **thrombocytopenia**: easy bruising, petechiae

Other features
· bone pain (2/2 bone marrow infiltration)
· splenomegaly   · hepatomegaly
· fever – up to 50% of new cases
· testicular swelling (2/2 spread)

Dx/Ix:
· FBC – ↓Hb, ↑WCC (in 50% pts), ↓neutrophils, ↓platelets
· peripheral blood – leukaemic lymphoblasts
· U&Es, uric acid, LDH, renal function, LFTs, coagulation profile
· Bone marrow aspiration and trephine biopsy
· Immunophenotyping, etc etc

Mx: chemotherapy

Prognosis · Better: t12;21, younger
· Worse: - age < 2yo or > 10yo
  - WBC > 20 at Dx
  - T or B cell surface markers
  - non-Caucasian   - male sex

Complications
· Neutropaenic sepsis – prevent with cotrimoxazole
· Revaccinate 6mo after chemo
· Hyperuricaemia: pre-treat with ↑fluid intake and allopurinol
· Poor growth
· Cancer elsewhere, esp CNS or 2nd leukemia (3% risk)

Febrile neutropaenia

Initial Mx
· Cultures and parenteral abx asap
  ↳ local guidelines
  ↳ NICE rec piptazo ± gentamicin
· Blood cultures (peripheral + central)
· MSU   · CXR if respi smx
· Swab all orifices + central line
· Swab for respi viruses
· Bloods & serology

Further Mx
· Mx in hospital by paeds oncology
· If Ix show viral or low-risk infxn, child may be discharged ± PO abx
· If blood culture is -ve, other tests inconclusive, child afebrile for >24h: continue abx for 5d
· If blood culture +ve, tx according to local guidelines
· If child continues to spike fevers or becomes more unwell, consider viral or fungal infxns or line infxn

Most likely Gram+ve (80%), likely coagulase-ve staph.

Complications
· Chest: bronchiectasis, granulomas, lymphoma
· GI: malabs, giardia, cholangitis, atrophic gastritis, colitis
· Liver: acquired hepatitis, chronic active hepatitis, biliary cirrhosis
· Blood: autoimmune haemolysis, ITP, anaemia of chronic disease, aplasia
· Eyes: keratoconjunctivitis, uveitis, granulomas, encephalitis
· Others: septic arthropathy, arthralgia, splenomegaly

Primary immunodeficiencies

D: group of disorders causing ↑risk of infxn and malignancy. Many are X-linked or AR genetic conditions

S/smx:
· Usually present after first months of life due to early protection from maternal antibodies
· Present with recurrent infxns
  - eg ≥2x pneumonia per year
  - ≥2x meningitis/sepsis ever
· Faltering growth
· FHx of PID / consanguinity
· Unusual pathogens in unusual locations
· Persistent candidiasis
· Non-healing wounds
· Complications with live vaccines
· Chronic sinusitis   · Absent tonsils
· Chronic diarrhoea

DDx: normal child can have ≤12 self-limiting infxns a year. Other conditions include atopy, allergic rhinitis, asthma, chronic disease (eg GORD with aspiration), acquired immunodeficiency (HIV, malignancy)

Dx/Ix: FBC + differential, blood film, U&Es, CRP/ESR, blood cultures, Ig levels, lymphocyte subsets (T and B cells, monocytes, NK cells), vaccine responses ± HIV tests

Mx: Ref to paeds immunologist
In general,
· Tx infxns promptly, aggressively
· Prophylactic abx
· Avoid live vaccines
· *Caution with blood products*
· Ig replacement
  - SE: HA, abd pain, anaphylaxis
  - prep adrenaline, hydrocortisone, antihistamines

Severe combined immunodeficiency

D: a group of inherited genetic disorders characterised by a profound deficiency in cellular and humoral immunity arising from one of many T-cell maturation defects in the bone marrow or thymus gland
· 1 in 50,000-75,000

R: FHx of SCID, FHx of infant death, Native Americans, Consanguinity

A: genetic mutations. 50% mutation in common γ chain on X chromosome that codes for IL receptors on T and B cells (X-linked recessive). Other mutations - JAC3, mutations leading to adenosine deaminase deficiency
P: Severe immunodeficiency leads to ↑susceptibility to opportunistic and recurrent infxns

S/smx: presentation as for PID
· Opportunitistic infxns can be severe and fatal, eg chickenpox, pneumocystis jirovecii, CMV

Omenn syndrome
· Rare cause of SCID (ΔRAG1/2)
· Erythroderma: red, scaly dry rash
· Alopecia   · Diarrhoea
· Failure to thrive
· Lymphadenopathy
· Hepatosplenomegaly

Mx: only definitive Tx is haematopoietic stem cell transplant
· Others: Ig therapy, sterile environment

Disorders

Neutrophil disorders	**B-cell disorders**
Chronic granulomatous disease	CVID
Chediak-Higashi syndrome	Bruton's agammaglobulinemia
Leukocyte adhesion deficiency	Selective IgA deficiency

Combined B&T disorders
SCID
Ataxic telangiectasia
Wiskott-Aldrich syndrome
Hyper IgM syndromes

T-cell disorders
DiGeorge syndrome

In IgA def, blood products should be given from IgA def donors, or use washed RBCs.

Diabetes mellitus

Type 1: metabolic disorder characterised by hyperglycaemia due to absolute insulin deficiency

R: genetics/FHx – risk is 5% with 1 affected family member

A/P: autoimmune pancreatic β-cell destruction in genetically susceptible individuals. When 80-90% β cells destroyed, hyperglycemia develops.

S/smx: • peak age of onset: 5 to 7
• Weeks of polyuria, polydipsia, lethargy, wt loss ± infxn, poor growth, DKA
  - 2ndary nocturnal enuresis
• If suspected in children, refer SAME DAY to paediatric diabetes MDT

Dx based on WHO criteria:
• smx + ↑BG ≥11.1mmol/L (random)
• smx + ↑BG ≥7mmol/L (fasting)
• ↑BG on 2 separate occasions
DDx: T2DM (obesity, Asian or black), Consider monogenic or mitochondrial DM in children if Dx in 1st year of life, absence of ketonaemia during hyperglycaemia, or syndromic features
Ix: diabetes-specific antibodies can be helpful. C-peptide levels low.

Mx: • give BG and ketone monitors
• education of child + caregivers!

Insulin regimens
• Basal bolus: combi of regular longer-acting insulin with 'carb counting' and short- or rapid-acting insulin before meals
• Continuous SQ: insulin pump
• 1-3 regular injections of mixed insulin

Insulin requirements: start with 0.5-0.75 U/kg/24h (total daily dose)
• If using basal-bolus, ÷TDD as 1/2 basal insulin + 1/2 in 3 doses before meals
• If using mixed insulins, give 2/3 pre breakfast, and 1/3 pre dinner
• Adjust based on general trends

HYPOGLYCAEMIA
• Smx: weakness, dizziness, shaking, palpitations, sweating, anxiety, hunger, vomiting. HA, confusion, blurred vision, lethargy, coma, convulsions
• Behavioural Δ: agitation, irritability
Mx:
• 10-20g of fast-acting glucose by mouth + complex carbs. If not possible, give oral glucose gel
  - 1tsp sugar moistened with water under tongue every 10-12min if nothing else available
• Or 5 mL/kg IV 10% glucose
• Severe out of hospital: glucagon 1mg IM (500 mcg if <8yo or <25kg)
• Expect quick return to consciousness: recheck BG <15min
  - if normal, possible post-ictal state after hypo fit – DO NOT give more glucose, may cause or worsen cerebral oedema

Maturity onset diabetes of the young
= autosomal dominant kind of non-ketotic diabetes. Single gene defect as opposed to T1/T2DM that have polygenic and environmental causes

MODY2 • mild, asmx. Drugs rarely needed, complications rare.

MODY3 • most common type.
• Severe hyperglycaemia after puberty → Dx of T1DM
• Sensitive to SU. Some children may be able to stop insulin
• Diabetic retinopathy and nephropathy often occur

MODY5: a/w pancreatic atrophy, renal abn, genital tract malforms

MODY1, 4, 6: rare

Diabetic ketoacidosis

D: acute metabolic complication of diabetes, with a biochemical triad of hyperglycaemia (or Hx of diabetes), ketonaemia, and metabolic acidosis

R: inadequate or inappropriate insulin therapy, infxn, MI, etc

A: ↓insulin + ↑glucagon, catecholamines, cortisol, growth hormone → metabolic derangements
P: leads to hyperglycemia, volume depletion, electrolyte imbalance
• insulin def leads to release of FFA from adipose tissue, hepatic fatty acid oxidation, formation of ketone bodies → ketonaemia + acidosis

S/smx: • abdominal pain
• polyuria, polydipsia, dehydration
• Kussmaul respiration (deep hyperventilation)
• acetone-smelling breath ('pear-drops' smell)

Dx: • glucose >11 or known DM
• pH <7.3   • bicarb <15 mmol/L
• ketones >3 or urine ketones ++
DDx: HHS (↑↑BG >30, little or no acidosis or ketones)

40 mmol of K for every 1L of NaCl given

Hourly rate = (48h maintenance + deficit - boluses given in excess of 20mL/kg) ÷ 48

Maintenance requirements
<10 kg: 2 mL/kg/h
10-40 kg: 1 mL/kg/h
>40 kg: 4 mL/kg/h

Deficit – estimate from pH
pH >7.1: 5% dehydration
pH <7.1: 10% dehydration
e.g. 20kg boy with severe DKA, deficit est at 100 mL/kg x 20 kg = 2000 mL

Mx: severity categorised by degree of acidosis – mild or mod (pH>7.1), severe pH<7.1
• Resus: fluids only if shocked (10 mL/kg 0.9 NaCl bolus)
  ↳ isotonic saline only
• Rapidly confirm Dx: BG, ABG, blood ketones, etc
• Monitor: GCS (q30min), ECG (look for hyperK)
• Start IVF: requirement = fluid deficit + maintenance fluids. Correct over 48h. Use lower fluid maintenance rates than APLS
  - K replacement: if K >5.5, no nil. If K 3.5-5.5, 40 mmol/L. if <3.5, senior review
• Formal Ix: wt, FBC, U&es, lab glucose, Ca, infxn screen
• start IV insulin only after 1-2h of fluids. DO NOT give insulin bolus; start fast-acting insulin infusion 0.1U/kg/h.
• once BG <14, start 10% dextrose inf at 125 mL/h in addition to 0.9% NaCl regimen

DKA resolution: pH >7.3 + blood ketones <0.6 + bicarb >15mmol/L
• Should resolve within 24h
  ↳ if not, need senior review
• If resolved, and pt E&D, switch to SQ insulin – stop infusion 30-60min after SQ insulin

Complications (from DKA or tx)
• gastric stasis
• thromboembolism
• arrhythmias 2/2 to hyperK or iatrogenic hypoK
• cerebral oedema (iatrogenic)
  - children esp vulnerable
  - esp 4-12h after tx starts. 1:1 nursing + neuro obs essential.
  - if suspicion, CTH + senior review
• ARDS   • AKI

Hypothyroidism ≈ cretinism

D: deficiency of thyroid hormones, which leads to a generalised slowing of metabolic processes
Congenital hypothyroidism
• Thyroid dysgenesis (85%)
• Dyshormonogenesis (15%)

Acquired hypothyroidism
• 1': prematurity, Hashimoto's (a/w Down's, T1DM, coeliac, Turner), I2 deficiency, drugs, irradiation, etc
• 2' hypopituitarism

S/smx: mostly late, .: screening !
• Prolonged neonatal jaundice
• Widely opened posterior fontanelle
• Poor feeding   • Hypotonia
• Dry skin
• ± Inactivity, ↑sleepiness, hoarse cry, constipation
Late signs: Flat nasal bridge, protuding tongue, umbilical hernia, slowly relaxing deep tendon reflexes, ↓pulse. If untreated, poor growth, cognitive disability

Dx: Day 5 dried blood spot – tests for ↑TSH to detect 1' hypothyroidism
Others: T4, thyroid imaging (for 2' or central hypothyroidism), thyroid antibody screen ± pituitary function

Mx: lifelong levothyroxine
• Neonates: start ~15 mcg/kg/d, adjust by 5 mcg/kg q2w to typical dose of 20-50 mcg/d.
• <2yo: start with 5 mcg/kg/d (max 50 mcg/d), adjust by 10-25 mcg q2w
• >2yo: start with 50 mcg/d, adjust by 25 mcg q2w
• Adjust according to growth and clinical state. Aim for high-normal T4 and low-normal TSH levels

See 06.01 for more

Hyperthyroidism

A: Graves, autoimmune thyroiditis (Hashimoto's), thyroid nodules, adenomas, carcinomas

S/smx: hyperactivity, irritability, ↑HR, palpitations, tremor, anxiety, heat intolerance, diarrhoea, hyperreflexia, wt loss despite ↑appetite, menstrual irregularity
Specific to Graves: exophthalmos, proptosis, lid lag, ophthalmoplegia

Mx:
1. Dose titration with antithyroid drugs (carbimazole or PTU), or
2. Block and replace – induce complete thyroid suppression, and replace with levothyroxine
3. (for multiple relapses) ablative tx with radioiodine or thyroid surgery

Transient neonatal thyrotoxicosis

A: maternal Graves disease
P: TSHR stimulating antibodies cross placenta and cause transient thyrotoxicosis in the newborn

S/smx: flushing, sweating, irritability, poor wt gain, ↑HR, heart failure
· Self-limiting, but antithyroid drugs and supportive tx prn

Hyperammonaemia

! medical emergency !

Complications: cerebral oedema, ↑ICP → neurodisability, death

S/smx: lethargy, vomiting, altered consciousness → coma
· early on, ↑RR + respi alkalosis

DDx: urea cycle defects, organic acidaemias, fat oxidation defects, non-IMD (liver failure, poor sampling)

Inherited metabolic diseases

D: conditions involving genetic defects (any mode of inheritance) that causes an enzyme in a cellular pathway to be dysfunctional or absent → causes a block in metabolic pathway ± toxic byproduct buildup
E: individual IMDs are rare, but incidence of combined IMDs is ~1:800

General s/smx: ! consider in DDx of acutely unwell child who does not have clear Dx or does not respond to standard therapy. Often misDx for sepsis !
► RED FLAGS ►
· neonatal presentation with ~few days of well-being/feeding prior to presentation
· Previous episodes triggered by illness or fasting, incl cyclical vomiting
· Δ in diet ppt illness (eg weaning)
· +ve FHx or consanguinity

Dx/Ix:	If IMD suspected,
· ABG	· discuss urgently with IMD centre
· Lactate	
· Glucose	· Consider: plasma, amino acids, acylcarnitine profile, urine organic acids
· Ketones	
· Ammonia	
· LFTs	
· CK	· ± DNA, skin biopsy

Mx: · stop feeds to contain potentially toxic substrate
· provide adequate energy to promote anabolism
· Dx and Mx of hyperammonia and hypoglycemia

Glycogen storage disorders

D: Conditions resulting from defects in enzymes required for synthesis and degradation of glycogen

A: genetic (mostly AR)
P: abn stores deposited in liver, muscle, heart or kidney ± CNS

Types:
· Cori disease
 - type III: hypoglycaemia, hepatomegaly, ↓growth
· Anderson disease (type IV)
· McArdle disease (type V)
 - most common GSD in teens
 - 2/2 myophosphorylase def → stiffness or myalgia after exercise
 - bloods after exercise: ↓lactate and pyruvate. ± myoglobinuria
 - biopsy: ↓phosphorylase
· Hers disease (type VI)
· Tauri disease (type VII)

Mx: depends on type
· Specialised diets
· Enzyme replacement therapy
· No extreme exercise
· Prevention of hypoglycemia, eg bedtime meal of slowly digested complex carbohydrates

Phenylalanine ketonuria

= phenylketonuria or phenylalanine hydroxylase (PAH) deficiency
D: autosomal-recessive inborn error of aa metabolism characterised by ↑blood phenylalanine (>6 mg/dL or >363 mmol/L)

R: +ve FHx, white

P: no PAH enzyme or defective PAH → ↑blood phe levels → ↑phe to brain → neurotoxicity
· Classic PKU leads to gradual cognitive impairment: ↓CNS dopamine, ↓protein synthesis, demyelination

S/smx: fair hair, fits, eczema, musty urine. ! ↓IQ (eg poor spelling, ↓cognition, inability to calculate)

Dx: newborn screening. Tests for ↑blood phenylalaine (>120 μmol/L)

Mx: tx started if >360 μmol/L
· Dietary restriction with phenylalanine-free protein substitute enriched in tyrosine and <300 mg to 8g of natural protein per day
 ↳ depends on severity
· Aim to keep levels <360 μmol/L
· Adherence may be poor, and other problems may arise (eg MH)

Maternal PKU: preconception counselling. Effects on baby: facial dysmorphism, microcephaly, growth retardation, ↓IQ

Lysosomal storage diseases

D: inherited disorders that arise from deficiency of enzymes required for the breakdown of products of intermediary metabolism

A: genetic mutations, usually AR, but some are sex-linked (eg Fabry's)

P: · accumulation of undegraded substrates
· enlargement of cells and organs
· ± ↑apoptosis of neurons
Specific disorders
· Fabry's: α-galactosidase deficiency
· Tay-Sachs: β-hexosamidase A def. Gangliosides accumulate in lysosomes, esp in neurons

Fabry's disease
· Torturing, lancinating pains in extremities ± abdomen
 - worse in cold, heat, exercise
 - 2/2 neuritis (vasculitis of the vasa nervorum)
· Angiokeratomata (clusters of dark, non-blanching, petechiae) in bathing trunk area, esp umbilicus and scrotum
· ± parasthaesia, corneal opacities, hypohidrosis, proteinuria, renal failure
· Mx: enzyme Rx ± carbamazepine

Tay-Sachs disease
· Infants: hyperacusia, macular 'cherry red spot'
· Juvenile form: optic atrophy, progressive dementia, ataxia, gait disturbance, failure to thrive, joint contracture, depression
· Young adults: psychosis, ataxia, dystonia, cataplexy
· more common in Ashkenazi Jews

Precocious puberty

D: condition where secondary sexual characteristics appear before 8yo in girls and 9yo in boys

R: brain tumours, cranial irradiation, McCune-Albright syndrome, gonadal tumours, congenital adrenal hyperplasia

A ÷ central (gonadotropin-dependent) or premature activation of the gonads or adrenal glands

P: centrally mediated PP
- HPG axis is prematurely activated → ↑serum gonadotrophins
- Pattern of endocrine Δ is same as normal puberty (consonant)
P: other causes
- secretion of sex steroids is autonomous (independent of hypothalamic GnRH pulse)
- loss of normal feedback regulation
- pubertal develop does not follow normal pattern (disconsonant)

S/smx: girls <8yo or boys <9yo with early signs of puberty

Dx: detailed hx + parental hx + social hx (adoption, abuse)
- Compare growth with growth charts
- Examination: Tanner's staging, Prader orchidometer
- Battery of blood tests

Mx of central PP:
- GnRH analogues given nasally, SC or IM – helps to suppress secretion of pituitary gonadotropins
  - helps to reversal gonadal maturation and ↓skeletal maturation

Delayed puberty

Refer if no signs of puberty
- Males >14yo
- Females >14yo with no breast development or absence of menarche ≥16yo

Congenital adrenal hyperplasia

D: family of inherited enzyme deficiencies that impair normal corticosteroid synthesis by the adrenal cortex

A: autosomal recessive disorder
- 21-hydroxylase deficiency
- 11-β-hydroxylase deficiency

- Cortisol production occurs in zona fasciculata of adrenal cortex
- ↓21H/11βH → ↓cortisol + ↑ACH & ACTH → adrenal hyperplasia and excess androgens
- Excess adrenal androgens block pituitary gonadotropins → gonadal dysfunction
- ↓↓21H can lead to insufficient aldosterone → salt wasting, cortisol deficiency + androgen excess

Classical CAH: salt-wasting
- Glucocorticoid and mineralocorticoid deficiency
- Most severe. 75% cases
- Can present with atypical genitalia in females
- Life-threatening adrenal crises and salt-wasting crises → vomiting and dehydration → ↓Na, ↑K, ↓glu
- Other s/smx: poor feeding, vomiting, dehydration, arrhythmias
- Hyperpigmentation
Classical CAH: simple virilising
- Moderate enzyme defects; retains ability to conserve salt
- Generally s/smx related to ↑androgen
- Females: tall, facial hair, absent periods, deep voice, early puberty
- Males: tall, deep voice, large penis, small testicles, early puberty
Non-classical CAH
- Mild to moderate enzyme deficiency
- S/smx of hyperandrogenism, but females do not have virilised genitalia at birth

Mx: cortisol replacement (hydrocort), aldosterone replacement (fludrocort). ± corrective surgery for virilised genitals in females

Genetic disorders

Disorders of chromosome number
- Trisomies
  - 21: Down syndrome
  - 13: Patau syndrome
  - 18: Edward syndrome
  - 47,XXY: Klinefelter syndrome
  - 47,XXX: Triple X syndrome
- Monosomies
  - 45,XO: Turner syndrome

Disorders of chromosome structure
- Microdeletions
  - 5p: Cri du chat syndrome
  - 22q11.2: DiGeorge syndrome
  - 7q11: Williams syndrome

Autosomal dominant inheritance
- Achondroplasia   · Marfan syndrome
- Huntington disease   · Myotonic dystrophy
- Neurofibromatosis   · Noonan syndrome
- Osteogenesis imperfecta (most forms)
- Otosclerosis   · Polyposis coli
- Tuberous sclerosis
- Familial hypercholesterolaemia (almost all cases)

Autosomal recessive inheritance
- Congenital adrenal hyperplasia
- Cystic fibrosis   · Friedreich ataxia
- Galactosaemia   · Hurler syndrome
- Glycoogen storage diseases
- Oculocutaneous albinism
- Phenylketonuria   · Sickle cell disease
- Tay–Sachs disease   · Thalassaemia
- Werdnig–Hoffmann disease (SMA1)

X-linked recessive inheritance
- Colour blindness (red–green)
- Duchenne and Becker muscular dystrophies
- Fragile X syndrome   · G6PD deficiency
- Haemophilia A and B   · Hunter syndrome

Imprinting and uniparental disomy
- 15q11-13 – paternal: Prader Willi syndrome
        maternal: Angelman syndrome

Developmental milestones

Avg age	Milestone	► Red flags ►
6w	· Smiles · Eyes follow an object past midline	· Strabismus persisting >3mo
4-6mo	· Sits with support · Rolls · Good head control · Reaches out for objects · Transfers objects from hand to hand · Starts babbling	At 6mo: · ↓eye contact · No smile · No grasp · Not rolling · Poor head control
6-9mo	· Crawls · Sits with support · Pulls to stand · Gives toy on request · Turns head to name · Responds to byebye · Gestures with babbling · First tooth	At 9mo: · No response to words · No gestures · No passing toys hand to hand · Unable to roll, crawl, or sit without support
7-12mo	· Walks with support or using furniture ("cruising") · Develops pincer grasp · Plays peekaboo · Waves goodbye	At 12mo: · Cannot pick up small items · Cannot crawl or bottom shuffle · Cannot pull self up · No babbled phrases
12-15mo	· Single words · Listens to stories · Drinks from cup	At 18mo: · Uninterested in playing w others · No clear words · Not walking without support · Not able to hold crayon · Unable to stack 2 blocks
18mo	· ≥6 words · Walk up steps · Names pictures · Walks independently · Scribbles · Builds with blocks	
1.5 to 2yo	· Kicks/throws ball · Runs · 2 word sentences · Follows 2 step command · Stacks 5-6 blocks · Turns pages · Uses spoon · Helps with dressing	At 2yo: · <50 words · Difficulty handling small objects · Cannot climb stairs · No interest in feeding/dressing

Speech delay

Causes of delayed speech
· Hearing impairment: esp chronic otitis media
· Familial: FHx
· Environmental: deprivation, poor social interaction, neglect, etc
· Neuropsychological: global developmental delay; ASD, acquired epileptiform aphasia

If <50 words at 3yo:
· Deafness
· Expressive dysphasia or speech dyspraxia
· Audio-premotor syndrome (APM)
  ↳ child is quiet, cannot hum/sing
· Respiro-laryngeal dysfunction
  ↳ voice is loud and rough
· Congenital aphonia (rare)
  ↳ thin effortful voice

If parents cannot understand most speech by 2.5yo:
· Deafness
· Articulatory dyspraxia. M>F 3:1
  - Tongue tie (may need surgery to frenulum and speech therapy)
· APM or RL dysfunction

If child is unable to understand simple phrases by 2.5yo (eg "get your shoes"):
· Deafness – if hearing is impaired, secretory otitis media is likely to be the cause
· Cognitive impairment
· Deprivation

Global developmental delay

D: delay in ≥2 dvp domains

Genetic: chromosomal disorders (eg Downs), DMD, metabolic (eg PKU)
Congenital brain abn: hydrocephalus, microcephaly
Prenatal cause: Teratogens (drugs, alcohol), congenital infxns (esp CMV, rubella, toxoplasmosis), hypothyroidism
Perinatal cause: extreme prematurity leading to IVH or periventricular leukomalacia, birth asphyxia, metabolic disorders or hypoglycemia
Postnatal cause: brain injury from suffocation, drowning, head injury, CNS infxn, hypoglycemia, hypothyroidism

Cerebral palsy

D: umbrella term referring to a non-progressive disease of the brain originating during the ante-, neo-, or early postnatal period → disorders of movement and posture development

R/A: prematurity, low birth wt, fetal birth asphyxia, multiple births, maternal illness, fetal brain malformation, major birth defects, familial metabolic or genetic disorder, neonatal complications, meningitis, maternal teratogen exposure, low socioeconomic status
· 70-80% ?antenatal causes
P: depends on cause

Classification according to motor impairment, anatomical distribution and functional level

÷ by movement disorder
· Spastic: velocity-dependent resistance to passive muscle stretch
  – ? pyramidal or UMN
  - further ÷ into monoplegia, hemiplegia, diplegia (bilateral lower limbs), quadriplegia
· Dyskinetic: uncoord, involuntary movements and postures – ? basal ganglia involvement
  - further ÷ into dystonia, chorea, athestosis. A/w kernicterus
· Ataxic: loss of muscular coordination with abn force and rhythm, decreased accuracy. Cerebellar.
· Mixed

÷ function by Gross Motor Function Classification System (levels)
1. walks, runs, climbs stairs without rail; speed, balance, coord limited
2. uses rail for stairs; walks but may use handheld or wheeled device for long distances or uneven terrain; minimal ability to run or jump
3. walks with handheld or wheeled device in most indoor settings, uses wheeled device for longer distances
4. mobility requires physical assist-ance or powered mobility in most settings
5. transported in manual wheelchair in all settings, limited anti-gravity head, trunk and limb control

S/smx:
· Abn tone in early infancy
· Delayed motor milestones
· Abn gait   · Feeding difficulties

A/w
· Learning difficulties (60%)
· Epilepsy (30%)   · Squints (30%)
· Hearing impairment (20%)

Mx: holistic with specialists
· Botulinum toxin may benefit children with spasticity
· Epidural cord, deep brain stimulation, intrathecal or oral baclofen

Prognosis: by 6yo, 80% hemiplegic or diplegic and 54% quadriplegic gain urinary continence

Muscular dystrophies

D: Inherited disorders characterised by muscle degeneration and weakness
· **Duchenne** muscular dystrophy (DMD): X-linked recessive. Most severe and rapidly progressive form
· **Becker** muscular dystrophy (BMD): milder form

R: FHx, males (∵ X-linked)

A: DMD & BMD are caused by mutation to the dystrophin gene
P: Absence of dystrophin protein → ↑instability and degeneration of skeletal muscle + replacement with adipose and connective tissue
· Brain cells & smooth muscle cells may be affected also

S/smx:
· Onset in childhood: DMD 5yo, BMD 10yo
· Progressive proximal muscle weakness
· Calf pseudohypertrophy,
· Gower's sign (child uses arms to stand up from squatted position)
· Intellectual impairment (esp in DMD)

Ix: CK ↑, genetic testing, rarely muscle biopsy (old method of testing)

Mx: · Supportive – ensuring pt has mobility aids, accessibility at home, etc
· No curative tx

P: DMD – most children cannot walk by 12yo, survive till 25-30yo. A/w dilated cardiomyopathy.

Down syndrome

D: trisomy 21. 1:800 births.

R: ↑maternal age (20yo 1:1500 risk; 40yo 1:100 risk), prev child with Down, parental karyotype with translocation

A: extra chromosome 21
P: may be due to non-disjunction of chromosome pairs during gamete formation, Robertsonian translocation or mosaicism

S/smx + associated conditions:
- Features in neonatal period
  - Hypotonia
  - Poor Moro reflex
  - Hyper-flexibility of joints
  - Extra skin on back of neck
  - Flat facial profile
  - Slanted palpebral fissures
  - Anomalous auricles
  - Hypoplasia of iliac wings
  - Short middle phalanx of the fifth finger
  - Single palmar crease
- GI abnormalities: duodenal atresia, Hirschsprung's disease
- Cardiac abnormalities
  - Atrioventricular septal defects (AVSD; 40%; most common)
  - VSD (30%)   - ASD (10%)
  - Tetralogy of Fallot (~5%)
  - Isolated PDA (~5%)
- Vision issues
  - Refractive errors more common
  - Strabismus (20-40%)
  - Cataracts (congenital or acquired)
  - Recurrent blepharitis
  - Glaucoma
- Hearing issues
  - Otitis media very common
- Haematological cancers: infants may be born with transient abnormal myelopoiesis (TAM) that may progress to ALL or AML
- Neurological issues
  - Learning difficulties
  - A/w Alzheimer's disease (onset in early 50s)
  - Epilepsy in 8%

Associated conditions (cont)
- Respiratory issues
  - Obstructive sleep apnoea
  - Recurrent infxns
- Thyroid disorders
  - Hypothyroidism more common
- Others
  - Atlantoaxial instability

Ix: chromosomal karyotype for Dx. Other tests according to complications (eg echocardiogram)

Mx:
- Ax + specialist consult
- Parental genetic counselling

P: avg life expectancy 50-60yo

Other trisomies

Patau syndrome
- D: Trisomy 13
- R: ↑maternal age
- A/P: as with Down's. Typically causes "midline" defects (eg cleft lip/palate)
- S/smx: - Microcephaly
  - Small or no eyes
  - Cleft lip or palate
  - Polydactyly
  - Scalp lesions
  - Cardiac abnormalities (any)
  - Other organ abnormalities
  - After infancy, pts have severe psychomotor disorder, failure to thrive, intellectual disability and seizures
- P: median survival 7-10d, 90% live for <1y

Edwards syndrome
- D: Trisomy 18
- R: ↑maternal age
- S/smx: - Micrognathia
  - Low-set ears
  - Rocker bottom feet
  - Overlapping of fingers
  - Cardiac defects in 90%
  - All organ systems may be affected
- P: median survival is 3-14d, 90-95% live for <1y

Klinefelter syndrome

D: ≥2 X chromosomes in a phenotypical male. 47,XXY is the most common form. ~1:1000 M.

R: ↑maternal & paternal age

S/smx:
- Often taller than average
- Genital abnormalities
  - Lack of 2ndary sexual characteristics
  - Small, firm testes
    ◊ ↑gonadotropins & low testosterone
  - Infertility
    ◊ most common presentation
- Gynaecomastia (a/w ↑risk of breast cancer)
- Intelligence usually in normal range, but some have educational and psychological problems

Triple X syndrome

D: trisomy X – 47,XXX. 1:1000 F.

S/smx:
- Wide range of phenotypes – estimated that only 10% are clinically Dxed (ie other 90% likely to be subclinical)
- At birth: hypotonia, clinodactyly (ie finger that curves to one side, eg pinky curving inward)
- Physical features: tall, epicanthal folds, widely spaced eyes (aka hypertelorism)
- Other associated conditions: genitourinary malformations, seizure disorder, intention tremor, congenital hip dysplasia, constipation or abdo pains
  - may only be Dxed in teens due to late menarche, menstrual irregularities or subfertility

Turner syndrome

D: Monosomy 45X; absence of the second sex chromosome in phenotypical females. ~1:5000 F.

R: no known risk factors

S/smx:
- Abnormal facies
  - Narrow or high arched palate
  - Short, broad / webbed neck
  - Low-set, anomalous pinnae (ears)
- Other phenotypic features
  - Short stature
    ↳ usually <5th percentile
    ↳ r/o other causes of poor growth
  - Shield chest, widely spaced nipples
  - Cystic hygroma
  - Short fourth metacarpal
  - Multiple pigmented naevi
- Cardiac abnormalities
  - Bicuspid aortic valve (15%)
  - Coarctation of the aorta (5-10%)
  - ↑risk of aortic dilation and dissection
- Endocrine abnormalities
  - Primary amenorrhea
  - ↑Gonadotropin levels
  - Hypothyroidism
- Renal: horseshoe kidney
- Lymphoedema in neonates
- ↑risk of autoimmune disease and Crohn's disease

May not be diagnosed until teens when pts present due to short stature and delayed puberty

Ix: karyotype for Dx

Mx: surveillance and preventative care
- Once pt has cyclical bleeding
  - Ovarian HRT: oral or transdermal oestrogen therapy, continued until ~50yo
- Education on reproductive issues
  - Most women with Turner's are infertile, but spontaneous menses and pregnancies occur in 2-3%
  - Will require genetic counselling

Prader-Willi syndrome   PWS

D: genetically inherited complex neurological disorder caused by absence of expression of **paternally** inherited imprinted genes on chromosome 15q11-q13

R: ↑maternal age (↑risk of maternal uniparental disomy), hydrocarbon exposure (in father), conception using assisted reproductive technology, sibling with PWS

A: 70% due to paternal deletion, 30% due to maternal disomy
P: attributed to hypothalamic dysfunction

S/smx: · Hypotonia in infancy
  - a/w breathing problems
- Dysmorphic features
- Short stature
- Learning difficulties
- Hypogonadism and infertility
- Hyperphagia + obesity in later childhood

P: shorter life expectancy mainly due to complications of hyperphagia and obesity

Angelman syndrome

D: neurodevelopmental disorder due to absence of expression of **maternally** inherited imprinted genes on chromosome 15q11-q13

S/smx:
- Severe intellectual disability
- Postnatal microcephaly
- Movement or balance disorder
  - Gait ataxia or tremor of limbs
- Behavioural abnormalities: apparent happy demeanor with emotional lability, excitable movement
- Seizure disorder, baseline EEG changes, and sleep disorder
- GI problems

Cri du chat syndrome

D: 5p microdeletion
- Most deletions occur de novo, 80-90% paternal

S/smx:
- High pitched cry in infancy
- Hypotonia
- Microcephaly and micrognathism
- Intellectual disability
  - severity depends on size of deletion
- Feeding difficulties

P: 10% survive >1y. Morbidity & mortality ↓ after first few years of life

DiGeorge syndrome

D: 22q deletion syndrome, aka velo-cardiofacial syndrome

R: FHx

A: 22q11.2 deletion
P: deletion → ↓TBX1, a key transcription factor for development of pharyngeal arches

S/smx: **CATCH-22**
- Conotruncal cardiac defects (eg tetralogy of Fallot)
- Abnormal facies
- Thymus a/hypoplasia
- Cleft palate
- Hypocalcaemia
- Others: intellectual disability, autism, ADHD

Mx: supportive tx of complications (no cure)

P: complete DGS (<1% pts) have very poor prognosis; most die by 1y. But depending on severity, pts can survive into adulthood

Williams syndrome

D: 7q11 microdeletion including the elastin gene

S/smx:
- Elfin-like facial features
- Supravalvular aortic stenosis
- Mild-to-mod learning difficulties
- Short stature
- Endocrine abnormalities: hypercalcaemia, hypothyroidism, delayed growth or early puberty

P: 50% chance of parents with Williams passing microdeletion to their children. If cardiac abnormalities are managed, pts can have a relatively normal life

Achondroplasia

D: autosomal dominantly inherited skeletal dysplastic disorder resulting in disproportionately short stature

R: FHx, ↑parental age (for de novo mutations)

A: de novo mutation in 70-80%
P: gain of function mutation in FGFR3 gene → inhibits chondrocyte proliferation → ↓endochondral bone formation, growth restriction, bone shortening, etc

S/smx:
- Distinctive craniofacial features
  - Macrocephaly
  - Frontal bossing
  - Midface retrusion
  - Saddle norse deformity
- Disproportionate short stature with shortening of arms & legs
- Shortening of fingers and toes (aka brachydactyly) + trident hands
- Kyphoscoliosis
- Accentuated lumbar lordosis

P: ↑mortality in childhood. Mean lifespan is ~61yo (~10y less than general population)

Marfan syndrome

D: autosomal dominant inherited disorder of connective tissue characterised by loss of elastic tissue. 1:3000 births.

R: FHx of Marfan's, FHx of aortic dissection or aneurysm, ↑paternal age (in de novo mutations)

A: inherited in 75%, de novo in 25%
P: mutation on FBN1 gene on chromosome 15 → ↓**fibrillin-1**

S/smx:
- Physical features
  - Tall with long arms
  - High-arched palate
  - Long fingers (aka arachnodactyly)
  - Pectus excavatum (dented chest)
  - Pes planus (flat foot)
  - Scoliosis >20°
- Cardiac conditions
  - Dilation of aortic sinuses (90%) – aortic aneurysms, aortic dissection, aortic regurgitation
  - Mitral valve prolapse (75%)
- Lungs: repeated pneumothoraces
- Eyes
  - Upward lens dislocation
  - Blue sclera   - Myopia
- Others
  - Dural ectasia (ballooning of dural sac at the lumbosacral level)

Ix:
- aortic root imaging: echo, thorax CT, or thorax MRI
- visualising the descending aorta: abdo US, CT, or MRI
- pneumothorax: CXR

Mx: • aortic monitoring
- In pts with aortic dilation, β-blocker used to prevent further dilation
  - if CI (eg due to asthma), losartan or verapamil may be used
  - If aortic diameter >4.5cm, or symptomatic (eg chest pain), consider surgery
- Orthopaedic correction for severe skeletal deformities

Noonan syndrome

D: autosomal dominant inherited disorder characterised by short stature and congenital heart disease. 1:1000-2500 births.

R: FHx, ↑paternal age

A: gain of function mutation in various genes
P: (not fully established)

S/smx ("male Turner's syndrome"):
- Physical features
  - Short stature
  - Webbed neck
  - Pectus carinatum or excavatum
  - Widely spaced nipples
- Facial features: ptosis, triangular-shaped face, low-set ears
- Cardiac conditions: pulmonary valve stenosis
- Haematological: factor XI deficiency

Ix: ECG + echo

Mx: • monitor for cardiac complications
- Cryptorchidism: ref to urology
- If poor growth, ref to endocrinology
  - may start on growth hormone

P: majority have normal lives; prog depends on type and severity of cardiac disease

Fragile X syndrome

D: X-linked recessive trinucleotide repeat disorder
↳ most common monogenic cause of autism spectrum disorder

R: FHx

A/P: CGG repetition within fragile X mental retardation 1 gene → ↓gene expression

S/smx:
- Not apparent in newborns; s/smx develop in early childhood (avg Dx 32mo ≈ 2yo 8mo)
- Characteristic facies: elongated, narrow face, broad forehead and philtrum, high-arched palate, protruding/large ears
- May present due to
  - Autistic behaviours (eg hand flapping, repetitive tasks)
  - Poor eye contact
  - Developmental delay
  - Seizures
  - Psych: anxiety, depression, ADHD
  - Sleep disturbance
  - Aggression
- In males, macro-orchidism is a hallmark of FXS
- Prader Willi phenotype may be observed as well

P: depending on severity, some pts can lead relatively normal lives
- Premutation carriers have less severe cognitive deficits BUT have high risk of developing Fragile X-associated tremor/ataxia syndrome (FXTAS)
  - presents in 6th decade of life
  - tremors, ataxia, neuropsych conditions

Neonatal sepsis

D: sepsis in premature babies.
÷ early onset (<72h after birth) or late onset

Early-onset sepsis

R • Mother known carrier of GBS from vagina or urine, or previous infant affected by this
  ↳ ** intrapartum abx!
• Intrapartum maternal pyrexia >38°C or suspected chorioamnionitis
• Prolonged (>18h) or pre-labour rupture of membranes
• Spontaneous preterm labour (<37w)
• Suspected maternal invasive bacterial infxn

A: organisms acquired from mother
• Usually GBS, E.coli or Listeria
• Others include HSV, Chlamydia, anaerobes and H.influenzae

Late-onset sepsis

R • Prematurity • Low birth wt
• Central lines and catheters
• Parenteral nutritions
• Congenital malformations
• Immunodeficiency

A: org acquired from environment
• coag-ve Staph, S.aureus, E.coli, GBS, viral, fungal, etc

S/smx: variable and can be subtle to collapse

Mx of collapse
• ABC - crystalloid 20mL/kg (caution if s/smx of HF)
• Fluid refractory shock: inotropes (eg dopamine 10 mcg/kg/min, intubate, ventilate)
• ABG, lactate, glucose, FBC, CRP, U&Es, clotting ± ammonia ± ECG
• Blood culture, CXR, urine (if >72h old), LP, skin swabs ± HSV PCR ± stool virology ± urine MCV PCR

Mx of sepsis/infection
• Abx according to Trust guidelines

Neonatal seizures

E: ~4/1000 births
• Most occur 12-48h after birth
• May be generalised, focal, tonic, clonic or myoclonic

Causes:
• Hypoxic-ischaemic encephalopathy
• Infxn (meningitis, encephalitis)
• ICH / infarction
• Structural CNS lesion
• Metabolic disturbance / disorder
• Neonatal withdrawal from maternal drugs or substance abuse
• Kernicterus
• Benign neonatal convulsions (aka 5th day fits, a Dx of exclusion)

Ix/Dx: cerebral function analysis monitoring (CFAM) or EEG to confirm seizure activity, video EEG

Mx: • ABC, glucose, turn on side if aspiration risk
• Single short seizure does not need to be treated with anticonvulsants
• If prolonged (>3-5 min) or repeated seizures, consider anticonvulsants
  - 1st: phenobarbital
  - 2nd: phenytoin
• If intractable, consider trials of pyridoxine or biotin supps
• Consider starting empirical abx
• Insert IV access, get bloods + ABG
• Imaging: US, MRI
• Other tests: toxicology, ammonia, urine organic acids, serum aa, karyotype, TORCH screen
• Treat the cause where identified

Neonatal respiratory distress

D: increased work of breathing in the newborn infant
• S/smx: ↑RR (>60 breaths/min), ↑work of breathing (chest wall recession, nasal flaring), expiratory grunting ± cyanosis

Aetiologies, risk factors, and pathophysiology
• Transient tachypnoea of the newborn (most common cause)
  - 2/2 ↑amniotic fluid in lungs (is transient as fluid is usually absorbed or expelled after a while)
• Meconium aspiration
  - Occurs in utero
  - R: post-term babies, fetal hypoxia
• Pneumonia
  - R: prolonged rupture of membranes, chorioamnionitis, low birthweight
• Pneumothorax (1-2% of births)
  - May occur 2/2 meconium aspiration, ARDS, or as a complication of mechanical ventilation
• Persistent pulmonary hypertension of the newborn
  - Can occur as a standalone condition or a/w hypoxic-ischaemic encephalopathy, meconium aspiration, sepsis or ARDS
• Milk aspiration
  - R: preterm infants, neurodisability, bronchopulmonary dysplasia, GORD, cleft palate
• Airway obstruction, eg choanal atresia
• Pulmonary hypoplasia
  - usually a/w syndromes
• Non-pulmonary causes
  - Congenital heart disease
  - Diaphragmatic hernia
  - Tracheo-oesophageal fistula
  - Hypoxic ischaemic encephalopathy
  - Severe anaemia
  - Metabolic acidosis   - Sepsis

Ix: CXR, bloods (for sepsis)

Mx: • Admit to neonatal unit
• Oxygen support depends on needs – may range from wafting oxygen, NIV (airvo, CPAP, etc), to mechanical ventilation and ECMO

Neonatal jaundice

D: Yellow discolouration of the skin and sclera of a neonate due to ↑bilirubin – clinically apparent when bilirubin ≥80 μmol/L.

! jaundice starting <24h after birth and/or persisting ≥2w is almost always pathological !

Jaundice starting <24h after birth
• Haemolytic disorders
  - Rh incompatibility
  - ABO incompatibility
  - G6PD deficiency
  - Spherocytosis, pyruvate kinase deficiency
• Congenital infection

Jaundice at 24h - 2w of age
• Physiological jaundice
  - occurs due to breakdown of fetal Hb + ineffective hepatic bilirubin breakdown in the first few days
• Breastmilk jaundice
  - ? 2/2 ↑entero-hepatic circulation of bilirubin
  - benign condition; can last ~3mo
• Infection, eg UTI
• Haemolytic causes (as above)
• Bruising
• Polycythaemia
• Crigler-Najjar syndrome

Jaundice at >2w of age
• Unconjugated bilirubin
  - Physiological or breastmilk
  - Infection, eg UTI
  - Hypothyroidism
  - Haemolytic causes (as above)
  - High GI obstruction, eg pyloric stenosis
• Conjugated bilirubin
  - Bile duct obstruction, eg biliary atresia
  - Neonatal hepatitis

Ix: Bilirubin charting to determine if baby has crossed threshold requiring treatment, and other Ix as required for determining cause (eg antenatal antibodies, LFTs, etc)

Mx:
• Phototherapy with blue-green light
  - converts bilirubin into water-soluble pigment excreted in urine
• Exchange transfusion required if bilirubin is very high
  - Baby's blood is taken, and replaced with donor blood

Complications
• Kernicterus: occurs when unconjugated bilirubin is deposited in the basal ganglia and brainstem nuclei
  - Baby's blood brain barrier is not completely formed, allowing this to occur
  - Results in encephalopathy, which can cause seizures, coma, and ultimately death
  - Long-term sequelae include choreoathetoid cerebral palsy, learning difficulties, sensorineural deafness

D: ischaemic necrosis of the intestinal mucosa

R: preterm (the more preterm the baby is, the higher the risk), IUGR, perinatal asphyxia

A/P: not fully understood, but thought to be a/w ischaemic injury and bacterial invasion of bowel wall and altered gut microbiome

S/smx:
- Early s/smx: feeding intolerance, vomiting (± bile stained), abdo distension, bloody stools
- Later on: abdo discolouration, shock (2/2 perforation), peritonism

Ix: XR – distended loops of bowel, thickening of bowel wall with intramural gas (aka pneumatosis intestinalis), portal venous gas, etc

Mx:
- Stop PO feeding, switch to parenteral nutrition
- Give broad spectrum abx (aerobic and anaerobic bacteria cover)
- Mechanical ventilation and circulatory support often required
- Surgical Mx if bowel perforation or failure of medical Mx

Complications
- 20% mortality
- Long-term sequelae: bowel strictures, malabsorption, ↑risk of poor neurodevelopmental outcome

D: (no fixed definition) <2.6mmol/L

Causes / risk factors
- May be transient in the first hours after birth (common)
- Preterm birth (<37w)
- Maternal DM
- IUGR
- Hypothermia
- Neonatal sepsis
- Inborn errors of metabolism
- Nesidioblastosis (diffuse islet cell hyperplasia arising from pancreatic ductal epithelium)
- Beckwith-Wiedemann syndrome (congenital overgrowth syndrome)

S/smx:
- May be asmx
- Autonomic smx: jittery baby, irritable, ↑RR, pallor
- Neuro smx: poor feeding / sucking, weak cry, drowsy, hypotonia, seizures
- Others: apnoea, hypothermia

Mx:
- If baby is still awake & able to, encourage PO feeding + monitor prefeeding sugars
- If baby is symptomatic or has very low blood glucose
  - IV infusion of 10% dextrose
  - Admit and monitor on neonatal unit

Causes: · Neonatal sepsis
- Werdnig-Hoffman disease (spinal muscular atrophy subtype)
- Hypothyroidism
- Syndromes: Down, Prader-Willi
- Maternal drug use (eg benzos)
- Maternal myasthenia gravis

Ix: very extensive to find cause (including bloods, genetics, MRI brain)

Mx: respi and feeding support as required

Infantile haemangioma
≈ aka strawberry naevus
- D: Benign vascular lesion that typically appears within the first few weeks of life
- R: low birth weight, prematurity, white ethnicity, F>M (5:1)
- S/smx: - 80% of these appear by first 3mo of life
  - Max size at ~9mo
  - flat or nodular lesion
  - Involution occurs with 90% completion by 4yo
  - Commonly appears on the face, scalp and back
  - Potential complications
    ◊ mechanical – rarely, if it develops in upper airway, can cause obstruction
    ◊ bleeding
    ◊ ulceration
    ◊ thrombocytopaenia
- Ix: generally not necessary unless doubt about Dx – Doppler US would be first line
- Mx: watch and wait unless large or over critical area (eg joint, eye)
  - propranolol to shrink

Umbilicus
- After birth, it should dry and separate by ~1w, but may persist for up to 3w
- Infection (omphalitis) is rare
- Granuloma: table salt application twice a day for 2 days usually results in complete resolution

Sticky eye
- Common in newborns
- Try applying mother's breast milk to the sticky eye or cleanse gently – should resolve
- If persistent, may be due to blocked tear duct
- Treat as infection if copious secretions, purulent discharge, or conjunctivitis

Red-stained nappy
- DDx: - urinary urate crystals (more likely when baby is dehydrated)
  - blood from cord
  - blood from baby's vagina (due to oestrogen withdrawal; "pseudo-menstruation")
- Generally not cause for concern if baby is systemically well

Miliaria crystallina
- D: cutaneous eruption due to retention of sweat due to occlusion or disruption of eccrine sweat ducts
- S/smx: - asymptomatic
  - clear vesicles that rupture easily
  - self-resolving problem
- Miliaria rubra – there is surrounding rash and pruritus
- Mx: ensure baby is not too warm, but problem is generally self-resolving (few hours to days)

Stork bites
- D: Benign areas of capillary dilation on the eyelids, forehead, or back of neck ("baby is held by a stork beak")
- S/smx: slight redness on those areas and fades within hours/days

Milia
- D: benign, transient, subepidermal keratin-filled cysts
- S/smx
  - White bumps, commonly on the face 1-2mm wide
  - Present in about half of newborns
  - Usually resolves spontaneously by 1mo old

Erythema toxicum neonatorum
- D: rash (reddish wheals with central white/yellow pustules) that is found in newborns
- A: ? reaction to meconium
- S/smx:
  - presents within 1st week of life
  - resolves within 7-14d
  - rash as above, may be exacerbated by heat
  - the majority of rashes are temporary, and they disappear within a few hours and reappear elsewhere

Harlequin colour change
- D: Transient, episodic, demarcated erythema on left or right, with contralateral blanching
- Benign and self-limiting

Developmental dysplasia of the hip
→ see MSK/Orthopaedics

Caput succedaneum
- D: Oedema of the scalp at the presenting part of the head
- S/smx: - Usually presents at birth
  - soft, puffy swelling due to localised oedema
  - Crosses suture lines
- Mx: watch and wait, self-resolving in days

Cephalohaematoma
- D: Haematoma 2/2 bleeding between periosteum and skull (typically at the parietal region)
- S/smx: Usually presents hours after birth
  - Swelling does not cross suture lines
- Ix: bilirubin + LFTs (jaundice may develop due to breakdown of Hb)
- Mx: watch & wait if not severe – may take up to 3mo to resolve
  - Other Mx dependent on how severe

Cradle cap
- D: Seborrhoeic dermatitis on the skull
- S/smx: - Usually develops in first few weeks of life
  - Erythematous rash + coarse yellow scales (can come in big patches)
  - Rash can appear on nappy area, face and limb flexures as well
- Mx: - Reassurance that it doesn't affect baby, will resolve in a few weeks
  - Massage topical emollient onto scalp to loosen scales, remove with soft brush and shampoo
  - If severe/persistent, topical imidazole cream trial
- P: Usually resolves by 8mo

See 16.09 for birth injuries.

Non-accidental injury   NAI

R: birthwt <2.5kg, mother <30yo, unwanted pregnancy, poverty, prematurity, multiple medical conditions, child <2yo, domestic abuse. Parental – substance and alcohol misuse, intellectual disability, Hx of childhood abuse, mental health problems

S/smx
- child may disclose it themselves
- story inconsistent with injuries
- repeated attendances at A&E
- delayed presentation
- child with a frightened, withdrawn appearance - 'frozen watchfulness'
- bruising
- fractures: particularly metaphyseal, posterior rib fractures or multiple fractures at different stages of healing
- torn frenulum: e.g. from forcing a bottle into a child's mouth
- burns or scalds
- failure to thrive
- STIs, eg gonorrhea, trichomonas

Ix of suspected physical abuse
- <2yo: skeletal survey, ophthalmology review (retinal haemorrhages indicate 71% of abusive head trauma in <3yo)
- head CT: for <1yo, consider in >1yo
- Bruising: clotting screen, FBC, film
- #: bone profile, vit D, PTH
- Consider urine tox if poisoning possible, and medical photography to document injuries

Information sharing: contact social services to check if pt/family known. Contact GP, health visitor, school.

DDx: osteogenesis imperfecta, ITP, leukaemia, HSP, coagulation disorder, scurvy, blue spots, osteoporosis

Mx: raise safeguarding issue. Document everything; differentiate fact and opinion.

Sexual abuse
- Adults often do not believe children's allegations of abuse
- Higher incidence in children with special needs
- Sexual activity <13yo is illegal in the UK even if child 'consents'
- Abusers: 30% father, 15% unrelated man, 10% older brother
- Possible presentations
  - pregnancy   - STIs
  - recurrent UTIs
  - sexually precocious behaviour
  - anal fissure   - bruising
  - reflex anal dilatation
  - enuresis and encopresis
  - behavioural problems, self-harm
  - recurrent symptoms e.g. headaches, abdominal pain
- Mx: raise safeguarding issue
  - Forensic evidence may be obtained up to 7d from vaginal intercourse
  - STI screening

Screening schedule

- Antenatal scans and other neonatal screening: should start by 12w of pregnancy
- Newborn: immediate physical external inspection after birth, then full physical exam by 72h
- Bloodspot screening: ideally day 5. Heel-prick blood test to test for
  - Hypothyroidism
  - Cystic fibrosis
  - Haemoglobinopathies
  - IMDs: PKU, MCADD, Maple syrup urine disease, isovaleric acidaemia, glutaric aciduria type 1, homocystinuria
- Newborn hearing screening programme: within 4-5w of birth
- 6-8w review (usually undertaken by GP): physical exam including CVS, hips, eyes, testes, discuss any concerns
- By 5yo: pre-school hearing screen + screening for visual impairment

Health and development reviews
- By 14d: f2f rv with both parents to review feeding, Ax maternal MH, discuss home safety, SIDS risk, promote sensitive parenting
- 2-2.5y review by health visitor

Sudden infant death syndrome

D: Sudden unexpected death of an apparently healthy infant under 1yo with the cause of death unclear after thorough investigation

! Odds ratios (OR) are additive – more than 1 risk factors ↑↑risk
Major risk factors
- Prone sleeping (3.5-9.3), ↑risk if baby not used to prone sleeping (sleeping on the tummy)
- Prenatal smoking (OR 5)
- Prematurity (OR 4)
- Bed sharing (OR 5.1)
- Hyperthermia or head covering
Other risk factors
- M>F   • Multiple births
- Lower socioeconomic status
- Maternal drug use   • Winter
Protective factors
- Breastfeeding
- Room sharing (but not bed sharing)
- Use of dummies / pacifiers

A/P: not fully understood; multifactorial – vulnerable infant + critical period + exogenous stressor → abnormal cardiorespiratory control → death

Mx: • Death must be referred to coroner
- Screen siblings for potential sepsis and inborn errors of metabolism

---

Vaccination schedule

Age	Vaccine	Dose
8w	• Diphtheria	1/5
	• Poliomyelitis	1/5
	• Tetanus	1/5
	• HiB	1/4
	• Pertussis	1/4
	• Hep B	1/3
	• MenB	1/3
	• Rotavirus	1/2
12w	• Diphtheria	2/5
	• Poliomyelitis	2/5
	• Tetanus	2/5
	• HiB	2/4
	• Pertussis	2/4
	• Hep B	2/3
	• Pneumococcal conjugate	1/2
	• Rotavirus	2/2
16w	• Diphtheria	3/5
	• Poliomyelitis	3/5
	• Tetanus	3/5
	• HiB	3/4
	• Pertussis	3/4
	• Hep B	3/3
	• MenB	2/3
1y	• MMR	1/2
	• MenB	3/3
	• Pneumococcal conjugate	2/2
	• HiB	4/4
2-3y	• Influenza	
40mo	• Diphtheria	4/5
	• Poliomyelitis	4/5
	• Tetanus	4/5
	• Pertussis	4/5
	• MMR	2/2
11y	• HPV	
13y	• MenA, MenC	
	• Diphtheria	5/5
	• Poliomyelitis	5/5
	• Tetanus	5/5
65y	• Pneumococcal polysaccharide	
70-79y	• Herpes zoster (live or recomb)	

Pre-pregnancy counselling

Immunisation: rubella

Stop smoking
- ↓ovulation, abn sperm production
- 2x miscarriage risk
- a/w preterm labour, fetal growth restriction, placenta praevia, abruption

Alcohol abstinence advised
- High levels cause fetal alcohol syndrome, ↑risk of miscarriage
- Minimal drinking (1-2u/w) has not been shown to adversely affect fetus, but crosses placenta and can affect fetal brain
- NICE rec <1u/24h; binge drinking (>5u/session esp harmful)

Recreational drugs a/w miscarriage, preterm birth, poor fetal development, intrauterine death

Wt loss: BMI >18.5 & <30
- Avoid contact sports please

Supplementation: folic acid
- Essential for DNA and RNA
- Causes of deficiency
  - Phenytoin   - MTX
  - Pregnancy   - Alcohol excess
- Consequences of deficiency
  - Megaloblastic anaemia
  - Neural tube defects
- Folic acid **0.4 mg daily >1mo preconception until ≥13w**
  - 5 mg/d if past neural tube defects, on antiepileptics, diabetic, obese, HIV+ve on co-trimox prophylaxis, or sickle cell disease

Supplementation: PO iron
- Only if anaemic – <105g/L in 1st trim or <115 g/L thereafter

Supplementation: Vitamin D
- 10 mcg/d for all women, esp in pts with darker skin or those who have covered skin

Supplementation: Vitamin A
- high doses (>700 mcg) are teratogenic; avoid eating liver

Pre-existing medical disorders
- Poorly controlled – same or worse
- Well controlled – same or better
- Refer for specialist help asap

Medication: Δ prior to conception to ↓risk of teratogenicity: antiepileptics, ACEI, immune-modulators
- Avoid OTCs as much as possible

Diet
- Avoid liver and Vit A
- Limit caffeine to 200 mg/d (≈2 cups of tea or coffee)
- Cook meat thoroughly
- Avoid cheese, shellfish & raw fish

Work
- Maternity rights and benefits
- Usually safe to continue working unless occupational hazards

Air travel
- Avoid after 37w for all singletons
- Avoid after 32w for multiples
- For complicated pregnancies, review risk factors and advice
- A/w ↑risk of VTE
  - Wear compression stockings!

Spontaneous miscarriage: 15-20% of all pregnancies, ↑ if extremes of age. Recurrent miscarriage = >3 consecutive miscarriages

Physiological changes in pregnancy

Hormonal changes
- Progesterone: ↓muscle excitability, ↑body temp
- Estrogens (90% estriol) ↑breast and nipple growth, water retention, protein synthesis
- Thyroid: ↑ in size
- Prolactin: ↑ throughout pregnancy
- Cortisol: ↑ output, but unbound levels constant

Genital changes
- Uterus: 100g → 1.1kg :0
  - hypertrophy occurs ≤20w, then stretching
- Vaginal discharge ↑ due to cervical ectopy, cell desquamation, ↑mucus production from vasocongested vagina

Haemodynamic changes
- Blood: plasma volume rises from 8 to 32w (50% >non-pregnant)
  - RBC ↑30% if supplements taken
  - ◊ Hb falls due to dilution
  - WCC, platelets, ESR, cholesterol, β-globulin, fibrinogen ↑
  - Albumin and GGT ↓
  - Urea and creatinine ↓
- Cardiovascular
  - CO↑ - SV ↑10%, HR ↑~15b/min
  - Peripheral resistance ↓
  - BP (esp DBP) ↓ during 2nd trim, then rises to non-pregnant levels by term
  - Varicose veins may form
- IVC compression from 20w will ↓CO by 30-40% (supine hypotension)
  ↳ left lateral position or tilt ~15' to the left to relieve this

Others
- Ventilation ↑40% 2/2 progesterone
  ↳ O2 ↑20% only   ↳ SOB common
- Gut motility ↓ - constipation, delayed gastric emptying, lax esophageal sphincter, heartburn
- Renal size ↑1cm in length, GFR ↑60% and ↑pressure on bladder → ↑micturition
- Skin pigmentation: linea nigra, nipples, chloasma, palmar erythema, spider naevi, striae
- Hair shedding in periperium
- Pregnancy tests: may be +ve from 9d post-conception (or from day 23 of a 28 day cycle). False +ve rate is low.

Antenatal care

1st antenatal (booking) visit
Full Hx taking
- FHx of DM, HTN, fetal abnormality, inheritable disease, twins?
- Concurrent illness, FGM ("cut"?), ↑risk for VTE (±LMWH)
- Is GDM a risk? 75g OGTT at 28w if BMI >30, previous macrosomia, 1st-degree family DM, ethnic risk
  - if previous GDM, screen at 16w and again at 28w
- Past mental illness? If serious (SCZ, bipolar, self-harm) or past postnatal depression: antenatal Ax by perinatal mental health team
- Women born outside UK: ↑Hb problems, BBV, pre-existing cardiac disease
- Unsupported women: ask about domestic violence, check for substance abuse

Examination: heart, lungs, BP, wt & BMI, abdomen. ? varicose veins
- ± pap smear   - FGM

Test: Hb, blood group, infectious disease, screen for sickle cell and thalassemia
- Offer screening for chromosomal and structural abnormalities
- 12w scan also confirms EDD

Advise on: (see counselling) + use of seat belts (above/below bump, not over it), offer antenatal classes, info on maternity benefits.
- Travel OK up to 36w but check with airline; avoid malarial areas
  - may require fit to fly letter >32w
- Intercourse ok if no bleeding

Later visits
- Discuss screening results, tx anaemia and UTI
- At each visit, check for protein, BP, fundal height
- Visits are at <12, 16, 25, 28, 31, 34, 36, 38, 40, 41 (preimp)
- 28w: Hb, Rh abs – give anti-D if needed

Structural abnormalities

- Most occur in low-risk patients with uncomplicated pregnancies
- Women at higher risk: previously affected child, pre-existing DM, epilepsy
- Everyone in UK to be offered tests
- ! tests are not diagnostic, and can be declined by the woman !

- US can detect pregnancy from approx 5w of gestation
- Used to date a pregnancy

Nuchal translucency (NT) at 11-13w
- Determines viability, dates pregnancy, Dx multiple pregnancy and chorionicity
- Screening for chromosomal abn by nuchal folds measurement + bloods
- ↑ fetal NT may reflect fetal heart failure, serious abn of heart and great arteries
- Bloods + NT - if risk <1:150, invasive testing is offered

Anomaly scan
- Detailed US at 18-22w to detect structural malformations
- About 30min to complete, sensitivity varies depending on many factors

Lethal anomalies
- Anencephaly
- Bilateral renal agenesis
- Some major cardiac abn
- Trisomies 13 and 18

Fetal echo: offered to those at high risk of fetal cardiac abn – FHx or personal Hx, NT >3.5mm, drugs in pregnancy (lithium), DM, mono-chorionic twins

Other types of scans
- Soft markers – slightly more common in chromosomally abn fetuses
- Fetal growth scans
- Doppler US – blood flow; useful in high-risk pregnancies

Aneuploidy & screening

Trisomy 21 (Down) →15.20
· 10% die before 5yo, life expectancy is 55yo. ↑rate of spontaneous miscarriage
· ↑maternal age → ↑risk <25yo 1:1500 vs 45yo 1:30
· Congenital cardiac malformations common, esp VSD or ASD, also duodenal atresia

Trisomy 18 (Edwards)
· Most die soon after birth; >1yo rare
· Small chin, low set ears, rocker bottom feet, VSD

Trisomy 13 (Patau)
· Most die soon after birth
· Microcephaly, holoprosencephaly, exomphalos, cleft lip/palate

Screening with **combined test**
· Uses NT + free hCG + pregnancy-associated plasma protein (PAPP-A) + woman's age
· w11 to 13+6
· Detects 90% of all aneuploidies
· Tests will return either a 'lower' or 'higher chance' – higher chance (>1:150) → counselling

Screening with **quadruple test**
· If women book later in pregnancy (w15-20)
· AFP, unconjugated estriol, hCG, inhibin A

	AFP	UcO	hCG	inhA
Down	↑	↓	↑	↑
Edwards/ Patau	↓	↓	↓	~
Neural tube defects	↑	~	~	~

Non-invasive prenatal screening (NIPT)
· Analyses small DNA fragments that circulate in the blood of a pregnant woman
· >99% sens+spec for chromosomal abn esp Down
· Private companies offer NIPT from 10w gestation

Invasive testing

Chorionic villus biopsy
· 10-13w; allows earlier termination than amniocentesis
· Placenta sampled via transabd or trans-cervical approach
· Risks: ↑miscarriage by 1-2%, ↑transmission of BBV, contamination by maternal cells, false +ve or -ve
· Not recommended for dichorionic multiple pregnancy

Amniocentesis
· 16w onwards
· Aspiration of fluid containing fetal cells shed from skin and gut via small needle passed transabdominally
· Fetal loss rate is ~1% at 16w
· Anti-D needed in all Rh-ve F
· Can Dx fetal infections such as CMV, ↓excess miscarriage rate

Use of anti-D

Dose - 250u for gestation <20w
    - 500u if >20w
· Give in deltoid IM
    - IV or SC if bleeding disorder
· From 20w, do Kleihauer test (FBC bottle of maternal blood, so can be counted to measure the bleed's volume) - do not give anti-D if already sensitised

Postnatal use: 500u normal dose
· Anti-D: for all Rh-ve women where baby's group cannot be determined, or if baby's group is unknown 72h post-delivery
· Do a Kleihauer test on all eligible for anti-D
· Any mother receiving anti-D prenatally should also receive it postnatally unless she delivers an Rh-ve baby

Anti-D in miscarriage in Rh-ve mums
· Give to all having surgical or medical terminations of pregnancy, evacuation of hydatidiform mole, and ectopic pregnancies, unless they are known to have anti-D abs
· Give where spontaneous miscarriage requires termination
· Anti-D should be given where spontaneous complete miscarriage occurs after 12w
· Threatened miscarriage ≥12w; if bleeding continues intermittently, give it q6w until delivery
· Routine anti-D not rec with threatened miscarriages before 12w

Anti-D in pregnancy in Rh-ve mums
· Take blood sample before 28w to look for antibodies
· Give anti-D 500u at 28 and 34w to Rh-ve women
· When significant transplacental haemorrhage may occur, use 250u before 20w gestation, 500u after 20w

Antenatal timetable

NICE recommendations
· 10 visits in 1st preg if uncomplicated
· 7 visits in subsequent if uncomp
· No need to be seen by consultant if uncomplicated

8-12w (ideally <10w)   **1st trim**
· Booking visit
· Booking bloods + urine culture (asymptomatic bacteriuria)

10 - 13+6w: early scan to confirm dates, exclude multiple pregnancies

11 - 13+6w: Down's syndrome screening including nuchal scan

16w: information on anomaly and blood results.   **2nd trim**
· If Hb <110 g/L, consider iron
· Routine care: BP and urine dipstick

18 - 20+6w: anomaly scan

25w (if premip)
· Routine care: BP, urine dipstick, symphysis-fundal height

28w · Routine care   **3rd trim**
· 2nd screen for anaemia and atypical red cell alloantibodies
    ↳ if Hb <105g/L, consider iron
· First dose of anti-D prophylaxis to rhesus -ve women

31w (if premip) · Routine care

34w · Routine care
· 2nd dose of anti-D (depending on local regime)
· Info on labour and birth plan

36w · Routine care
· Check presentation: offer external cephalic version if indicated
· info on breastfeeding, vitamin K, baby-blues

38w · Routine care

40w (if premip) · Routine care
· Discussion about options for prolonged pregnancy

41w – same as 40w visit

Offer screening for these:
· Anaemia
· Bacteriuria
· Blood group, Rhesus status and anti-RBC antibodies
· Down's syndrome
· Fetal anomalies
· Hepatitis B
· HIV
· Neural tube defects
· Risk factors for pre-eclampsia
· Syphilis

Screening depending on Hx:
· Placenta praevia
· Psychiatric illness
· Sickle cell disease
· Tay-Sachs disease
· Thalassaemia

Do not offer screening routinely:
· Bacterial vaginosis
· Chlamydia
· Cytomegalovirus
· Fragile X
· Hepatitis C
· Group B Streptococcus
· Toxoplasmosis

- HA, palpitations, fainting
  - 2/2 dilated peripheral circulation, ↑sweating and feeling hot
  - Mx: ↑fluid intake, stand slowly
- Urinary frequency
  - 2/2 pressure of fetal head on bladder in later pregnancy, ↑GFR
  - exclude UTI
- Abdominal pain
- Breathlessness – r/o VTE
- Constipation
  - 2/2 ↓gut motility
  - Mx: ↑fluids, high fibre diet
  - Avoid stimulant laxatives
- GORD
  - 2/2 progesterone-mediated pyloric sphincter relaxation + fetal pressure
  - Mx: avoid triggers; eat small meals; antacids, H2RA or PPI; use more pillows and prop up
- Symphysis pubis dysfunction
  ≈ pelvic girdle pain
  - 2/2 pelvic ligament and muscle relaxation
  - Mx: analgesia, physio
- Carpal tunnel syndrome
  - 2/2 fluid retention
  - Mx: wrist splints
- Itch / itchy rashes (up to 25%)
  - 2/2 common causes or pruritic eruption of pregnancy
    ◊ PEP - intensely itchy papular/plaque rash on abd + limbs; common in primip >35w
  - Mx: emollients, weak topical steroids; delivery is the cure
  - If vesicles present, think of pemphigoid gestationis – can cause fatal heat loss and cardiac failure. Refer early. May recur.
- *Ankle oedema*
  - Measure BP, check urine for protein, check legs for DVT – Mx: rest, leg elevation
  - Reassure that harmless unless in pre-eclampsia
- Leg cramps (33%)
  - Mx: ↑fluids, bananas, tonic water
  - Can be difficult to treat
- Chloasma: patch of darker pigmentation
- Nausea: 80%, vomitting 50% – can start at 4w, ↓over following weeks

D: persistant N/V in pregnancy causing wt loss >5%, dehydration and electrolyte imbalance

R: ↑hCG (multiple pregnancies, trophoblastic disease), nulliparity, obesity, FHx or PMH of HG
Smoking ↓risk of HG

S/smx for admission / referral
- Continued N/V, unable to keep down liquids or oral antiemetics
- Continued N/V, with ketonuria and/or wt loss >5%, despite tx with oral antiemetics
- A confirmed or suspected comorbidity (e.g. unable to tolerate oral abx for a UTI)

Criteria for Dx
- ≥5% pre-pregnancy wt loss
- dehydration
- electrolyte imbalance
Pregnancy-Unique Quantification of Emesis (**PUQE**) score to classify severity of HG

Ix: Urine dip for ketones, UTI
- FBC, U&Es, LFTs
- If refractory HG, check TFTs, LFTs, calcium, phosphate, amylase (r/o pancreatitis), ABG
- US to Dx multiple pregnancy and r/o trophoblastic disease

Mx:
- simple measures: rest; avoid triggers; bland foods; ginger; wrist acupuncture
- medications
  - cyclizine or promethazine
  - prochlorperazine or chlorpromazine
  - combination doxylamine/pyridoxine – not available in UK
- medications
  - ondansetron: in first trim, a/w small risk of cleft lip/palate.
  - metoclopramide or domperidone – do not use >5d ∴ extrapyramidal SE

- Admission if refractory for tx
  - IVF – normal saline +K or Hartmann's for rehydration
    ◊ do not give glucose as can precipitate Wernicke's
- If vomiting still intractable, consider steroids (prednisolone 40-50 mg od or hydrocortisone 100 mg/12h IV)
- Prescribe high dose folic acid 5mg/d, thiamine to prevent Wernicke's. In hospital, give enoxaparin 40 mg od and anti-VTE stockings (dehydration ↑risk for VTE)

Complications
- AKI   • Wernicke's encephalopathy
- Esophagitis, Mallory-Weiss tear
- VTE
- Fetal outcome: HG is a/w small ↑ in preterm birth and low birth weight

General advice
- Avoid immobility and dehydration
- Risk ↑ from early in first trim to 6w postpartum

Risk factors for VTE
- ► HIGH RISK → give antenatal LMWH
  - Hx of ≥2 VTE
  - Unprovoked or oestrogen-related VTE
  - Single provoked VTE + thrombophilia or FHx
  - Antithrombin III def (30% risk)
- Intermediate risk → consider
  - Thrombophilia but no VTE
  - Single provoked VTE
  - Medical comorbidities, eg cancer, inflammatory conditions, significant cardiac or respi conditions, SLE, sickle cell disease, nephrotic syndrome, IVDU, any antenatal surgery
- Other risks (if ≥3, consider)
  - age >35   - obesity
  - parity ≥3   - smoker
  - large varicose veins
  - current infxn   - pre-eclampsia
  - immobility   - dehydration
  - multiple pregnancy
  - assisted reproduction techniques
- Postpartum risk factors
  - mid-cavity or rotational instrumental delivery
  - PPH + blood transfusion

Indications for VTE
- See risk factors
- If pt gets antenatal LMWH, it must be continued until 6w post-partum (pp)
- Emergency LCSC: 7d pp

Dosing of LMWH
- Depends on body wt
- Enoxaparin 40 mg SC for 50-90kg, 60 mg if 91-130 kg, 80 mg if 131-170kg OD
- Wait 4h after siting epidural or removal
- DO NOT give if PPH ongoing (duh)
- Otherwise can give immediately

E: 0.1-0.2% of all pregnancies
- DVT 3x more common than PE
- Untreated DVT leads to PE in 16%
- DVT more common postnatally

Ix
- Bloods: FBC, U&Es, LFTs, clotting
- If PE suspected, ABG, ECG, CXR
- D-dimers: useful only if -ve (to r/o) (ie don't routinely order)

Imaging
- DVT: compression or duplex US of deep veins
- If high clinical suspicion, continue tx dose of LMWH + repeat imaging in 1w
- In PE, CXR → if (normal) US of deep veins
  - if still -ve, use V/Q scanning
  - ? spiral CT or MRI

Mx - start asap if suspected
- Massive PE
  - immediate senior help
  - thrombolysis or percutaneous catheter thrombus fragmentation
  - consider UFH
  - take blood for APTT 6h post-loading dose; aim for 1.5-2.5x lab control value
- Generally, use LMWH
  - BD dosing for LMWH (ref to BNF)
  - Ref to haematology for f/u
  - Consider switching to warfarin post-delivery
  - Must be continued for ≥6w pp
- During labour
  - Stop LMWH
  - keep well hydrated
  - Avoid regional anaesthesia until ≥12h after last dose of prophylactic LMWH or ≥24h after tx dose
  - Wait >4h until epidural catheter removed until next dose
  - Do not remove catheter until >12h after last dose
  - Those at high risk on stopping anticoagulation: consider UFH ± IVC filter

Hypertension

Normal course of BP in pregnancy
- ↓ in early pregnancy till about 24w
- Then ↑ thereafter (↑stroke volume
- ► >160/110 = EMERGENCY

Chronic hypertension

- HTN before 20w gestation or high booking BP (>130/80) → likely to develop chronic HTN
- in 3-5% pregnancies
- Risks - pre-eclampsia
  - fetal growth restriction
  - placental abruption

- Pre-conception Mx
  - Change drug to labetalol, nifedipine, hydralazine or methyldopa
    ↳ ! ACEI/ARBs are teratogenic
- Antenatal Mx
  - Aim BP <150/90 but with DBP≥80
  - Aspirin 75mg OD until baby born
  - Admit if >160/110
  - Fetal US q4w from 28w to Ax fetal growth, amniotic fluid volume and umbilical artery Dopplers
  - If fetal activity abnormal, CTG
  - Aim to induce around EDD
- Intrapartum Mx
  - Monitor BP qhly if BP <159/109, continuously if ≥160/110
  - If high BP refractory to tx, advise operative delivery
  - Give oxytocin alone at 3rd stage of labour (! ergometrine CI)
- Postnatal Mx
  - check BP on every day days 1-5, and at 2w
  - Change methyldopa to other antiHTN as risk of postnatal depression
    ↳ avoid diuretic if bfding

Pregnancy-induced hypertension (PIH)

- HTN (>140/90) in second half of pregnancy in the *absence* of proteinuria or other features of pre-eclampsia
- 6-7% pregnancies

Anaemia in pregnancy

- Defined as Hb < 105 g/L
- Antenatal screening at booking + 28w
- Cut offs for tx with PO Fe:
  - 1st trim: <110 g/L
  - 2nd/3rd: <105 g/L
  - Post-partum: <100 g/L
- Offer PO ferrous sulfate 200 mg bd PO with orange juice. If unable to tolerate: every other day, or 2x/w. Avoid with tea, Ca, metal-containing supplements
  - continue for 3mo after identified to allow stores to be replenished
- Thalassemia: refer to specialists
- Sickle cell: aim for Dx at birth (cord blood) for penicillin pneumococcal prophylaxis

Antenatal Mx
- Urine testing for proteinuria or ACR testing to r/o pre-eclampsia
- If mild, check urine and BP weekly
  - 4wkly fetal growth scans
- >150/100, start tx + check 2x/w
- ≥160/110, admit,
  - measure BP every 6h
  - check urine 6hlr
  - check FBC, U&Es, AST/ALT, bilirubin at presentation & wkly
  - if refractory, make plans for delivery
- Aim for delivery after 37w unless pre-eclampsia develops
Intrapartum Mx
- Continue antihypertensives
- Monitor BP qhly; continuously if >160/110 - advise C-sec
Postnatal Mx
- Continue Rx until BP <130/80
- Review at 2w and 6w
- If tx still needed at 6w, refer to cardiologists

Diabetes in pregnancy

DM in 5% of pregnancies:
87.5% GDM, 7.5% T1, 5% T2

R: BMI >30, previous macrosomia (≥4.5kg), previous GDM, 1st FHx, ethnicity

Screening: OGTT
- If prev GDM, OGTT asap after booking, and at 24-28w.
- If other risk factors, OGTT within 24-28w
- NICE rec early self-monitoring using blood glucose early on

Dx: fasting glucose ≥ 5.6 mmol/L
2h-OGTT ≥ 7.8 mmol/L

Mx of newly Dx GDM:
- joint DM-antenatal clinic w/in 1w
- teach self-monitoring of BGC
- advice – diet, exercise
- if fasting glucose <7, offer to trial diet and exercise
  - if targets not met w/in 1-2w, start metformin
  - if targets not met, + insulin
- if fasting glucose ≥7 at Dx, start short-acting insulin
  - if glucose 6-6.9 + evidence of complications, start insulin

Mx of previous DM
- wt loss if BMI >27
- stop hypoglycaemics except metformin, start insulin
  - tight glycaemic control ↓complications
- folic acid 5 mg/d pre-conception to 12w gestation
- detailed anomaly scan at 20w including four-chamber view of the heart and outflow tracts
- tx retinopathy as can worsen during pregnancy

C: 50% of women with GDM develop T2DM – check fasting glucose 6w postpartum or HbA1c at 13w pp: screen annually

Hyperthyroidism in pregnancy

- Usually Graves' disease, can be a/w infertility, prematurity, fetal loss, malformations.
- Mx with PTU (↓crossing placenta)
- Partial thyroidectomy if severe
- Monitor ≥monthly
- TSH-receptor stimulating abs can cause fetal thyrotoxicosis (1%) after 24w. Many complications.
  - test TFTs in affected babies frequently
  - usually resolves spontaneously in 2-3mo
- Thyroid storm can be ppt by labour – urgent tx required

Jaundice in pregnancy

- Occurs in 1:1500 pregnancies
- Dx urgently – travel Hx, DHx, BBV

Obstetric cholestasis (0.7% prev)
- Pruritus (palms, soles) in 2nd half, no rash. Worse at night.
- Dx of exclusion – r/o BBV, autoimmune diseases, US of liver
- Weekly LFTs. Give Vitamin K 10mg/24h if abn clotting screen, and 1mg to baby at birth
- Typically induced at 37w
- Ursodeoxycholic acid ↓itch
- Smx resolve w/in 1w of delivery
- Can recur with COCP and ≤70% subsequent pregnancies

Acute fatty liver of pregnancy
- Rare but serious
- Abn pain, jaundice, HA, vomitting ± thrombocytopaenia, pancreatitis
- a/w pre-eclampsia in 30-60%
- Complications: coma, death
- Mx in HDU/ITU – supportive tx.
  Expedite delivery
  - ! epidural, regional anaesthesia contraindicated

Other causes of jaundice:
- Viral   • Severe pre-eclampsia →16.08
- HELLP syndrome →16.08
- Anaesthesia (halothane)

Malaria in pregnancy

S/smx: in any woman who presents with odd behaviour, fever, jaundice, sweating, DIC, fetal distress, premature labour, seizures, or LOC → ask could this be malaria??
→ do thick and thin films
→ seek expert help

- Advice against travelling to endemic areas, or to use preventative measures (eg mosquito nets, insect repellants)

Renal disease in pregnancy

Asymptomatic bacteriuria
- 2% of sexually active women
- ≤7% pregnant women, ↑in DM, renal transplants. 30% develop into pyelonephritis
- If present on MSU, abx given
  - cefalexin 500 mg PO for 5d
  - trimethoprim (avoid in 1st)
  - nitrofurantoin (avoid in 3rd)

Pyelonephritis
- 1-2% of pregnant women
- do blood and urine culture
- IV abx eg cefuroxime 1.5g/8h, consider stat dose gentamicin
- Continue IV abx for at least 24h, PO abx for 2-3w
- Repeat MSU to check eradication
- If ≥2 confirmed UTIs in pregnancy, do renal US, consider abx prophylaxis for rest of pregnancy

AKI related to pregnancy
- 2/2 sepsis, haemolysis (eg HELLP syndrome), hypovolaemia, volume contraction (eg pre-eclampsia), drugs (esp NSAIDs)
- Monitor UO and fluid balance (catheterisation needed). Aim for >30 mL/h output. + renal bloods
- Ref to specialist if needed

Drugs used in psychiatry and epilepsy

- Risk vs benefit
- Consult with specialists esp in severe depression, bipolar, SCZ
  - high risk of rapid postpartum relapse a/w significant risks to mother and infant, esp in bipolar disorder (up to 50%)

Antidepressants
- SSRIs, usually **sertraline**
  - small risk of persistent fetal pulmonary HTN and neonatal withdrawal
  - Avoid paroxetine
  - Bfding ok unless detrimental to maternal well-being

Mood stabilisers (AEDs)
- ✗ valproate and carbamazepine CI in WoCA
  - valproate has 10% malformation rate with NTDs, craniofacial abn, 30-40% neurodevelopmental problems
    ↳ carbamazepine 2.2%
    ↳ lamotrigine 2.1%
- Avoid all in bfding also

Lithium a/w teratogenecity, neonatal thyroid abn, floppy baby syndrome
- only prescribe if no other choice
- offer specialist fetal echo
- monitor drug levels q4w to 36w, then wkly; do not change brands
- signs of toxicity: tremor, drowsiness, visual disturbances
- stop Li during labour
- check 12h post-dose level, restart Li based on this result
- No bfding ∵ neonatal toxicity

Antipsychotics
- rates of fetal abn ↑ in SCZ even in those taking no drugs
- women on antipsychotics a/w wt gain should have OGTT
- if on clozapine, do not BF ∵ risk of fetal agranulocytosis
- avoid depot meds in WoCA

Benzos a/w cleft lip/palate – avoid.
- Avoid diazepam in delivery ∵ risk of neonatal withdrawal

WoCA = women of childbearing age

Epilepsy in pregnancy

D: ~0.5% F of childbearing age
Other causes of seizures: eclampsia, cerebral vein thrombosis, intracranial mass, stroke, metabolic abn, drugs and withdrawal, etc

Before pregnancy
- Optimise tx – aim for lowest dose
- **Folic acid 5mg for >3mo prior to conception**
- Counsel about ↑risk of epilepsy in children (4-5% if either parent, 15-20% if both parents)
- Specific points on drugs
  - **Lamotrigine**: possibly lower rates of congenital malformations than other AEDs. May need to ↑dose
  - Valproate a/w neural tube defects
  - Carbamazepine: considered the least teratogenic of older AEDs
  - Phenytoin a/w cleft palate

During pregnancy
- Consultant-led clinic with aim for vaginal delivery
- Nuchal thickness and anomaly scans (±fetal echo) and then serial growth scans in 3rd trim (↑risk of SGA fetus)
- 5mg folic acid daily for 1st trim
- Routine drug level testing not rec
- Stress and sleep deprivation ↑risk of seizures – AVOID

Intrapartum
- Delivery in hospital, continue AEDs
- Pain relief: epidural safe
- Benzos if seizure not self-terminating (eg lorazepam 4 mg IV)
- Seizures more common intrapartum and postpartum due to ↓sleep

Postpartum
- Vitamin K 1mg to baby
- Inpt for 24h postpartum – ↑risk
- Advise on strategies to avoid dropping baby if seizure occurs, eg changing baby on floor
- Encourage bfding and review AED dose w/in 10d of delivery to avoid tox
- Discuss contraception
  - CI estrogen-containing drugs; ↑risk of seizures with lamotrigine

Connective tissue disease in pregnancy

Rheumatoid arthritis
- 75% improve during pregnancy, but 90% have flare in puerperium
- Medications
  - MTX not safe; stop ≥6mo before conception
  - Leflunomide not safe
  - Sulfasalazine, HCQ – safe
  - TNF α-blockers – ?safe
  - low dose corticosteroids may be used to control smx
  - paracetamol ⚬ for pain relief
  - NSAIDs ok until 32w; risk of early closure of ductus arteriosus
- Refer to obstetric anaesthetist due to risk of atlanto-axial subluxation

SLE
- Flares commoner in pregnancy and periperium – can ↑risk to baby
- Planned pregnancies during remission have better outcomes (similar to general population)
- Disease flares should be Mxed with corticosteroids + HCQ
- Aspirin 75-150 mg from +ve pregnancy test till delivery
- If mother is Ro+ve, 2% risk of congenital heart block and 5% transient neonatal cutaneous lupus

Antiphospholipid syndrome
- If untreated, <20% pregnancies proceed to live birth due to 1st trim loss or placental thrombosis
- ↑risk of pre-eclampsia and IUGR
- Mx
  - Uterine artery Dopplers at 20-24w
  - If high risk, 4wkly fetal growth scans including umbilical artery Dopplers from 28w
  - Aspirin 75-150mg OD if no previous adverse outcomes (live birth rate 70-80%)
  - If previous fetal loss + LMWH (enoxaparin 40 mg SC) when fetal heart identified (~6w) throughout pregnancy
  - Postpartum: heparin or warfarin

HIV in pregnancy →08.06

HIV in pregnancy
- without intervention, 15% of babies acquire HIV if mother is +ve
- 2/3 vertical transmission occurs during pregnancy, but bfding 2x rate
- ↑risk with longer membrane rupture, viral load >400, seroconversion during preg, advanced disease, pre-term labour, HCV
- ≤1% risk with maternal HAART, elective C-sec, bottle feeding
  - vaginal delivery rec if viral load <50 at 36w, otherwise C-sec
  - start zidovudine inf 4h before C-sec
- Screening at booking, 28w; if status unknown at labour, perform rapid test. Mx accordingly

Rubella in pregnancy →08.06

Maternal s/smx – absent in 50%
- Prodrome: fever
- Maculopapular rash starting from face, spreading to body
- Lymphadenopathy

- Fetus most at risk in first 16w
  - 80% of fetuses are affected if maternal primary infxn is in first 12w
- Miscarriage or stillbirth may occur
Congenital rubella syndrome
- Sensorineural deafness
- Congenital cataracts (a/w infxn at 8-9w)
- Congenital heart disease, eg patent ductus arteriosus (a/w infxn at 5-10w)
- Growth retardation
- Hepatosplenomegaly
- Purpuric skin lesions
- 'Salt and pepper' chorioretinitis
- Microphthalmia
- Cerebral palsy

Ix: take abs 10d apart, look for IgM abs 4-5w from incubation period or date of contact
- If infxn confirmed in 1st trim, **TOP** is offered without invasive prenatal Dx

TOP = termination of pregnancy. See 17.03

Measles in pregnancy →08.05

Maternal s/smx
- Prodromal phase: irritable, cough, conjunctivitis, fever
- Koplik spots (appear before rash)
- Rash – starts behind ears then spreads to the whole body
  - discrete maculopapular rash becomes blotchy and confluent
- Diarrhoea in 10%

Ix: IgM abs detected >4d and <1mo of rash onset. Viral RNA in saliva.

Implications on pregnancy
- A/w fetal loss and pre-term delivery
- No congenital infxxn or abn
- If maternal rash appears 6d pre- or post-delivery, give human normal IG immediately after birth or exposure to child to prevent neonatal subacute sclerosing panencephalitis

Complications
- Encephalitis: typically occurs 1-2w following the onset of the illness
- Subacute sclerosing panencephalitis: very rare, may present 5-10y after illness
  - S/smx: Δ behaviour, myoclonus, choreoathetosis, dystonia, dementia, coma, death
- Febrile convulsions

Intrauterine syphilis →08.08

- 🦠 *Treponema pallidum*

Maternal s/smx →08.08

Fetal or neonatal s/smx
- Rhinitis & snuffles · Rash
- Hepatosplenomegaly
- Lymphadenopathy
- Anaemia · Jaundice
- Ascites · Hydrops
- Nephrosis · Meningitis
- Keratitis · SNHL

Ix · XR: perichondritis
- Nasal discharge exam: spirochetes
- CSF: ↑monocytes and proteins with +ve serology

Mx
- Maternal: benzylpenicillin 600 mg/24h IM for 10d
- Neonate (per BNFC): benzylpenicillin 50,000 U/kg as a single dose
  - OHCS says benzylpenicillin 30 mg/kg/12h IV for 7d, then 8hly for 10d
  - use Trust guidelines

Parvovirus B19 →08.06

- 🦠 DNA virus 💨 respiratory droplets
- E: 50% women in UK are immune

Maternal s/smx: usually asmx
- If smx: 'slapped cheek' rash, maculo-papular rash, fever, arthralgia
- Usually no complications for mother
- If mother is immunocompromised or otherwise susceptible (eg sickle cell),
  ❗ sudden haemolysis may occur, requiring transfusion

Fetal s/smx: affects 30% fetuses
- Fetal suppression of erythropoiesis and cardiac toxicity → HF and fetal hydrops
- 10% of fetuses affected at <20w will die
- No teratogenicity

CMV in pregnancy →08.05

- 🦠 CMV (subtype of *Herpes*)
- 5:1000 live births infected
  - 20% develop late and usually minor problems (1:1000)
  - 10% are smx – 1/3 die, 2/3 long-term problems (congenital CMV)

Maternal s/smx ≈ CMV mononucleosis
- flu-like smx: ↑T°, lymphadenopathy, rash and sore throat

Fetal smx ≈ congenital CMV
- growth retardation
- pinpoint petechial 'blueberry muffin' skin lesions
- microcephaly
- sensorineural deafness
- encephalitis (seizures)
- hepatosplenomegaly → jaundice
- chorioretinitis

Ix: generally, refer to lab
- Amniocentesis at >20w + shell viral culture can detect fetal transmission
- Throat swab, urine culture, baby's serum after birth

Prevention
- Avoid exposure to toddler's urine

Ix: paired samples in the acute and convalescent phases (>10d apart) - IgM abs appear, and IgG titres ↑

Mx: serial US looking for signs of fetal anaemia (fetal hydrops and abnormal MCA Dopplers)
- If fetus develops anaemia, manage in tertiary fetal medicine unit, consider in utero RBC infusion

Toxoplasmosis →04.05, 08.07

- 🦠 *Toxoplasma gondii*
- 💨 Oocytes in cats, rats ↦ GIT, lungs, broken skin
- Affects 2-7:1000 pregnancies; 40% of fetuses are affected if mum has illness
- The earlier in pregnancy, the more damage it causes, but the less transmissible it is

Maternal s/smx: similar to glandular fever ± fever, rash, eosinophilia

Fetal s/smx: >90% asmx
↳ picked up by serology
- If severe, intracranial calcifi cation, hydrocephalus, choroidoretinitis
- Others: encephalitis, epilepsy, mental and physical developmental delay, jaundice, hepatosplenomegaly, thrombocytopenia, and skin rashes

Ix: Dx by reference lab IgG and IgM

Maternal Mx
- If <18w gestation, start spiramycin 1g PO q8h asap
- In smx non-immune women, test every 10w through pregnancy
- If infected, consider amniocentesis to see if fetus is infected
- If ≥18w and fetal infxn confirmed, give mother
  - Pyrimethamnine 50 mg BD on d1, then 1mg/kg/d thereafter
  - and sulfadiazine 50 mg/kg/12h,
  - and calcium folinate 15mg twice weekly until delivery

Prevention:
- Avoid eating raw meat
- Wash hands if raw meat touched
- Wear gloves if gardening or dealing with cat litter
- Avoid sheep during lambing time

Listeria

- 🦠 Gram +ve rod *Listeria monocytogenes*
- 💨 Soil, food contamination (esp in soft cheeses, unpasturised milk, deli meats, deli salads, meat spreads, pâté [?ground meat] etc
  ↳ Rarely spreads vertically
- Affects 6-15:100,000 pregnancies

Maternal s/smx:
- Fever, shivering, myalgia, HA, sore throat, cough, vomiting, diarrhoea, vaginitis
- Rarely, miscarriage (± recurrent), premature labour, stillbirth

Fetal s/smx:
- 20% affected are stillborn
- Fetal distress in labour is common
- Early postnatal: respi distress from pneumonia
- Others: convulsions, hepatospleno-megaly, pustular or petechial rashes, conjunctivitis, fever, leukopenia, meningitis

Maternal Ix/Dx:
- **Blood cultures** in any pregnant pt with unexplained fever for ≥48h ▶
- Serology, vaginal and rectal swabs do not help :(

Fetal Ix/Dx:
- **Blood cultures** ± CSF, meconium, placenta cultures

Mx:
- ❗ Isolate baby
- Tx with ampicillin 50 mg/kg/6h IV and gentamicin 3mg/kg/12h until 1w after fever subsides
- Monitor levels of abx

Hepatitis B in pregnancy →03.03

- 🦠 DNA virus
- 💨 Blood, bodily fluids, vertically
- Affects 6-15:100,000 pregnancies

Maternal infection
- Can be asmx. If mother develops acute infxn in mid or 3rd trimester, there is a high risk of perinatal infxn
- Risk of death 0.5-3%
- All mothers should be screened for HBsAg (then whole hepatitis panel)
  - carriers have HBsAg for >6mo
  - HBeAg +ve indicates ↑infectivity

Fetal infection
- Without immunisation, 95% of babies born to these mums develop Hep B; 93% are chronic carriers at 6mo
- Most infxns occur at birth, some are transplacental (→ results in apparent failure of vaccination)
- In infected infants, lifetime risk of developing HCC is 50% for M, 20% for F – most will develop cirrhosis :(

Mx
- Immunoglobulin (200U IM) + vaccinate babies of carriers and infected mothers at birth
- In uncomplicated HepB, anti-HBc and anti-HBe abs will develop, and antigens will disappear ~3mo
- Do serology of vaccinated baby at 12-15mo; if HBsAg-ve and anti-HBs +ve, the child is protected

Also, · HepB is not transmitted by bfding
- little evidence to suggest C-sec ↓ vertical transmission rates

Hepatitis E →03.03

Maternal infxn
- ↑risk of maternal mortality - 25% in 3rd trimester
- Can cause fulminant hepatic failure, coma, massive PPH → death :(

Fetal infxn
- 33-50% babies become infected

Herpes simplex →08.05, 08.08

🦠 HSV1, HSV2

Maternal infxn
- Prevalence of past infxn is 25%
- Recurrence in pregnancy rare
- If mother develops **primary genital herpes** in pregnancy
  - Ref to GUM to screen for other STIs + confirm primary infxn
    ↳ Dx confirmed by PCR
  - If in 3rd trim, **PO aciclovir** or valaciclovir
  - ± elective C-sec if 1' infxn within 6w of due date
- If mother has primary infection lesions *at time of delivery*
  - LSCS recommended
  - If vaginal delivery, give mother and newborn high-dose aciclovir
  - Avoid fetal blood sampling, scalp electrodes, and instrumental delivery

Fetal infxn
- If vaginal delivery, risk of infxn to baby is 41% → high-dose aciclovir
- Do PCR for baby at birth
- Neonatal infxn appears at 5-21d
  - Grouped vesicles/pustules on a red base
    ◇ tends to be on presenting part or sites of trauma (eg scalp electrode)
  - ± Periocular and conjunctival lesions
  - ± Non-vesicular rash
- Complications: blindness, ↓IQ, epilepsy, jaundice, respi distress, DIC, death (in 30%, even with tx)

Varicella zoster →09.07

🦠 DNA virus (part of HSV group)

Maternal infxn
- Smx as per normal VZV
- 5x ↑risk of pneumonitis

Risks to baby when mother is infected:
- Fetal varicella syndrome
  - 1% risk if before 20w gest
  - skin scarring, eye defects (microphth-almia, limb hypoplasia, microcephaly, learning disabilities
- shingles in infancy: 1-2% risk if maternal exposure in 2nd/3rd trim
- severe neonatal varicella: fatal in 20% cases
  - risk if mother develops rash btwn 5d before and 2d after birth → due to ↑↑risk of transmission

VZV prophylaxis/Mx in pregnancy
- if in doubt, check maternal blood for varicella antibodies urgently
- if ≤20w and not immune,
  - give VZIG asap – effective 10d post-exposure
- if >20w and not immune,
  - either VZIG
  - or PO antivirals from day 7 to 14 post-exposure

Mx of chickenpox in pregnancy
- Ref to specialist
- RCOG suggest PO aciclovir if ≥20w and presenting within 24h of rash onset
- If woman is <20w, PO aciclovir considered with caution

Chlamydia trachomatis →08.08

🦠 *Chlamydia trachomatis*

Fetal infxn/complications
- A/w low birthwt, premature membrane rupture, fetal death
- 30% of infected mother have affected babies
- Conjunctivitis develops 5-14d after birth (late) – inflammation / pus
- Complications: chlamydia pneumonitis, pharyngitis, otitis media

Mx: · Local cleansing of eye
- Erythromycin 12.5 mg/kg/6h PO for 3w eliminates lung organisms
- Give parents erythromycin or azithromycin 1g PO single dose

Gonorrhea →08.08

🦠 *Neiserria gonorrhoeae*

Fetal infxn/complications
- Occurs within 4d of birth (early), with purulent discharge and lid swelling ± corneal hazing, corneal rupture, panophthalmitis
- 50% concurrent chlamydial infxn

Mx of infants of mums with known gonorrhea
- Within 1h of birth
  - Cefotaxime 100 mg/kg IM stat
  - Chloramphenicol 0.5% eye drops
Mx of infants who have active gonococcal infxn
- Benzylpenicillin 50 mg/kg/12h IM
- Chloramphenicol 0.5% eye drops every 3h for 7d
- Isolate baby

Clostridium perfringes →08.02

D: Gram +ve bacilli

R: illegal termination of pregnancy (improperly cleaned equipment)

S/smx: endometritis → septicaemia, gangrene → myoglobinuria → renal failure → death
- In utero death of fetus
- Local infxn of anaerobic site (eg haematomas)

Ix/Dx: swab genital site - intracellular encapsulated Gram +ve rods

Mx: · Surgically debride all devitalised tissue
- Hyperbaric O2
- High dose IV benzylpenicillin (erythromycin if serious pen allergy)

TB →02.03

- BCG vaccination after birth for
  - all babies born into households with TB
  - mums from areas with high TB prevalence
  - all who will travel to such areas
- Give all other vaccinations per normal schedule; avoid BCG arm for 3mo
- Separate babies from mums with active or open TB until she has had 2w of tx and is sputum -ve
- Vaccinate baby with BCG and tx with isoniazid until he/she has +ve skin reaction (Mantoux)
- Consider CXR in pregnant women with cough, fever or wt loss
- Encourage bfding

Group B Strep →08.03

📧 Mother to child
  ↳ 20-40% mothers have GBS in their bowel flora
Risk factors for transmission
- Premature birth
- Prolonged rupture of membrane
- Previous sibling GBS infxn
- Maternal pyrexia

Fetal infxn/complications
- Severe, early onset – 20% mortality
- Pneumonia, meningitis, septicaemia

Mx – give all women IV abx if
- +ve GBS high vaginal swab at any time in this or previous pregnancy
- Any documented GBS bacteriuria in this pregnancy
- Gestation <37w
- Any intrapartum fever
- Mum is GBS+ve with prelabour rupture of membranes at term
  - induce labour
- Culture results unknown and rupture of membranes >18h

Abx - benzylpen 3g IV loading dose, then 1.5g q4h throughout labour
- If pen allergic, clindamycin 900 mg IV q8h

Ophthalmia neonatorum

D: purulent discharge from eye of a neonatal <21d

A: blocked lacrimal glands, infxn (chlamydia, herpes virus, staph, strep, pneumococci, E.coli)

Dx: swab for bacterial and viral culture, microscopy (look for intra-cellular gonococci) and Chlamydia

Mx: · Tx infxn
- Bathe eyes with cooled boiled water or expressed breast milk

Abdominal pain in pregnancy

Pregnancy-related causes

- LABOUR?
- ► Pre-eclampsia
  - esp in later half of pregnancy
- ► Cardiac causes
  - chest, back, or epigastric pain
  - severe enough for opioids
  - full cardiac workup
- ► Abruption
  - Triad: abd pain + uterine rigidity / tenderness + vaginal bleeding
    ↳ clinical Dx (don't rely on US)
  - 1 in 80-200 pregnancies
  - Fetal loss high if >50% of placenta affected
  - Live viable fetus → rapid delivery
  - Prepare for DIC (33-50%), PPH
- ► Uterine rupture
- Uterine fibroids
- Uterine torsion
- Ovarian tumours

Other causes

- Appendicitis
  - ~1:1000 pregnancies; ↑mortality, ↑perforation
  - Fetal mortality 1.5% simple, ~30% in perforation
  - Clinical s/smx may be different due to shift in position of appendix
  - DON'T DELAY SURGERY: lap
- Cholecystitis
  - ~1-6:10,000 pregnancies
  - S/smx similar to non-pregnant: subcostal pain, N&V
  - US confirms stones
  - Usually resolves on its own, but if surgery is required, lap chole is safe
- Gastroenteritis (common)
  - If otherwise well, Mx at home
  - ORS + rest.   Beware sepsis !
- Rectus sheath haematoma (rare)
  - Dx: US
  - Mx: lap if Dx is in doubt or if pt is in shock
- Pancreatitis (rare)
  - ↑mortality. Dx: serum amylase
- UTI and pyelonephritis →16.04

Pre-eclampsia

D: disorder of pregnancy characterised by
- new-onset HTN (SBP ≥140 and/or DBP ≥90 mmHg) after 20w
- proteinuria (≥300 mg protein in 24h urine collection, or dipstick reading ≥2+, or protein:creatinine ratio ≥30mg/mmol)
- where proteinuria is absent,
  - thrombocytopaenia (platelets <100)
  - renal insufficiency (SrCr >90μmol/L)
  - impaired liver function
  - pulmonary oedema
  - new onset HA not attributable to other conditions

High risk factors:
- HTN disease in previous pregnancy
- Chronic hypertension
- CKD   • T1/T2DM
- Autoimmune disease (eg SLE)
Moderate risk factors:
- Nulliparity (ie first pregnancy)
- ≥40yo   • prev pregnancy >10y ago
- BMI ≥35 at booking visit
- FHx of pre-eclampsia   • Twins

A/P: failure of normal trophoblast invasion → maladaptation of maternal spiral arterioles + vasoconstriction and capillary leaking → HTN + complications

S/smx (if severe):
- HTN (typically >160/110)
- Proteinuria   • HA
- Visual disturbances, papilloedema
- RUQ/epigastric pain
- Hyperreflexia   • HELLP syndrome

Complications: • Eclampsia
- Fetal: intrauterine growth restriction, prematurity
- Liver involvement   • Heart failure
- Haemorrhage (placental abruption, intra-abdo haemorrhage, ICH)

Ix: urinalysis + bloods (for Dx and to check for complications), fetal US, umbilical artery Doppler velocimetry, amniotic fluid Ax

Mx:
- Prevention of complications
  - in women with ≥1 high risk factors or ≥2 moderate risk factors
  - Aspirin 75-150 mg OD from 12w gestation until birth
- If new onset pre-eclampsia suspected, refer for emergency secondary care Ax
  - if BP ≥160/110, pt is likely to be admitted and observed
  - If BP remains high after anti-hypertensives started, pt may need prophylactic Mg sulphate
- For Mx of HTN (>150/100)
  - ⊙ PO labetalol
  - ⊙ Nifedipine (eg if asthmatic) and hydralazine
- Plan for baby's birth

HELLP syndrome

= Haemolysis, Elevated Liver enzymes, and Low Platelets

R: white ethnicity, mother >35yo, obesity, chronic HTN, DM, autoimmune disorders, migraine, abnormal placentation (eg molar pregnancy), prev pregnancy with pre-eclampsia

A/P: thought to be a severe form of pre-eclampsia (about 10-20% pts with severe pre-eclampsia will develop HELLP)

S/smx: • NV, RUQ pain, lethargy

Ix: FBC with differential including platelets (↓Hb, thrombocytopaenia), peripheral blood smear (haemolysis will show up as schistocytes), liver enzymes (AST >70, ALT >70; or >2x ULN), urinalysis, clotting screen

Mx: • If suspected, start IV Mg sulphate to prevent seizures
- Start dexamethasone
- Definitive Mx is to deliver the baby

Oligohydramnios

D: reduced amniotic fluid
- amniotic fluid index ≤5cm (or <5th centile)

Causes
- Idiopathic (although cause may be found after baby is born)
- Maternal causes
  - uteroplacental insufficiency, eg pre-eclampsia
  - medications (eg NSAIDs)
- Placental causes
  - Abruption
  - Placenta thrombosis / infarction
- Fetal causes
  - Chromosomal abnormalities, eg Potter sequence (bilateral renal agenesis + pulmonary hypoplasia → baby is not producing as much urine → ↓amniotic fluid)
  - Growth restriction or death
  - Post-term gestation
  - Ruptured fetal membranes

Polyhydramnios

D: excessive amniotic fluid
- Suspect if uterine size is large for gestational age
- Amniotic fluid index ≥24cm

Causes
- Idiopathic (although cause may be found after baby is born)
- Fetal structural anomaly that impedes swallowing, eg esophageal atresia, cleft lip, etc
- Fetal neuromuscular disorder that impedes swallowing
- Genetic syndromes, eg Trisomies, Prader-Willi, etc
- High fetal cardiac output state, eg severe anaemia
- Maternal diabetes mellitus
- Macrosomia
- Hydrops fetalis

Small for gestational age

D: <10th centile for gestational age or abdominal circumference <10th centile

R: maternal age >40, smoker, cocaine use, prev SGA baby, prev stillbirth, maternal or paternal SGA, chronic HTN, DM, renal impairment, antiphospholipid syndrome, heavy antepartum bleeding, echogenic bowel, pre-eclampsia, low PAPP-A

A: abnormal trophoblast invasion tends to cause asymmetrical growth restriction (head sparing, ↓abdo circumference). Genetic abnormal-ities (eg trisomies), congenital abnormalities and infxns usually cause symmetrically small fetus

Screening:
- Mums with risk factors should be monitored more closely
- If <10th centile or static growth → refer for fetal US

Mx:
- Once identified, serial measurements of fetal size
  - umbilical artery Doppler from 26-28w + every 2-3w
- If Dopplers remain normal, aim for induction of labour at 37w
- If Dopplers abnormal, other factors will determine urgency of delivery
  - may require C-sec
- Offer corticosteroids for fetal lung maturity up to 35+6w
- After birth
  - Temperature regulation important
  - Feed within 2h of birth + monitor for hypoglycemia

P: In adulthood, ↑risk of HTN, coronary artery disease, T2DM, autoimmune thyroid disease

Prematurity

D: infant born before 37w gestation
· extreme premarurity: <28w
· term infants = 37-41w

R: intrauterine infxn, preterm premature rupture of membranes, pre-eclampsia or pregnancy-induced hypertension, placental abruption, antepartum haemorrhage

Risks that need to be managed for premature infants
· Extreme prematurity a/w highest risks for mortality
· Respiratory distress syndrome
 - 2/2 immature lungs and surfactant deficiency
 - Mx with antenatal corticosteroids and postnatal surfactant
 - ↑risk of bronchopulmonary dysplasia or chronic lung disease
· Sepsis
 - ↑risk with ↓age and need for invasive procedures
· Anaemia of prematurity
 - tx with adequate nutrition and iron supplementation
· Nutritional deficiencies
 - tx with early introduction of breast milk feeds or use of premature formula
· Jaundice
 - 2/2 inadequate GI losses of bilirubin + poor enteral nutrition
 - Mx with phototherapy
· Intraventricular haemorrhage and white matter injury
 - 2/2 immature blood vessels in brain. A/w high mortality and neuro-developmental dysfunction
· Necrotising enterocolitis
 - Mx with antenatal corticosteroids and breast milk ± probiotics
· Patent ductus arteriosus
· Retinopathy of prematurity
 - a/w excessive O2 exposure
 - maintain O2 sats 85-93% until 32w post-menstrual age
 - regular ophth screening
· Cerebral palsy and neurodevelop-mental impairment
· ADHD / other behavioural sequelae
· ↑risk of abuse/neglect

Postmaturity

D: infant born after 42w pregnancy

R: previous prolonged pregnancy

Risks to baby & mum
· Intrapartum deaths (4x risk)
· Early neonatal deaths (3x risk)
· ↑rates of induction of labour and operative delivery
· ↑risk of placental insufficiency
· Macrosomia (>4kg), shoulder dystocia, fetal injury
· Fetal skull more ossified, less mouldable
· ↑ meconium passage in labour
 - ↑risk of meconium aspiration
· ↑fetal distress in labour
· ↑C-sec rates

Mx
· At 38w visit, discuss plan + arrange for visit at 41w if not delivered
· Membrane sweep
 - Finger inserted through cervix and membrane is palpated. Thought to induce natural prostaglandins
 - Offer at 40- and 41w visit
· Induction at 41w reduces fetal death: vaginal prostaglandin + oxytocin
· If mum declines induction, then arrange twice-weekly cardiotocography + estimation of amniotic fluid depth → detects fetuses who may be becoming hypoxic

Large for gestational age
· D: >95th centile in wt for gestation
· R: FHx of LGA babies, maternal DM, obesity
· Mx:
 - Prep for shoulder dystocia delivery
 - Babies are prone to hypoglycaemia and hypocalcaemia – prompt feeding and monitor electrolytes
 - Left colon syndrome may develop self-limiting condition clinically mimicking Hirschsprung disease)

Birth injuries

Moulding (not an injury)
· Overriding of skull bones

Cephalhaematoma
· Subperiosteal swelling on fetal head
· Limited by suture lines + fluctuant
· May take weeks to spontaneously resolve, and may contribute to jaundice

Caput succedaneum
· Oedematous swelling of scalp, superficial to cranial periosteum
· Swelling not limited by suture lines
· Pressure during labour → venous congestion + exuded serum
 - known as a chignon when caused by ventouse cup
· Gradually resolves in first few days after birth

Erb's palsy
· Brachial trunk nerve damage
· S/smx: flaccid arm + hand in fixed posture. Most resolve.
· Exclude fractured clavicle, and arrange for physio. If not resolved by 6mo, unlikely to improve further

Subaponeurotic haematoma
· Blood between aponeurosis and periosteum
· A/w vaccum extractions. May contribute to anaemia or jaundice

Skull fractures
· A/w difficult forceps delivery or after second-stage C-sec delivery where head is impacted
· Parietal or frontal bones most commonly affected
· Check for CNS signs → consult neurosurgery

Intracranial injuries
· Intracranial haemorrhage a/w difficult or fast labour, instrumental delivery or breech delivery, esp in premature babies
· Anoxia may cause intraventricular haemorrhage
· Asphyxia causes ICH and may result in cerebral palsy
 - may present as extradural, subdural or subarachnoid haemorrhages
 - supportive Mx

Fetal laceration
· Occurs in 1-2% C-sec deliveries
 - More common in breech C-sec delivery and C-sec after membrane rupture
· Most are superficial and heal without scarring
· Warn parents when taking consent for C-sec

See 15.23 for minor neonatal problems

Normal labour

D: Onset of regular and painful contractions a/w cervical dilation and descent of the presenting part
- Occurs after 37w gestation
- Results in spontaneous delivery of baby within 24h of onset of spontaneous contractions
- ÷ 3 stages

Pre-labour (signs)
- "Show": shedding of cervical mucus plug and a little blood (as membranes strip from the os)
- ± Rupture of membranes

Stage 1: from onset of true labour to when cervix is fully dilated (~8-18h in premip; 5-12h in multip)
- Latent phase
  - painful + irregular contractions
  - cervix shortens + dilates to 3cm*
- Established phase
  - regular contractions with dilation from 3cm,* normally 1cm/h

Stage 2: from full dilation to delivery of fetus (~3h in premip, 2h in multip)
- Passive phase: complete cervical dilation but no pushing
  - 1-2h of passive stage recommended in women with epidural anaesthesia to ↓instrumental delivery rate
- Active phase: pushing with abdo muscles and Valsava manoeuvre
  - Encourage mother to adopt comfortable position
  - If contractions wane, oxytocin augmentation may be needed
  - Active phase ~1h; if >1h, consider Ventouse extraction, forceps delivery or C-sec

Stage 3: delivery of placenta
- Uterus contracts to <24w size after baby is born
- Placenta separates from uterus, buckles, and a small amount of retroplacental haemorrhage aids its removal

* Passmed says 3cm, OHCS says 4cm

Induction of labour

Indications
- Post-maturity pregnancy (ie 1-2w after est date of delivery)
- Prelabour premature rupture of membranes where labour does not start spontaneously
- Maternal medical problems
  - Diabetic mother >38w
  - Pre-eclampsia
  - Obstetric cholestasis
- Rhesus disease
- Intrauterine fetal death

Contraindications
  ↳ consider C-sec instead
- Malpresentations (incl breech)
- Fetal distress
- Placenta praevia   · Vasa praevia
- Cord presentation
- Pelvic tumour, eg cervical fibroid

Modified Bishop score
- ≥8 indicates cervix is favourable – high chance of spontaneous labour or response to interventions made to induce labour
- <5: labour unlikely to start without induction

Mx:
- If Bishop ≤6: vaginal prostaglandins or oral misoprostol
  - Consider mechanical methods (eg balloon catheter) if woman is at higher risk of hyperstimulation or has had previous C-sec
- If Bishop >6: amniotomy and IV oxytocin infusion

Methods of induction
- Membrane sweep
  - ? adjunct to induction
  - examining finger is inserted through the cervix and rotated against the wall of the uterus to separate the chorionic membrane from the decidua
  - can be done by midwife at antenatal clinic
    ◊ premip: offered at 40w, 41w
    ◊ multip: offered at 41w
- Vaginal prostaglandin E2 (aka dinoprostone) – pessary or gel
  - CTG monitor of fetus before and for 30min post insertion
- Oral prostaglandin E1 (aka misoprostol)
- Maternal oxytocin infusion (aka Syntocinon)
- Amniotomy ("breaking of waters") – a little rod-hook device is inserted into the vaginal canal and used to rupture the amniotic membrane
- Cervical ripening balloon – balloon is passed through endocervical canal, and gently inflated to dilate the cervix

Complications
- Uterine hyperstimulation (1-5%)
  = prolonged and frequent uterine contractions (≈ tachysystole)
  - Can cause fetal hypoxemia and acidaemia, and uterine rupture
  - Mx: remove vaginal prostaglandins and stop IV oxytocin ± tocolysis

Pain relief in labour

Non-pharmacological methods
- Education on labour process
- Transcutaneous electrical nerve stimulation (TENS)
- Water birth – rec by NICE
  - Water temp must be <37.5°C to prevent maternal pyrexia

Pharmacological options
- Nitrous oxide (Entonox; 50% in O2)
  - CI: pneumothorax
  - Short onset of action
  - SE: NV, feeling faint
- Opiate analgesia
  - Eg pethidine 50-150mg IM
  - Limited pain relief, but significant SE (drowsiness, NV; baby may have short-term respi depression and drowsiness)
  - If given IM or IV, give with antiemetic (eg cyclizine 50mg IM)
  - CI: water birth (cannot be given <2h before entering birthing pool)
- Pudendal nerve block (S2-4)
  - Eg 8-10 mL 1% lidocaine
  - Useful for instrumental delivery
- Local anaesthesia (lidocaine) – injected into perineum, used before epiostomy at time of delivery, and before suturing vaginal tears
- Regional anaesthesia
  - Epidural analgesia
  - Combined spinal epidural anaesthesia
  - Spinal anaesthesia

Regional anaesthesia (continued)
- Epidural analgesia
  - targets pain fibres in T10-S5
  - aim for L3/4 epidural space
  - can be topped up every 2h
  - complications
    ◊ failure to site / patchy block
    ◊ hypotension
    ◊ dural puncture (<1:100)
    ◊ post-dural puncture HA
    ◊ transient or permanent nerve damage (very rare)
    ◊ ↑risk of operative vaginal delivery
  - can cause transient fetal bradycardia; recovers with IV fluids administration
- Spinal anaesthesia
  - used for most C-secs (easier to insert than epidural)
  - needle is inserted into subarachnoid space, single dose
  - ↑risk of profound hypotension compared to epidural
- Combined spinal epidural anaesthesia
  - quicker pain relief
  - can be used in C-sec where there is risk of prolonged procedure
- LMWH in regional anesthesia
  - wait 12h after prophylactic heparin/ LMWH given to insert block or remove catheter
  - wait 24h if pt on therapeutic dose
  - wait ≥4h after block siting for next dose of LMWH

	0	1	2	3
Cervical position	Posterior	Intermediate	Anterior	-
Cervical consistency	Firm	Intermediate	Soft	-
Cervical effacement	0-30%	40-50%	60-70%	80%
Cervical dilation	<1cm	1-2cm	3-4cm	>5cm
Fetal station	-3	-2	-1, 0	+1, +2

Monitoring in labour
- Fetal heart rate monitored every 15min (or continuously via CTG)
- Contractions assessed every 30min
- Maternal HR assessed every 1h
- Maternal BP and temp every 4h
- Vaginal exam should be offered every 4h to check progression of labour
- Maternal urine should be checked for ketones and protein every 4h

Twins 1:105 pregnancies
Triplets 1:10,000 pregnancies

R: previous twins, FHx, ↑maternal age, ↑oculation/IVF, race origin (eg Japanese, Nigerian Yoruba)

A/P: • Zygote = fertilised ovum
• Dizygotic / fraternal twins (develop from separate ova → 2 zygotes that were fertilised at the same time)
• Monozygotic (develop from one zygote that splits into two embryos)
  - Dichorionic & diamniotic: both babies have their own amniotic sac and placenta
  - Monochorionic & diamniotic: babies share the same placenta but have their own amniotic sac
  - Monochorionic & monoamniotic: babies share the same placenta and amniotic sac (cosy)

S/smx: • large uterus
• hyperemesis
• >2 poles felt, multiplicity of fetal parts felt, 2 fetal heart rates heard
• polyhydramnios (later on)

Complications during pregnancy
• Polyhydramnios
• Pre-eclampsia (30% in twins)
• Anaemia
• ↑risk of antepartum haemorrhage
  - 2/2 ↑risk of abruption and placenta praevia (due to large placenta)
• Gestational diabetes
• Operative delivery

Fetal complications
• ↑perinatal mortality
• Prematurity
  - mean gestation for twins is 37w, for triplets 33w
• Growth restriction
• ↑rates of malformation (esp if monozygotic)
• Twin-twin transfusion syndrome
  - in monochorionic twins
  - due to placental vascular anasta-moses – one twin acts as donor, the other as recipient

Fetal complications (cont)
• Fetal papyraceous: fetus dies in utero, shrinks, and mummifies

Complications during labour
• PPH (2x risk in twins)
• Malpresentation is common
• Vasa praevia rupture
• Cord prolapse
• Placental abruption
• Cord entanglement

Preparations for labour
• Give aspirin >12w if there other risk factors for pre-eclampsia
• Tell mother how to identify pre-term labour, and what to do
• Offer elective birth at 37w for uncomplicated dichorionic twins
• Offer elective birth at 36w for uncomplicated monochorionic twins
• Offer elective birth at 35w + steroids for uncomplicated triplets
• Have paediatricians (1 per baby) at delivery in case resus needed

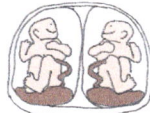

Dichorionic + Diamniotic

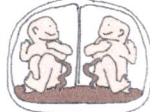

Monochorionic + Diamniotic

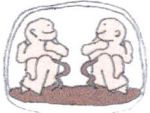

Monochorionic + Monoamniotic

D: baby presenting for delivery with the buttocks or feet first rather than head
• 25% of pregnancies at 28w
• 3% of pregnancies at or near term

R: prematurity, SGA, nulliparity, fetal congenital anomalies, previous breech delivery, uterine malforma-tions or fibroids, abn amniotic fluid volume (oligo/poly), placental abn (eg placenta praevia)

Classification
• Frank or extended breech (65-70% breeches)
  - baby's buttocks lead the way into the birth canal
  - hips flexed, knees extended, feet close proximity to head
• Complete breech (15%)
  - baby presents with buttocks first
  - hips and knees flexed; baby may be sitting cross-legged
• Incomplete or footling breech
  - Baby's foot/feet lie below the breech, so the foot or knee is lowermost in the birth canal
  - a/w ↑risk of cord prolapse (5-20%)

Mx • If <36w, many fetuses will turn spontaneously
• If at 36w still breech, offer external cephalic version
  - obstetrician places hands on mother's abdomen and applies pressure to turn the baby
  - at 36w for nullip women, at 37w for multip women
  - contraindicated if
    ◊ C-sec delivery required
    ◊ antepartum haemorrhagae within the last 7d
    ◊ abnormal cardiotocography
    ◊ major uterine abnormality
    ◊ ruptured membranes
    ◊ multiple pregnancy
• Pt education
  - planned C-sec has ↓risk of perinatal & neonatal mortality
  - how baby is born does not influence long-term health in breech presentation

Meconium = baby's first poop

Meconium-stained liquor
• If passed in late pregnancy, it stains the amniotic fluid dull green
• May be passed as part of normal labour or as a sign of distress → transfer to consultant-led unit, commence continuous FHR monitoring
• ► Prelabour rupture of membranes with meconium-stained liquor – request immediate induction of labour in consultant-led unit with advanced neonatal life support available

Meconium aspiration syndrome
• D: respiratory distress in the newborn due to the presence of meconium in the trachea
  - occurs in 1:1000 deliveries
• R: >42w preg, pregnancy-induced HTN, maternal DM, maternal drug abuse or smoking, fetal distress, oligohydramnios, chorioamnionitis
• Mx:
  - only suction airway if there is thick meconium in oropharynx and baby requires resus – this should be done only by neonatalists
  - babies may require O2 therapy ± ventilation, abx (eg ampicillin and gentamicin)

Fun(?) fact: liquor is latin for "fluid". Liquor amnii refers to amniotic fluid, which is the likely reason as to why this is referred to as meconium-stained liquor (amniotic fluid)

RFM

Normal(?) movements
• Mothers should start feeling move-ments between 18-20w
  - first onset of recognised fetal movements is known as quickening
• ↑strength and freq until about 32w, then regular pattern until delivery

Reduced movements
• Any reduction is a potentially important clinical sign of impending fetal demise – ►►►
• R: fetal growth restriction, SGA, placental insufficiency, congenital malformations
• Ask mother to lie on left lateral position, and focus on fetal movements for 2h; if <10 movements in same period, go to maternal A&E asap – requires same-day Ax

Mx if <28w
• Handheld Doppler to confirm fetal heartbeat
• If no fetal heartbeat detectable, offer immediate US
• If fetal heartbeat present, CTG for ≥20min to monitor FHR
• If concerns remaining despite CTG, urgent US to Ax abdominal circum-ference, estimate fetal wt, amniotic fluid volume measurement

Mx if 24-28w, or <24w and previous fetal movements have been felt
• Handheld Doppler

Mx if <24w and no previous fetal movements
• Ref to maternal fetal medicine unit

P: • In 70% pregnancies with single episode of RFM, no further complications
• 40-55% of women who suffer from stillbirth have RFM

Retained placenta

D: Placenta that is not delivered by 30min with active Mx, or by 60min with physiological birth

R (or a/w): prev retained placenta or uterine surgery, preterm delivery, maternal age >35yo, placental wt <600g, parity >5, induced labour, pethidine used during labour

Mx:
· Avoid excessive cord traction (cord may snap or uterus may invert)
· Check that placenta is not in vagina
· Palpate the abdomen and try to precipitate a contraction
· Oxytocin
  - Encourage bfding (natural ↑)
  - 20IU oxytocin in 20 mL saline into umbilical vein + clamp cord proximally to injection site
· Empty bladder
· If placenta still not delivered in further 30min, offer exam to see if manual removal is needed
  - Stop if painful
  - Transfer to theatre for regional anaesthesia and prep for manual removal
  - IV access + FBC, G&S + consent

Manual removal
· Lithotomy position
· One hand on abdomen to stabilise uterus
· Other hand inserted through cervix into the uterus. Work around the placenta, and separate it from the uterus, then pull on the cord to remove
· Ensure complete removal of placenta
· Give oxytocin + 1 dose of abx
· If still not separated (placenta accreta), senior help asap

C: main complication is haemorrhage; do not delay manual removal if needed as may precipitate PPH

Instrumental vaginal delivery

Indications for use
· Maternal
  - prolonged 2nd stage for any reason
  - maternal exhaustion
  - medical avoidance of pushing (eg severe cardiac disease)
  - pushing not possible
· Fetal
  - suspected fetal distress
  - for after-coming head in breech delivery

Forceps
· Curved blades that fit around the fetal head. Traction can be applied by pulling on the handles
· ↓maternal effort for delivery as compared to ventouse
· safer for baby, but can cause significant maternal genital tract trauma
· Complications for fetus (rare)
  - facial nerve palsy
  - skull fractures   - orbital injury
  - intracranial haemorrhage

Ventouse
· Suction device to suck fetal scalp tissues into a ventous cup
· Causes swelling of the head (known as a chignon) which can take 24-48h to resolve
  ↳ warn mother about this
· A/w ↓maternal genital tract trauma but ↑risk of fetal trauma. Also more likely to fail
· Complications for fetus
  - cephal-haematoma (common)
  - retinal haemorrhage
  - scalp lacerations and scalp avulsions (more common if >3 pulls used)

Other notes
· Avoid sequential use of instruments
· When to abandon use
  - no descent with each subsequent pull
  - delivery not imminent after 3 pulls
  - head impacted in pelvis + difficult to deliver → emergency C-sec

Caesarean section CS

D: delivery of fetus through incision in the abdominal wall and uterus
· 25% of nullip deliveries
· <5% of multip if no previous CS
· Greater predictor of CS is having a previous CS

Indications
· Fetal compromise, eg fetal bradycardia, scalp pH <7.20, cord prolapse
· Failure to progress in labour, or failed induction of labour
· Malpresentation, eg transverse lie
· Severe pre-eclampsia
· IUGR with absent or reversed end-diastolic flow
· Twin pregnancy with non-cephalic presenting twin
· Placenta praevia

Types of CS
· Lower segment Caesarean section, LSCS
  - Incision may be transverse or vertical but they are lower down
  - Most commonly used due to better outcomes, lower risks
· Classical – rarely used now, almost like a laparotomy

Categories of CS
· Category 1 (crash)
  - immediate threat to life of woman or fetus
  - baby should be delivered within 30min of decision for CS
  - eg placental abruption
  - if ↑risk of maternal bleeding, G&S + crossmatch (2u for placental abruption, 6u for placenta praevia)
· Category 2
  - maternal or fetal compromise but not immediately life-threatening
  - deliver baby within 75 min
  - eg failure to progress
· Category 3
  - semi-elective, eg pre-eclampsia
· Category 4
  - elective, eg term singleton breech
  - carried out after 39w, unless risk changes to cat 1 to 3

Risks to mother
· Frequent risks
  - persistent wound, abdo discomfort (may last months post-op)
  - ↑risk of repeat CS
  - readmission to hospital
  - haemorrhage
  - infection (wound, endometritis)
· Serious risks
  - emergency hysterectomy
  - need for further surgeryat later date (eg curettage to remove retained placental tissue)
  - admission to ITU
  - thromboembolic disease
  - bladder or ureteric injury
  - death (1:12,000)
· Serious risks in future pregnancies
  - ↑risk of uterine rupture
  - ↑risk of antepartum stillbirth
  - ↑risk of placenta praevia and placenta accreta

Risks to baby
· Lacerations (1-2:100)

Vaginal birth after CS (VBAC)
· Planned VBAC is an appropriate method of delivery for pregnant women at ≥37w with single previous CS
· Successful in 70-75%
· Contraindications
  - previous uterine rupture
  - if classical CS scar

Stillbirth Intrauterine fetal death

D: death in utero >24w
· <24w is classified as miscarriage
· Occurs in 1:200 births

Causes: · No cause found in 28%
· Placental cause 12%
· Ante-/intrapartum haemorrhage 11%
· Major congenital anomaly 9%
· Others: infection, HTN, renal disease, diabetes, IUGR, etc

R: multiple pregnancy, social depri-vation, ↑maternal age, smoking, previous CS, IVF, obesity

S/smx: · ↓fetal movements

Ix/Dx: · Handheld Doppler: RFM
· US: absent heartbeat – requires 2 independent practitioners to confirm
· Repeat US if mother requests

Ix for cause
· Kleihauer + other bloods
· Blood culture, viral screen, MSU
· Thrombophilia screen
· Antibodies   · Cervical swab
· Fetal tests - fetal and placental swab + request parental permission for postmortem

Mx:
· If mother is Rh-ve, give anti-D
· Do Kleihauer on all women to Dx fetomaternal haemorrhage (FMH)
  - test to screen maternal blood for presence of fetal RBCs
  - Ax / quantifies severity of FMH
  - Repeat at 48h if large FMH – ensure all fetal RBCs cleared
· Advice delivery for pre-eclampsia, abruption, sepsis, coagulopathy, or membrane rupture
· Mother may deliver spontaneously, or may require induction of labour
· See OHCS (5th edition) pp78-79 for how to help parents during and after labour
· Arrange f/u with obstetrician to discuss cause if known, and implications for future pregnancy

For Miscarriage, see Gynae 17.03

Placenta problems

Velamentous insertion (1%)
= umbilical vessels travel within the membranes before placental insertion

Placental succenturia (5%)
= separate (succenturiate) lobe away from the main placenta which may fail to separate normally; can cause PPH or puerperal sepsis

Vasa praevia
= malformation of fetal vessels where they run through the free placental membranes
· Risk of fetal haemorrhage when membranes rupture
· Requires C-sec
  - urgent if fetal compromise
  - elective if detected antenatally

Placenta membranacea
= thin placenta surrounds baby
· Predisposes to antepartum haemorrhage, PPH, IUGR
· Not much mentioned in literature regarding Mx; case reports on use of C-sec

Placenta accreta
= abnormal adherence of all or part of the placenta to the uterus
· Placenta **increta** if myometrium infiltrated
· Placenta **percreta** if serosa or perimetrium infiltrated
· R: prev C-sec, placenta praevia
· Dx on colour Doppler US or MRI
· All 3 types predispose to PPH :(
· Mx (RCOG recommendations):
  - planned delivery at 35-36w with elective C-sec
  - G&S + X-match in prep for potential haemorrhage
  - Hysterectomy (with placenta left in situ) seems to be the standard of care, but experienced surgeons may attempt uterus preserving surgery

Placenta praevia
· D: placenta overlying the cervical os. Found in ~0.5% pregancies
  - "low-lying placenta" refers to placenta <2cm from cervical os but not directly covering os
· R (or a/w): prev C-sec; multiparity; multiple pregnancy
· A/P: exact cause unknown; in some cases uterine scarring may interfere with process of placentation
· S/smx:
  - shock in proportion to visible blood loss
  - lie and presentation may be abnormal
  - NO pain, no uterine tenderness
    ↳ "painless praevia"
  - coagulation problems rare, fetal heart usually normal
· Ix
  - ! US first; do NOT perform digital vaginal exam before US as this may provoke haemorrhage
  - usually picked up on routine 20w abdominal US; transvaginal US is better (safe and ↑accuracy)
· Classical grading
  - I: placenta reaches lower segment but not internal os
  - II: placenta reaches internal os but does not cover it
  - III: covers internal os before dilation, but not when dilated
  - IV (major): placenta completely covers internal os
· Mx:
  - if identified at 20w, rescan at 32w
  - no need to limit activity or intercourse unless bleeding
  - if still present at 32w, rescan q2w
  - final US at 36-37w to determine method of delivery
    ◊ elective C-sec for grades III/IV between 37-38w
    ◊ trial of vaginal delivery if grade I
  - if pt has known placenta praevia and goes into labour before elective C-sec, perform emergency C-sec to prevent PPH
  - ➤ placenta praevia with bleeding
    ◊ Admit + ABCDE stabilisation
    ◊ If pt cannot be stabilised, or if in labour or term reached, perform emergency C-sec

Perineal tears

Classification
· 1st degree: superficial, no muscle involvement; generally do not require repair
· 2nd degree
  - injury to perineal muscle
  - does NOT involve anal sphincter
  - requires sutures (on ward)
· 3rd degree
  - injury to anal sphincter muscle
  - 3a: external sphincter <50% thickness torn
  - 3b: >50% thickness torn
  - 3c: both external and internal anal sphincters torn
  - requires repair in theatre + abx
· 4th degree
  - injury to anal sphincter and rectal mucosa
  - requires repair in theatre under epidural or GA + abx

R: primigravida, large babies, precipitous labour (very quick birth), shoulder dystocia, forceps delivery

Mx:
· Grade III & IV will require repair in theatre with intraop abx cover
· Advise high-fibre diet and laxatives for 10d to avoid constipation
· Arrange pelvic floor physio and obstetric clinic f/u at 6-12w postnatally
· If pain or incontinence develops, ref to specialist gynae or colorectal surgeon for endoanal US or manometry

Episiotomy
· Cut to the perineum to enlarge cervical outlet to allow baby to born more quickly (eg in fetal distress)
· Tissues cut: vaginal epithelium, perineal skin, bulbocavernous muscle, superficial, and deep transverse perineal muscles
· Complications: bleeding, infxn, breakdown, haematoma formation
· Post-cut Mx: ice pack, salt baths, rectal diclofenac

Physiological changes
· Uterus: 1kg → 100g. While it shrinks, there may be afterpains (esp during bfding)
· Cervix becomes firm over 3d
· Internal os closes by 3d
· External os closes by 3w
· Lochia (endometrial slough, red cells, white cells) passed per vaginum: red → yellow → white, until 6w
· Colostrum for first 3d → milk; breasts are swollen and tender with engorgement at 3-4d

Puerperal psychosis
· 1:500 births
· S/smx:
  - high suicidal drive, mania, severe depression, rarely schizophrenic smx with delusions
  - presents by 7d postpartum in 50%, by 3mo in 90%
  - sudden onset + rapid deterioration
· Mx:
  - admit + ref to perinatal psych team or psych liaison
  - ideally specialist mother and baby unit if possible
· 25-50% risk of recurrence in following pregnancies

Sepsis in the puerperium

D: life-threatening organ dysfunction caused by a dysregulated host response to an infection

More common causes
- Most common generally: Group A Strep and E. coli
- Chorioamnionitis: mixed Gram-ve and Gram+ve organisms
- UTI, preterm prolonged rupture of membranes and cervical cerclage: Gram-ve bacilli

S/smx:
- As per other infxns
- Specifically in pregnancy
  - abdominal or pelvic pain
  - offensive vaginal discharge
    ◊ smelly ≈ anaerobes
    ◊ serosanguinous ≈ Strep
- Sepsis Dx criteria – may develop later in pregnant women
  - Temp >38°C or <36°C
  - HR >100   · RR >20
  - SBP <90 or MAP <70 mmHg
  - Impaired mental state
  - ↑inflammatory markers
  - ↑lactate (>4 mmol/L)

Ix/Mx:
- Mx is similar to that of sepsis for any other pt
- Sepsis is a/w preterm labour; alert neonatal unit
- If chorioamnionitis is suspected, expedite delivery
- Lower threshold for transfer to ITU
- In labour,
  - continuous fetal monitoring in labour is recommended
  - avoid spinal and epidural analgesia; use GA for C-sec

Eclampsia

D: seizures in a/w pre-eclampsia:
- Pregnancy-induced HTN, and
- Proteinuria, and
- Tonic-clonic seizures

R: as per pre-eclampsia; 1% of pre-eclampsia develops into eclampsia

S/smx: tonic clonic seizure
- May be the first presentation of eclampsia / pre-eclampsia
- 38% fit antenatally, 18% during labour, 44% postnatally

Mx: · Call for help asap
- ABCDE stabilisation
- **Magnesium sulfate** to prevent and tx seizures – 4g IV over 5-10 min, then 1g/h for 24h
  - continue for 24h after last seizure or delivery
  - treat further seizures with 2g bolus + diazepam
  - stop if RR <12/min, loss of tendon reflexes, or UO <20 mL/h
  - if MgSO4 toxicity (respi depression), give calcium gluconate over 10min
- Mx of BP
  - if >160/110 or MAP >125, use labetalol 20 mg IV increasing after 10min intervals to 40mg, then 80mg
  - switch to hydralazine is still uncontrolled
  - alternatively, use hydralazine first then labetalol if still uncontrolled
- R/o intracranial haemorrhage
- Catheterise for hourly UO, take obs every 15min
- Restrict fluids to 80 mL/h until clinically and biochemically improving
  ↳ unless haemorrhaging
- Monitor fetal HR with CTG
- Deliver once mother is stable
  - C-sec quickest, but vaginal delivery is not contraindicated
  - Mx 3rd stage with oxytocin; other drugs contraindicated

Placental abruption

D: premature separation of a normally located placenta from the uterine wall that occurs before delivery of the fetus. 1:200 pregnancies

R: chronic HTN, pre-eclampsia, smoking, cocaine use, trauma, chorioamnionitis, uterine malformations, prior placental abruption, oligohydramnios

A: direct or indirect trauma, cocaine use (→ vasospasm → bleeding)
P: unknown

S/smx:
- Shock *out of keeping* with visible loss of blood
- Constant pain, tender and tense uterus
- Coagulation problems (eg DIC)
- Baby is usually in normal lie and presentation, but fetal heart sounds may be absent or distressed

Ix: fetal monitoring, Hb+Hct, coagulation studies, US

Mx: stabilise mum & baby
- Resus as needed, blood transfusion if evidence of anaemia
- Anti-D Ig in Rh-ve women
- >34w + baby stable: vag delivery
- >34w + baby or mum unstable: C-sec delivery
- <34w + baby & mum stable: aim to manage conservatively and delay delivery
- <34w + baby or mum unstable: deliver (vag or C-sec)

P: for baby, depends on age at which abruption occurs (younger a/w worse outcomes). For mum, monitor subsequent pregnancies carefully (5.8% recurrence); also a/w lifetime ↑risk for cardiovascular and cerebrovascular disease

Cord prolapse

D: presentation of the umbilical cord before the fetal presenting part

R: 2nd twin, footling breech, pre-maturity, polyhydramnios, unengaged head, transverse or unstable lie, M>F

A/P: cord compression and vasospasm from exposure of the cord causes fetal asphyxia :(

S/smx:
- May be obvious if cord can be seen
- However, fetal bradycardia or variable fetal heart decelerations may be the only sign

Ix: fetal monitoring

Mx: · Get senior help + 2222
- Minimise cord compression and vasocompression
  - presenting part of the fetus may be pushed back into uterus to avoid compression
  - if cord is past the level of the external opening of the vaginal canal: minimal handling + keep warm (prevents vasospasm)
  - tell pt to go on "all fours" or left lateral position (knees to chest) until prep for C-sec is done
  - tocolytics may be used to ↓contractions
  - retrofilling bladder with 500 mL of saline may help to elevate presenting part
    ↳ bladder then needs to be emptied before delivery

Other causes of antepartum haemorrhage (APH)
- APH = genital tract bleeding from 24w gestation. 3-5% pregnancies.
- **Placental abruption** (painful)
- **Placenta previa** (painless)
- Vasa previa   · Cervical polyps
- Erosions and carcinomas
- Cervicitis   · Vaginitis
- Vulval varicosities

Shoulder dystocia

D: delivery requiring additional obstetric manouevres to release the shoulders after gentle downward traction has failed. 1:200 pregnancies

R: large/post-mature fetus, maternal BMI >30, induced labours, prolonged 1st or 2nd stage, assisted vag delivery, previous shoulder dystocia

Mx (SPEED IS KEY)
- Get senior++ help
- Episiotomy gives space for internal manoeuvres
- **McRoberts' manoeuvre**
  - flexion + abduction of maternal hips to bring mother's thighs towards her abdomen (aka hyperflexed lithotomy)
  - this rotation ↑ relative anterior-posterior angle of pelvis and helps delivery (90% success)
- Suprapubic pressure helps to displace the anterior shoulder
- Enter pelvis for internal manoeuvres – rotate the fetal shoulders, or 180° to make posterior shoulder anterior, or deliver posterior shoulder first
- Roll mother on all fours if these fail
- Other measures
  - Maternal symphysiotomy
  - Zavanelli manoeuvre (essentially replaces baby back into uterus + C-sec)
- If baby dies before delivery, cut through both clavicles to allow for delivery
- ! Check baby for damage, eg Erb's palsy or fractured clavicle
- Beware PPH or 3rd/4th vaginal tears in the mother

Complications
- Mum: PPH in 11%, perineal tears in 3.8%
- Baby: brachial plexus injuries 4-16% (1:2300 live births UK) – 10% left with permanent disability
- ?? common cause of litigation
  - Parents need to be counselled about this risk for vaginal deliveries + informed that C-sec is not an option if shoulder dystocia happens

Uterine rupture

D: Complete division of all 3 layers of the uterus (endometrium, myometrium and perimetrium)
· Uterine dehiscence is the incomplete division of the uterus that does not penetrate all layers

R: previous C-sec (~70% of UK ruptures due to dehiscence of C-sec scars), prev uterine rupture, prev cervical or uterine surgery, induction of labour

S/smx:
· Abnormal fetal heart rate
· Abdo pain – sudden onset, but may be masked by epidural anaesthesia
· ± vaginal bleeding
· Baby may be partially extruded through rupture
· Haematuria if rupture extends into bladder
· Haemodynamic instability
  - there may not be much blood vaginally as most of the blood is intraperitoneal
· Changes in contraction patterns
· Postpartum: pain + persistent vag bleeding despite use of uterotonic agents ± haematuria

Mx:
· Stabilise pts (resus)
· Notify anaesthesia, neonatology
· Crossmatch 6u + prep for fast transfusion
· Laparotomy
  - Hysterectomy if no choice
  - Or attempt uterine repair
  - ± Bladder repair if trauma

P: maternal mortality 5%, fetal mortality 30%

Postpartum haemorrhage   PPH

D: blood loss of >500 mL after vaginal delivery
· primary PPH occurs within 24h after delivery; 2ndary >24h
· Massive obstetric haemorrhage: >1000-1500 mL loss

R: previous PPH or retained placenta, BMI >35, maternal Hb <85 before labour, antepartum haemorrhage, multiparity >4, maternal age >35, uterine malformations, large placenta & uterus, placental abruption, labour complications

A (÷4Ts)
· **Tone: uterine atony (90%)**
· Tissue: retained products of conception (more a/w 2ndary)
· Trauma: genital tract trauma
· Thrombin: clotting disorders

Mx: · Book mothers with risk factors for obstetric unit delivery
· Call for help – all hands on deck
· Resus pt – ABC
  - intubate if ↓consciousness
  - X match 4-6u + transfuse 1u packed RBC to 1u FFP
· Deliver placenta, empty uterus of clots or retained tissue
· Massage uterus to generate contraction, or perform bimanual compression
· Drugs to contract uterus
  - syntometrine
  - oxytocin
  - ergometrine
  - misoprostol
  - *carboprost*
· Repair vaginal or cervical tears
· If bleeding still not stopping, exam under anaesthesia ± laparotomy
  - Insertion of intrauterine balloon tamponade
· May require subtotal or total hysterectomy

P: 2 deaths per year in the UK, 125,000 deaths worldwide.

Amniotic fluid embolism

D: Condition arising from entry of amniotic fluid or fetal cells into maternal circulation

R: multiple pregnancy, maternal age >35, C-sec, instrumentation, eclampsia, polyhydramnios, placental abruption, uterine rupture, induction of labour

A/P: likely due to immune-mediated (over)reaction to fetal cells; likened to an anaphylactic like response

S/smx:
· Dyspnoea, chest pain, hypoxia, respi arrest → ARDS (may be the first sign)
· Hypotension   · Fetal distress
· Seizures (20%)   · ↓consciousness
· Cardiac arrest
· Almost all develop DIC within 48h

Mx:
· Prevent death from respi failure
  - high flow + 100% O2
  - call anaesthetist asap; intubation and ventilation may be necessary
  - transfer to ITU asap
· CPR if indicated
· Deliver baby via C-sec; aids resus of mother as well
· Monitor for fetal distress
· If hypotensive
  - IV fluids, dobutamine
  - Pulmonary artery catheterisation to guide Mx
  - After initial hypotension corrected, only give maintenance fluid required to avoid pulmonary oedema from ARDS
· Mx DIC with *fresh whole blood, packed* RBC, or FFP

P: most mortality occurs within first hour; 26-61% mortality. If mum survives, 85% have neurological damage. Request to perform autopsy asap

DIC & coagulation defects

D: acquired syndrome characterised by activation of coagulation pathways, resulting in formation of intravascular thrombi and depletion of platelets and coagulation factors

A: disease states that trigger systemic activation of coagulation, e.g. obstetric disorders, sepsis

P: continuous generation of intravascular fibrin and consumption of procoagulants and platelets. Also mutual potentiation between inflam-matory and coagulation pathways

S/smx:
· oliguria, ↓BP, ↑HR
· pupura fulminans, gangrene, acral cyanosis, petechiae, ecchymosis, oozing, haematuria
· delirium, coma

Dx scoring / criteria
· ↓platelets
  - moderate: <100 x 10⁹/L
  - severe: <50 x 10⁹/L
· ↑fibrin degredation products (eg D-dimer)
· ↑prothrombin time
  - moderate: >3s but <6s
  - severe: >6s
· ↓fibrinogen <2.94 mmol/L
· blood film may show schistocytes due to microangiopathic haemolytic anaemia

Mx: · Tx underlying cause asap
· Mx shock – O2, IV fluids
· *Blood products: tranexamic acid,* vitamin K (esp if prolonged PT), platelets, fibrinogen concentrate

P: <1% mortality if due to placental abruption, 50-80% if due to infxn

Combined oral contraceptive pill

- MOA: inhibits ovulation
- 99% effective if used correctly

Contraindications
UKMEC 4: unacceptable risk
- Current breast cancer
- PMH of VTE, MI, or stroke
- Antiphospholipid antibodies +ve
- Uncontrolled hypertension
- Migraine with aura (↑risk of stroke)
- >35yo + smoking ≥15 cigs/day
- Breastfeeding <6w post-partum
- Major surgery with prolonged immobilisation
UKMEC3: risks outweigh benefits
- PMH or FHx of breast cancer (or gene mutation carrier)
- FHx of VTE (1st degree relatives)
- Controlled hypertension
- >35yo + smoking <15 cigs/day
- BMI >35
- Immobility, incl wheelchair use
- Current gallbladder disease
UKMEC 2: benefits outweigh risks
UKMEC 1: no restrictions

Risks
- ↑risk of VTE, stroke, MI
- ↑risk of breast and cervical cancer
Benefits
- ↓risk ovarian, endometrial and colorectal cancer
- Often helps with acne, ovarian cysts, and can make periods regular, lighter, and less painful

How to take
- Ideally within first 5 days of first day of period → then no additional contraception required
- If started at any other point in the cycle, use alternative contraception for the first 7d (eg condoms)
- Take same time every day

How to take (continued)
- Method 1: 21d + 7d-pill-free break
  - Mimics physiological menses
  - No medical benefit from withdrawal bleed; entirely based on pt preference
- Method 2 (tricycling): 3x 21d packs then 4 or 7d-pill-free break
- Sexual intercourse during pill-free period is only safe if next pack is started on time

Special situations
- Vomiting: if pt vomits within 2h of taking COCP, repeat dose
- Antibiotic use – generally ok to take together; caution only with enzyme-inducing abx (eg rifampicin)
- Drug interactions – check on BNF

Missed pills
1 missed pill (at any time in cycle)
- Take last pill asap, even if it means taking 2 in one day, then continue taking pills daily, one per day
- No emergency contraception required
≥2 missed pills
- Take last pill asap, even if it means taking 2 in one day
- In week 1, emergency contraception if UPSI in pill-free week or day1-7
- In week 2, emergency contraception not required
- In week 3, finish all pills in current pack, then omit pill-free interval
- In general, another method of contraception (eg condoms) recommended until pills have been taken 7d in a row

Combined contraceptive patch

- = Evra patch
- MOA: inhibits ovulation
- 99% effective if used correctly

How to use
- 1 patch per week for 3w, then no patch worn for 1w (= 4w cycle)

Missed patches
After week 1 or 2
- If delay in changing patch for <48h, change asap + no further precautions needed
- If delay >48h, change asap + use barrier method for next 7d
  - If UPSI during "patch-free interval" or last 5d, use emergency contraception
After week 3
- If delay in removing patch, remove asap + apply new patch asap (skip patch-free week) + no further pre-cautions needed
At the start of week 1
- If delayed, use barrier contraception for first 7d

Combined contraceptive ring

- = NuvaRing (etonogestrel and ethinylestradiol)
- MOA: inhibits ovulation

How to use
- Insert within first 5 days of start of cycle + no additional contraception
- If inserted at any other time of cycle, use barrier contraception for first 7d
- 1 ring will last for 3w, then remove → ring-free week → start next cycle
- Check that the ring is present regularly
- Ring can be kept in during sex or when using tampon

Expelled rings
- See patches (but change "patch" for "ring") – similar Mx

Condoms

- MOA: physical barrier
- Only method that protects against STIs
- 98% effective if used correctly, but lower efficacy in younger people as not used correctly

Progestogen-only pill POP aka mini pill

- MOA: thickens cervical mucus
- 99% effective if used correctly

Side effects
- Common: irregular vaginal bleeding

How to take
- Ideally within first 5 days of first day of period → no additional contraception required
- If started at any other point in the cycle, use alternative contraception for the first 2d (eg condoms)
- No pill-free break
- Take same time every day

Special situations
- Diarrhoea and vomiting: repeat dose ± barrier contraception if "≥3h late"
- Check with pharmacist for enzyme inducing drugs (incl some abx)

Missed pills
- If <3h late, continue as normal
- If >3h late, take missed pill asap (even if it means taking 2 in the same day), and use barrier contraception for next 48h
- For desogestrel (Cerazette), the grace period is 12h

Injectable contraceptive

- = Medoxyprogesterone acetate (Depo Provera)
- MOA: inhibits ovulation and thickens cervical mucus

Side effects
- Irregular bleeding   · Weight gain
- ↑risk of osteoporosis
- Not easily reversible; fertility make take up to 1y to return to baseline
Contraindications
- Current breast cancer; high risk also with PMH of breast cancer

How to use
- IM injection once every 12-14 weeks
- Beyond 14w, barrier contraception must be used

Implantable contraceptives

- = Nexplanon / Implanon (etonogestrel)
- MOA: inhibits ovulation and thickens cervical mucus
- Most effective form of contraception

Side effects
- Irregular or heavy bleeding – may need to take COCP at first to manage this
- HA, nausea, mastalgia
Contraindications
- UKMEC4: current breast Ca
- UKMEC3: stroke, MI, unexplained vaginal bleeding, PMH of breast Ca, severe liver cirrhosis, liver Ca

How to use
- If inserted in first 5d of cycle, no additional contraception required
- If inserted after, use barrier contraception for first 7d
- Effective for 3 years

Intrauterine system (IUS)

- Releasing levonorgestrel
  - Mirena **8y**, Jaydessa 3y, Kyleena 5y
- MOA: prevents endometrial proliferation + thickens cervical mucus

Side effects
- Common: bleeding and spotting initially then becomes more light; some women become amenorrhoeic
- Infection (esp in first 3w after insertion)
- Expulsion – 1 in 20 risk, ↑risk in first 3mo
- Rarely, uterine perforation (more common in breastfeeding women)
- Relative ↑risk of ectopic pregnancies (as compared to other contraceptives)
  - Overall risk is very low as most pregnancies are prevented

How to use
- Inserted in clinic; pt should be taught on how to check that IUS is still in place
- Use barrier contraception for first 7d after insertion

Copper IUD

- Aka intrauterine device (IUD)
- MOA: ↓sperm motility and survival

Side effects
- Heavier, longer and more painful periods
- Risks similar to IUS: infection, expulsion, uterine perforation and relative ↑risk of ectopic pregnancies

How to use
- Inserted in clinic; pt should be taught on how to check that IUS is still in place
- Effective immediately after insertion
- Effective for 5 to 10y

Emergency contraception

Levonorgestrel
- Single dose = 1.5 mg
  - Double dose if BMI >26 or wt >70 kg
- Efficacy 84% (more effective the sooner it is taken after UPSI)
- Can be taken up to **72h** after UPSI
  - If vomiting within 3h of taking, repeat the dose
  - Can be used more than once in menstrual cycle if needed
- Less effective if taken after ovulation
- SE: disturbance of current menstrual cycle, vomiting (1%)
- Can use hormonal contraception immediately after using levonorgestrel for emergency contraception
- No issues with breastfeeding

Ulipristal acetate
- Single dose = 30 mg
- Can be taken up to **120h** after UPSI
  - Can be used more than once in menstrual cycle if needed
- Avoid in pts with severe asthma
- Less effective if taken after ovulation
- Hormonal contraception (pill, patch or ring) – (re)start 5d after ulipristal
  - Use with levonorgestrel not rec
- Breastfeeding: delay for 1w after taking ulipristal

Copper IUD
- Most effective method of emergency contraception – should be offered first. 99% effective
- Must be inserted within **5d** of UPSI, or up to **5d** after likely ovulation date, whichever is later in the cycle
- Can be given with prophylactic abx if pt considered to be high risk of STIs
- Can be left in situ for long-term contraception

See also FRSH guidelines on emergency contraception

Postpartum contraception

- Women require contraception after day 21 postpartum

Lactational amenorrhea
- 98% effective if women is fully breast-feeding with no supplementary feeds, is amenorrhoiec, and is <6mo postpartum

POP
- Can be started any time postpartum
- If started after day 21, use barrier contraception for first 2d
- Safe for breastfeeding – small amount of progestogen released in breastmilk

COCP
- Absolutely contraindicated in first 6 weeks postpartum
  - ↑risk of VTE
- Pros outweigh cons between 6w and 6mo postpartum
- When started, use barrier contraception for first 7d

IUS
- Can be inserted within 48h of childbirth (no additional contraception needed), or after 4 weeks postpartum (use barrier contraception for first 7d)
- Can be inserted during C-section

Copper IUD
- Can be inserted within 48h of childbirth or after 4 weeks postpartum (effective immediately)
- Can be inserted during C-section

Contraception for >40yo

- Most methods ok

COCP
- Slight ↑risk in >40yo – consider ↓dose
- Benefits: maintains bone mineral density, ↓menopause symptoms
- Can be continued up to 50yo, thereafter switch to non-hormonal or progestogen-only method

POP, implant, IUS
- Continue for ≥1y with amenorrhea, stop when FSH ≥30 µL or at 55yo
- If not amenorrheic, consider investigating abnormal bleeding pattern

Depo-Provera (injectable)
- Small loss in bone mineral density, usually recovered after stopping
- Continue for ≥1y with amenorrhea, stop when FSH ≥30 µL or at 55yo
- If not amenorrheic, consider investigating abnormal bleeding pattern

Non-hormonal methods
- If <50yo, stop after 2y of amenorrhea
- If ≥50yo, stop after 1y of amenorrhea

Contraception in obese pts

COCP
- UKMEC3: BMI ≥35 (risks > benefits)
- UKMEC2: BMI 30-34 (benefits >risks)

Combined contraceptive patch
- Less effective in pts >90kg

Others
- Oral contraception cannot be used in pts who have had gastric sleeve, bypass or duodenal switch surgery

Contraception in epilepsy

Phenytoin, carbamazepine, barbiturates, primidone, topiramate, oxcarbazepine
- No restrictions: Depo-Provera, copper IUD and IUS
- Benefits > risks: Nexplanon implant
- Risks > benefits: COCP, POP

Lamotrigine
- No restrictions: POP, implant, Depo-Provera, copper IUD and IUS
- Risks > benefits: COCP

Contraception in transgender and non-binary people

In pts assigned female at birth (AFAB) or with a uterus
- POP and non-hormonal methods are most effective as they do not affect testosterone therapy
- Testosterone therapy does not provide protection against pregnancy
- If pts become pregnant, testosterone therapy is contraindicated (teratogenic)
- If pts are on testosterone, oestrogen-containing regimes are **not** recommended (interference)
- If emergency contraception is needed, all forms are ok

In pts assigned male at birth (AMAB) or with male reproductive organs
- There is ↓sperm production with
  - Oestradiol   - GnRH analogues
  - Finasteride   - Cyproterone
- However, this is NOT a reliable means of preventing pregnancy
- Use condoms

This page has been left blank intentionally.

Female genital mutilation

D: removal or partial removal of external female genitalia or injury to other internal female genital organs
- Illegal in the UK
  - Engage child safeguarding
  - Any new cases in <18yo must be reported to police
- Traditionally practised in Africa, some parts of India and Indonesia; not limited to any particular cultural or religious group

WHO classification
- Type I: partial/total removal of clitoris and/or prepuce
- II: partial/total removal of clitoris and labia majora ± excision of labia majora
- III: narrowing of vaginal orifice with creation of covering seal by cutting and appositioning the labia minora and/or majora ± excision of clitoris (=infibulation)
- IV: any other harmful procedures to the female genitalia for non-medical purposes, eg pricking, piercing

Complications
- Acutely: death, blood loss, sepsis, pain, urinary retention, infxns (HIV, hepatitis, tetanus)
- Long-term: inability to have sexual intercourse (= apareunia), superficial dyspareunia, anorgasmia, sexual dysfunction, chronic pain, scarring, slow urination, UTIs, etc
- Maternal consequences: PPH, ↑risk of C-sec, episiotomy, fistula, difficulty in examining and catheterising, etc

Mx:
- Defibulation (reconstructive surgery of infibulated scar) – may be done antenatally
  - If not done antenatally, deliver in unit with emergency obstetric care
  - Offer epidural if vag exam poorly tolerated / episiotomy anticipated
- Screen for hep C
- Repair post-delivery should control bleeding. Re-infibulation is illegal.

Primary amenorrhoea

D: failure to start menstruating by
- 15yo in girls with normal sexual characteristics, or
- 13yo in girls with no secondary sexual characteristics

A/P:
- In those with normal sexual characteristics
  - Physiological causes
  - Genito-urinary malformations, eg imperforate hymen
  - Endocrine disorders
    ◊ Hyper/hypothyroidism
    ◊ Hyperprolactinaemia
    ◊ Cushing's syndrome
- In those with no secondary sexual characteristics, amenorrhoea is due to primary ovarian insufficiency
  - Chromosomal irregularities, eg Turner's syndrome
  - Hypothalamic-pituitary dysfunction, eg stress, wt loss

Ix: • Exclude pregnancy (bHCG)
- FBC, U&Es, coeliac screen, thyroid function test
- Gonadotrophins
  - ↓LH/FSH ≈ hypothalamic cause
  - ↑LH/FSH ≈ ovarian problem or gonadal dysgenesis (eg Turner's)
- Prolactin • Oestradiol
- Androgen – may be ↑ in PCOS

Mx: • Treat underlying cause
- If pt has primary ovarian insuff due to gonadal dysgenesis, they may benefit from HRT

Secondary amenorrhea

D: Cessation of menstruation
- For 3-6mo in women with previously normal and regular menses
- For 6-12mo in women with previous oligomenorrhea

Causes
- In those with no features of androgen excess
  - Physiological causes (eg pregnancy, lactation, menopause)
  - Hypothalamic dysfunction, eg due to chronic illness or stress, excessive exercise
  - Hyper/hypothyroidism
  - Primary ovarian insufficiency, eg due to chemo, radiotherapy
  - Sheehan syndrome (postpartum hypopituitarism due to necrosis of pituitary gland)
  - Asherman syndrome (intrauterine adhesions)
- In those with features of androgen excess (eg hirsutism, acne, virilisation)
  - PCOS
  - Cushing's syndrome
  - Late-onset congenital adrenal hyperplasia
  - Androgen-secreting tumours of the ovary or adrenal gland

Ix: as per primary amenorrhea

Mx: exclude pregnancy, lactation, and menopause (in ≥40yo)
- Treat underlying cause

Polycystic ovarian syndrome

D: condition of ovarian dysfunction involving hyperandrogenism, oligo-menorrhoea, and polycystic ovaries

R: FHx, early onset of pubic/axillary hair and apocrine sweat gland development (=adrenarche), obesity

A/P: unknown, ?inheritance, ?insulin resistance, overlap with metabolic syndrome

S/smx:
- Obesity (PCOS does not cause obesity, but many women with PCOS are obese)
- Subfertility and infertility
- Menstrual disturbances
  - Oligomenorrhea and amenorrhea
- Features of hyperandrogenism
  - Hirsutism   - Acne
- Acanthosis nigricans (due to insulin resistance)

Ix:
- Pelvic US looking for ovarian cysts
- Baseline bloods: FSH, LH, TSH, prolactin, testosterone, sex hormone-binding globulin (SHBG)
  - Prolactin and testosterone may be normal or mildly elevated
  - SHBG is normal to low in PCOS
- Check for impaired glucose tolerance

Rotterdam Dx criteria (≥2 of 3):
- Polycystic ovaries (≥12 follicles or ovarian volume >10 cm3 on US)
- Oligo-ovulation or anovulation
- Clinical and/or biochemical signs of hyperandrogenism
  - eg ↑LH:FSH ratio

Mx: *wt loss*
- Hirsutism and acne
  - COCP (third gen); balance with risk of VTE
  - If no response, trial of topical eflornithine, or other drugs under specialist supervision
- Infertility
  - medications: clomifene (induces ovulation), metformin, or combination
  - ovarian drilling for those who don't respond to clomifene
  - use of COCP to control bleeding and ↓risk of endometrial cancer

Day	Hormonal change	Ovarian cycle	Uterine cycle
0-4			Menses
4-14	LH/FSH stimulate follicular maturation. Estradiol secreted by maturing follicle.	Follicular phase Maturation of dominant follicle into Graafian follicle (mainly FSH driven)	Proliferative phase; laying down new endometrial layer (estrogen driven)
14	GnRH surge → LH just before ovulation	* Ovulation *	
14-28	Progesterone secreted by corpus luteum. LH/FSH levels decrease	Luteal phase: post-ovulation corpus luteum (LH/FSH helps formation of corpus luteum)	Secretory: endometrium receptive to implantation (progesterone supported)

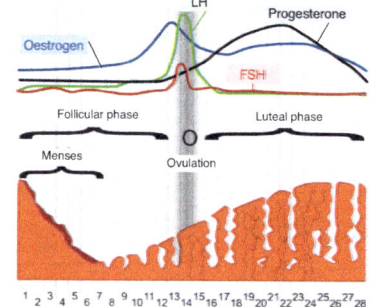

Menorrhagia

D: heavy menstrual bleeding that interferes with quality of life

Causes
- Dysfunctional uterine bleeding (ie menorrhagia in the absence of under-lying pathology)
- Anovulatory cycles
- Uterine fibroids
- Hypothyroidism
- Intrauterine devices (copper coil)
- Pelvic inflammatory disease
- Bleeding disorders

Ix:
- FBC, haematinics if anaemic, TSH, cervical smear, STI screen – as indicated by history
- If risk factors for endometrial cancer or hx suggestive endometrial pathology, refer for outpatient hysteroscopy ± biopsy
- Imaging: US

Mx:
- Mirena IUS: ↓bleeding by releasing levonorgestrel into the uterus, causing atrophy
  - SE: irregular bleeding for first 4-6mo, and progestogenic effects
- COCP effective in ↓bleeding but many CI
- 3rd line: progestogens IM, eg medroxyprogesterone
- If pt does not require contraception,
  - mefenamic acid (useful if there is dysmenorrhoea also)
  - tranexamic acid
  - start either on first day of period
- Surgery
  - Indications: fibroids >3cm, inadequate response to prev tx, declined medical Mx
  - Endometrial ablation
  - Myomectomy
  - Hysterectomy

Premenstrual syndrome

D: repetitive, cyclical, physical, and behavioural symptoms occurring in the luteal phase of the normal menstrual cycle

A/P: serotonin and GABA seem to be implicated

S/smx: anxiety, stress, fatigue, mood swings, bloating, breast pain

Mx:
- Mild: lifestyle changes
  - regular sleep, exercise, smoking cessation, ↓alcohol intake
  - regular, frequent, small, balanced meals rich in complex carbs
- Moderate: new gen COCP (eg Yasmin)
- Severe: SSRI – can be taken continuously or only during luteal phase (eg days 15-28 of cycle)

Premenstrual dysphoric disorder
- Most severe form of PMS
DSM5 criteria
- ≥1 following smx must be present
  - Mood swings, sudden sadness
  - Anger, irritability
  - Sense of hopelessness, depressed mood, self-critical thoughts
  - Tension, anxiety, feeling on edge
- ≥5 total smx
  - Difficulty concentrating
  - Change in appetite
  - Diminished interest in usual activities
  - Easy fatiguability, ↓energy
  - Feeling overwhelmed
  - Breast tenderness (cyclical mastitis), bloating, wt gain, joint/muscle aches
  - Sleeping too much or not enough

Menopause

D: period of waning fertility leading up to the last period
- Average age in UK is 52yo
- Retrospective Dx when menses has ceased for ≥12 consecutive months, not attributable to other reasons
- Premature menopause: <40yo
- Perimenopause: period of time marked by menstrual irregularity, ends 12mo after final menstrual period

R: 40-60yo (tends to occur earlier in Asian women; in 40s), cancer tx, smoking (2y earlier), ovarian surgery

A: natural process that is triggered by declining number of oocytes
P: ↓ovarian production of progeste-rone, estradiol and testosterone
- ↓hormones → various s/smx

S/smx:
- Vasomotor smx (80%):
  - hot flushes (may occur every few minutes for >10yo)
  - night sweats
  - palpitations
- Urogenital changes (35%): vaginal dryness and atrophy, urinary frequency, atrophy of breasts and skin also
- Psychological: 10% have anxiety and depression ± short-term memory impairment
- Long-term complications
  - ↑risk of cardiovascular disease
  - ↑risk of osteoporosis

Mx: • Confirm menopause (r/o thyroid & psychiatric problems)
- Diet and exercise changes
- Menorrhagia: Mirena coil
  - Consider ref for hysteroscopy if smx suggestive of endometrial pathology
- Use contraception until >1y amenorrhea if >50yo, >2y if <50yo
- Vaginal dryness: oestrogen cream 0.1% PV every night for 2w, then 2x per week as required
- HRT (see HRT section)

Hormone replacement therapy

D: oestrogen + progesterone replacement

Indications
- Menopausal smx: vasomotor smx, mood disorders, urogenital smx
- Premature menopause
  - Primarily for the prevention of osteoporosis
  - Continue until 50yo

Benefits
- ↓vasomotor smx due to oestrogen, benefit by ~4w, max effect in 3mo
- urogenital smx: benefit may take several months to be apparent; continue for long term
- ↓risk of osteoporotic fractures: sustained & life-long tx necessary
- ↓risk of colorectal cancer

Risks
- Breast cancer risk ↑ by 2.3% per year; dependent on duration and type of HRT. Risk ↓ to baseline 5y after stopping.
  - highest risk with combined HRT (but not seen in those who start HRT for premature menopause)
- Endometrial cancer (RR 2.3) if use of only oestrogen in those with uterus (ie unopposed oestrogen); risk remains for ≥5y after stopping
- HRT ↑risk of VTE (≥2x), but absolute risk remains small. Most likely to occur in first year of taking HRT. Lower risk with patches.

Contraindications
- Breast cancer (past or present)
- Oestrogen-dependent cancer
- Undiagnosed vaginal bleeding
- Untreated endometrial hyperplasia
- Previous idiopathic or current VTE, unless already on anticoagulation
- Active or recent arterial thromboembolic disease (eg MI)
- Active liver disease with abnormal liver function tests
- Pregnancy
- Thrombophilic disorder

Legalities (UK specific) – TOP is allowed if
- pregnancy <24w + continuation of pregnancy is riskier than TOP (physical or mental health risk to woman or existing children)
- *TOP necessary to prevent grave permanent injury to physical or mental health of pregnant woman
- *Continuation of pregnancy will involve risk to life of pregnant woman greater than TOP risks
- *Substantiated risk that if the child were born, it would suffer from serious handicaps from physical or mental abnormalities
- For asterisked points (*), no time limit on term of pregnancies

Other legal points
- Requires 2 doctors to sign off
  - In emergencies, only 1 Dr needs to sign off
- If <16yo presents for TOP, try to get parents' consent or involve parents or other responsible adult
- TOP after 24w can only be carried out in NHS hospitals
  - TOP can only be done by licensed medical practitioner

Choice of procedure + other issues
- If <9w, usually medical methods are used at home
  - Still 5% chance of needing to use surgical procedure after that
- If >9w, there is still a choice between medical and surgical methods
- In terminations later than 21+6w, it is essential that fetus is born dead (unless it is a lethal fetal abnormality) – use 3mL intracardiac 15% potassium chloride & confirm asystole with US
- If born after 24w, the dead fetus is considered a stillbirth and needs to be registered
  - If signs of life, then a death certificate is required

Medical/drug options
- Mifepristone followed 48h later by prostaglandin (eg misoprostol)
  - Doses depend on gestational
  - "Mimicking a miscarriage"
- May be done at home depending on gestation; timings are not predictable
- Requires "multi-level pregnancy test" (with bHCG levels) in 2w to confirm that pregnancy has ended

Surgical options
- Vacuum aspiration (MVA)
- Electric vacuum aspiration (EVA)
- Dilation and evacuation (D&E)
- Cervical priming with misoprostol ± mifepristone used before procedures
- Various anaesthetic options can be used (including LA or GA)
- Intrauterine contraceptive can be inserted immediately following procedure

Before TOP
- Offer counselling + support
- US to confirm gestation and identify non-viable or ectopic pregnancies
- Screen for STIs
- Give abx prophylaxis if surgical option is to be used
- Discuss contraception
- If ≥10w, do Rhesus testing and give anti-D prophylaxis if Rh-ve
  - Dose depends on gestation

Complications of TOP
- Failed TOP <1:100, medical TOP failure rate higher than surgical
- Infection ~2:100
- Haemorrhage <1:1000, higher risk if ≥20w
- Uterine perforation 1-4:000 (surgical risk only)
- Uterine rupture <4:1000
- Cervical trauma 1:100
- Retained products of conception 1:100
  → will require surgical evacuation

D: involuntary, spontaneous loss of pregnancy before 24w (in the UK)
- >24w is classified as stillbirth
- Miscarriage occurs in up to 1/3 of pregnancies

Descriptive terms
- Threatened miscarriage: painless vaginal bleeding occurring <24w
  - typically occurs at 6-9w
  - bleeding often less than menses
  - cervical os is closed
  - complicates ≤25% pregnancies
- Inevitable: heavy bleeding with clots and pain with open cervical os
- Incomplete: when not all products of conception have been expelled
  - pain and vaginal bleeding
  - open cervical os
- Complete
- Missed / delayed: gestational sac containing a dead fetus before 20w without smx of expulsion
  - closed cervical os
  - usually painless. Light vaginal bleeding may be present
- Recurrent: spontaneous loss of ≥3 consecutive pregnancies before 24w

R: older age (a/w occurrence of chromosomal abnormalities), uteirne malforamtion, bacterial vaginosis, thrombophilia, parental chromoso-mal anomaly, vitamin D def

A: primary embryonic disease, disorder or damage; chromosomal abnormalities; maternal genital tract dysfunctions or exposre to high doses of toxic agents
P: unclear

S/smx:
- Vaginal bleeding ± clots
- ± Pain (suprapubic or low back pain)
- Recent post-coital bleed (2x odds of miscarriage in women who report bleeding after sexual intercourse during pregnancy)

For Stillbirth, see Obstetrics 16.12

Ix
- Transvaginal US will differentiate between stages and types of miscarriage
  - Consider miscarriage if gestational sac has mean diameter ≥25mm with no visible yolk sac or fetal pole; also likely when crown-rump length ≥7mm with no obvious fetal heart activity
- Serum bHCG titres if uncertain about miscarriage status
  - >50% drop in 48h suggestive of failing pregnancy → refer for clinical review in early pregnancy Ax service within 24h
  - Rise of ≥50% in 48h suggestive of possible ongoing pregnancy
- Other bloods (FBC, Rhesus, anti-bodies) or vaginal swab as clinically indicated

Mx ÷ 3 types
Expectant Mx
- ≈ waiting for spontaneous miscarriage. Generally preferred.
- If unsuccessful or following risk factors present, then offer medical/surgical Mx
  - ↑risk of haemorrhage (late in first trimester or coagulothopathies)
  - previous adverse ± traumatic experience a/w pregnancy
  - evidence of infection
Medical Mx
- Missed miscarriage: PO mifepristone, then misoprostol PV, PO or sublingual 48h later
  - If no bleeding within 48h of misoprostol, tell them to come back
- Incomplete miscarriage: single dose of misoprostol PV, PO or sublingual
- Offer antiemetics and pain relief
- Perform pregnancy test 3w later
Surgical Mx
- Vacuum aspiration (suction curettage) can be performed under local anaesthetic as outpatient
- Surgical Mx in theatre has to be done under GA (= evacuation of retained products of conception)

D: loss of ≥3 consecutive pregnancies before 24w with the same biological father

R: the more miscarriages, the worse the prognosis

Ix is guided by likely causes
- Infection
  - Bacterial vaginosis a/w 2nd trimester loss; screening & tx rec for those with previous mid-trim miscarriage
- Parental chromosome abnormality
  - Parents may be phenotypically normal but 60-75% of their gametes may be affected
  - Refer to clinical geneticist
  - Karyotype fetal products on 3rd and subsequent fetal losses – if unbalanced chromosomal abn is identified, karyotype peripheral blood of both parents
- Antiphospholipid syndrome
  - APS abs (lupus, phospholipid and anticardiolipin abs)
    ↳ APS dxed if 2 tests abs +ve taken 12w apart
  - Present in 15% of women with recurrent miscarriage
  - Mx with aspirin from day of +ve pregnancy test + LMWH (eg enoxaparin) as soon as fetal heart is seen on US
  - A/w high risk of other complications (eg pre-eclampsia); pregnancy should be monitored by experienced obstetrician
- Thrombophilia
  - Blood tests to determine
  - Heparin helps to ↓risk of miscarriage
- Alloimmune causes
- Uterine malformations
  - Previous uterine surgery ↑risk of uterine rupture

Ectopic pregnancy

D: implantation & growth of a fertilised ovum outside the uterine endometrial cavity
· 96% in fallopian tube (most in the ampulla: more dangerous if in isthmus), ~3% ovaries, ~1% in abdomen

R: previous ectopic pregnancy, prev tubal sterilisation surgery, IUD use, prev genital infxns (& its risk factors including multiple sexual partners), chronic salpingitis, endometriosis, infertility, smoking, IVF

A/P: causes broadly ÷ into conditions that hamper transfer of fertilised oocyte to uterine cavity, and conditions that predispose to premature implantation

S/smx:
· Hx of amenorrhea – smx generally appear 6-8w after last normal menstrual period
· Abdo pain (due to tubal spasm) – constant and classically unilateral
· Vaginal bleeding – less than normal period, dark brown in colour
· Peritoneal bleeding (2/2 ruptured ectopic pregnancy) may present as shoulder tip pain or pain on defecation or urination
· ↑blood loss (2/2 rupture) may present as anaemia (dizziness, fainting, syncope)
· Smx of pregnancy (eg breast tenderness) may be reported
· Examination findings
  - Cervical motion tenderness
  - Adnexal mass / tenderness
  - If uterine cervix dilated, this may suggest a miscarriage

Ix:
· Serum bHCG >1500 suggestive of ectopic pregnancy
· High res transvaginal US to determine location of pregnancy
  - "bagel sign" refers to empty gestational sac
  - if pregnancy cannot be located, this is referred to as pregnancy of unknown location
  - transabdo US is less sensitive
· If pt is in shock (or getting there), order FBC + X-match 6u bloods + get senior help asap

Mx dependent on how pt presents
· Expectant Mx
  - if low risk, haemodynamically stable and asmx women + evidence that ectopic pregnancy is resolving
  - size <35 mm, hCG <1000 IU/L
  - Involves closely monitoring over next 48h, taking serial bHCG levels to ensure decline
· Medical Mx
  - similar criteria to expectant Mx, but cannot be used if there is another intrauterine pregnancy
  - size <35 mm, hCG <1500 IU/L
  - Methotrexate given to pt
  - Can only be done if pt is willing to attend follow-up
· Surgical Mx
  - if >35 mm, ruptured, pain, visible fetal heartbeat, and/or hCG >5000 IU/L
  - Involves salpingectomy or salpingotomy
  - Salpingectomy (removal of fallopian tube): first-line if no other risk factors for infertility
  - Salpingotomy (removal of ectopic pregnancy from tube only) – consider if woman has other factors for infertility (eg contralateral tube damage)
    ↳ 20% will require further tx such as methotrexate or salpingectomy

Gestational trophoblastic disease aka molar pregnancy

D: Group of conditions including tumours arising from placental trophoblasts
· Hydatidiform moles: pregnancies with chromosomal abnormalities that have the potential to become malignant
· Gestational trophoblastic neoplasia (GTN): persistent locally invasive and/or metastatic trophoblastic tumour (different subtypes)

R: extremes of maternal age (<20yo or >35yo), prior molar pregnancy

A/P: presence of excess paternal chromosomes ± other mechanisms. Eg empty egg is fertilised by single sperm that duplicates its own DNA; all 46 chromosomes are of paternal origin
· Complete moles do not have any evidence of fetal parts, fetal circulation or fetal RBCs
· Partial moles have histological or macroscopical evidence of the above
· Both types of moles will produce very high levels of hCG due to abnormal and hydropic chorionic villi

S/smx:
· Bleeding in 1st or early 2nd trim
· Exaggerated smx of pregnancy, eg hyperemesis
· Uterus large for dates
· Very high levels of hCG
· ± HTN and hyperthyroidism
  - Hyperthyroidism may develop as hCG mimics the action of TSH

Ix: serum hCG (very high), pelvic US ("snowstorm appearance of mixed echogenecity in complete moles), histological exam of placental tissues

Mx: · Urgent ref to specialist centres; need to evacuate the uterus under general anaesthesia
  - Risk of thyroid storm after op
  - Give anti-D if Rh-ve
· Monitor hCG levels for ≥6mo
  - Levels should return to normal by 6mo; avoid pregnancy until hCG normalises
  - If levels do not normalise, either mole was invasive or has given rise to choriocarcinoma

Indications for chemotherapy
· hCG ≥20,000 IU/L ≥4w post evacuation
· Static or rising hCG after evacuation in absence of new pregnancy
· Raised hCG 6mo post evacuation, even if levels dropping
· Heavy vaginal bleeding, or GI or intraperitoneal bleeding
· Evidence of brain, liver or GI metastases, or lung opacities >2cm
· Histology of choriocarcinoma

P: 15-20% of women with complete molar pregnancies and up to 5% with partial molar pregnancies develop GTN. However, cure rate >95%

Pregnancy of unknown location
· Dxed when there is no sign of intrauterine or ectopic pregnancy or retained products of conception in the presence of a +ve pregnancy test (serum hCG >5IU)
· DDx of PUL
  - Early intrauterine pregnancy (too early to seen on scan)
  - Complete miscarriage
  - Failing pregnancy (cannot be seen on scan, but will resolve on its own)
  - Ectopic pregnancy (10%)
  - Persistent PUL
  - hCG-secreting tumour
· Mx according to smx

Pelvic inflammatory disease PID

D: spectrum of inflammatory disorders of the upper female genital tract, including any combination of endometritis, salpingitis, tubo-ovarian abscess, and pelvic peritonitis

R: prior infxn with chlamydia or gonorrhoea, young age of onset of sexual activity, unprotected sex with multiple partners, PMH of PID, IUD use (first 3w post-insertion)

A: polymicrobial infxn – **chlamydia** and **gonorrhoea** and mycoplasma most common
P: cervical infxn ascending to upper genital tract

S/smx:
· Lower abdo / pelvic pain – constant or intermittent, uni or bilateral
· Fever (may be afebrile if chronic)
· Deep dyspareunia, intermenstrual or postcoital bleeding
· Dysuria   · ± Irregular menses
· Vaginal or cervical discharge
· Cervical excitation

Ix: pregnancy test (r/o ectopic), FBC (↑WBC), high vaginal swab (often -ve), screen for chlamydia and gonorrhoea (NAAT/PCR)

Mx: · Low threshold for treating
· PO ofloxacin + metronidazole
  or IM ceftriaxone + PO doxycycline
  + PO metronidazole
· Differing guidelines on whether IUD should be removed (if present)

Complications
· Perihepatitis (Fitz-Hugh-Curtis syndrome): inflammation of liver capsule with "violin string-like" adhesions. Occurs in ~10%
  - S/smx: RUQ pain
  - Mx: same as PID
· Infertility due to tubal blockage (↑risk with ↑episodes)
· Chronic pelvic pain
· Ectopic pregnancy

Endometriosis

D: presence of endometrial glands and stroma outside the endometrial cavity and uterine musculature (most commonly in the pelvic peritoneum and ovaries)

R: FHx, nulliparity, mullerian anomalies (in pre-menarcheal girls)

A/P: various theories eg retrograde mensturation, genetic predisposition, altered immune response, etc

S/smx:
· Chronic pelvic pain
  - Cyclical if 2/2 endometrial tissue responding to menstrual cycle
  - Constant if 2/2 adhesions from chronic inflammation
· 2ndary dysmenorrhea (pain often starts days before menses)
  - May be debilitating (inability to go to school or work)
· Deep dyspareunia
· Subfertility
· Urinary smx: dysuria, urgency, haematuria, painful bowel movements
· Anxiety and depression due to smx
· On pelvic exam: ↓organ mobility, tender nodularity in the posterior vaginal fornix ± visible vaginal endometrial lesions

Ix: Laparoscopy. Little row for US or other Ix as direct visualisation is needed for Dx

Mx   · Medical
  - NSAIDs + paracetamol
  - COCP or progesterone only pill if analgesics are ineffective
  - GnRH analogues (said to induce pseudomenopause)
· Surgery
  - Laparoscopic excision or ablation of endometriosis ± adhesions
    ↳ ↑chances of conception
  - Ovarian cystectomy (for endometriomas)

P: mean of 10y delay from onset of smx to therapeutic interventions :(

Fibroids Uterine leiomyomata

D: benign tumours of the uterus primarily composed of smooth muscle and fibrous connective tissue

R: ↑BMI, age ~40s, black ethnicity, ↓vitamin D

A/P: ?monoclonal tumours, promoted by hormonal changes

S/smx: · May be asmx
· Menorrhagia ± iron deficiency anaemia
· Mass effect (due to ↑size of fibroids)
  - Lower abdo pain: cramping pains, often during menses
  - Bloating
  - Urinary smx: frequency
· Subfertility
· Rarely, polycythaemia due to autonomous production of erythropoietin

Ix: transvaginal US

Mx: · If asmx, watch & wait
· Menorrhagia
  - Levonorgestrel intrauterine system – useful if woman also wants contraception, but cannot be used if there is distortion of uterine cavity
  - COCP, progesterone (PO or IM)
  - NSAIDs, eg mefenamic acid
  - Tranexamic acid (↓bleeds)
· To shrink or remove fibroids
  - GnRH agonists (short-term effect only due to side effects + loss of bone mineral density)
  - Ulipristal acetate (not often used due to risks of liver toxicity)
  - Myomectomy via laparotomy, laparoscopy or hysteroscopy
  - Hysteroscopic endometrial ablation
  - Hysterectomy
  - Uterine artery embolization

P: fibroids generally regress after menopause. Fibroids may rarely undergo red degeneration during pregnancy, where they haemorrhage

Chronic pelvic pain

· Descriptive term for lower abdo pain >6mo not exclusively a/w menses, intercourse or pregnancy
· DDx: endometriosis, PID, fibroids, adenomyosis, adhesions, pelvic congestion, Mittelschmerz
  - non-gynae DDx: irritable bowel syndrome, interstitial cystitis
· Ix guided by smx: laparoscopy may reveal course but is normal in 30%
· Mx: if pain is cyclical, consider COCP to suppress ovaries
  - GnRH analogues can also be used to induce temporary menopause to see if smx are related to hormones

Mittelschmerz

· D: Mid-cycle menstrual pain around the time of ovulation
· Usually affects teenagers and older women
· Mx: analgesics (NSAIDs, paracetamol)

Adenomyosis

· D: endometrial glands and stroma are present within the myometrium, causing myometrial hypertrophy
· Can be asmx or causing dysmenorrhea, menorrhagia ± uterine enlargement / boggy
· Ix: transvaginal ultrasound / MRI
· Mx: if smx, tranexamic acid for menorrhagia, trial of GnRH agonists or uterine artery embolism
  - definitive Mx: hysterectomy

Dyspareunia

· D: pain during intercourse
· DDx of superficial dyspareunia
  - Infection (ulcers, discharge)
  - Vaginal dryness (postmenopause, breastfeeding)
  - Lack of sexual stimulation
  - Scarring (FGM, postpartum perineal repair)
  - Dermatographism (itchy vulval wheals after dermatographometer application)
· DDx of deep dyspareunia
  - Endometriosis
  - Pelvic infections

Male subfertility

Causes
· Semen abnormality
  - Idiopathic oligo-astheno-terato-zoospermia
  - Testicular cancer
  - Alcohol, smoking, other drugs
  - Varicocele
· Azoospermia
  - Pretesticular, eg anabolic steroid use, Kallmann syndrome
  - Non-obstructive, eg cryptorchidism, orchitis, Klinefelter syndrome, chemo
  - Obstructive, eg congenital bilat absence of the vas deferens, vasectomy, chlamydia, gonorrhoea
· Immunological
  - Anti-sperm antibodies
· Coital dysfunction
  - Erectile dysfunction with normal sperm function
    ◊ Some drugs can cause ED, eg beta-blockers, antidepressants
  - Hypospadias, phimosis, etc
  - Retrograde ejaculation
  - Failure in ejaculation 2/2 other causes, eg multiple sclerosis, spinal cord injury

Ix
· Detailed history + examination
· Testicular US
· Hormones – LH, FSH, testosterone
· Genetic tests (karyotyping, etc)

Mx
· Lifestyle modifications
· Consider changing medications
· Consider starting multivitamin containing zinc, selenium & vit C, then repeat semen analysis in 3mo
· Intracytoplasmic sperm injection if refractory to conservative Mx

Semen analysis see next page

Subfertility

D: no strict definition; major guidelines agree that fertility is "delayed" if a woman of reproductive age has not conceived after 1y of unprotected vaginal sexual intercourse or therapeutic donor insemination

Causes
- Anovulation 21% [→17.01]
  - 2/2 premature ovarian failure, Turner syndrome, surgery, chemo, PCOS, endocrine issues, Kallman syndrome, hyperprolactinaemia
- Male factor 25% [→17.05]
- Tubal factor 15-20%
- Endometriosis 6-8%
- Unexplained 28%

Ix
- Detailed histories from both male and female partner
- STI screening
- Baseline hormonal profile, TSH, prolactin, testosterone
- Day 21 progesterone level to confirm ovulation ("mid cycle progesterone)
  - blood sample taken 7d before expected period
- Semen analysis
  - If abnormal, ask male to make lifestyle changes and start multivitamin containing selenium, zinc and vitamin C, then repeat semen analysis in 3mo
- Transvaginal US
  - r/o masses, fibroids, polyps
  - helps to confirm PCOS if present
- Hysterosalpingogram
  - contrast XR – shows uterine anatomy and tubal patency
  - may cause period-like cramps and tubal spasm, causing false +ve
  - Can be done as an US instead
- Laparoscopy and dye test
  - Gold standard for Ax of tubal patency
  - 1st line if strong clinical suspicion of tubal abnormality
  - Dye is injected, and tubes are visualised with laparoscope

Mx

Lifestyle modifications
- Normalise wt, healthy diet
- Stop smoking / recreational drugs
- Drink within recommended limits
- Regular exercise
- Aim to have regular intercourse every 2-3d
- No need for ovulation monitors (↑stress, no proven benefit)

Medical Mx: Ovarian induction
- Wt loss/gain
- Clomifene citrate on d2-6 of cycle
  - 10% multiple pregnancies
  - Can cause hot flushes, labile mood. If severe HA or visual disturbance, stop immediately
  - Should only be used for 6-12 cycles (linked to ovarian cancer)
  - Requires follicular monitoring by US (risk of hyperstimulation)
- Laparoscopic ovarian drilling
  - Only for pts with PCOS
  - Small holes drilled into each ovary to ↓LH and restore feedback mechanisms
  - Successful in 50%, effect lasts for 12-18mo
- Gonadotrophins
  - Used for clomifene-resistant PCOS or low oestrogen with normal FSH
- Metform (unlicensed)
  - Used in women with PCOS
  - Not as effective as losing wt

Surgical Mx
- Tubal disease – tubal catheterisation or hysteroscopic cannulation
  - High rates of ectopic pregnancy
- Endometriosis – surgical Mx
- Intrauterine adhesions: hysteroscopic adhesiolysis

In vitro fertilisation
- D: Process of fertilisation where an oocyte is combined with a sperm in vitro (outside the body)
  - Oocyte production is stimulated, and the oocytes are collected
  - The oocytes are then fertilised with harvested sperm
    ◊ Intra-cytoplasmic sperm injection: sperm is directly inserted into the egg cytoplasm using micropipette
    ◊ Older method where oocyte and sperm are just placed in a petri dish and we wait
  - Once egg is fertilised, the embryo is reintroduced into uterus
  - Embryos may be screened for specific genetic disorders using pre-implantation genetic diagnosis
    ◊ May be offered to pts that have terminated a pregnancy previously due to serious genetic disease, personal or FHx of serious genetic disease
    ◊ There is risk to the embryo
  - Luteal support via progestogens
  - Woman should do a pregnancy 2w later
- Indications
  - Tubal disease
  - Male factor subfertility
  - Endometriosis
  - Anovulation not responding to clomifene
  - Subfertility 2/2 ↑maternal age
  - Unexplained subfertility >2y
- Requirements (under NHS)
  - Woman must be <43yo, had regular unprotected penetrative sexual intercourse for 2y with no resultant pregnancy
    ↳ <35 in some other countries
  - No current children
  - Non-smokers
  - BMI <30
  - No gamete donation required
    ◊ if woman is >45yo, and previous IVF attempts have failed, egg donation may be an option
    ◊ other options: adoption, fostering
    ◊ surrogacy: controversial, speak to your lawyer please

Other options
- Donor insemination
  - Sperm is donated from someone else, and that sperm is then used to inseminate the oocyte
  - Uses: male partner azoospermia, failed surgical sperm retrieval, those at high risk of transmitting genetic disorder or HIV, female with no male partner
- Intrauterine insemination: sperm is directly injected into womb
  - Uses: male factor subfertility, coital difficulties, unexplained subfertility, same-sex couples
  - Can be combined with ovarian stimulation
- In vitro maturation
  - Immature eggs are collected from ovaries and matured in lab. Sperm is then injected for fertilisation
  - Uses: women with PCOS (avoids risk of ovarian hyperstimulation)
- Ooplasmic transfer or nuclear transfer procedure
  - Nucleus of one oocyte is inserted into the cytoplasm of another oocyte (with its mitochondrial DNA)
  - Uses: female couples
- Percutaneous epididymal sperm aspiration: removal of sperm with needle into epididymus
- Pregnancy by ovary transplant

Semen analysis
- Should be performed between 3-5d abstinence, and sample needs to be delivered to lab within 1h
- Normal semen results
  - Volume >1.5mL
  - pH >7.2
  - Concentration >15 million/mL
  - Vitality (live sperm) >58%
  - Normal forms >4%
  - Progressive motility >32%
  - Total motility >40%

See male subfertility on previous page

Ovarian hyperstimulation syndrome   OHSS

D: A systemic disease that is a complication of ovulation induction or superovulation

R: young age, low BMI, polycystic ovaries, previous OHSS
- Less seen with clomifene
- More with gonadotrophin or hCG tx

A/P: Vasoactive products (esp vascular endothelial growth factor), oestrogens and progesterone are present in higher concentrations as a result of ovulation induction
- This results in ↑membrane permeability and loss of fluid from the intravascular compartment → ↑concentration of blood and hypercoagulability
- Fluid accumulates in the peritoneal and pleural spaces

S/smx ÷ according to RCOG:
- Mild: abdo pain, abdo bloating
- Mod: + NV, US evidence of ascites
- Severe: + clinical evidence of ascites, oliguria, Hct > 45%, hypoproteinaemia
- Critical: + thromboembolism, ARDs, anuria, tense ascites

Mx
- If mild or moderate, outpt tx ok
  - Analgesia but avoid NSAIDs
  - Avoid strenuous activities and intercourse due to risk of ovarian torsion
  - Continue with progesterone luteal support, avoid hCG
  - Review by assisted conception unit every 2-3d
- If severe, may need to admit
  - Daily bloods, strict fluid balance
  - Daily Ax of ascites, wt, legs
  - Thromboprophylaxis (stockings, LMWH)
  - Paracentesis for ascites ± IV replacement of albumin
- If critical, admit asap + senior help + consider ITU

Vulva problems

Pruritus vulvae (= vaginal itch)
- Causes: allergy (eg to washing powder, dyes), skin disease (eg psoriasis, lichen sclerosis), infxn (eg candida), infestations (eg scabies), or vulval dystrophy
- Mx: treat cause if possible
  - Avoid sensitisers
  - Advice showers rather than baths as baths may make it worse
  - Clean vulval area with emollients
  - Clean only 1x/d
  - Short course of topical steroids ± topical antifungal may help
  - If no response to tx, Ix for vulval intraepithelial neoplasia or carcinoma

Lichen sclerosis
- D: autoimmune condition characterised by skin atrophy and hypopigmentation, most commonly affecting genitalia
- Affects F>M, elderly; 40% develop other autoimmune disorders
- S/smx: itchy white patches ± scarring ± pain (during intercourse or urination)
  - "Bruised" red, purpuric signs may appear at first (may be mistaken for abuse)
- Ix: clinical Dx ± biopsy if doubt (no response to tx or cancer suspected)
- Mx: topical steroids and emollients
  - topical tacrolimus if no response
  - long-term monitoring required as these are premalignant lesions

Leukoplakia
- D: white vulval patches due to skin thickening and hypertrophy
  - may appear on other mucosal surfaces, eg mouth
- S/smx: white patches that do not rub off + itchy
- Ix: biopsy (premalignant lesion)
- Mx: topical corticosteroids
  - other options: UV phototherapy methotrexate, ciclosporin

Lichen planus
- D: chronic inflammatory dermatosis resulting from keratinocyte apoptosis. Can affect various body parts including genitalia
- R: hepatitis C infxn
- S/smx: **p**ain > itch (planus for pain)
  - In mouth and genital area, it can be erosive; appears with well-demarcated glazed appearance around introitus
- Ix: clinical Dx
- Mx: topical potent corticosteroid
  - tacrolimus
  - American College of O&G rec graded vaginal dilators in conjunction to prevent vaginal adhesions and stenosis

Lichen simplex (chronicus)
- D: a neurodermatitis; cutaneous disorder characterised by well-circumscribed erythematous, often hyperpigmented, plaques of thickened lichenified skin
  - May develop as a primary disorder, or 2/2 chronic rubbing and scratching from other pruritic disorder
- S/smx: chronic intractable itching, esp at night
  - non-specific inflammation of vulva ± mons pubis and inner thighs
  - exacerbated by stress, sensitising chemicals, low body iron stores
- Ix: clinical Dx ± biopsy if unsure
- Mx: vulval care
  - steroids to break itch-scratch cycle ± antihistamines

Vulval intraepithelial neoplasia
- D: non-invasive squamous lesion; precursor to squamous cell carcinoma of vulva
- R: HPV 16 & 18, smoking, HSV2, lichen planus
- S/smx: itching/burning of vulva
  - raised, well defined skin lesions
- Mx: surveillance + biopsy of suspicious lesions (recurrence is common)
  - Imiquimod cream may help to regress disease. Cream has to be applied 2-3x/w for 12w

Genital warts
- HPV 6 & 11 most common
  HPV 16, 18, 33 cancer

S/smx: small (2-5mm) fleshy protuberances, slightly pigmented; may bleed or itch

Mx: • if multiple, non-keratinised warts: topical podophyllum
- solitary, keratinised: cryotherapy
  topical imiquimod
- Genital warts are can be resistant and recurrent
- Most clear without intervention within 1-2y

Genital herpes
- HSV1, HSV2

S/smx: • painful genital ulceration
- a/w dysuria and pruritus
- Primary infection is often more severe than recurrent episodes
  - systemic features (HA, fever, malaise) more common in primary infxn
- ± tender inguinal lymphadenopathy, urinary retention

Ix: NAAT, ?HSV serology

Mx:
- Strong analgesia (eg lidocaine gel)
- Salt baths (+ peeing in bath)
- Aciclovir helps to shorten duration of smx
  - Higher doses if immunocomp
- If >6x/year, consider suppressive aciclovir for 6-12mo

Pregnancy
- elective C-sec if first episode occurs during pregnancy within 6w of due date or during time of delivery
- high dose aciclovir required to ↓risk of fetal infxn

Vulval carcinoma

D: cancer of the vulva – 80% squamous cell carcinomas, 5% vulva melanoma

R: ↑age, HPV infxn (16, 18, 33), vulval intraepithelial neoplasia, lichen sclerosis, immunosuppresion

S/smx:
- Lump/ulcer on labia majora
- Inguinal lymphadenopathy
- ± itching or irritation (or pt may be asmx)
- Vulva melanoma: often present late, with bleeding, mass, ulceration

Ix: biopsy + histology

Mx: surgical excision ± adjuvant radiation and/or chemotherapy

Other vulval lumps and bumps
- Urethral caruncle
  - small red swelling at urethral orifice 2/2 meatal prolapse
  - may be tender + pain on urination
  - Mx: excision or diathermy
- Bartholin's cyst and abscess
  - Bartholin's gland located under labia minora
  - If the duct blocks → painless cyst
  - If infected → abscess (very painful, pt cannot sit down, hot red labium)
  - Mx: incise + drain the abscess
- Vulval ulcers
  - painless genital ulcer from primary syphilis (ie a chancre)
  - condylomata lata (2ndary syphilis)
- Local varicose veins
- Uterine prolapse
- Uterine polyp
- Inguinal hernia
- Molluscum contagiosum

Vaginal discharge

Physiological discharge 2/2 pregnancy, sexual arousal, puberty, COCP

Bacterial vaginosis

🦠 anaerobic *Gardnerella vaginalis*

MOA: overgrowth of *G. vaginalis* leads to fall in aerobic lactobacilli producing lactic acid → ↑pH → problems :(

Ansel's criteria for Dx of BV (≥3 of 4)
- thin, white homogenous discharge
- clue cells on microscopy: stippled vaginal epithelial cells
- vaginal pH > 4.5
- +ve whiff test (addition of KOH results in fishy odour)

Mx: PO metronidazole for 5-7d
- 70-80% initial cure, relapse >50% within 3mo
- 🔹 topical metronidazole or topical clindamycin

Complications – in pregnancy
- Preterm labour, low birth weight, chorioamnionitis, late miscarriage
- Tx still low dose PO metronidazole

Trichomonas vaginalis

S/smx:
- Vaginal discharge: offensive, yellow/green, frothy
- Vulvovaginitis – **strawberry cervix**
- pH >4.5
- In males: asmx or urethritis

Ix: microscopy of wet mount shows mobile trophozoites

Mx: PO metronidazole 5-7d or one-off 2g metronidazole

Chlamydia

🦠 obligate intracellular *Chlamydia trachomatis*

S/smx: asmx in 70%F. Incubation 7-21d
- Cervicitis (discharge, bleeding), dysuria

Ix: 🔹 vulvovaginal swab in F
- Carried out 2w post-exposure

Mx: 🔹 doxycycline 7d
🔹 azithromycin 3d
- if pregnant: azithromycin, erythromycin or amoxicillin
- Partner notification, treating most recent sexual partner, then testing (based on exposure)

Complications
- PID → perihepatitis (FHC)
- endometritis
- ↑risk ectopic pregnancies
- infertility
- reactive arthritis

Gonorrhoea

🦠 Gram-ve diplococcus *Neisseria gonorrhoeae*

S/smx: · GU, rectal, pharynx
- Incubates 2-5d
- Cervicitis, vaginal discharge
- Rectal and pharyngeal: asmx

Ix: swabs (NAAT and culture)

Mx: 🔹 IM ceftriaxone 1g
🔹 PO cefixime 400mg
+ PO azithromycin 2g

Complications:
- Disseminated gonococcal infxn
  - tenosynovitis
  - migratory polyarthritis
  - dermatitis (maculopapular or vesicular)

Candidiasis (thrush)

🦠 C. albicans (95%) or C. glabrata

R: DM, drugs (abx, steroids), pregnancy, HIV

S/smx: · cottage cheese discharge that does not smell offensive
- Vulvitis: vulva and vagina may be red, fissured and sore; may cause superficial dyspareunia and dysuria
- Itchy
- Pt may have thrush elsewhere (eg mouth)

Ix: clinical Dx; high vag swab *not* routinely indicated

Mx: 🔹 fluconazole 150 mg PO single dose
🔹 clotrimazole 500 mg intravaginal pessary if PO therapy CI (eg pregnancy)
- If vulval smx, consider adding topical imidazole
- If recurrent (≥4 episodes / year)
  - Ensure compliance to tx
  - Confirm Dx with high vag swab ± check for DM
  - r/o other similar diseases eg lichen sclerosis
  - Induction-maintenance regime
    ◊ induction with fluconazole PO every 3 days for 3 doses
    ◊ maintenance with fluconazole PO weekly for 6mo

Discharge in children
- May be infxn from faecal flora a/w prepubertal atrophic vaginitis
- Likely causative agents: Staph, Strep, threadworms (pruritus)
- Always consider sexual abuse
- Ix: vulval ± vaginal swab, MSU (checking for DM)
- Mx: hygiene ± abx (erythromycin)

Urinary incontinence

D: involuntary loss of urine

÷ clinical classification
- Stress inco: leakage on effort, exertion, sneezing or coughing
- Urgency inco: accompanied by or immediately preceded by urgency
- Overactive bladder (detrusor overactivity): urgency ± frequency ± incontinence
- Mixed inco
- Nocturia: sleep interruption to urinate ≥1x per night
- Nocturnal enuresis: involuntary loss of urine occurring during sleep
- Continuous inco
- Overflow inco: leakage from over-distended bladder
- Functional inco: pt is unable to get to a bathroom in time (eg dementia, hemiplegia)

R: ↑age, prev pregnancy & child-birth, high BMI, hysterectomy, FHx

Ix: r/o UTI, urodynamics to confirm Dx (will guide Mx options)

Mx (general)
- Avoid excessive fluid intake, caffeine, fizzy, squash, alcohol (bladder irritants)

Mx of urge incontinence:
- Bladder retraining – ↑intervals between voiding; ≥6w training
- Antimuscarinics (eg oxybutynin, tolteridine or darifenacin)
- Mirabegron useful if concerns about anticholinergic SE in frail elderly people

Mx of stress incontinence:
- Pelvic floor muscle training – ≥8 contractions performed 3x/d for ≥3mo
- Surgical, eg retropubic mid-urethral tape procedures
- If woman declines surgical option, offer duloxetine (SNRI)

Pelvic organ prolapse

Aka urogenital prolapse, the general term encompassing the following
- Cystocele (bladder prolapse)
- Rectocele (prolapse of rectum or large bowel)
- Enterocele (small bowel prolapse)
- Uterine prolapse (prolapse of uterus)

R: vaginal delivery (↑risk for more births), ↑age, ↑BMI, prev surgery for prolapse, FHx, white ancestry, spina bifida

A/P: damage to pelvic musculature, ligaments and nerves → weakness of pelvic floor muscles ± levator ani

S/smx: · May be asmx
- Sensation of pressure & heaviness, dragging feeling, feeling of a lump coming down
- Others: dyspareunia, backache
- Urinary smx: incontinence, frequency, urgency, incomplete bladder emptying
- Rectocele: constipation, difficulty with defecation

Ix: · Exam to r/o pelvic masses
- Urodynamic studies if urinary incontinence

Mx:
- Conservative: wt loss, pelvic floor muscle exercise, don't strain
- Pessaries
  - Usually in the form of rings
  - Placed between posterior aspect of the symphysis pubis and posterior fornix of vagina
  - Change every 6mo
- Surgery
  - Indicated if severe smx, sexually active, pessaries no effect
  - Redundant tissues may be excised + strengthen support
  - May result in reduced vaginal width
  - Meshes have been banned due to high complication rate
  - Severity will guide options

Cervical cancer screening

D: Procedure via which a cell sample from the junction of the ectocervix and endocervix is collected and analysed (aka pap smear)
- A speculum is inserted into the vaginal canal, and the cells are collected with a brush
- In the UK, the sample is first tested for high risk strains of HPV
- If this is +ve, the sample is then sent for cytological exam

Who?
- All women 25-64yo are offered screening
- 25-49yo: every 3y
- 50-64yo: every 5y
- In Scotland, 25-64yo: every 5y
- If pregnant, cervical screening is delayed till 3 months post-partum
- If woman has never been sexually active, they have a very low risk of developing cervical cancer (due to ↓risk of getting HPV), and therefore can opt out

What happens next?
- If HPV -ve, continue normal schedule
- If HPV +ve & cytology normal
  - repeat smear in 12mo
  - if HPV -ve in 12mo, continue normal schedule
  - if HPV +ve in 12mo, colposcopy
- If HPV +ve & deranged cytology
  - refer for colposcopy
  - if colposcopy is -ve, continue normal schedule
  - if CIN grade I is detected, repeat smear in 12mo
  - if CIN II or III, refer for large loop excision of transformation zone (LLETZ)
- If smear shows moderate dyskaryosis with CIN being treated, repeat smear in 6mo as test of cure
- If cervical cancer is detected, refer for colposcopy 2ww !
- If sample is inadequate, repeat sample in 3mo
  - If 2 consecutive samples are inadequate, ref for colposcopy

Cervical cancer

D: HPV-related malignancy of the uterine cervical mucosa
- 80% SCC, 20% AC
- 2 peaks in ages – 30s and >70yo

R: HPV (16, 18, 33 are the highest risk), HIV, early onset of sexual activity, multiple sexual partners, ↑no of kids, COCP, smoking, lower socio-economic status, immunosupp

A/P: HPV activates oncoproteins which drive CIN and eventually result in invasive cancer

S/smx:
- Asmx; incidental finding on tx of CIN
- Postcoital ± postmenopausal bleeding or watery vaginal discharge
- Features of advanced disease:
  - Heavy vaginal bleeding
  - Ureteric obstruction
  - Wt loss   - Bowel disturbance
  - Vesicovaginal fistula   - Pain

Ix: pap smear, biopsy

Mx depends on stage and functional status
- If Stage I (confined to cervix), hysterectomy + lymphadectomy
- If Stage II (local spread to vagina), chemoradiotherapy needed
- If Stage IV (spread to bladder, rectum or distant organs), palliative radiotherapy may be indicated to control bleeding

P: 5-year survival is ~67% (best prognosis for stage I – 91%). Most recurrences happen within 2-3y

Vaginal cancer

D: Cancer of the vagina
- Most are due to metastatic spread from cervical, uterine or vulva Ca
- If true primary vaginal cancer, mostly SCC, mean age 60yo

R: similar risk factors to cervical cancer (especially HPV)

S/smx: - Many are asmx
- Vaginal bleeding (usually postcoital or postmenopausal)
- Vaginal mass

Ix: biopsy

Mx: as per cervical cancer
- Lower stage tumours may be amenable to resection, but higher stages will require chemoradiotherapy

Endometrial hyperplasia

D: abnormal proliferation of the endometrium – may be a precursor to endometrial cancer
÷ EH without atypia and with atypia
  - With atypia, aka endometrial intraepithelial neoplasia (EIN) = precancerous lesions on endometrium
÷ further divided into simple or complex

S/smx: EIN usually presents with abnormal uterine bleeding; Ix as per endometrial cancer

Mx of EIN: Hysterectomy due to high risk of concurrent or progression to endometrial carcinoma
- If not surgical candidate, progesterone therapy is indicated

Endometrial cancer

D: epithelial malignancy of the uterine corpus mucosa, usually an adenocarcinoma

R: - ↑age (>50yo)
- Excess oestrogen
  - nulliparity   - early menarche
  - late menopause
  - unopposed oestrogen
    ↳ if pt is on oestrogen, progesterone will help to ↓risk
- Metabolic syndrome
  - obesity   - DM   - PCOS
- Tamoxifen
- Hereditary non-polyposis colerectal carcinoma (HNPCC / Lynch)

Protective factors: multiparity, COCP, smoking (??)

S/smx
- Postmenopausal bleeding
  - slight, intermittent → heavier
- If premenopausal, may present as menorrhagia or intermenstrual bleeding
- Pain – may indicate extensive disease
- Vaginal discharge – not common
- ► If ≥55yo with postmenopausal bleeding – 2ww referral to gynae

Ix: ⬍ transvaginal US (normal endometrial thickness <4mm has -ve predictive value)
- Hysteroscopy with endometrial biopsy

Mx
- Localised disease: total abdominal hysterectomy with bilat salpingo-oophorectomy
- ± Adjuvant radiotherapy
- In later stage disease: chemo, immunotherapy ± radiotherapy
- If not candidate for surgery, progesterone therapy may be used

Ovarian cancer

D: neoplasm of the ovaries
• 90% – epithelial ovarian cancer

R: BRCA1, BRCA2, other genetic mutations, HNPCC, ↑age, FHx (ovarian cancer, breast cancer), never used combined oral contraceptives, early menarche, late menopause, nulliparity

Protective: pregnancy, bfding, COCP, tubal ligation

S/smx are usually very vague
• Abdo distention + bloating
• Abdo + pelvic pain
• Urinary smx, eg urgency
• Early satiety
• Diarrhoea

Ix: Ca125 – if ≥35 IU/mL, refer for urgent US of abdomen and pelvis
 - DO NOT use Ca125 as screening tool as there are false +ve due to menses, benign ovarian cysts, etc
• Transvaginal US
• CXR, CT to look for mets
• May require diagnostic laparotomy to confirm Dx

Mx:
• Full staging laparotomy involves
 - Mildline laparotomy
 - Hysterectomy
 - Bilat salpingo-oophorectomy
 - Omentectomy
 - Para-aortic and pelvic lymph node sampling
 - Peritoneal washings + biopsies
• If young + desiring fertility + low stage, the uterus and other ovary might be left
• Chemotherapy is recommended for Stage Ic and upwards

Ovarian cysts

D: fluid-filled sac in the ovarian tissue ÷ physiological/functional cysts, benign germ cell tumours, and benign epithelial tumours

Functional cysts
÷ follicular and corpus luteum cysts
• Most common type of cysts
 - Considered normal if <5cm
• Follicular cysts form due to non-rupture of dominant follicle, or failure of atresia in a non-dominant follicle
• Corpus luteum cysts form due to persistence of corpus luteum after the menstrual cycle – may become filled with blood or fluid
 - Can present with intraperitoneal bleeding
• Usually regress after 2-3 menstrual cycles

Benign germ cell tumours
↳ Dermoid cysts, aka mature cystic teratomas, arising from primitive germ cells
↳ May contain well-differentiated tissue (hair, teeth); 20% bilateral
• Most common benign ovarian tumour in woman <30yo
• Usually asmx, but can cause ovarian torsion

Benign epithelial tumours
• Arise from ovarian surface epithelium
• Serous cystadenomas
 - Develop papillary growths
 - Cyst may appear solid, bilateral in 20-30%
 - 30% turn malignant
• Mucinous cystadenomas
 - Commonest large ovarian tumours (become enormous ± multilocular)
 - ~5% malignant
 - If they rupture, they may cause pseudomyxoma peritonei

General Mx of ovarian cysts
• Complex / multi-loculated ovarian cysts should be biopsied to r/o malignancy
• In premenopausal women
 - r/o malignancy, aim to preserve fertility
 - if asmx + simple cyst <5cm: discharge
 - if asmx + simple, but 5-7cm: yearly scan
 - if smx, or >7cm, or multiloculated: laparoscopic ovarian cystectomy
• If postmenopausal women
 - calculate risk of malignancy index
 - if low risk cyst <5cm: repeat trans-vaginal cycle and Ca125 every 4mo ◊ if no change in 1y, discharge
 - if mod risk cyst: bilateral oophorectomy
 - if high risk cyst: refer to cancer centre for staging laparotomy

Risk of malignancy index (RMI)
= U x M x Ca125

U = US Score
(0 if no features, 1 if 1 feature, 2 if ≥2 features)
• Multilocularity
• Solid areas   • Metastases
• Ascites   • Bilaterality of lesions
M = menopausal status
• 1 = premenopausal
• 3 = postmenopausal
Ca125 = serum level (U/L)

Overall risk
• Low: RMI <25, <3% risk of cancer
• Mod: RMI 25-250, ~20% risk
• High: RMI >250, 75% risk

Pseudomyxoma peritonei
• D: clinical syndrome characterised by diffuse mucinous peritoneal involvement, often a/w a ruptured mucinous appendiceal lesion
 → causes thick, jelly-like deposits throughout the abdomen
• Mx with surgical debulking for symptomatic relief + chemo

Ovarian torsion

D: twisting of the ovary around its ligamentous supports, aka adnexal torsion

R: ovarian neoplasm, non-functional ovarian cyst, pregnancy, ovarian hyperstimulation syndrome

A: underlying anatomical abnormalities, ovarian mass, ↑size of ovary
P: Rotation of ovary on ligament →
↓blood supply to ovary ± fallopian tube
→ ischaemia, necrosis, haemorrhage

S/smx:
• Sudden onset deep colicky pain in the pelvis/abdomen
 - May radiate to back, flank, groin
• Nausea, vomiting, diarrhoea
• Palpable adnexal mass + tenderness

Ix: r/o pregnancy, US (free fluid or whirlpool sign)

Mx: ! surgical emergency
• Go to theatres asap
• Surgical detorsion preferred, generally done as laparoscopy
• Salpingo-oophorectomy if ovary is non-viable or malignancy present
• Consider oophoropexy

Printed in Great Britain
by Amazon